**LIBRARY**

College of Physicians and Surgeons
of British Columbia

# Respiratory Medicine

*Series Editor:*
Sharon I.S. Rounds

For further volumes:
http://www.springer.com/series/7665

Keith C. Meyer • Steven D. Nathan
Editors

# Idiopathic Pulmonary Fibrosis

## A Comprehensive Clinical Guide

Humana Press

*Editors*
Keith C. Meyer, M.D.
Department of Internal Medicine
Section of Allergy, Pulmonary
    and Critical Care Medicine
University of Wisconsin School of
    Medicine and Public Health
Madison, WI, USA

Steven D. Nathan, M.D.
Advanced Lung Disease and Lung
Transplant Program
Department of Medicine
Inova Fairfax Hospital
Falls Church, VA, USA

ISBN 978-1-62703-681-8        ISBN 978-1-62703-682-5 (eBook)
DOI 10.1007/978-1-62703-682-5
Springer New York Heidelberg Dordrecht London

Library of Congress Control Number: 2013949784

Printed on acid-free paper

Humana Press is a brand of Springer
Springer is part of Springer Science+Business Media (www.springer.com)

Keith Meyer and Steve Nathan dedicate this
book to their families, mentors, and patients.
They both would like to especially dedicate
this book to their respective mothers.
Idella Ruby Kortbein Meyer provided the
nurturing, loving support, and inspiration
that allowed Keith to embark on an
educational voyage that led to his eventual
pursuit of an academic career in science
and medicine. The late Professor Carmen
Nathan, a legal academic, Dean of her Law
Faculty, and author of numerous texts
and books, continues to be an inspiration
through her spirit of challenging the status
quo and being prepared to step outside
the bounds of academic comfort.

# Preface

The term, idiopathic pulmonary fibrosis (IPF), first appeared in the medical literature in the mid-twentieth century. However, the disorder described by this term has undergone a metamorphosis from a loosely defined diagnostic entity that encompassed a number of fibrotic interstitial lung diseases (ILDs) to what we now (as of the twenty-first century) recognize as a tightly defined fibrotic lung disorder that is characterized by the presence of usual interstitial pneumonia (UIP) that is not linked to the presence of a connective tissue disorder (CTD) or caused by an inhaled agent (such as asbestos) or drug-induced lung injury.

This book is intended to provide readers with a comprehensive understanding of the definition and changing perceptions of IPF as a clinical and pathologic entity. Chapter 1 provides a historical perspective of the evolution from what was perceived as the clinical entity of IPF in the middle of the twentieth century to what we now recognize as a specific disease that stands apart from other forms of ILD including the non-IPF idiopathic interstitial pneumonias (IIPs). Drs. Olga Tourin, Jeffrey Swigris, and Amy Olson provide a comprehensive and up-to-date review of our current knowledge of the epidemiology and natural history of IPF in Chap. 2, and Dr. Jeffrey Myers provides an in-depth review of the key histopathologic features of IPF in Chap. 3 and contrasts findings in UIP/IPF with non-IPF entities that can have similar clinical presentations. Imaging via high-resolution computed tomography (HRCT) of the thorax has emerged as a critical diagnostic test that can frequently allow a confident diagnosis of IPF and differentiate it from other forms of ILD. However, HRCT imaging may also be indeterminate such that surgical lung biopsy is still needed to attain a confident IPF diagnosis. Drs. Jonathan Chung and Jeffrey Kanne review the current and evolving role of thoracic imaging in the diagnosis of IPF in Chap. 4.

Making a confident diagnosis of IPF requires a thorough examination of all available clinical data and ensuring that non-IPF forms of ILD are not diagnosed as cases of IPF. Drs. Anish Wadhwa and Kevin Flaherty review key diagnostic criteria that are required to make a confident diagnosis of IPF in Chap. 5. When a diagnosis of IPF has been made, accurate physiologic assessment of pulmonary function plays a key role in providing a prognosis, clinical decision making, and assessing responses to potential therapeutic interventions in clinical trials. Dr. Athol Wells provides an erudite and extremely useful review of current approaches to pulmonary function testing in Chap. 6.

Chapters 7 and 8 discuss current and evolving concepts of the pathogenesis of IPF. Dr. Steven Duncan discusses a variety of observations that have linked adaptive immunity and associated lung inflammation to the onset and progression of IPF in Chap. 7, and Dr. Nathan Sandbo discusses current concepts concerning the genesis and progression of tissue fibrosis in Chap. 8. Chapters 10 and 11 discuss phenotypes of IPF and the overlap of IPF with CTD-associated ILD. Subgroups of patients diagnosed with IPF have features of their disease that can significantly alter their course and prognosis, and Dr. Steven Nathan examines evolving concepts of IPF phenotypes in Chap. 10. An often difficult issue for both clinicians and researchers is deciding whether patients with UIP and features that suggest the presence of an autoimmune disorder have UIP associated with CTD or IPF with isolated autoimmune phenomena that do not allow one to make a diagnosis of CTD. Indeed, some patients with apparent UIP/IPF can develop a specific autoimmune disorder such as rheumatoid arthritis or scleroderma months to years after an apparent diagnosis of IPF has been assigned. Drs. Joshua Solomon and Aryeh Fischer discuss features that distinguish CTD-ILD from IPF and other IIP in Chap. 11.

Advancing age has been strongly linked to an increased risk for developing IPF, and gastroesophageal reflux (GER) has also been recognized as a risk factor for the development and progression of IPF. Drs. Moises Selman, Yair Romero, and Annie Pardo discuss features of the aging process that may predispose elderly patients to develop IPF in Chap. 12, while Drs. Stephenie Takahashi, Karen Patterson, and Imre Noth examine the link between GER and risk for developing IPF in Chap. 13.

Treating IPF has proved to be extremely frustrating for both patients and clinicians, and current approaches to the management of patients with IPF are given in Chaps. 14–18. Drs. Paolo Spagnolo, Fabrizio Luppi, Gloria Montanari, and Luca Richeldi provide a comprehensive review of the clinical trials to evaluate pharmacologic therapies that have been performed to data in Chap. 14. Drs. Teng Moua and Jay Ryu highlight the prevalence and management of comorbidities that are frequently present in IPF patients in Chap. 15 and underscore the importance of being aware of these in the comprehensive management of IPF patients. Chapter 16, authored by Drs. Anne Holland and Jeffrey Swigris, provides an overview of the role and benefits of pulmonary rehabilitation and oxygen therapy, both of which have been associated with significant improvement in the quality of life of patients with IPF.

A substantial number of patients will develop an unpredictable episode of abrupt deterioration in lung function due to an acute exacerbation of IPF, and this event can occur in patients with relatively good physiologic function and apparently mild disease. Drs. Joyce Lee and Harold Collard discuss the clinical features, diagnosis, and management of such acute exacerbations in Chap. 17. Finally, as discussed by Drs. Daniela Lamas and David Lederer in Chap. 18, the only intervention that has been shown to prolong survival and improve quality of life for patients with advanced IPF is lung transplantation. However, relatively few patients qualify for placement on the transplant waiting list, and many wait-listed patients never receive transplants due to a persistent shortage of donor lungs.

Chapters 19–21 discuss newer approaches that will hopefully facilitate our attempts to discover newer therapies and improve our ability to evaluate such therapies in clinical trials. Genomic profiling holds the promise of applying such technology to improve diagnosis (differentiate IPF from other forms of fibrotic ILD), to detect signals that can be used as biomarkers to predict disease progression with greater precision, and to identify targets for new drug therapies. Drs. Jose Herazo-Maya and Naftali Kaminski discuss the promise and potential impact of genomics on the diagnosis and treatment of IPF in Chap. 19. Despite the completion of a relatively large number of clinical trials with new agents that appeared to hold potential therapeutic benefit for patients with IPF, unequivocal efficacy of a specific pharmacologic agent has yet to be demonstrated. The structure of a clinical trial (including the selected endpoints) can be critical to demonstrating a meaningful benefit for a specific therapy, and Dr. Fernando Martinez discusses clinical trial design and endpoint choices in Chap. 20. Finally, Drs. Carmen Mikacenic and Ganesh Raghu provide a road map for future directions that are needed for both basic and translational research. It is hoped that lessons learned will help pave future paths to the development of effective therapies that have a significant impact on the natural history of IPF and prevent the inevitable, progressive, and usually relentless loss of lung function that is a defining feature of this disease.

It is our hope that this book will not only improve readers' knowledge of all aspects of the disease that we recognize as IPF but also inspire readers to engage in meaningful basic and clinical research. We are indebted to the authors who were gracious enough to contribute chapters, and we believe that this compendium of knowledge and wisdom provides a firm foundation that will hopefully lead to the discovery of effective therapies for patients with this devastating disease.

Madison, WI                                                                                  Keith C. Meyer, M.D.
Falls Church, VA                                                                         Steven D. Nathan, M.D.

# Contents

# Contributors

**Jonathan H. Chung, M.D.** Department of Radiology, National Jewish Health, Denver, CO, USA

**Harold R. Collard, M.D.** Department of Medicine, University of California, San Francisco, CA, USA

**Sonye K. Danoff, M.D., Ph.D.** Department of Medicine, Division of Pulmonary and Critical Care Medicine, Johns Hopkins University School of Medicine, Baltimore, MD, USA

**Steven R. Duncan, M.D.** Department of Pulmonary, Allergy, and Critical Care Medicine, University of Pittsburgh Medical Center, Pittsburgh, PA, USA

**Aryeh Fischer, M.D.** Division of Rheumatology, Department of Medicine, Autoimmune and Interstitial Lung Disease Program, National Jewish Health, Denver, CO, USA

**Kevin R. Flaherty, M.D., M.S.** Department of Internal Medicine, Division of Pulmonary and Critical Care Medicine, University of Michigan Health System, Ann Arbor, MI, USA

**Jose D. Herazo-Maya, M.D.** Pulmonary, Critical Care and Sleep Medicine, Yale School of Medicine, New Haven, CT, USA

**Anne E. Holland, B.App.Sc., Ph.D.** Department of Physiotherapy, Alfred Health and La Trobe University, Melbourne, VIC, Australia

**Cheilonda Johnson, M.D., M.H.S.** Department of Medicine, Johns Hopkins University, Baltimore, MD, USA

**Naftali Kaminski, M.D.** Pulmonary, Critical Care and Sleep Medicine, Yale School of Medicine, New Haven, CT, USA

**Jeffrey P. Kanne, M.D.** Department of Radiology, University of Wisconsin School of Medicine and Public Health, Madison, WI, USA

**Daniela J. Lamas, M.D.** Pulmonary and Critical Care Medicine, Harvard University, Massachusetts General Hospital, Boston, MA, USA

**David J. Lederer, M.D., M.S.** Lung Transplantation Program, Columbia University Medical Center, New York, NY, USA

Interstitial Lung Disease Program, Columbia University Medical Center, New York, NY, USA

Division of Pulmonary, Allergy, and Critical Care Medicine, Columbia University Medical Center, New York, NY, USA

**Joyce S. Lee, M.D.** Department of Medicine, Interstitial Lung Disease Program, University of California, San Francisco, CA, USA

**Fabrizio Luppi, M.D., Ph.D.** Center for Rare Lung Diseases, University Hospital Policlinico of Modena, Modena, Italy

**Fernando J. Martinez, M.D., M.S.** Division of Pulmonary and Critical Care Medicine, Department of Internal Medicine, University of Michigan Health System, Ann Arbor, MI, USA

**Keith C. Meyer, M.D., M.S.** Department of Internal Medicine, Section of Allergy, Pulmonary and Critical Care Medicine, University of Wisconsin School of Medicine and Public Health, Madison, WI, USA

**Carmen Mikacenic, M.D.** Division of Pulmonary and Critical Care Medicine, University of Washington Medical Center, Seattle, WA, USA

**Gloria Montanari, M.D.** Center for Rare Lung Diseases, University Hospital Policlinico of Modena, Modena, Italy

**Teng Moua, M.D.** Division of Pulmonary and Critical Care Medicine, Mayo Clinic, Rochester, MN, USA

**Jeffrey L. Myers, M.D.** Divisions of Anatomic Pathology and MLabs, Department of Pathology, University of Michigan, Ann Arbor, MI, USA

**Steven D. Nathan, M.D.** Advanced Lung Disease and Lung Transplant Program, Department of Medicine, Inova Fairfax Hospital, Falls Church, VA, USA

**Imre Noth, M.D.** Department of Medicine, Section of Pulmonary and Critical Care, University of Chicago Medical Center, Chicago, IL, USA

**Amy L. Olson, M.D., M.S.P.H.** Division of Pulmonary and Critical Care Medicine, National Jewish Health, Interstitial Lung Disease Program and Autoimmune Lung Center, Denver, CO, USA

**Annie Pardo, Ph.D.** Facultad de Ciencias, Laboratorio de Bioquímica, Universidad Nacional Autónoma de México, México D.F., Mexico

**Karen C. Patterson, M.D.** Department of Medicine, Section of Pulmonary and Critical Care, University of Chicago Medical Center, Chicago, IL, USA

**Ganesh Raghu, M.D.** Division of Pulmonary and Critical Care Medicine, University of Washington Medical Center, Seattle, WA, USA

The Center for Interstitial Lung Diseases, University of Washington Medical Center, Seattle, WA, USA

Scleroderma Clinic, University of Washington Medical Center, Seattle, WA, USA

**Luca Richeldi, M.D., Ph.D.** Chair of Interstitial Lung Disease, University Hospital Southampton, Southampton, United Kingdom

**Yair Romero, M.Sc.** Facultad de Ciencias, Laboratorio de Bioquímica, Universidad Nacional Autónoma de México, México D.F., Mexico

**Jay H. Ryu, M.D.** Division of Pulmonary and Critical Care Medicine, Mayo Clinic, Rochester, MN, USA

**Nathan Sandbo, M.D.** Division of Allergy, Pulmonary, and Critical Care, University of Wisconsin, Madison, WI, USA

**Moisés Selman, M.D.** Dirección de Investigación, Instituto Nacional de Enfermedades Respiratorias, Ismael Cosio Villegas, México D.F., Mexico

**Joshua J. Solomon, M.D.** Department of Medicine, Autoimmune and Interstitial Lung Disease Program, National Jewish Health, Denver, CO, USA

**Paolo Spagnolo, M.D., Ph.D.** Center for Rare Lung Diseases, University Hospital Policlinico of Modena, Modena, Italy

**Jeffrey J. Swigris, D.O., M.S.** Autoimmune Lung Center and Interstitial Lung Disease Program, National Jewish Health, Denver, CO, USA

**Stephenie M. Takahashi, B.A., M.D.** Department of Medicine, Section of Pulmonary and Critical Care, University of Chicago Medical Center, Chicago, IL, USA

**Olga Tourin, M.D.** University of Calgary, Adult Respirology Residency Program, Rockyview General Hospital, Calgary, AB, Canada

**Anish Wadhwa, M.D.** Division of Pulmonary and Critical Care Medicine, University of Michigan Health System, Ann Arbor, MI, USA

**Simon Ward, B.Sc., Hons.** Lung Function Unit, Royal Brompton and Harefield NHS Trust, London, UK

**Athol U. Wells, M.D.** Interstitial Lung Disease Unit, Royal Brompton Hospital, London, UK

# Chapter 1
# Idiopathic Pulmonary Fibrosis:
# A Historical Perspective

Keith C. Meyer

**Abstract** The term "idiopathic pulmonary fibrosis" (IPF) began to appear in the medical literature in the mid-1900s and was initially used by clinicians and radiologists to refer to fibrosing pneumonitis of unknown cause. However, the entities that we now recognize as idiopathic interstitial pneumonias (IIPs) and other entities with similar clinical presentations, such as interstitial lung disease (ILD) associated with connective tissue disorders (CTD) or fibrotic hypersensitivity pneumonitis (HP), were often identified as cases of IPF by clinicians due to similar clinical presentation and radiographic appearance. As our knowledge of fibrosing ILD expanded over the last three decades of the twentieth century, it became clear that histopathologic patterns could be found that paved the way to our current clinicopathologic classification of the IIPs, with the term "IPF" used exclusively to designate patients with idiopathic usual interstitial pneumonia (UIP). This introductory chapter will review how terminology and concepts of the disorder that we now recognize as IPF have evolved over the decades such that IPF has become the preferred diagnostic term for patients diagnosed with UIP of unknown cause.

**Keywords** Pulmonary fibrosis • Idiopathic pulmonary fibrosis • Cryptogenic fibrosing alveolitis • Idiopathic interstitial pneumonia • Usual interstitial pneumonia • Lung transplant • Interstitial lung disease

K.C. Meyer, M.D., M.S. (✉)
Department of Internal Medicine: Section of Allergy, Pulmonary
and Critical Care Medicine, University of Wisconsin School of Medicine
and Public Health, K4/910 Clinical Science Center, 600 Highland Avenue,
Madison, WI 53792-9988, USA
e-mail: kcm@medicine.wisc.edu

K.C. Meyer and S.D. Nathan (eds.), *Idiopathic Pulmonary Fibrosis: A Comprehensive Clinical Guide*, Respiratory Medicine 9, DOI 10.1007/978-1-62703-682-5_1,

# Introduction

Hippocrates, recognized in his time as a master physician and thorough observer of human diseases, described fibrotic changes in the lungs in the fifth century BC. Descriptions of pulmonary fibrosis were, however, sparse until the early twentieth century, and pulmonary fibrosis was thought to be a rare form of lung disease. Over the past century, our knowledge of interstitial lung disease (ILD) and pulmonary fibrosis has grown in leaps and bounds. With the lack of today's more sophisticated diagnostic tools, the term "idiopathic pulmonary fibrosis" (IPF) allowed a broad net to be cast such that many other forms of ILD, such as CTD-associated ILD, fibrotic hypersensitivity pneumonitis (HP), pneumotoxic drug reaction, and other forms of idiopathic interstitial pneumonias (IIP) were often captured under this umbrella term. Over the past 50 years, the clinical evaluation of patients in the context of multidisciplinary interactions by pulmonologists, pathologists, and radiologists has led to the recognition of IPF as a diagnosis that applies exclusively to patients who have a usual interstitial pneumonia (UIP) histopathologic pattern of pulmonary fibrosis that is not associated with any of the aforementioned entities. This introductory chapter will review various investigations that have led to the recognition of the characteristics of the entity that we currently recognize as IPF.

# Early Perceptions and Terminology for Interstitial Lung Disease and Pulmonary Fibrosis

In the early 1900s pathologists began to recognize that some patients had bilateral lung disease at autopsy that was not related to more common causes of death such as infection or malignancy. These lungs were observed to be scarred, shrunken, and cystic, with these changes appearing to be most prominent peripherally and at the lung bases with relative sparing of the apices and more central areas. What appeared to be smooth muscle could be seen in some cases, and the term "muscular cirrhosis" of the lung was coined. Additionally, the presence of cysts was referred to as "honeycomb change" or "honeycomb lung."

In 1935, Hamman and Rich described four previously healthy patients who developed what appeared to be fulminant lung disease of rapid onset that relentlessly progressed to respiratory failure within 1–3 months from their initial presentation. Advanced lung fibrosis and honeycomb change was found at autopsy, and this was recognized as an entity that became known as the "Hamman–Rich syndrome." The term "IPF" first appeared in the medical literature in the late 1940s, but many other terms were used to denote what was likely the same entity (e.g., bronchiolar emphysema, pulmonary muscular hyperplasia, cystic pulmonary cirrhosis, idiopathic

## Histopathology Classification of
## Interstitial Pneumonias: 1975-2002

| 1975 Liebow | 1993 Katzenstein | 2002 ATS Statement |
|---|---|---|

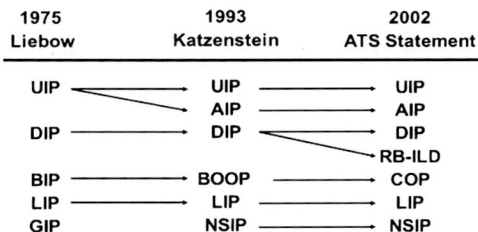

Fig. 1.1 The changing classification of interstitial pneumonias from 1975 to 2002. *AIP* acute interstitial pneumonia, *ATS* American Thoracic Society, *BIP* bronchiolitis obliterans with interstitial pneumonia, *BOOP* bronchiolitis obliterans organizing pneumonia, *COP* cryptogenic organizing pneumonia, *DIP* desquamative interstitial pneumonia, *GIP* giant cell interstitial pneumonia, *LIP* lymphoid interstitial pneumonia, *NSIP* nonspecific interstitial pneumonia, *RB-ILD* respiratory bronchiolitis interstitial lung disease, *UIP* usual interstitial pneumonia

interstitial fibrosis, idiopathic diffuse interstitial pulmonary fibrosis, honeycomb lung, diffuse interstitial pneumonitis, interstitial pneumonitis-fibrosis, and diffuse fibrosing alveolitis).

The pathologist Averill Liebow took interest in these interstitial lung disorders and published a classification scheme in 1975 for cases in which diffuse interstitial pneumonia was present without any findings to suggest infection or malignancy. He referred to the five different histopathologic patterns (Fig. 1.1) that he described as idiopathic interstitial pneumonias (IIP), a term that has persisted through the decades. The five histopathologic patterns that Liebow described were UIP, desquamative interstitial pneumonia (DIP), bronchiolitis obliterans with interstitial pneumonia (BIP), lymphoid interstitial pneumonia (LIP), and giant cell interstitial pneumonia (GIP). Liebow coined the term "UIP" because it was the most common of the histopathologic patterns recognized. He also noticed that UIP tended to occur in older adults and appeared to affect lobules in a highly variable fashion.

A European classification system was evolving simultaneously, and the term "idiopathic fibrosing alveolitis" appeared in the medical literature in the early 1970s. The term "cryptogenic fibrosing alveolitis" (CFA) was eventually adopted by the Europeans to describe a histopathologic pattern that was essentially the same as UIP. The European system also used the term "cryptogenic organizing pneumonia" (COP) to describe interstitial inflammation with polypoid aggregates of fibroblasts in alveolar spaces that was essentially the equivalent of the BIP lesion described by Liebow. Additionally, the concept of "lone CFA" versus CFA associated with CTD gradually evolved. As the study of the interstitial pneumonias progressed through the 1980s and into the late 1990s, clinicians tended to increasingly recognize and discern the various forms of IIP, enabling a more precise understanding of IPF as a distinct entity.

## The Evolving Role of Imaging in the Diagnosis of ILD

The routine chest X-ray was the only radiologic imaging that was available from the early 1900s for the clinical evaluation of patients until the advent of computed axial tomography (CAT) in the 1970s. As the CAT scan became increasingly available and applied in the clinical evaluation of patients with suspected ILD, patterns were discerned and correlated with histopathology obtained at autopsy or on surgical lung biopsy. As image resolution improved over time, the ability of high-resolution computed tomography (HRCT) of the thorax was exploited to more confidently identify radiologic patterns such as honeycomb change, reticular markings, ground-glass opacities, and consolidation (as well as emphysematous changes, parenchymal nodules, and adenopathy).

Other imaging techniques also became available over time, including nuclear medicine modalities such as gallium scanning and magnetic resonance (MR) imaging. The use of gallium scanning to detect active "alveolitis" reached its zenith in the 1980s. However, it was eventually recognized that such imaging was not particularly accurate in determining "activity" of disease, and its use for evaluating patients with ILD waned in the early 1990s. On the other hand, MR imaging continues to evolve and may eventually provide an alternative to HRCT, which has become the imaging modality of choice for the diagnostic evaluation of suspected ILD or to assess responses to therapeutic interventions. One advantage of MR imaging would be the avoidance of ionizing radiation that patients receive from currently utilized HRCT imaging techniques.

## Flexible Bronchoscopy as a Diagnostic Clinical Tool

The flexible bronchoscope, pioneered and introduced into clinical use in the 1970s, allowed sampling of lung tissue via endobronchial or transbronchial biopsy. Although such biopsies have proven to be quite useful for diagnosing disorders such as sarcoidosis, diagnostic tissue sampling for other forms of ILD remains problematic. The concept of bronchoalveolar lavage (BAL) was introduced into the clinical arena in the 1980s by Herbert Reynolds and colleagues; this procedure was increasingly accepted as a clinical tool that could gauge the "alveolitis" of ILDs. However, it gradually became apparent that the ability of BAL to discern immune cell profiles that were diagnostic for specific forms of ILD was limited and actually somewhat disappointing. Nonetheless, certain patterns such as lymphocytosis in the absence of evidence of infection can be highly suggestive of diagnoses, such as sarcoidosis or hypersensitivity pneumonitis, and provide useful information when considered in the context of the clinical presentation and thoracic imaging studies.

## IPF in the Twenty-First Century

In the 1990s, a considerable body of clinical data pertaining to ILD and IIP had developed in the literature, and the pathology of IIP was revisited and correlated with clinical features. Anna-Louisa Katzenstein described the entity of nonspecific interstitial pneumonia (NSIP) and together with Jeffrey Myers published a manuscript in 1998 in which clinical features were correlated with the histopathologic patterns of acute interstitial pneumonia (AIP), UIP, DIP, respiratory bronchiolitis-associated ILD (RB-ILD), and NSIP. This landmark manuscript underscored the concept that various forms of IIP that had previously been lumped together and termed "IPF" or "CFA" by clinicians were actually fairly distinct clinico-pathologic entities. This set the stage for the term "IPF" to be redefined as idiopathic UIP in the ATS 2000 statement on IPF and the 2002 statement on IIP. Subsequently, other terms, including CFA, gradually disappeared from the medical literature as IPF became the preferred term for idiopathic UIP that usually occurs in older individuals.

The ATS 2011 clinical practice guideline on the diagnosis and management of IPF was the next landmark document to be published. Importantly, this expert panel, using evidence in the published medical literature, recognized that a confident diagnosis of IPF could be established in a substantial number of patients on the basis of a consistent clinical presentation and characteristic HRCT imaging. However, surgical lung biopsy showing changes compatible with UIP would still be required for a confident diagnosis of UIP/IPF if the HRCT was indeterminate.

## Management of IPF: From Corticosteroids to Lung Transplantation

Margaret Turner-Warwick and colleagues published their observations from a large series of patients in England who were diagnosed with CFA in 1980; their report suggested that some had significant clinical improvement when treated with corticosteroids. Further analysis indicated that "responders" were younger, had cellular histology on lung biopsy specimens, and had increased numbers of lymphocytes in their BAL fluid. A subsequent study performed in the United States (27 patients) by Raghu and colleagues was published in 1991 and suggested that adding azathioprine to corticosteroids provided a survival benefit versus corticosteroids alone for patients with IPF (as IPF was defined during that era). It has become clear with the passage of time that these and other studies enrolled a mix of patients. Substantial numbers of patients with what is now recognized as NSIP, DIP, AIP, CTD-associated ILD, and even COP were likely enrolled in these studies and labeled as having IPF or CFA. In the 2000 ATS IPF statement, despite acknowledgement of the lack of sufficient clinical evidence to support the notion that any therapy provided benefit for patients with IPF, it was nonetheless suggested that corticosteroids plus a cytotoxic agent (azathioprine or cyclophosphamide) could be prescribed for and potentially might help patients with the disease. Patients with IPF were therefore widely treated with these therapies as the committee's suggestions were taken as "recommendations," despite the lack of evidence from robustly powered and rigorously performed clinical trials.

It has more recently become apparent from clinical experience that immunosuppressive/anti-inflammatory therapies did very little, if anything, to arrest the disease process. Therefore, therapies targeted against the fibrotic process began to be evaluated through the implementation of robust, randomized, controlled clinical trials in the early 2000s. Indeed, there has been an explosion of interest, and subsequent drug studies have been undertaken and completed in the intervening decade between ATS statements. These studies have provided a wealth of information concerning the natural history of IPF, but, unfortunately, agents such as interferons beta and gamma, etanercept, imatinib, and the endothelin receptor antagonists have been demonstrated to be ineffectual. Indeed, when the ATS/ERS/JRS/ALAT Clinical Practice Guideline on the diagnosis and treatment of IPF was published in 2011, the expert panel reviewed all available publications and concluded that there was insufficient data supporting the use of any specific agent. The strongest recommendation that was afforded any medical therapy was a "weak negative" for monotherapy with either $N$-acetylcysteine or pirfenidone. In addition, this most recent statement recanted the prior suggestion that immunosuppressive therapy may be beneficial, not based on any new data, but rather in recognition of the level of evidence required to provide consensus support for any therapy. This stance was subsequently validated by the results of the NIH-sponsored PANTHER study, which demonstrated that immunosuppressive therapy with azathioprine not only did not help but actually appeared to harm patients with IPF.

Human lung transplantation was first attempted in the 1960s, and a transiently successful lung transplant for a patient with CFA was reported in 1971. However, lung transplantation for patients with advanced, progressive lung disease that was unresponsive to nonsurgical therapies did not enter into the clinical arena as a relatively accepted therapy until the 1980s when potent immunosuppressive agents became available. In 2007, IPF surpassed COPD as the leading indication for lung transplantation in the United States, and lung transplant is currently viewed as a preferable treatment option for patients with advanced IPF. However, due to the inability to meet criteria for lung transplantation, only a relatively small subset of IPF patients are able to meet the necessary criteria to enable placement on a lung transplant waiting list. Indeed, less than 1,000 transplants are performed for IPF per year, which is in part due to a persistent paucity of donor organ availability. Interestingly, recurrent UIP in lung allografts has never been reported, despite a growing number of long-term IPF transplant survivors.

## Summary and Conclusions

The use and definition of the term "IPF" has changed considerably over the decades since the term was first applied to pulmonary fibrosis of unknown cause. IPF is now used to signify a diagnosis that is based upon clinical, radiologic, and (if necessary) histopathologic data that indicate the presence of UIP not associated with other known fibrogenic entities. The causes of this disorder remain elusive, and treatment responses to a variety of pharmacologic agents have been mostly disappointing. At this time, lung transplantation is the only therapeutic option that is universally acknowledged as having a beneficial impact on quality of life and survival in select patients. However, with the growing interest and understanding of this disease, and with the plethora of agents in various stages of drug development, it is the belief of the editors that it is just a matter of time before there are effective medical therapies available for this devastating condition. We hope that this book and the many outstanding, provocative chapters from world-renowned authorities in the field will serve as a platform and spur even more interest in this enigmatic disease.

## Suggested Readings

1. American Thoracic Society. Idiopathic pulmonary fibrosis: diagnosis and treatment. International consensus statement. American Thoracic Society (ATS), and the European Respiratory Society (ERS). Am J Respir Crit Care Med. 2000;161(2 Pt 1):646–64.
2. American Thoracic Society; European Respiratory Society. American Thoracic Society; European Respiratory Society. American Thoracic Society/European Respiratory Society International Multidisciplinary Consensus Classification of the Idiopathic Interstitial Pneumonias. Am J Respir Crit Care Med. 2002;165(2):277–304.
3. Ander L. Idiopathic interstitial fibrosis of the lungs. I. Prognosis as indicated by radiological findings. Acta Med Scand. 1965;178:47–58.
4. Brown CH, Turner-Warwick M. The treatment of cryptogenic fibrosing alveolitis with immunosuppressant drugs. Q J Med. 1971;40(158):289–302.
5. George TJ, Arnaoutakis GJ, Shah AS. Lung transplant in idiopathic pulmonary fibrosis. Arch Surg. 2011;146(10):1204–9.
6. Gottlieb AJ, Spiera H, Teirstein AS, Siltzbach LE. Serologic factors in idiopathic diffuse interstitial pulmonary fibrosis. Am J Med. 1965;39:405–10.
7. Hamman L, Rich AR. Fulminating diffuse interstitial fibrosis of the lungs. Trans Am Clin Climatol Assoc. 1935;51:154–63.
8. Hugh-Jones P, Macarthur AM, Cullum PA, Mason SA, Crosbie WA, Hutchison DC, et al. Lung transplantation in a patient with fibrosing alveolitis. Br Med J. 1971;3(5771):391–8.
9. Idiopathic Pulmonary Fibrosis Clinical Research Network, Raghu G, Anstrom KJ, King Jr TE, Lasky JA, Martinez FJ. Prednisone, azathioprine, and N-acetylcysteine for pulmonary fibrosis. N Engl J Med. 2012;366(21):1968–77.

10. Katzenstein AL, Fiorelli RF. Nonspecific interstitial pneumonia/fibrosis. Histologic features and clinical significance. Am J Surg Pathol. 1994;18(2):136–47.
11. Katzenstein AL, Myers JL. Idiopathic pulmonary fibrosis: clinical relevance of pathologic classification. Am J Respir Crit Care Med. 1998;157(4 Pt 1):1301–15.
12. Liebow AA. Definition and classification of interstitial pneumonias in human pathology. Prog Respir Res. 1975;8:1–31.
13. Malmberg R, Berglund E, Ander L. Idiopathic interstitial fibrosis of the lungs. II. Reversibility of respiratory disturbances during steroid administration. Acta Med Scand. 1965;178:59–66.
14. Meyer KC, Raghu G, Baughman RP, Brown KK, Costabel U, du Bois RM, et al. An official American Thoracic Society clinical practice guideline: the clinical utility of bronchoalveolar lavage cellular analysis in interstitial lung disease. Am J Respir Crit Care Med. 2012;185(9):1004–14.
15. Montgomery CH. Idiopathic interstitial pulmonary fibrosis (Hamman-Rich syndrome): report of a case and survey of the literature. Harv Dent Alumni Bull. 1964;19:48–68.
16. Nathan SD, Shlobin OA, Weir N, Ahmad S, Kaldjob JM, Battle E, et al. Long-term course and prognosis of idiopathic pulmonary fibrosis in the new millennium. Chest. 2011; 140(1):221–9.
17. Peikert T, Daniels CE, Beebe TJ, Meyer KC, Ryu JH, Interstitial Lung Diseases Network of the American College of Chest Physicians. Assessment of current practice in the diagnosis and therapy of idiopathic pulmonary fibrosis. Respir Med. 2008;102(9):1342–8.
18. Raghu G, Collard HR, Egan JJ, Martinez FJ, Behr J, Brown KK, et al. An official ATS/ERS/JRS/ALAT statement: idiopathic pulmonary fibrosis: evidence-based guidelines for diagnosis and management. Am J Respir Crit Care Med. 2011;183(6):788–824.
19. Raghu G, Depaso WJ, Cain K, Hammar SP, Wetzel CE, Dreis DF, et al. Azathioprine combined with prednisone in the treatment of idiopathic pulmonary fibrosis: a prospective double-blind, randomized, placebo-controlled clinical trial. Am Rev Respir Dis. 1991;144(2):291–6.
20. Reid JM, Cuthbert J, Craik JE. Chronic diffuse idiopathic fibrosing alveolitis. Br J Dis Chest. 1965;59(4):194–201.
21. Robbins LL. Idiopathic pulmonary fibrosis; roentgenologic findings. Radiology. 1948;51(4): 459–67.
22. Sheridan LA, Harrison Jr EG, Divertie MB. The current status of idiopathic pulmonary fibrosis (Hamman-Rich syndrome). Med Clin North Am. 1964;48:993–1010.
23. Stack BH, Choo-Kang YF, Heard BE. The prognosis of cryptogenic fibrosing alveolitis. Thorax. 1972;27(5):535–42.
24. Stack BH, Grant IW, Irvine WJ, Moffat MA. Idiopathic diffuse interstitial lung disease. A review of 42 cases. Am Rev Respir Dis. 1965;92(6):939–48.
25. Wildevuur CR, Benfield JR. A review of 23 human lung transplantations by 20 surgeons. Ann Thorac Surg. 1970;9(6):489–515.

# Chapter 2
# Idiopathic Pulmonary Fibrosis: The Epidemiology and Natural History of Disease

Olga Tourin, Jeffrey J. Swigris, and Amy L. Olson

**Abstract** Idiopathic pulmonary fibrosis (IPF) was once thought to be a rare disease and has been classically described as a disease that progresses in a "relentless and often insidious manner." However, recent epidemiologic studies have revealed the true burden of this disease on society and identified risk factors for the development of disease that may ultimately allow for not only disease prevention but also further insight into the pathobiology of this—as of yet—idiopathic disease. At the same time, recent cohort studies and clinical trials have better defined the natural history of this disease. In this manuscript, we will review recently acquired epidemiologic data and summarize the current understanding of the natural history of IPF.

**Keywords** Idiopathic pulmonary fibrosis • Natural history • Clinical course • Epidemiology • Risk factors • Mortality • Incidence • Prevalence

O. Tourin, M.D.
University of Calgary, Adult Respirology Residency Program,
Rockyview General Hospital, Calgary, AB, Canada

J.J. Swigris, D.O., M.S.
Autoimmune Lung Center and Interstitial Lung Disease Program,
National Jewish Health, 1400 Jackson Street, Denver, CO 80238, USA

A.L. Olson, M.D., M.S.P.H. (✉)
Division of Pulmonary and Critical Care Medicine, National Jewish Health,
Interstitial Lung Disease Program and Autoimmune Lung Center, 1400 Jackson Street,
Denver, CO 80238, USA
e-mail: olsona@njhealth.org; amy.olson@ucdenver.edu

K.C. Meyer and S.D. Nathan (eds.), *Idiopathic Pulmonary Fibrosis: A Comprehensive Clinical Guide*, Respiratory Medicine 9, DOI 10.1007/978-1-62703-682-5_2,
© Springer Science+Business Media New York 2014

# Introduction

Idiopathic pulmonary fibrosis (IPF) has been classically described as a disease that progresses in a "relentless and often insidious manner," with median survival estimates of 2–3 years from the time of diagnosis [1, 2]. However, research over the past two decades has improved our understanding of the natural history of IPF. Although some patients experience steadily progressive respiratory decline, it is now recognized that the clinical course for others is marked by rapid progression and/or acute episodes of worsening that do not infrequently result in death. At the group level, clinical factors associated with an increased risk of mortality have been identified, but predicting the course of disease in an individual patient is challenging, if not impossible. Whether differences in the clinical course result from varying phenotypes of IPF or from other factors (e.g., differences in the type, degree, or intensity of environmental exposures or ethnic and racial differences) is unclear [2, 3]. While certain investigators were generating research that refined understanding of how IPF behaves over time, others were performing epidemiologic studies that better defined the societal burden of IPF and identified environmental exposures associated with an increased risk for developing disease. In this chapter, we review recently acquired epidemiologic data on IPF and describe the variable natural history of this disease that continues to confound clinicians and researchers alike.

# The Epidemiology of IPF

## Background

Investigators have used epidemiologic studies to determine the societal burden of IPF and to identify possible exposures/risk factors (predominantly through case–control studies) for disease development. These studies have revealed that IPF is not as rare as it was once believed to be, underscoring the need for more resources to advance research for this devastating condition. Results from additional epidemiologic studies have identified specific risk factors for IPF, providing insight into possible pathobiologic mechanisms for disease. Hopefully, these studies will prove useful as investigators search for approaches to limit disease occurrence [4].

Prior to the 1990s, factors that kept investigators from conducting large-scale epidemiologic studies in IPF included the supposed rarity of disease, the evolving (changing) case definition of IPF, and the lack of a specific International Classification of Diseases (ICD) diagnostic code. Since then, three developments have changed the landscape of epidemiologic research in IPF: (1) the ninth revision of the ICD coding (ICD-9) system (which for the first time assigned a diagnostic code for IPF and occurred at the end of the 1970s), (2) large population databases (including death certificate data and healthcare claims data), and (3) both regional and multicenter collaborative efforts to determine both the extent of and risk factors for disease.

**Table 2.1** The prevalence of IPF by age strata and gender in Bernalillo County, New Mexico, from 1988 to 1993 [5] compared to a healthcare claims processing system of a large United States health plan from 1996 to 2000 using the broad case definition [6] (see text)[a]

| Idiopathic pulmonary fibrosis (prevalence, per 100,000 persons) | | | | |
|---|---|---|---|---|
| | 1988–1993 | | 1996–2000 | |
| Age strata (years) | Men | Women | Men | Women |
| 35–44 | 2.7 | – | 4.9 | 12.7 |
| 45–54 | 8.7 | 8.1 | 22.3 | 22.6 |
| 55–64 | 28.4 | 5.0 | 62.8 | 50.9 |
| 65–74 | 104.6 | 72.3 | 148.5 | 106.7 |
| ≥75 | 174.7 | 73.2 | 276.9 | 192.1 |

[a]Adapted from Table 4 in [5] and Fig. 1 in [6]

## Prevalence, Incidence, and Secular Trends

Prevalence is a ratio defined as the number of persons with a disease at a specific point in time divided by the total population at that time. Incidence is a rate, defined as the number of new cases (that have developed over a given period of time) divided by the number of persons at risk for developing disease over that period of time.

Coultas and colleagues performed the first regional epidemiologic investigation in the USA to determine the prevalence and incidence of interstitial lung disease (ILD) [5]. Using multiple case-finding methods (including primary care and pulmonary physician's records, histopathology reports, hospital discharge diagnoses, death certificates, and autopsy reports), these investigators established a population-based ILD registry in Bernalillo County, New Mexico—a county with a population of nearly one-half million at the time of this study. Based on data from 1988 to 1993, the overall prevalence of IPF was 20.2 cases per 100,000 population in men and 13.2 cases per 100,000 population in women. When these data were stratified by age and gender, the prevalence of IPF increased with increasing age and was higher for men than for women in each age strata (Table 2.1). The incidence of IPF was 10.7 per 100,000 persons/year in men and 7.4 per 100,000 persons/year in women. Again, when stratified by age and gender, the incidence of IPF generally increased with increasing age and was typically higher for men than for women (Table 2.2).

Raghu and colleagues determined the prevalence and incidence of IPF from 1996 to 2000 using data from a large US healthcare plan's claims system [6]. Using a broad definition for IPF (age >18 years, one or more medical encounters coded for IPF, and no medical encounters after that IPF encounter with a diagnosis code for any other type of ILD), these investigators estimated the prevalence and annual incidence of the disease to be 42.7 and 16.3 per 100,000 people, respectively. A narrow case definition (broad definition plus at least one medical encounter with a procedure code for a surgical lung biopsy, transbronchial biopsy, or computed tomography [CT] of the thorax) yielded a prevalence and annual incidence of 14.0 per 100,000 people and 6.8 per 100,000 people, respectively. In their dataset, both prevalence and incidence increased with increasing age, and rates were higher in

**Table 2.2**[a]   The incidence of IPF by age strata and gender from Bernalillo County, New Mexico, from 1988 to 1993 [5] compared a healthcare claims processing system of a large United States health plan from 1996 to 2000 using the broad case definition [6] (see text)

| Idiopathic pulmonary fibrosis (incidence, per 100,000 persons/year) | | | | |
|---|---|---|---|---|
| | 1988–1993 | | 1996–2000 | |
| Age strata (years) | Men | Women | Men | Women |
| 35–44 | 4.0 | – | 1.1 | 5.4 |
| 45–54 | 2.2 | 4.0 | 11.4 | 10.9 |
| 55–64 | 14.2 | 10.0 | 35.1 | 22.6 |
| 65–74 | 48.6 | 21.1 | 49.1 | 36.0 |
| ≥75 | 101.9 | 57.0 | 97.6 | 62.2 |

[a]Adapted from Table 5 in [5] and Fig. 2 in [6]

men than women (see Tables 2.1 and 2.2). Results from these two studies suggest that rates have increased over time; however, their limitations limit these studies as only being hypothesis generating.

Fernández-Pérez and colleagues performed a population-based, historical cohort study in Olmsted County, Minnesota, of patients evaluated at their center between 1997 and 2005. They had three aims for their study: (1) determine the prevalence and incidence of IPF, (2) determine if incidence changed over time, and (3) predict the future burden of disease [7]. For 2005, using narrow case-finding criteria [usual interstitial pneumonia (UIP) pattern on surgical lung biopsy or definite UIP pattern on high-resolution CT (HRCT)], the age- and sex-adjusted prevalence (for people over the age of 50 years) was 27.9 cases per 100,000 persons (95 % CI = 10.4–45.4); using broad case-finding criteria (UIP pattern on surgical lung biopsy or definite *or possible* UIP pattern on HRCT), it was 63 cases per 100,000 persons (95 % CI = 36.4–89.6). Over the 9 years of this study, the age- and sex-adjusted incidence (for those over the age of 50) was 8.8 cases per 100,000 person-years (95 % CI = 5.3–12.4) and 17.4 cases per 100,000 person-years (95 % CI = 12.4–22.4) for the narrow and broad case-finding criteria, respectively. In contrast to the incidence rates reported by Coultas and Raghu [8, 9], results here suggest significantly decreasing incidence rates over the last 3 years of the study to 6.0 or 11.0 per 100,000 person-years using the narrow or broad case-finding criteria, respectively ($p < 0.001$). Despite the estimated declining incidence, given the aging US population, these investigators projected that the annual number of new cases will continue to rise, with 12,000–21,000 new IPF cases by 2050. Several limitations, including the small total number of incident IPF cases (only 47 based on the broad case criteria), detract from the confidence that these results accurately reflect national trends.

Large-scale epidemiologic studies from the UK also suggest an increase in the incidence of IPF over time. Gribbin and colleagues analyzed a large longitudinal general practice database in the UK from 1991 to 2003 and found that overall the incidence of IPF more than doubled over this time period [10]. The overall crude incidence of IPF was 4.6 per 100,000 person-years, and the annual increase in the incidence of IPF was 11 % (rate ratio 1.11, 95 % CI = 1.09–1.13, $p < 0.0001$)

after adjusting for sex, age, and geographic region. As in the studies described above, these investigators found the incidence of IPF was higher in men than women and increased with age (until >85 years of age). They could not determine if the trends observed were from increased case ascertainment—due to either the expanding routine use of HRCT scanning or simply increased awareness perhaps stemming from globally visible consensus statements and multinational IPF drug trials.

Recently, Navaratnam and colleagues extended the work of Gribbin and colleagues [11]. Using the same longitudinal primary care database from the UK, these investigators determined the incidence of what they called the IPF clinical syndrome (IPF-CS) (defined by the following diagnostic codes: idiopathic fibrosing alveolitis, Hamman–Rich syndrome, cryptogenic fibrosing alveolitis, diffuse pulmonary fibrosis, and idiopathic fibrosing alveolitis NOS, excluding connective tissue disease, extrinsic allergic alveolitis, asbestosis, pneumoconiosis, and sarcoidosis) from 2000 to 2008. In their study, the overall crude incidence of IPF-CS was 7.44 per 100,000 person-years (nearly double the rate that Gribbin and colleagues reported for the prior decade); it was higher in men than women and generally increased with age. After adjusting for age, sex, and health authority, the incidence of IPF-CS increased by 5 % annually from 2000 to 2008 (rate ratio 1.05, 95 % CI = 1.03–1.06).

The majority of these data suggest the incidence of IPF is increasing. In IPF, because the disease is lethal within a relatively short period of time, mortality rates should mirror incidence rates, making mortality rate studies an additional, potentially rich source of data on these trends.

## Mortality Rates and Secular Trends

Mortality rates for a condition are calculated as the number of deaths per year from the condition of interest, divided by the number of persons alive in the midyear population. Death certificate and census recording can provide data for such calculations. Because the validity of IPF death certificate data is largely unknown, studies using these data should be interpreted with caution. In the era of ICD-9 coding, when IPF (ICD-9 code 516.3) was coded on a death certificate, it was generally accurate. However, because a significant proportion of decedents with IPF were coded as 515—the code for post-inflammatory pulmonary fibrosis (PIPF)—IPF (whose ICD-9 code is 516.3) was typically under-recorded as the cause of death [12, 13]. In 1998, the ICD-10 coding system combined both IPF and PIPF into one diagnostic code (J84.1). In some studies, investigators have used this code—and made concerted efforts to exclude decedents with codes for known causes of ILD— to capture a cohort most likely to have IPF. Other investigators have conducted similar studies and either intentionally or unintentionally included decedents with coexisting conditions associated with pulmonary fibrosis (e.g., connective tissue disease), leaving cohorts they labeled as having pulmonary fibrosis (PF) or IPF clinical syndrome (IPF-CS) [11, 14, 15]. Regardless of the term used, a great many decedents in these studies had IPF, and all almost certainly had progressive fibrotic lung disease that has resulted in death.

In the first large-scale study of mortality rates from IPF, Johnston and colleagues examined ICD-9-coded death certificates from 1979 to 1988 and found that mortality rates from IPF (ICD-9 code 516.3) in England and Wales more than doubled over this time period [12]. Although more men than women died of IPF (60 % of decedents), over the study period, mortality rates increased in both men and women (after standardization for age) and were greater among the aged. Specifically, the mortality rate in those aged ≥75 years was eight times that of those aged 45–54. They identified higher mortality rates in the industrialized central areas of England and Wales, raising occupational or environmental exposures as potential risk factors for the disease. Confirming and expanding the findings of Johnston and colleagues, Hubbard and colleagues examined ICD-9-coded death certificates and found that mortality rates from IPF rose in England, Wales, Scotland, Australia, and Canada from 1979 to 1992 [16].

Mannino and colleagues examined US death certificate data and found that, from 1979 to 1991, age-adjusted mortality for pulmonary fibrosis (PF) increased 4.7 % in men (from 48.6 deaths per million to 50.9 deaths per million) and 27.1 % in women (from 21.4 deaths per million to 27.2 deaths per million). Again, PF-associated morality increased with increasing age [14]. Higher mortality rates were identified in the West and Southeast, and lower mortality rates occurred in the Midwest and Northeast.

Using the same database as Mannino and colleagues, our group found that, from 1992 to 2003, PF-associated mortality rates increased 29.4 % in men (from 49.7 deaths per million to 64.3 deaths per million) and increased 38.1 % in women (from 42.3 deaths per million to 58.4 deaths per million) (Fig. 2.1). Mortality rates increased with advancing age and were consistently higher in men than in women; however, mortality rates increased at a faster pace in women than in men over this period of time [15].

Similar trends in mortality were recently reported in the UK; the overall age- and sex-adjusted mortality rate from IPF-CS from 2005 to 2008 was 50.1 per million person-years. The overall annual increase in mortality was approximately 5 % per year (RR = 1.05, 95 % CI = 1.04–1.05) from 1968 to 2008, which equated to a six-fold increase in mortality over this study period [11]. These studies suggest mortality from IPF is increasing, and IPF is an important and growing public health concern, particularly in the aging population.

## Risk Factors

### Definitions and Limitations

Most studies of risk factors for IPF have been retrospective and subject to a number of limitations. Because the disease status and the exposure are assessed at the same time, temporality cannot be established. Further, systematic biases resulting from both recall and diagnostic misclassification are possible. Recall bias exists when

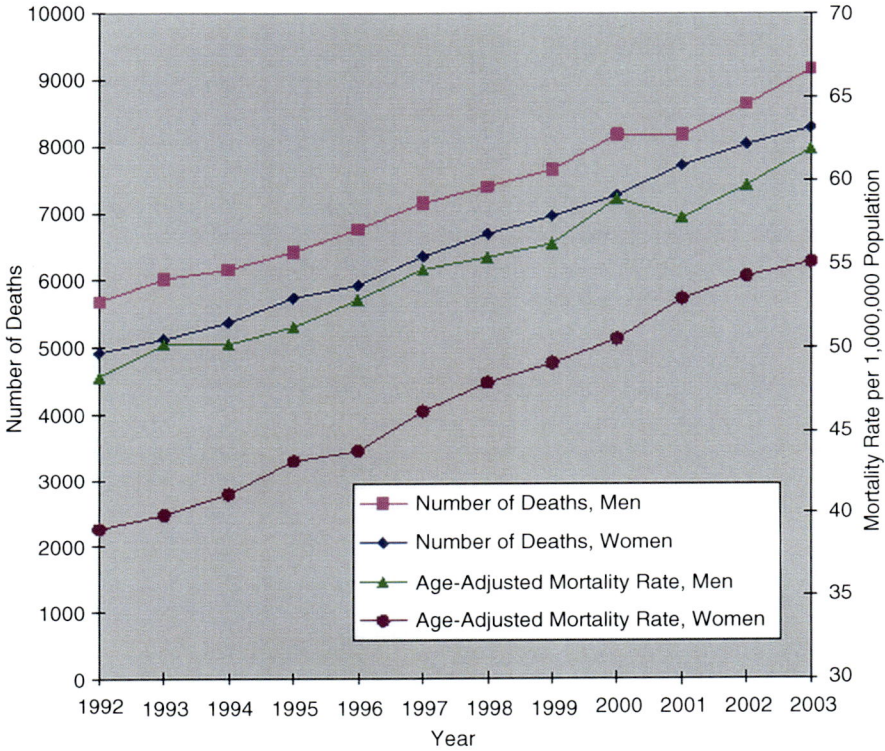

**Fig. 2.1** Actual number of deaths per year (first *y*-axis) and age-adjusted mortality rates (second *y*-axis) in decedents with PF per 1,000,000 population from 1992 to 2003 in the USA. Mortality rates are standardized to the 2000 US Census Population (Reprinted with permission of the American Thoracic Society. Copyright© 2012 American Thoracic Society. Olson AL, Swigris JJ, Lezotte DC, Norris JM, Wilson CG, Brown KK. Mortality from pulmonary fibrosis increased in the USA from 1992 to 2003. Am J Respir Crit Care Med. 2007;176:277–284. Official Journal of the American Thoracic Society)

cases recall past exposures differently than controls—and the net effect results in an exaggeration of risk [17]. Diagnostic misclassification bias arises when cases are incorrectly diagnosed with the disease or when controls have subclinical and undiagnosed disease. These scenarios have likely occurred in IPF, specifically in the time period before the routine use of HRCT scanning and consensus statements on the classification of idiopathic interstitial pneumonias (IIP) and IPF [1, 18]. The net effect of this type of error results in bias towards the null (a reduction in the strength of the association between exposure and disease). When identified, dose–response relationships strengthen the likelihood of a significant risk for the development of disease.

## Cigarette Smoking

In a number of case–control studies, cigarette smoking has been identified as a risk factor for IPF and for familial pulmonary fibrosis (FPF). In the USA, Baumgartner and colleagues performed an extensive analysis of the risk of IPF associated with smoking [19]. From 1989 to 1993, they compared 248 IPF patients at any of 16 referral centers with 491 controls matched on age, sex, and geography. They found that a history of ever smoking was associated with a 60 % increase in risk for the development of IPF (OR = 1.6, 95 % CI = 1.1–2.2). Additional analysis revealed that former smoking was associated with a 90 % increased risk for the development of IPF (OR = 1.9, 95 % CI = 1.3–2.9), whereas current smoking was not associated with an elevated risk (OR = 1.06, 95 % CI = 0.6–1.8). A dose–response relationship was not identified: compared to subjects with a less than 20-pack-year history, those who smoked 21–40 pack-years had an increased risk of IPF (OR = 2.26, 95 % CI = 1.3–3.8), while those who smoked more than 40 pack-years did not (OR = 1.12, 95 % CI = 0.7–1.9). However, among former smokers, those who had recently stopped smoking possessed the highest risk for the development of IPF (for those who stopped smoking less than 2.5 years prior, OR = 3.5, 95 % CI = 1.1–11.9; for those who stopped smoking 2.5–10 years prior, OR = 2.3, 95 % CI = 1.3–4.2; for those who stopped smoking 10–25 years prior, OR = 1.9, 95 % CI = 1.1–3.2; and for those who stopped smoking more than 25 years ago, OR = 1.3, 95 % CI = 0.7–2.3). Similar to Baumgartner and colleagues, Miyake and colleagues compared 102 cases of IPF to 59 controls in Japan and found an increased risk of IPF only in those who smoked between 20 and 40 pack-years (OR = 3.23, 95 % CI = 1.01–10.84) compared to never smokers [20].

Taskar and colleagues [21] conducted a meta-analysis that included these two and three additional case–control studies from the UK [22, 23] and Japan [24]. Ever smoking was associated with a 58 % increase in the risk for the development of IPF (OR = 1.58, 95 % CI = 1.27–1.97). Given the high prevalence of smoking, these investigators determined that 49 % of IPF cases could be prevented by entirely eliminating smoking within the population. The results from two other case–control studies from Mexico, not included in the meta-analysis, also suggest smoking is a risk factor for IPF (OR adjusted = 3.2, 95 % CI = 1.2–8.5 and OR adjusted = 2.5, 95 % CI = 1.4–4.6) [25, 26]. An association between smoking and lung fibrosis has also been identified in FPF. Steele and colleagues compared 309 cases of FPF with 360 unaffected family members from 111 families and found that, after adjustment for age and sex, ever smoking was associated with a greater than threefold odds of developing disease (OR = 3.6, 95 % CI = 1.3–9.8) [27].

## Occupational Exposures

Case–control studies have also found an association between a number of dusts and/ or dusty environments and the development of IPF.

## Metal Dusts

In a meta-analysis of five case–control studies published between 1990 and 2005, investigators found a significant association between metal dust exposure and the development of IPF (OR = 2.44, 95 % CI = 1.74–3.40) [20–24, 28]. Baumgartner and colleagues identified a dose–response relationship between metal dust exposure and IPF. For subjects with less than 5 years of metal dust exposure, there was no association (OR = 1.4, 95 % CI = 0.4–4.9); however, for those with more than 5 years of metal dust exposure, the risk for the development of IPF was elevated over twofold (OR = 2.2, 95 % CI = 1.1–4.7) [28].

Hubbard and colleagues analyzed data from the pension fund archives of a metal engineering company and identified more deaths within this cohort than would be expected from national mortality data [29]. Among all decedents with IPF and records available, there was not an increased risk of IPF associated with metal dust exposure. However, there was a dose–response relationship: for those with more than 10 years of exposure, there was an increased risk of IPF (OR = 1.71, 95 % CI = 1.09–2.68).

Pinheiro and colleagues analyzed mortality data from 1999 to 2003 and found an increased proportionate mortality ratio (PMR) and mortality odds ratio (MOR) among decedents with ICD-10 for pulmonary fibrosis whose records also contained a code for "metal mining" (PMR = 2.4, 95 % CI = 1.3–4.0; MOR 2.2, 95 % CI = 1.1–4.4) and "fabricated structural metal products" (PMR = 1.9, 95 % CI = 1.1–3.1; MOR 1.7, 95 % CI = 1.0–3.1) [30]. In contrast, in a recent study from Sweden, investigators did not identify an association between metal dust exposure and IPF among patients on oxygen therapy (OR = 0.8, 95 % CI = 0.43–1.44) [31].

## Wood Dust

Results from two of five case–control studies (one from the UK and one from Japan) and a meta-analysis of these studies suggest an association between wood dust exposure and IPF (OR summary = 1.94, 95 % CI = 1.34–2.81) [20–23, 28, 32]. Discrepancies in results between individual studies may result from differences in the type of wood exposure. In a case–control study, investigators in Sweden found an association between both birch (OR = 2.4, 95 % CI = 1.18–4.92) and hardwood dust (OR = 2.5, 95 % CI = 1.06–5.89) and IPF, but not fir dust (OR = 1.4, 95 % CI = 0.82–2.52) [31].

## Agriculture (Farming and Livestock)

Farming and livestock exposures have been linked to an increased risk of IPF. In each of two case–control studies (one from the USA and one from Japan), investigators found a significant association between farming or residing in an agricultural region and IPF (summary OR = 1.65, 95 % CI = 1.20–2.26) [21, 24, 28]. In the Japanese study, exposure to agricultural chemicals was also associated with an increased risk of IPF (OR = 3.32, 95 % CI = 1.22–9.05) [24].

Results from two case–control studies, one from the USA and one from the UK, suggest an association between livestock and IPF (summary OR = 2.17, 95 % CI = 1.28–3.68) [21, 22, 28]. In the US study, investigators observed a dose–response relationship between exposure to livestock and IPF: for subjects with less than 5 years of exposure, no association was identified (OR = 2.1, 95 % CI = 0.7–6.1), but subjects with more than 5 years of exposure to livestock had a greater than threefold risk for IPF (OR = 3.3, 95 % CI = 1.3–8.3) [28].

Sand, Stone, and Silica

Results from a meta-analysis of four studies with contrasting results show a significant association between stone, sand, and silica dusts and IPF (summary OR = 1.97, 95 % CI = 1.09–3.55) [20–22, 28, 32].

**Miscellaneous Exposures**

After adjusting for age and cigarette smoking, Baumgartner and colleagues found an association between IPF and hairdressing (OR = 4.4, 95 % CI = 1.2–16.3) or raising birds (OR = 4.7, 95 % CI = 4.7, 95 % 1.6–14.1) [28]. The latter association raises the possibility that some patients with chronic hypersensitivity pneumonitis might have been inadvertently diagnosed as IPF. Residing in an urban/polluted area is another risk factor for IPF that emerged from a case–control study in Japan (OR = 3.33, 95 % CI = 1.26–8.79) [24].

# The Natural History of IPF

## *Background*

Historically, IPF has been described as a disease marked by inexorable progression [1, 2]. For patients with steadily progressive disease (i.e., moderately worsening lung function with each passing year), symptoms of breathlessness typically precede the diagnosis of IPF by 1–3 years [33–35], and median survival ranges from 2 to 3 years from the time of diagnosis [1, 2, 33–36]. However, careful inspection of results reveals significant heterogeneity in survival rates within cohorts [1, 37, 38]. In the last handful of years, investigators have drilled deep into their datasets in an attempt to better understand this heterogeneity; although some of it may result from differences in disease severity at the time of diagnosis, it has become clear to the ILD field that there are actually different IPF phenotypes that can be defined by

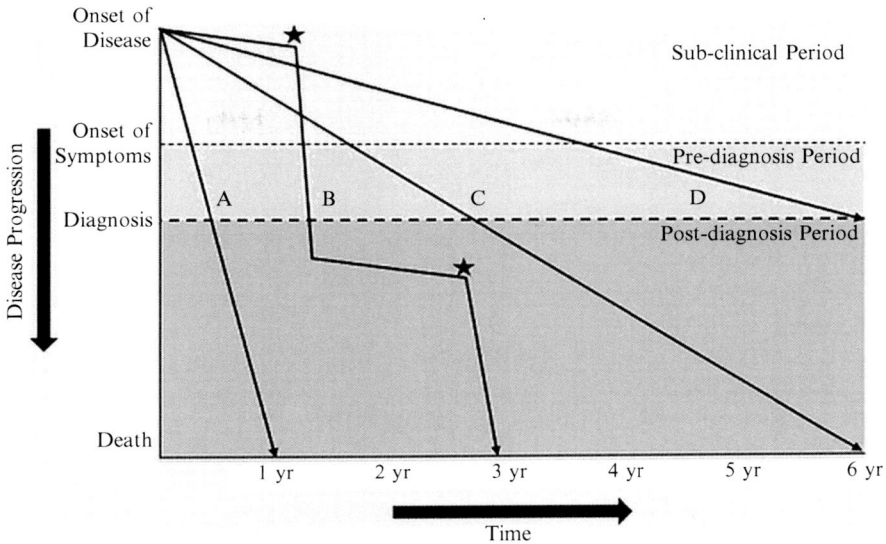

**Fig. 2.2** Schematic representation of potential clinical courses of IPF. The *y*-axis represents disease progression from the onset of disease with a likely subclinical/asymptomatic period, which is followed by a period of symptoms that precede a formal diagnosis and then followed by the period of diagnosis through death with the *x*-axis representing time. As noted in the text, disease progression may be accelerated (**a**), relatively stable (**c** or **d**), or alternate between periods of relative stability marked by acute worsening (*stars*) (**b**) (Reprinted with permission of the American Thoracic Society. Copyright©2012 American Thoracic Society. Ley B, Collard HR, King TE Jr. Clinical course and prediction of survival in idiopathic pulmonary fibrosis. Am J Respir Crit Care Med. 2011;183:431–440. Official Journal of the American Thoracic Society)

disease behavior over time (Fig. 2.2). For example, in every IPF study, there is a subgroup of long-term survivors; a significant minority of IPF patients will suffer one or more acute exacerbations of IPF; and investigators are finding more and more patients with subclinical disease. What drives the phenotypic expression is unknown, but the current theory holds that it results from complex interactions involving the age and genetic makeup of the host and environmental exposures.

## Predicting Survival

Nathan and colleagues examined data from their center collected over the past decade and found that for 357 IPF patients, the median survival was 45.9 months (3.8 years) from the time of their initial pulmonary function test. When stratified on disease severity, patients with percent predicted forced vital capacity (FVC%) $\geq 70$ %, 55–69 %, OR <55 % had median survival values of 55.6 months (4.6 years), 38.7 months (3.2 years), and 27.4 months (2.3 years), respectively [38].

In addition to FVC, a number of other individual clinical, radiographic, physiologic, and pathologic variables as well as various biomarkers correlate with survival [39]. Several investigators have generated prognostic models that incorporate combinations of these variables collected at the time of diagnosis [34, 35]. For example, King and colleagues used data from 183 patients with biopsy-proven IPF and found that survival was dependent on a combination of age, smoking status, clubbing, extent of interstitial abnormalities, and presence of evidence of pulmonary hypertension on chest radiograph, total lung capacity (TLC), and abnormal gas exchange during maximal exercise [35]. Based on this model with these clinical, radiological, and physiological (CRP) determinants, 5-year survival ranged from 89 % in patients with lower scores to <1 % in patients with higher CRP scores. Although this and other similar models [40, 41] reveal that differences in survival depend on baseline characteristics, none have been formally externally validated, and each has limited ability to predict disease behavior in an individual patient.

Collard and colleagues determined that after adjustment for baseline values, 6 and 12 months' change in any of a number of variables including dyspnea score, TLC, FVC, partial pressure of arterial oxygen, peripheral oxygen saturation, and alveolar–arterial oxygen gradient predicted survival time [37]. As with baseline predictors, these seem to perform well at the group level [42, 43], but may not at the patient level.

## Rate of Decline in FVC

Data from the placebo arms of several therapeutic trials reveal that the annual decline in absolute FVC ranges from 0.15 to 0.22 L [44–51] (Table 2.3). Given inclusion criteria (which typically seek to identify patients with earlier/milder disease) and exclusion criteria (which typically exclude patients with significant comorbid conditions) [38], these estimates of disease progression are unlikely to apply to the general population of IPF patients.

## The Underlying Cause of Death

For the majority of patients with IPF, the underlying cause of death (UCD) is respiratory failure [14, 15, 39, 52]. Panos and colleagues reviewed series of cases with mortality data published from 1964 to 1983: among 326 deaths, respiratory failure was the UCD in 38.7 % [52]. Using US death certificate data from 1979 to 1991, Mannino and colleagues found that in patients with pulmonary fibrosis, the UCD was the disease itself in 50 % of decedents [14]. Our group extended the work of Mannino and colleagues by examining US death certificate data from 1992 to 2003

**Table 2.3** Recent randomized, placebo-controlled trials in which the absolute decline in forced vital capacity (FVC) for the placebo group was reported over the study period [44–51]

| Study | Drug | Baseline FVC, L (FVC%) | Absolute decline in FVC, L | Time of assessment (weeks) | Annual rate of decline in FVC, L/year |
|---|---|---|---|---|---|
| TOMORROW [44] | Nintedanib | 2.70 (77.6 %) | −0.19 | 52 | −0.19/year |
| BUILD-3 [45] | Bosentan | 2.66 (73.1 %) | −0.18 | 52 | −0.18/year |
| Imatinib [46] | Imatinib | 2.54 (65.5 %) | −0.14 | 48 | −0.15/year |
| Shionogi [47] | Pirfenidone | 2.47[a] (79.1 %)[a] | −0.16[a] | 52 | −0.16/year[a] |
| Etanercept [48] | Etanercept | NR (63.0 %) | −0.20 | 48 | −0.22/year |
| Shionogi [49] | Pirfenidone | NR (78.4)[a] | −0.13[a] | 36 | −0.19/year[a] |
| IFIGENIA [50] | NAC | 2.36[a] (66.6 %)[a] | −0.19[a] | 52 | −0.19/year[a] |
| GIPF-001 [51] | Interferon Gamma-1b | NR (64.1 %) | −0.16 | 48 | −0.17/year |

In those studies that were less than 52 weeks in duration, the annual rate of decline was determined from available data by assuming a constant rate of decline

*NR* not reported

[a]Studies actually reported vital capacity (VC)

and found that pulmonary fibrosis was the UCD in 60 % of decedents with IPF [15]. Among IPF subjects in therapeutic trials, the UCD is a respiratory cause in nearly 80 % [39, 46, 48, 53, 54]. Taken together, these data reveal that over the past 50 years, the proportion of patients with IPF who are dying from, rather than with, the disease has grown. These trends may reflect advances in diagnostic accuracy. However, another potential explanation is that effective therapies for some of the more common comorbid conditions (e.g., cardiovascular disease) result in them being more likely to die from IPF than these other treatable conditions (Table 2.4).

Besides disease progression, UCDs in patients with IPF include coronary artery disease (CAD), pulmonary embolism, and lung cancer. While the proportion dying from cardiovascular disease has declined over time (see Table 2.4), patients with IPF appear to be at greater risk for CAD than patients with chronic obstructive pulmonary disease (COPD) (or other respiratory diseases requiring transplantation) [56–58] or people in the background population [59–61]. Thromboembolic disease and pulmonary embolism occur more often in patients with IPF than those with COPD, lung cancer, or in people in the background population [55, 60, 62]. Furthermore, IPF decedents with a code for thromboembolic disease on their death certificates died younger [74.3 vs. 77.4 years in females ($p < 0.0001$) and 72.0 vs. 74.4 years in males ($p < 0.0001$)] than IPF decedents without codes for thromboembolic disease [55]. Compared with the background population, the risk for lung cancer is significantly elevated in patients with IPF, and this appears to be independent of smoking history [63, 64]; however, its overall effect on survival in this population remains unknown [65].

**Table 2.4** The underlying cause of death in patients with idiopathic pulmonary fibrosis (see text) [14, 15, 52, 55]

| Underlying cause of death study | Respiratory pulmonary fibrosis | Respiratory pneumonia | Respiratory COPD | Respiratory PE | Lung cancer | Cardiovascular disease | Other |
|---|---|---|---|---|---|---|---|
| Panos (1964–1983) | 39 % | 2.8 % | NR | 3.4 % | 10.4 % | 27.0 % | 14.1 % |
| Mannino (1979–1991) | 50.0 % | NR | 22.6 % | NR | 4.8 % | 22.6 % | NR |
| Olson/Sprunger[a] (1992–2003)/ (1998–2007)[a] | 60.0 % | 2.4 % | NR | 1.74 %[a] | 2.9 % | 9.6 % | 23.4 % |

NR not reported

[a] combined data

## Phenotypic Subgroups

### Long-Term Survivors

In studies conducted prior to the development of the current IIP classification system [18], nearly 30 % of subjects with IPF were alive at 10 years from diagnosis [66, 67]. It has been assumed that, in retrospect, these long-term survivors had diseases other than IPF [e.g., nonspecific interstitial pneumonia (NSIP)]. However, using the ATS/ERJ criteria for the diagnosis of IPF [1] and data from the past decade, Nathan and colleagues found that approximately one-quarter of their IPF patients ($n = 357$) survived more than 5 years from the time of diagnosis, and survival time was not necessarily associated with baseline FVC [38].

### Rapid Progression from Diagnosis

Some patients with IPF follow a rapidly progressive clinical course from the onset (see Fig. 2.2). Selman and colleagues compared IPF patients with ≤6 months of symptoms (rapid progressors) to those with symptoms for ≥24 months (slow progressors) prior to first presentation. They found that despite the absence of differences between groups in baseline age, physiology, or gas exchange parameters, compared with slow progressors, rapid progressors had a significantly increased risk of death (HR = 9.0, 95 % CI = 4.48–18.3) and were more likely to be male (OR = 6.5, 95 % CI = 1.4–29.5) and either former or current smokers (OR = 3.04, 95 % CI = 1.1–8.3) [68]. Further, in rapid progressors, the authors found a distinctive gene expression pattern marked by overexpression of genes involved in morphogenesis, oxidative stress, and migration and proliferation of fibroblasts and smooth muscle cells.

Boon and colleagues examined gene expression profiles in surgical lung biopsy specimens and identified 134 transcripts that sufficiently distinguished relatively stable disease from progressive IPF [69]. They commented that similar to human cancers, genes related to cell proliferation, migration, invasion, and morphology were over represented in subjects with progressive disease. These findings highlight the heterogeneity of IPF at the transcriptional level and probably explain in large part the varying clinical courses among patients with disease.

### Stable Disease Followed by Accelerated Disease

Still other IPF patients follow a relatively stable or mildly progressive course for months to years, and then their disease accelerates. Using data from the placebo arm of a large therapeutic trial, Martinez and his coinvestigators observed that among patients who survived to the end of the 72-week study (78.6 %), the mean FVC% decreased from $64.5 \pm 11.1$–$61 \pm 14.1$, the mean DLCO% decreased from

$37.8 \pm 11.1 - 37.0 \pm 19.9$ %, and there was little worsening in dyspnea [53]. However, among 36 subjects who succumbed (21.4 %), death was IPF related in 32 patients (89 %) and the result of disease progression in 20 patients (56 %). Of those deaths resulting from progressive IPF, 47 % were acute (deterioration over 4 weeks or less) and 50 % were subacute (progression over weeks to months), thus demonstrating that disease progression accelerates prior to death in some.

## Acute Exacerbations of IPF

In Japan, it has been recognized for over 30 years that some patients with IPF experience acute respiratory decline [70, 71]. Until recently, this was thought to be a rare phenomenon in Western countries [72]. However, sudden respiratory decline in a previously stable patient is now a well-recognized phenomenon in IPF patients around the world. When these events are idiopathic, they are termed acute exacerbations (AEx) of IPF and are associated with significant morbidity and mortality [73].

To help unify research efforts, Collard and colleagues proposed the following definition for AEx: (1) a previous or concurrent diagnosis of IPF, (2) unexplained development of dyspnea or worsening within 30 days, (3) high-resolution computed tomography (HRCT) with new bilateral ground-glass abnormality and/or consolidation superimposed on a background pattern consistent with IPF, (4) no evidence of pulmonary infection by endotracheal aspirate or bronchoalveolar lavage, and (5) exclusion of alternative causes including left heart failure, pulmonary embolism, and identifiable causes of acute lung injury [73].

Since these criteria were proposed, two retrospective analyses have better defined the incidence of, risk factors for, and mortality from these events. Kondoh and colleagues retrospectively studied 74 patients with IPF and observed that the 1-year, 2-year, and 3-year incidences of AEx were 8.6 % (95 % CI = 1.7–12.6 %), 12.6 % (95 % CI = 4.5–20.0 %), and 23.9 % (95 % CI = 12.9–33.5 %), respectively [74]. In a multivariate analysis, they found that a decline of 10 % in FVC at 6 months, a higher BMI, and greater dyspnea at baseline were significant risk factors for AEx. The survival time in subjects with an AEx was significantly shorter (median 26.4 months) compared to those without an AEx (median 52.8 months). Song and colleagues reviewed records of 461 patients with IPF with a median follow-up time of 22.9 months and observed that 96 patients (20.8 %) had either a definite (using Collard's criteria) or suspected AEx [75]. Further, 17 of these patients (17.7 %) experienced multiple episodes of AEx. The 1-, 2-, and 3-year incidences (excluding patients who presented concurrently with a new diagnosis of IPF and an AEx) were 11.6 %, 16.3 %, and 18.2 %, respectively. In a multivariate analysis, a lower FVC% and never smoking were significant risk factors for an AEx, and AEx were associated with poor outcomes: 50 % of patients died during hospitalization for the AEx, 90 % of those who required mechanical ventilation died, and 60 % of patients died within 90 days. For those who lived past 90 days, the median survival was 15.5 months, compared with 60.6 months for those without an AEx ($p < 0.001$). Clearly, AEx are not as rare as once believed and are associated with poor survival.

Additional data from recent prospective therapeutic trials have reported AEx frequencies ranging from 1.7 % over 96 weeks to 14.2 % over 36 weeks [8, 9, 44–47, 49, 51, 53, 54, 76] (Table 2.5). Differences in baseline patient populations, diagnostic criteria used, and case-finding methods likely account for some of the variability in reported frequency of AEx. These discordant data confirm that additional research regarding AEx of IPF is needed.

## Subclinical Disease

Based largely on studies of family members of patients with familial FPF, it is apparent that asymptomatic/subclinical disease precedes the development of symptomatic IPF. Some asymptomatic relatives from FPF kindreds have evidence of alveolar inflammation on bronchoalveolar lavage [77] or evidence of pulmonary fibrosis (with a UIP of injury) on either imaging or based on surgical lung biopsy [27, 78].

Among 417 unaffected (by self-report) family members from 111 families with FPF, 28 (6.7 %) had possible disease (based on chest radiographs), and 33 persons (7.9 %) had either probable (based on HRCT abnormalities) or definite (based on either surgical lung biopsy or autopsy evidence of an IIP) disease [27]. Rosas and colleagues evaluated 143 asymptomatic subjects from 18 kindreds with FPF and found that 31 subjects (22 %) had HRCT changes (including increased septal lines, peribronchovascular thickening, reticulation, and ground-glass opacities) consistent with ILD [78]. Compared with affected family members, those with HRCT evidence of ILD but without symptoms were younger (46 years vs. 67 years, $p < 0.001$). These findings suggest that progression of asymptomatic to symptomatic disease may occur over a period of decades; however, to date, the proportion of people who will progress, over what time frame progression occurs, and which variables predict progression are unknown.

In 1982, Bitterman and colleagues assessed 17 clinically unaffected family members of three families with FPF and found that 8 (47 %) had evidence of alveolar inflammation on lavage studies [77]. Two of these patients were reassessed 27 years later. One had developed symptomatic IPF, and the other was asymptomatic but did have evidence of early IPF on HRCT, suggesting that in some cases, there is a latency period of two to three decades from asymptomatic alveolar inflammation to overt disease [79].

Additional evidence suggesting that subclinical disease precedes IPF and clouding our understanding of the natural history of IPF is found in reports of AEx in the subclinical period. Case reports and series have described patients without known ILD who present with acute respiratory failure [clinical adult respiratory distress syndrome (ARDS)] and histopathologic findings of diffuse alveolar damage (DAD) superimposed on a UIP pattern—the same pattern observed in AEx of IPF [75, 80–82].

Patients with subclinical IPF and lung cancer who undergo lobectomy appear to be at an increased risk of AEx. In a review of 1,148 patients with lung cancer who underwent thoracotomy, investigators found 15 patients who developed postoperative ARDS. Of these, 11 patients (73 %) had both interstitial abnormalities on

**Table 2.5** Recent randomized, placebo-controlled trials in which the incidence or percentage of patients with acute decompensation and/or an acute exacerbation was reported [8, 9, 44–47, 49, 53, 54, 76]

| Study | Drug | Placebo cohort (n) | FVC (L or % predicted) | Definition | Incidence or percentage reported | Study period |
|---|---|---|---|---|---|---|
| ACE-IPF [76] | Warfarin | 73 | 58.7 % | Acute exacerbation[a] | 2.7 % | 28 weeks (mean follow-up) |
| TOMORROW [44] | Nintedanib | 87 | 2.70 L | Acute exacerbation[b] | 15.7 per 100 patient-years | 52 weeks |
| BUILD-3 [45] | Bosentan | 209 | 2.66 L | Acute exacerbation[c] | 2.9 % | 80 weeks (mean study duration) |
| STEP-IPF [8] | Sildenafil | 91 | 58.7 % | Acute exacerbation[d] | 4.4 % | 12 weeks |
| STEP-IPF [8] | Sildenafil | 91 | 58.7 % | Acute exacerbation[d] | 7.7 % | 24 weeks (last 12 weeks on therapy) |
| Imatinib [46] | Imatinib | 60 | 2.54 L | Acute worsening[e] | 1.7 % | 96 weeks |
| Shionogi [47] | Pirfenidone | 104 | 2.47 L | Acute exacerbation[f] | 3.8 % | 52 weeks |
| INSPIRE [54] | INF-γ | 275 | 73.1 % | Acute decompensation[g] | 8.7 % | 77 weeks (mean study duration) |
| INSPIRE [54] | INF-γ | 275 | 73.1 % | Acute exacerbation[g] | 5.4 % | 77 weeks (mean study duration) |
| BUILD-1 [9] | Bosentan | 83 | 69.5 % | Acute decompensation[h] | 3.6 % | 54 weeks (mean study duration) |
| Shionogi [49] | Pirfenidone | 35 | 78.4 % | Acute exacerbation[i] | 14.2 % | 36 weeks |
| GIPF-001 [51, 53] | Interferon gamma-1b | 168 | 64.1 % | Death from either progression of IPF or acute respiratory distress syndrome after a period of decompensation lasting <4 weeks | 4.8 % | 76 weeks (median observation period) |

Definitions from the study for acute exacerbation, acute worsening, or acute decompensation are given below

[a] Acute exacerbation was determined via adjudication as part of the study

[b] Acute exacerbation definition: progression of dyspnea over several days to 4 weeks, new parenchymal ground-glass abnormalities on X-ray or HRCT, and a decrease in $PaO_2$ ≥10 mmHg or increase in alveolar–arterial oxygen gradient, within a 1-month period that could not be otherwise explained

cAcute exacerbation definition: unexplained rapid deterioration of condition within 4 weeks with increasing dyspnea requiring hospitalization and $O_2$ supplementation

dAcute exacerbation definition: (1) unexplained worsening of dyspnea or cough within 30 days, triggering medical care with no clinical suspicion or overt evidence of cardiac event, pulmonary embolism, deep venous thrombosis to explain worsening of dyspnea, or pneumothorax; (2) one of the following radiologic or physiologic findings: (a) new ground-glass opacity or consolidation on CT scan or new alveolar opacities on chest X-ray or (b) decline of $\geq$5 % in resting room air $SpO_2$ from last recorded level or decline of $\geq$8 mmHg in resting room air $PaO_2$ from last recorded level and (3) no clinical or microbiologic evidence of infection

eAcute worsening was not otherwise specified

fAcute exacerbation definition: worsening clinical features within 1 month including progression of dyspnea, new radiographic/HRCT ground-glass abnormalities without pneumothorax or pleural effusion, a decrease in $PaO_2$ by 10 mmHg or more, and exclusion of obvious causes including infection, cancer, pulmonary thromboembolism, malignancy, or congestive heart failure

gAcute respiratory decompensation: evidence of all of the following must be present within a 4-week period: worsening $PaO_2$ or new or significant increase in the use of supplemental oxygen. clinically significant worsening of dyspnea, and new or worsening radiographic abnormalities on chest radiograph or HRCT. Acute exacerbation=evidence of all of the following must be present within a 4-week period: worsening $PaO_2$ at rest ($\geq$8 mmHg drop from most recent pre-worsening value), clinically significant worsening of dyspnea, new ground-glass opacities on HRCT, and all other causes, such as cardiac, thromboembolic, aspiration, or infectious processes, have been excluded

hAcute decompensation definition: unexplained rapid deterioration over 4 weeks with increased dyspnea requiring hospitalization and oxygen supplementations of $\geq$5 L/min to maintain a resting oxygen saturation by blood gas of $\geq$90 % or $PaO_2$ $\geq$55 mmHg (sea level) or $PaO_2$ $\geq$50 mmHg (above 1,400 m)

iAcute exacerbation definition: worsening clinical features within 1 month with progression of dyspnea over a few days to less than 5 weeks, new radiographic/HRCT parenchymal abnormalities without pneumothorax or pleural effusion, a decrease in $PaO_2$ by 10 mmHg or more, and exclusion of apparent infection by absence of Aspergillus and pneumococcus antibodies in blood, urine for Legionella pneumophila, and sputum cultures

preoperative CT and a UIP pattern in resected lung tissue. The risk of postoperative ARDS was significantly higher in those with evidence of subclinical IPF on CT imaging (8.8 %) compared to those without ILD (0.4 %) ($p < 0.001$) [83]. Fukushima and colleagues found subpleural fibrosis in 127 of 776 patients (16.4 %) who underwent lobectomy for lung cancer. Three patients progressed acutely following surgery, and another seven progressed to classic IPF over a period of 5 years [84].

Araya and colleagues reviewed 14 autopsy cases of idiopathic DAD [acute interstitial pneumonia (AIP)] and found that 50 % of cases also had evidence of subpleural fibrosis, suggesting that some cases of AIP may in fact be the result of an AEx of subclinical IPF [85]. Although subclinical disease is becoming increasingly recognized [86], many questions concerning the clinical significance of subclinical disease remain. Longitudinal studies are needed to determine risk factors for disease progression, the time period over which the transition from subclinical to clinically relevant disease occurs, and whether early interventions can improve outcomes.

## Specific Clinical Phenotypes of Disease

Identifying specific clinical phenotypes of disease is paramount, because doing so may provide insight into the pathobiology of disease [87]. Patients with IPF and either disproportionate pulmonary hypertension or concurrent emphysema are believed by some experts to represent distinct clinical phenotypes of disease, and investigation of these concurrent processes has furthered our understanding of the heterogeneous clinical course.

## IPF + Pulmonary Hypertension

The development of pulmonary hypertension in patients with IPF was once believed to be due to vascular obliteration from pulmonary fibrosis. However, in several studies, investigators have not found a clear association between the severity of fibrosis and the presence or severity of pulmonary hypertension, suggesting that additional factors are involved [88–90]. Regardless of the underlying mechanisms that lead to the development of pulmonary hypertension, its presence negatively impacts survival [35, 89, 91, 92].

## Combined Pulmonary Fibrosis and Emphysema

There is increasing recognition of the coexistence of pulmonary fibrosis and emphysema—a syndrome termed combined pulmonary fibrosis and emphysema (CPFE)—within individual patients. CPFE is characterized by relatively preserved static and forced lung volumes, a disproportionately reduced diffusing capacity, and a high prevalence of pulmonary hypertension [93, 94]. In patients with apparent IPF, concurrent evidence of emphysema on HRCT imaging ranges from 18.8 % to

50.9 %, and the median survival in such patients is estimated at 2.1–8.5 years [95]. At this point, it is unclear if patients with CPFE have a worse survival compared to those with IPF alone. Mejía and colleagues suggested that the reduced survival among subjects with CPFE compared to IPF subjects was due to the presence of pulmonary hypertension in patients with CPFE [96].

## Summary

Over the past two decades, results from multiple studies have advanced our understanding of the natural history of IPF. It has become evident that IPF, once thought to be a steadily progressive disease in all patients, may actually follow any number of different courses. This heterogeneity makes it impossible to confidently determine how the disease will behave over time in an individual patient. However, given this knowledge, investigators may now embark on studies to explain this variability and tease out the pathobiologic mechanisms that drive it. Epidemiologic studies suggest that IPF should no longer be considered an orphan disease, especially considering that mortality rates are similar to those associated with some common malignancies. Case–control studies have revealed potential exposures for disease development, but these studies are subject to a number of potential biases. Maintaining the momentum and propelling the field forward will require carefully planned, well-designed studies to further decipher disease heterogeneity, identify additional risk factor for disease development, and determine how to prevent and treat this devastating disease.

## References

1. American Thoracic Society. Idiopathic pulmonary fibrosis: diagnosis and treatment. International consensus statement. American Thoracic Society (ATS), and the European Respiratory Society (ERS). Am J Respir Crit Care Med. 2000;161:646–64.
2. Raghu G, Collard HR, Egan JJ, Martinez FJ, Behr J, Brown KK, et al. An official ATS/ERS/JRS/ALAT statement: idiopathic pulmonary fibrosis: evidence-based guidelines for diagnosis and management. Am J Respir Crit Care Med. 2011;183:788–824.
3. Swigris JJ, Olson AL, Huie TJ, Fernandez-Perez ER, Solomon J, Sprunger D, Brown KK. Ethnic and racial differences in the presence of idiopathic pulmonary fibrosis at death. Respir Med. 2012;106:588–93.
4. Gordis L. The epidemiologic approach to disease and intervention. In: Gordis L, editor. Epidemiology. 3rd ed. Philadelphia, PA: Elsevier Saunders; 2004. p. 1–14.
5. Coultas DB, Zumwalt RE, Black WC, Sobonya RE. The epidemiology of interstitial lung diseases. Am J Respir Crit Care Med. 1994;150:967–72.
6. Raghu G, Weycker D, Edelsberg J, Bradford WZ, Oster G. Incidence and prevalence of idiopathic pulmonary fibrosis. Am J Respir Crit Care Med. 2006;174:810–6.
7. Fernández-Pérez ER, Daniels CE, Schroeder DR, St Sauver J, Hartman TE, Bartholmai BJ, et al. Incidence, prevalence, and clinical course of idiopathic pulmonary fibrosis. Chest. 2010;137:129–37.

8. Idiopathic Pulmonary Fibrosis Clinical Research Network, Zisman DA, Schwarz M, Anstrom KJ, Collard HR, Flaherty KR, Hunninghake GW. A controlled trial of sildenafil in advanced idiopathic pulmonary fibrosis. N Engl J Med. 2010;363:620–8.

9. King Jr TE, Behr J, Brown KK, du Bois RM, Lancaster L, de Andrade JA, et al. BUILD-1: a randomized placebo-controlled trial of bosentan in idiopathic pulmonary fibrosis. Am J Respir Crit Care Med. 2008;177:75–81.

10. Gribbin J, Hubbard RB, Le Jeune I, Smith CJ, West J, Tata LJ. Incidence and mortality of idiopathic pulmonary fibrosis and sarcoidosis in the UK. Thorax. 2006;61:980–5.

11. Navaratnam V, Fleming KM, West J, Smith CJ, Jenkins RG, Fogarty A, Hubbard RB. The rising incidence of idiopathic pulmonary fibrosis in the UK. Thorax. 2011;66:462–7.

12. Johnston I, Britton J, Kinnear W, Logan R. Rising mortality from cryptogenic fibrosing alveolitis. BMJ. 1990;301:1017–21.

13. Coultas DB, Hughes MP. Accuracy of mortality data for interstitial lung disease in New Mexico, USA. Thorax. 1996;51:717–20.

14. Mannino DM, Etzel RA, Parrish RG. Pulmonary fibrosis deaths in the United States, 1979–1991. Am J Respir Crit Care Med. 1996;153:1548–52.

15. Olson AL, Swigris JJ, Lezotte DC, Norris JM, Wilson CG, Brown KK. Mortality from pulmonary fibrosis increased in the United States from 1992 to 2003. Am J Respir Crit Care Med. 2007;176:277–84.

16. Hubbard R, Johnston I, Coultas DB, Britton J. Mortality rates from cryptogenic fibrosing alveolitis in seven countries. Thorax. 1996;51:711–6.

17. Raphael K. Recall bias: a proposal for assessment and control. Int J Epidemiol. 1987;16:167–70.

18. American Thoracic Society; European Respiratory Society. American Thoracic Society/ European Respiratory Society International Multidisciplinary Consensus Classification of the Idiopathic Interstitial Pneumonias. This joint statement of the American Thoracic Society (ATS), and the European Respiratory Society (ERS) was adopted by the ATS board of directors, June 2001 and by the ERS Executive Committee, June 2001. Am J Respir Crit Care Med. 2002;165:277–304.

19. Baumgartner KB, Samet JM, Stidley CA, Colby TV, Waldron JA. Cigarette smoking: a risk factor for idiopathic pulmonary fibrosis. Am J Respir Crit Care Med. 1997;155:242–8.

20. Miyake Y, Sasaki S, Yokoyama T, Chida K, Azuma A, Suda T, et al. Occupational and environmental factors and idiopathic pulmonary fibrosis in Japan. Ann Occup Hyg. 2005;49:259–65.

21. Taskar VS, Coultas DB. Is idiopathic pulmonary fibrosis an environmental disease? Proc Am Thorac Soc. 2006;3:293–8.

22. Scott J, Johnston I, Britton J. What causes cryptogenic fibrosing alveolitis? A case–control study of environmental exposure to dust. BMJ. 1990;301:1015–7.

23. Hubbard R, Lewis S, Richards K, Johnston I, Britton J. Occupational exposure to metal or wood dust and aetiology of cryptogenic fibrosing alveolitis. Lancet. 1996;347:284–9.

24. Iwai K, Mori T, Yamada N, Yamaguchi M, Hosoda Y. Idiopathic pulmonary fibrosis: epidemiologic approaches to occupational exposures. Am J Respir Crit Care Med. 1994;150:670–5.

25. García-Sancho Figueroa MC, Carrillo G, Pérez-Padilla R, Fernández-Plata MR, Buendía-Roldán I, Vargas MH, Selman M. Risk factors for idiopathic pulmonary fibrosis in a Mexican population. A case–control study. Respir Med. 2010;104:305–9.

26. García-Sancho C, Buendía-Roldán I, Fernández-Plata MR, Navarro C, Pérez-Padilla R, Vargas MH, et al. Familial pulmonary fibrosis is the strongest risk factor for idiopathic pulmonary fibrosis. Respir Med. 2011;105:1902–7.

27. Steele MP, Steer MC, Loyd JE, Brown KK, Herron A, Slifer SH, et al. Clinical and pathologic features of familial pulmonary fibrosis. Am J Respir Crit Care Med. 2005;172:1146–52.

28. Baumgarter KB, Samet JM, Coutas DB, Stidley CA, Hunt WC, Colby TV, Waldron JA. Occupational and environmental risk factors for idiopathic pulmonary fibrosis: a multicenter case–control study. Am J Epidemiol. 2000;152:307–15.

29. Hubbard R, Cooper M, Antaoniak M, Venn A, Khan S, Johnston I, et al. Risk of cryptogenic fibrosing alveolitis in metal workers. Lancet. 2000;355:466–7.

30. Pinheiro GA, Antao VC, Wood JM, Wassell JT. Occupational risks for idiopathic pulmonary fibrosis mortality in the United States. Int J Occup Environ Health. 2008;14:117–23.
31. Gustafson T, Dahlman-Höglund A, Nilsson K, Ström K, Tornling G, Torén K. Occupational exposure and severe pulmonary fibrosis. Respir Med. 2007;101:2207–12.
32. Mullen J, Hodgson MJ, DeGraff CA, Godar T. Case–control study of idiopathic pulmonary fibrosis and environmental exposures. J Occup Environ Med. 1998;40:363–7.
33. Nicholson AG, Colby TV, du Bois RM, Hansell DM, Wells AU. The prognostic significance of the histologic pattern of interstitial pneumonia in patients presenting with the clinical entity of cryptogenic fibrosing alveolitis. Am J Respir Crit Care Med. 2000;162:2213–7.
34. King TE, Schwarz MI, Brown K, Tooze JA, Colby TV, Waldron Jr JA, et al. Idiopathic pulmonary fibrosis: relationship between histopathologic features and mortality. Am J Respir Crit Care Med. 2001;164:1025–32.
35. King Jr TE, Tooze JA, Schwarz MI, Brown KR, Cherniak RM. Predicting survival in idiopathic pulmonary fibrosis. Am J Respir Crit Care Med. 2001;164:1171–81.
36. Rudd RM, Prescott RJ, Chalmers JC, Johnston ID, Fibrosing Alveolitis Subcommittee of the Research Committee of the British Thoracic Society. British Thoracic Society Study on cryptogenic fibrosing alveolitis: response to treatment and survival. Thorax. 2007;62:62–6.
37. Collard HR, King TE, Bartelson BB, Vourlekis JS, Schwarz MI, Brown KK. Changes in clinical and physiologic variables predict survival in idiopathic pulmonary fibrosis. Am J Respir Crit Care Med. 2003;168:538–42.
38. Nathan SD, Shlobin OA, Wier N, et al. Long-term course and prognosis of idiopathic pulmonary fibrosis in the new millennium. Chest. 2011;140:221–9.
39. Ley B, Collard HR, King Jr TE. Clinical course and prediction of survival in idiopathic pulmonary fibrosis. Am J Respir Crit Care Med. 2011;183:431–40.
40. Wells AU, Desai SR, Rubens MB, Goh NS, Cramer D, Nicholson AG, et al. Idiopathic pulmonary fibrosis: a composite physiologic index derived from disease extent observed by computed tomography. Am J Respir Crit Care Med. 2003;167:962–9.
41. Ley B, Ryerson CJ, Vittinghoff E, Ryu JH, Tomassetti S, Lee JS, et al. A multidimensional index and staging system for idiopathic pulmonary fibrosis. Ann Intern Med. 2012;156:684–91.
42. Hanson D, Winterbauer RH, Kirtland SH, Wu R. Changes in pulmonary function test results after 1 year of therapy as predictors of survival in patients with idiopathic pulmonary fibrosis. Chest. 1995;108:305–10.
43. Du Bois RM, Weycker D, Albera C, et al. Ascertainment of individual risk of mortality for patients with idiopathic pulmonary fibrosis. Am J Respir Crit Care Med. 2011;184(4):459–66.
44. Richeldi L, Costabel U, Selman M, Kim DS, Hansell DM, Nicholson AG, et al. Efficacy of a tyrosine kinase inhibitor in idiopathic pulmonary fibrosis. N Engl J Med. 2011;365:1079–87.
45. King Jr TE, Brown KK, Raghu G, du Bois RM, Lynch DA, Martinez F, et al. BUILD-3: a randomized controlled trial of bosentan in idiopathic pulmonary fibrosis. Am J Respir Crit Care Med. 2011;184:92–9.
46. Daniels CE, Lasky JA, Limper AH, Mieras K, Gabor E, Schroeder DR, Imatinib-IPF Study Investigators. Imatinib treatment for idiopathic pulmonary fibrosis: randomized placebo-controlled trial results. Am J Respir Crit Care Med. 2010;181:604–10.
47. Taniguchi H, Ebina M, Kondoh Y, Ogura T, Azuma A, Suga M, et al. Pirfenidone in idiopathic pulmonary fibrosis. Eur Respir J. 2010;35:821–9.
48. Raghu G, Brown KK, Costabel U, Cottin V, du Bois RM, Lasky JA, et al. Treatment of idiopathic pulmonary fibrosis with etanercept: an exploratory, placebo controlled trial. Am J Respir Crit Care Med. 2008;178:948–55.
49. Azuma A, Nukiwa T, Tsuboi E, Suga M, Abe S, Nakata K, et al. Double-blind, placebo-controlled trial of pirfenidone in patients with idiopathic pulmonary fibrosis. Am J Respir Crit Care Med. 2005;171:1040–7.
50. Demedts M, Behr J, Buhl R, Costabel U, Dekhuijzen R, Jansen HM, et al. High-dose acetylcysteine in idiopathic pulmonary fibrosis. N Engl J Med. 2005;353:2229–42.

51. Raghu G, Brown KK, Bradford WZ, Starko K, Noble PW, Schwartz DA, et al. A placebo-controlled trial of interferon gamma-1b in patients with idiopathic pulmonary fibrosis. N Engl J Med. 2004;350:125–33.
52. Panos R, Mortenson RL, Nicolli SA, King Jr TE. Clinical deterioration in patients with idiopathic pulmonary fibrosis: causes and assessment. Am J Med. 1990;88:396–404.
53. Martinez FJ, Safrin S, Weycker D, Starko KM, Bradford WZ, King Jr TE, et al. The clinical course of patients with idiopathic pulmonary fibrosis. Ann Intern Med. 2005;142:963–7.
54. King Jr TE, Albera C, Bradford WZ, Costabel U, Hormel P, Lancaster L, et al. Effect of interferon gamma-1b on survival in patients with idiopathic pulmonary fibrosis (INSPIRE): a multicentre, randomised, placebo-controlled trial. Lancet. 2009;374:222–8.
55. Sprunger DB, Olson AL, Huie TJ, Fernandez-Perez ER, Fischer A, Solomon JJ, et al. Pulmonary fibrosis is associated with an elevated risk of thromboembolic disease. Eur Respir J. 2012;39:125–32.
56. Nathan SD, Basavaraj A, Reichner C, Shlobin OA, Ahmad S, Kiernan J, et al. Prevalence and impact of coronary artery disease in idiopathic pulmonary fibrosis. Respir Med. 2010;104:1035–41.
57. Izbicki G, Ben-Dor I, Shitrit D, Bendayan D, Aldrich TK, Kornowski R, Kramer MR. The prevalence of coronary artery disease in end-stage pulmonary disease: is pulmonary fibrosis a risk factor? Respir Med. 2009;103:1346–9.
58. Kizer JR, Zisman DA, Blumenthal NP, Kotloff RM, Kimmel SE, Strieter RM, et al. Association between pulmonary fibrosis and coronary artery disease. Arch Intern Med. 2004;164:551–6.
59. Ponnuswamy A, Manikandan R, Sabetpour A, Keeping IM, Finnerty JP. Association between ischaemic heart disease and interstitial lung disease: a case control study. Respir Med. 2009;103:503–7.
60. Hubbard RB, Smith C, Le Jeune I, Gribbin J, Fogarty AW. The association between idiopathic pulmonary fibrosis and vascular disease: a population-based study. Am J Respir Crit Care Med. 2008;178:1257–61.
61. Heart disease and stroke statistics – 2004 update. Coronary heart disease, acute coronary syndrome and angina pectoris. Am Heart Assoc. 2004. 6:9–12.
62. Sode BF, Dahl M, Nielsen SF, Nordestgaard BG. Venous thromboembolism and risk of idiopathic interstitial pneumonia: a nationwide study. Am J Respir Crit Care Med. 2010;181:1085–92.
63. Hubbard R, Venn A, Lewis S, Britton J. Lung cancer and cryptogenic fibrosing alveolitis: a population based study. Am J Respir Crit Care Med. 2000;161:5–8.
64. Le Jeune I, Gribbin J, West J, Smith C, Cullinan P, Hubbard R. The incidence of cancer in patients with idiopathic pulmonary fibrosis and sarcoidosis in the UK. Respir Med. 2007;101:2534–40.
65. Aubry MC, Myers JL, Douglas WW, Tazelaar HD, Washington Stephens TL, Hartman TE, et al. Primary pulmonary carcinoma in patients with idiopathic pulmonary fibrosis. Mayo Clin Proc. 2002;77:763–70.
66. Turner-Warwick M, Burrows B, Johnson A. Cryptogenic fibrosing alveolitis: clinical features and their influence on survival. Thorax. 1980;35:171–80.
67. Carrington CB, Gaensler EA, Coutu RE, FitzGerald MX, Gupta RG. Natural history and treated course of usual and desquamative interstitial pneumonia. N Engl J Med. 1978;298:801–11.
68. Selman M, Carrillo G, Estrada A, Mejia M, Becerril C, Cisneros J, et al. Accelerated variant of idiopathic pulmonary fibrosis: clinical behavior and gene expression pattern. PLoS One. 2007;2:e482.
69. Boon K, Bailey NW, Yang J, Steel MP, Groshong S, Kervitsky D, et al. Molecular phenotypes distinguish patients with relatively stable from progressive idiopathic pulmonary fibrosis. PLoS One. 2009;4:e5134.
70. Kondo A, Saiki S. Acute exacerbation in idiopathic interstitial pneumonia (IIP). In: Harasawa M, Fukuchi Y, Morinari H, editors. Interstitial pneumonia of unknown etiology. Tokyo: University of Tokyo Press; 1989. p. 33–42 [Intractable Diseases Research Foundation Publication No. 27].

71. Kondoh Y, Taniguchi H, Kawabata Y, Yokoi T, Suzuki K, Takagi K. Acute exacerbation in idiopathic pulmonary fibrosis: analysis of clinical and pathologic findings in three cases. Chest. 1993;103:1808–12.
72. Colby TV. Interstitial lung disease. In: Colby TV, Lombard CM, Yousem SA, et al., editors. Atlas of pulmonary surgical pathology. Philadelphia, PA: WB Saunders; 1991. p. 227–306.
73. Collard HR, Moore BB, Flaherty KR, Brown KK, Kaner RJ, King Jr TE, et al. Acute exacerbations of idiopathic pulmonary fibrosis. Am J Respir Crit Care Med. 2007;176:636–43.
74. Kondoh Y, Taniguchi H, Katsuta T, Kataoka K, Kimura T, Nishiyama O, et al. Risk factors of acute exacerbation of idiopathic pulmonary fibrosis. Sarcoidosis Vasc Diffuse Lung Dis. 2010;27:103–10.
75. Song JW, Hong SB, Lim CM, Kim DS. Acute exacerbation of idiopathic pulmonary fibrosis: incidence, risk factors, and outcome. Eur Respir J. 2011;37:356–63.
76. Noth I, Anstrom KJ, Clavert SB, de Andrade J, Flaherty KR, Glazer C, et al. A placebo-controlled randomized trial of warfarin in idiopathic pulmonary fibrosis. Am J Respir Crit Care Med. 2012;186:88–95.
77. Bitterman PB, Rennard SI, Keogh BA, Wewers MD, Adelberg S, Crystal RG. Familial idiopathic pulmonary fibrosis. Evidence of lung inflammation in unaffected family members. N Engl J Med. 1986;314:1343–7.
78. Rosas IO, Ren P, Avila NA, Chow CK, Franks TJ, Travis WD, et al. Early interstitial lung disease in familial pulmonary fibrosis. Am J Respir Crit Care Med. 2007;176:698–705.
79. El-Chemaly S, Ziegler SG, Wilson K, Gahl WA, Moss J, Gochuico BR. Familial pulmonary fibrosis: natural history of preclinical disease. Am J Respir Crit Care Med. 2010;181:A2980.
80. Sakamoto K, Taniguchi H, Kondoh Y, Ono K, Hasegawa Y, Kitaichi M. Acute exacerbation of idiopathic pulmonary fibrosis as the initial presentation of the disease. Eur Respir Rev. 2009;18:129–32.
81. Parambil JG, Myers JL, Ryu JH. Histopathologic features and outcome of patients with acute exacerbation of idiopathic pulmonary fibrosis undergoing surgical lung biopsy. Chest. 2005;128:3310–5.
82. Kim DS, Park JH, Park BK, Lee JS, Nicholson AG, Colby T. Acute exacerbation of idiopathic pulmonary fibrosis: frequency and clinical features. Eur Respir J. 2006;27:143–50.
83. Chida M, Ono S, Hoshikawa Y, Kondo T. Subclinical idiopathic pulmonary fibrosis is also a risk factor of postoperative acute respiratory distress syndrome following thoracic surgery. Eur J Cardiothorac Surg. 2008;34:878–81.
84. Fukushima K, Kawabata Y, Takashi U, Yuzuki N. Prognosis of possible development into diffuse interstitial pneumonia for 127 patients with localized usual interstitial pneumonia. Nihon Kokyuki Gakkai Zasshi. 1999;37:177–82 [Japanese].
85. Araya J, Kawabata Y, Jinho P, Uchiyama T, Ogata H, Sugita Y. Clinically occult subpleural fibrosis and acute interstitial pneumonia a precursor to idiopathic pulmonary fibrosis. Respirology. 2008;13:408–12.
86. Doyle TJ, Hunninghake GM, Rosas IO. Subclinical interstitial lung disease: why you should care. Am J Respir Crit Care Med. 2012;185:1147–53.
87. Fell CD. Idiopathic pulmonary fibrosis: phenotypes and comorbidities. Clin Chest Med. 2012;33:51–7.
88. Nathan SD, Nobel PW, Tudor RM. Idiopathic pulmonary fibrosis and pulmonary hypertension: connecting the dots. Am J Respir Crit Care Med. 2007;175:875–80.
89. Kawut SM, O'Shea MK, Bartels MN, Wilt JS, Sonett JR, Arcasoy SM. Exercise testing determines survival in patients with diffuse parenchymal lung disease evaluated for lung transplantation. Respir Med. 2005;99:1431–9.
90. Nathan SD, Shlobin OA, Ahmad S, Urbanek S, Barnett SD. Pulmonary hypertension and pulmonary function testing in idiopathic pulmonary fibrosis. Chest. 2007;131:657–63.
91. Lettieri CJ, Nathan SD, Barnett SD, Ahmad S, Shorr AF. Prevalence and outcomes of pulmonary arterial hypertension in advanced idiopathic pulmonary fibrosis. Chest. 2006;129:746–52.
92. Nadrous HF, Pellikka PA, Krowka MJ, Swanson KL, Chaowalit N, Decker PA, Ryu JH. Pulmonary hypertension in patients with idiopathic pulmonary fibrosis. Chest. 2005; 128:2393–9.

93. Cottin V, Nunes H, Brillet PY, Delaval P, Devouassoux G, Tillie-Leblond I, et al. Combined pulmonary fibrosis and emphysema: a distinct underrecognised entity. Eur Respir J. 2005; 26:586–93.
94. Cottin V, Le Pavec J, Prévot G, Mal H, Humbert M, Simonneau G, Cordier JF, GERM"O"P. Pulmonary hypertension in patients with combined pulmonary fibrosis and emphysema syndrome. Eur Respir J. 2010;35:105–11.
95. Jankowich MD, Rounds SI. Combined pulmonary fibrosis and emphysema syndrome. Chest. 2012;141:222–31.
96. Mejía M, Carrillo G, Rojas-Serrano J, Estrada A, Suárez T, Alonso D, et al. Idiopathic pulmonary fibrosis and emphysema: decreased survival associated with severe pulmonary arterial hypertension. Chest. 2009;136:10–5.

# Chapter 3
# Histopathology of IPF and Related Disorders

Jeffrey L. Myers

**Abstract** Histopathologic classification schemes provide the underpinnings for separating idiopathic interstitial pneumonias into clinically meaningful groups. A number of multidisciplinary position papers and guidelines published over the last decade have cemented usual interstitial pneumonia (UIP) as the defining feature of idiopathic pulmonary fibrosis (IPF). Surgical lung biopsy is an important diagnostic tool in patients for whom imaging studies are inconclusive. Diagnosis of UIP on a surgical lung biopsy remains the single most important predictor of outcome at the time of diagnosis in patients with otherwise unexplained diffuse lung disease. Identifying patients with respiratory bronchiolitis interstitial lung disease (RBILD), desquamative interstitial pneumonia (DIP), and nonspecific interstitial pneumonia (NSIP) is more challenging and requires careful correlation of lung biopsy findings with other clinical and radiological data.

**Keywords** Idiopathic interstitial pneumonia • Usual interstitial pneumonia • UIP • Nonspecific interstitial pneumonia • NSIP • Pulmonary fibrosis

## Introduction

Idiopathic interstitial pneumonias are an important subset of the broader category of diffuse, nonneoplastic interstitial lung diseases [1–3]. Common to all idiopathic interstitial pneumonias is expansion, and potentially distortion, of distal lung interstitium by some combination of inflammation and/or fibrosis. Fibrosis, when

J.L. Myers, M.D. (✉)
Divisions of Anatomic Pathology and MLabs, Department of Pathology,
University of Michigan, 1500 East Medical Center Drive, 2G332UH,
Ann Arbor, MI 48109, USA
e-mail: myerjeff@umich.edu

K.C. Meyer and S.D. Nathan (eds.), *Idiopathic Pulmonary Fibrosis: A Comprehensive Clinical Guide*, Respiratory Medicine 9, DOI 10.1007/978-1-62703-682-5_3,
© Springer Science+Business Media New York 2014

present, takes the form of increased numbers of fibroblasts and myofibroblasts and/or collagen deposition. These changes are usually seen in patients with breathlessness or cough, diffuse radiological abnormalities, and evidence of physiologic dysfunction.

Averill Liebow pioneered the notion that morphologic classification of idiopathic interstitial pneumonias is useful in separating them into distinct clinical categories [4]. Since then a number of classification schemes have been proposed. In 2002 an international committee, sponsored by the American Thoracic Society (ATS) and the European Respiratory Society (ERS), proposed a classification scheme reflecting consensus of a large multidisciplinary group of experts [5]. This statement has had a profound impact, influencing management of patients with suspected idiopathic interstitial pneumonias, driving study design for clinical trials, and creating opportunities for research to challenge areas in which evidence was weak. An updated statement highlights substantial changes that have occurred in the intervening decade that impact the role of biopsy in patients with idiopathic interstitial pneumonia including more refined criteria for identifying patients with nonspecific interstitial pneumonia (NSIP) and the importance of acute exacerbation in our revised understanding of the natural history of untreated idiopathic pulmonary fibrosis (IPF) [6]. The purpose of this review is to briefly summarize the relationship between clinical, radiological, and histopathologic features of the idiopathic interstitial pneumonias, focusing primarily on usual interstitial pneumonia (UIP) and IPF. Other forms of diffuse lung disease typically included with the idiopathic interstitial pneumonias are briefly discussed to highlight those features that set them apart from UIP in surgical lung biopsies.

## Histopathologic Classification of Idiopathic Interstitial Pneumonias

The previously referenced 2002 consensus classification proposed seven categories of idiopathic interstitial pneumonia, ordering them by relative frequency and separating *histologic patterns* from *clinical-radiologic-pathologic diagnoses* (Table 3.1) [5]. Katzenstein has popularized a simplified approach that uses a single unifying terminology and omits cryptogenic organizing pneumonia (COP), also termed idiopathic bronchiolitis obliterans organizing pneumonia (BOOP), and lymphoid interstitial pneumonia (LIP) [2]. The rationale for omitting idiopathic COP is that pathologically it is predominantly an air space, rather than interstitial, process and clinically mimics infectious pneumonias rather than diffuse interstitial pneumonia. LIP is omitted because it represents a form of lymphoproliferative disorder more closely allied to follicular bronchiolitis on one hand and low-grade lymphoma on the other. Katzenstein's classification scheme serves as a framework for this overview. Acute interstitial pneumonia (AIP), a form of rapidly progressive diffuse lung disease first described by Hamman and Rich in the 1930s and 1940s, is not included in this review, which is focused instead on the chronic forms of idiopathic interstitial pneumonia [7, 8].

**Table 3.1** Classification of idiopathic interstitial pneumonias

| Katzenstein [2] | International consensus classification clinical-radiologic-pathologic diagnoses [5] |
|---|---|
| Usual interstitial pneumonia (UIP) | Idiopathic pulmonary fibrosis (IPF) |
| Desquamative interstitial pneumonia (DIP)/respiratory bronchiolitis interstitial lung disease (RBILD) | Desquamative interstitial pneumonia (DIP) |
|  | Respiratory bronchiolitis interstitial lung disease (RBILD) |
| Acute interstitial pneumonia (AIP) | Acute interstitial pneumonia (AIP) |
| Nonspecific interstitial pneumonia (NSIP) | Nonspecific interstitial pneumonia (NSIP) |
|  | Cryptogenic organizing pneumonia (COP) |
|  | Lymphoid interstitial pneumonia (LIP) |

## *Usual Interstitial Pneumonia*

UIP is the most common of the idiopathic interstitial pneumonias, accounting for about 60 % of biopsied patients [9–12]. An ATS consensus statement published in 2000 cemented the link between UIP and IPF by defining the latter as, "a specific form of chronic fibrosing interstitial pneumonia limited to the lung and associated with histologic appearance of UIP on surgical (thoracoscopic or open) lung biopsy" [13]. A more recent revision published as a multidisciplinary guideline for diagnosis and management of IPF affirmed UIP as the defining feature of IPF [14]. As these statements imply, UIP and IPF are nearly synonymous terms, potential exceptions being those patients with underlying systemic connective tissue diseases or occupational/environmental exposures that may suggest an etiology for their lung disease (e.g., asbestosis). UIP is also the most common finding in patients with familial interstitial pneumonia [15, 16].

### Clinical Features

The clinical features of UIP/IPF are detailed elsewhere in this text (see Chap. 2). Briefly, patients with surgical lung biopsy diagnoses of UIP usually present in the sixth or seventh decade of life with slowly progressive dyspnea and nonproductive cough. Men are affected more commonly than women by a ratio of nearly 2:1. Physical findings include bibasilar inspiratory crackles, a nonspecific but characteristic finding in nearly all patients. Pulmonary function studies show restrictive abnormalities in most patients accompanied by a reduction in the diffusion capacity for carbon monoxide (DLCO) with hypoxemia at rest and/or with exercise (see Chap. 6). No single pharmacologic agent or combination of drugs has shown consistent efficacy in patients with UIP, although a number of novel therapies are being investigated in clinical trials (see Chap. 14). Lung transplantation is an option for some patients, but its application is limited due to older age and frequent comorbidities. In most patients UIP pursues a progressive course with median survivals from the time of diagnosis of about 3 years in retrospective, observational case-based studies [9, 17].

Occasional patients present with a more acute onset of respiratory symptoms that may mimic the clinical presentation of AIP [18, 19]. This syndrome has been termed *acute exacerbation of IPF* (or *accelerated UIP*) and occurs in as many as 14 % of untreated patients and about half of those who die from respiratory failure (see Chap. 17) [20, 21]. Histopathologic findings consistent with acute exacerbation are common at autopsy in UIP patients [22]. Acute exacerbation is defined as the sudden onset of rapid clinical deterioration without an identifiable cause in patients with IPF [18]. Diagnosis depends on exclusion of other known and potentially treatable causes of clinical worsening, such as cardiac disease, pulmonary embolism, and infection. Most patients are known to have UIP at the time of acute worsening, but some patients with clinically occult IPF present with an acute exacerbation without a previously established diagnosis of fibrotic lung disease [19]. The prognosis is grim, with short-term mortality rates in excess of 50 % in the majority of reported series.

The relative role of imaging studies and surgical lung biopsies in patients with UIP has changed over the last decade, as reflected in the most recently published guideline for diagnosis [14]. High-resolution computed tomography (HRCT) scans have greatly improved diagnostic accuracy over conventional chest radiography, revolutionizing the role of radiology in managing patients with diffuse interstitial lung diseases (see Chap. 4). HRCT scans in about half of patients show a characteristic combination of peripheral (subpleural), irregular, linear ("reticular") opacities involving predominantly the lower lung zones with associated architectural distortion in the form of traction bronchiectasis and bibasilar honeycomb change [23–26]. Experienced radiologists can make a specific diagnosis of UIP with a high degree of accuracy in patients with this combination of findings, thus obviating the need for lung biopsy. Lung biopsy is increasingly limited to those patients with atypical radiological findings, meaning that there is a growing selection bias toward reserving surgical lung biopsy for patients with potentially "discordant" or atypical radiological findings. It is this change that has created confusion concerning the relative roles of clinicians, radiologists, and pathologists in the evaluation of biopsied patients. In this context, most of the evidence indicates that a biopsy diagnosis of UIP remains the single most important predictor of outcome at the time of diagnosis and thus remains a diagnostic "gold standard" of sorts [23, 27].

## Pathologic Features

UIP is a specific morphologic entity defined by a combination of (1) fibrosis, (2) a heterogeneous ("patchwork") distribution of qualitatively variable abnormalities, (3) architectural distortion in the form of honeycomb change and/or scars, and (4) fibroblast foci [1, 2, 28–30]. The histologic hallmark of UIP in surgical lung biopsies is a heterogeneous or variegated appearance resulting from irregularly distributed fibrotic scarring, honeycomb change, interstitial inflammation, and relatively unaffected lung (Fig. 3.1). This distinctive "patchwork" appearance is fundamental to recognizing UIP at low magnification.

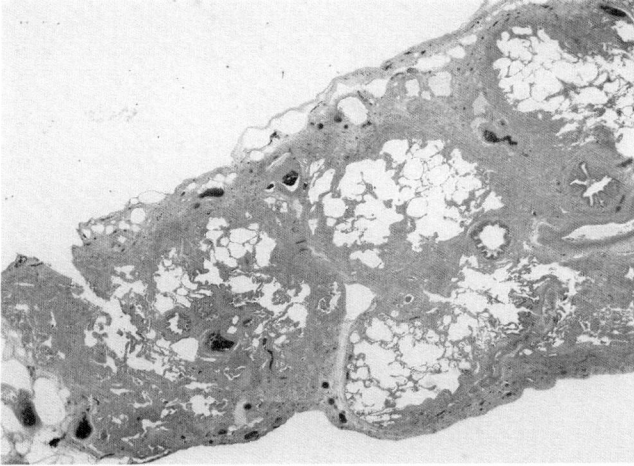

**Fig. 3.1** Low-magnification photomicrograph of surgical lung biopsy showing UIP (hematoxylin and eosin stain; original magnification ×20). There is patchy fibrosis affecting subpleural and paraseptal parenchyma, as well as bronchovascular bundles, leaving intervening lung tissue relatively unaffected. The fibrosis is paucicellular with minimal associated inflammation

Fibrosis predominates over inflammation in classical UIP and comprises dense eosinophilic collagen deposition, which is often accompanied by smooth muscle hyperplasia. Fibroblast foci are invariably seen and represent small interstitial foci of acute lung injury in which fibroblasts and myofibroblasts are arranged in a linear fashion within a pale staining matrix (Fig. 3.2) [31]. Overlying epithelium consists of hyperplastic pneumocytes or columnar non-ciliated bronchiolar cells. Fibroblast foci, although seen in other conditions, are characteristic of UIP and represent an important diagnostic feature when seen in the context of patchy fibrosis and honeycomb change. The presence of these microscopic zones of acute lung injury set against a backdrop of chronic scarring accounts for the *temporal heterogeneity* typical of UIP.

Honeycomb change is present in most surgical lung biopsies and is another important diagnostic feature. Honeycomb change comprises cystic dilatation of air spaces that are frequently lined by columnar respiratory epithelium in scarred, fibrotic lung tissue (Fig. 3.3). The honeycomb spaces primarily affect peripheral subpleural lung, which results in a characteristic *cobblestone* appearance of the visceral pleural surface that resembles cirrhotic liver (Fig. 3.4). Fibrotic scars that obscure the underlying lung architecture without associated honeycomb change are another form of architectural distortion that is characteristic of UIP (Fig. 3.5). Smooth muscle hyperplasia is commonly seen in areas of fibrosis and honeycomb change, and this finding can be striking in some patients.

The histopathologic findings described for patients with sporadic IPF are indistinguishable from the findings seen in patients with familial disease [15, 16].

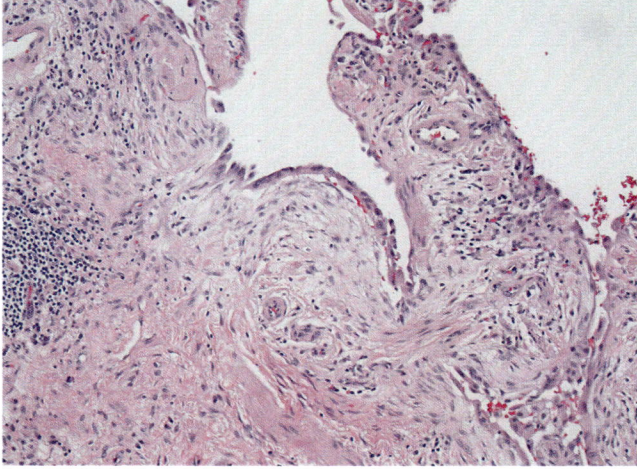

**Fig. 3.2** High-magnification photomicrograph showing fibroblast focus in UIP (hematoxylin and eosin stain; original magnification ×200). A small area of subepithelial stromal pallor demonstrates plump fibroblasts and myofibroblasts arranged in a vaguely linear fashion. The fibroblast focus is sandwiched between overlying type 2 pneumocytes and adjacent fibrotic scar

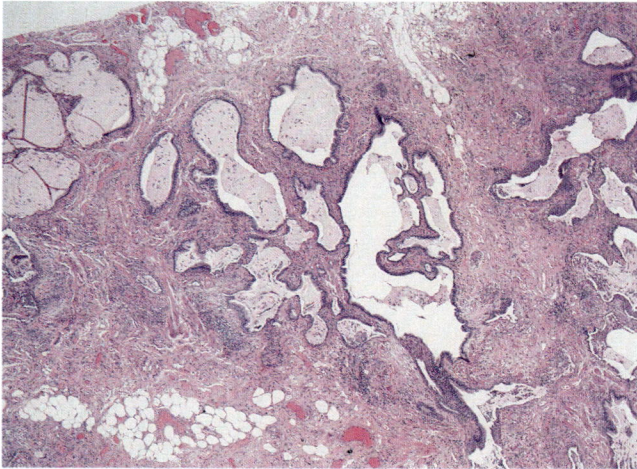

**Fig. 3.3** Low-magnification photomicrograph showing honeycomb change in a surgical lung biopsy from a patient with UIP/IPF (hematoxylin and eosin stain; original magnification ×40). Cystic spaces situated in densely scarred subpleural lung (visceral pleural surface at *upper left*) are lined by bronchiolar epithelium

Similarly, UIP in IPF patients cannot be reliably separated from UIP in patients with underlying systemic connective tissue diseases on the basis of histology alone. Lymphoid hyperplasia in the form of peribronchiolar lymphoid aggregates ("follicular bronchiolitis") is more common in patients with underlying rheumatoid

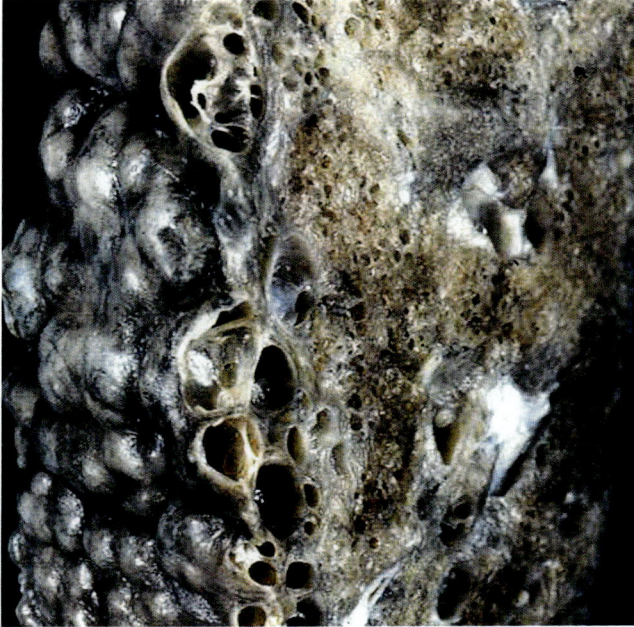

**Fig. 3.4** Photograph showing visceral pleural surface (*left*) and cut surface (*right*) of autopsy lung from a patient with UIP/IPF. Peripheral, subpleural honeycomb change results in a *cobblestone* appearance of the lung surface

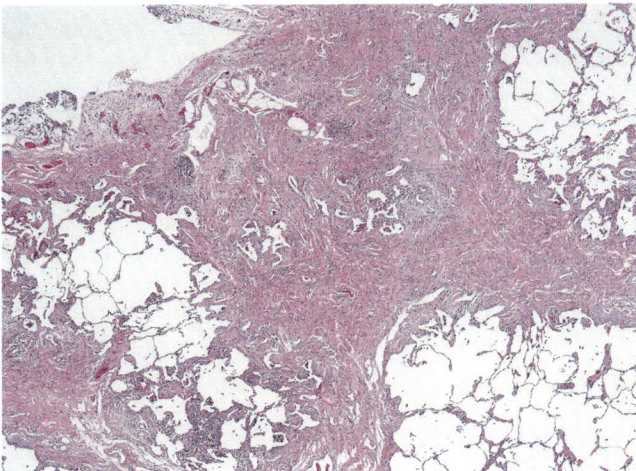

**Fig. 3.5** Low-magnification photomicrograph showing area of subpleural scarring without well-developed honeycomb change in a patient with UIP (hematoxylin and eosin stain; original magnification ×40). The area of scarring effaces the lung architecture and is characterized by a combination of dense collagen deposition and smooth muscle hyperplasia with minimal inflammation

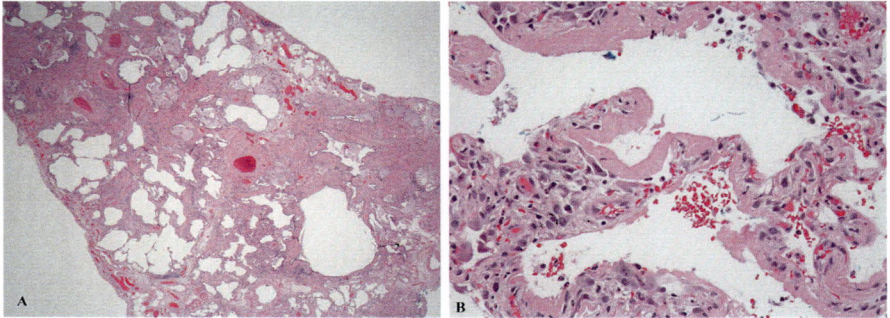

**Fig. 3.6** (a) Low-magnification photomicrograph showing combination of "patchwork fibrosis" and honeycomb change typical of UIP in a patient with IPF (hematoxylin and eosin stain; original magnification ×20). (b) High-magnification photomicrograph from different area of same biopsy showing an area of diffuse alveolar damage (hematoxylin and eosin stain; original magnification ×400). Alveolar septa show a scant inflammatory infiltrate, myofibroblasts, and a few residual pneumocytes associated with distinct eosinophilic hyaline membranes. Hyaline membranes are the histologic hallmark of diffuse alveolar damage, establishing the diagnosis of acute exacerbation in a patient with IPF for whom there is no other identifiable cause for acute respiratory distress

arthritis but also occurs, albeit less commonly, in patients with IPF [31]. For that reason, the presence or absence of associated lymphoid hyperplasia in an individual surgical lung biopsy demonstrating otherwise typical UIP cannot by itself be used to separate IPF from connective tissue disease-associated pulmonary fibrosis.

Biopsies from patients with acute exacerbation usually show a combination of UIP and superimposed diffuse alveolar damage (DAD) (Fig. 3.6) [18, 19]. The features of DAD may be patchy and typically include some combination of confluent alveolar septal thickening and distortion by fibroblasts and myofibroblasts with minimal associated inflammatory cells, marked hyperplasia of cytologically atypical type 2 pneumocytes, hyaline membranes, fibrin thrombi in small vessels, and squamous metaplasia of bronchiolar epithelium. In other patients the superimposed pattern of acute lung injury more closely resembles organizing pneumonia.

No single histologic finding consistently predicts prognosis in individual patients with UIP. Patients with more extensive fibroblast foci have experienced shorter mean survivals in some studies [33–36], while other investigators have failed to demonstrate the same relationship in patients without clinical or histologic evidence of acute exacerbation [17, 37].

## Desquamative Interstitial Pneumonia/Respiratory Bronchiolitis Interstitial Lung Disease

Desquamative interstitial pneumonia (DIP) and respiratory bronchiolitis interstitial lung disease (RBILD) are two highly related and overlapping forms of diffuse interstitial lung disease typically grouped with the idiopathic interstitial pneumonias.

Katzenstein has proposed collapsing the two into a single category for reasons described later. DIP/RBILD is uncommon, accounting for only a small minority of surgical lung biopsies from patients with idiopathic interstitial pneumonias [9–11]. They are separated from UIP/IPF because of marked differences in natural history and prognosis [38, 39].

## Clinical Features

DIP/RBILD affects younger patients, with a mean age at diagnosis in the fourth or fifth decade of life [1, 2]. Nearly all patients have strong histories of cigarette smoking, prompting many to consider DIP/RBILD a form of smoking-related lung disease rather than an idiopathic condition [24, 40]. Pulmonary function tests in most patients show evidence of mild restrictive disease accompanied by a moderate decrease in diffusing capacity. HRCT scans typically show patchy ground-glass opacities, often with a lower lung zone distribution without the traction bronchiectasis and honeycomb change typical of UIP.

DIP/RBILD is associated with a significantly better prognosis than UIP. Overall survival is nearly 90 %, ranging from around 70 % to 80 % in older studies to 100 % in more recently published series [1, 39]. Higher survival rates in more recent studies may reflect a trend toward assigning cases with associated fibrosis to the category of NSIP. RBILD is associated with an equally good or better prognosis [39, 41, 42]. Retrospective case series suggest smoking cessation as an important therapeutic strategy, but the impact on outcome is controversial [41].

## Pathologic Features

DIP/RBILD is characterized by the presence of pigmented ("smokers") macrophages within the lumens of distal airways (i.e., respiratory bronchioles) and air spaces. The macrophages are distinctive in that they have abundant cytoplasm containing finely granular, dusty brown pigment. In RBILD the changes are patchy at low magnification and limited to the airways with only minimal or mild interstitial inflammation or fibrosis (Fig. 3.7). The appearance is indistinguishable from isolated respiratory bronchiolitis (RB), a common, incidental finding in otherwise asymptomatic cigarette smokers who lack clinical evidence of restrictive lung disease. RBILD may include mild fibrotic thickening of alveolar septa without architectural distortion that is immediately adjacent to the visceral pleura and bronchovascular bundles in some patients (Fig. 3.8) [43]. This pattern of concomitant fibrosis has been referred to using a variety of terms [most recently, smoking-related interstitial fibrosis (SRIF)], and like respiratory bronchiolitis, this pattern does not by itself predict clinically or physiologically significant lung disease [44].

Historically, DIP was defined not only by the airway-centered changes described in RBILD but also by uniform alveolar septal thickening that is due to a combination of mild fibrosis and inflammation (i.e., interstitial pneumonia). The advent of SRIF as a form of fibrosis in patients who otherwise fit comfortably into the

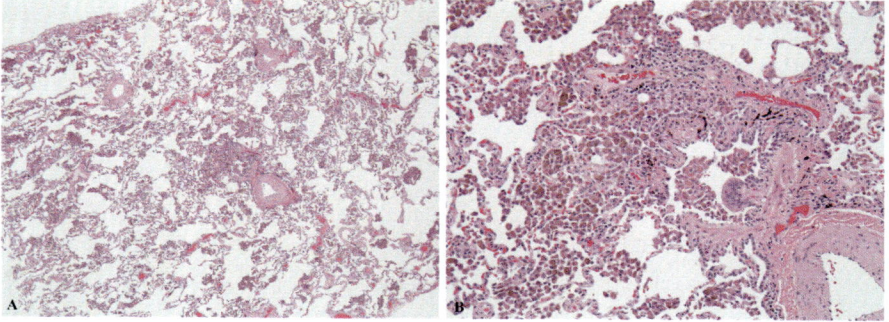

**Fig. 3.7** (a) Low-magnification photomicrograph showing respiratory bronchiolitis (hematoxylin and eosin; original magnification ×40). Pigmented alveolar macrophages are clustered within the lumens of distal bronchioles and peribronchiolar air spaces without the fibrosis or architectural distortion typical of UIP. (b) High-magnification photomicrograph from same biopsy illustrated in A showing respiratory bronchiolitis (hematoxylin and eosin; original magnification ×400). Pigmented ("smoker's") macrophages are loosely clustered within the lumen of a respiratory bronchiole and peribronchiolar alveolar spaces

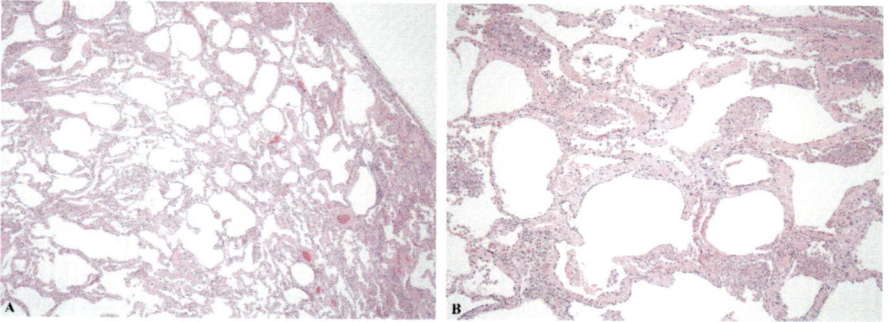

**Fig. 3.8** (a) Low-magnification photomicrograph showing subpleural, smoking-related interstitial fibrosis (SRIF) in a patient with RBILD (hematoxylin and eosin stain; original magnification ×40). Subpleural alveolar septa are mildly and diffusely thickened by paucicellular, eosinophilic collagen deposition without architectural distortion in the form of tissue-destructive scarring or honeycomb change. (b) Intermediate-magnification photomicrograph illustrating uniform alveolar septal thickening by dense eosinophilic collagen deposition with minimal associated interstitial inflammation in SRIF complicating RBILD (hematoxylin and eosin stain; original magnification ×100)

category of RBILD, plus the recognition of NSIP as a form of interstitial pneumonia distinctly different from UIP, have combined to effectively eliminate DIP as a modern category of idiopathic interstitial pneumonia. Patients historically labeled as having DIP are increasingly assigned to the categories of either RBILD (with SRIF) or NSIP. As originally defined, the key feature that separated DIP from UIP was that the interstitial changes were more uniform at low magnification with a focally bronchiolocentric distribution but without honeycomb change or fibrotic scarring (Fig. 3.9) [4, 45].

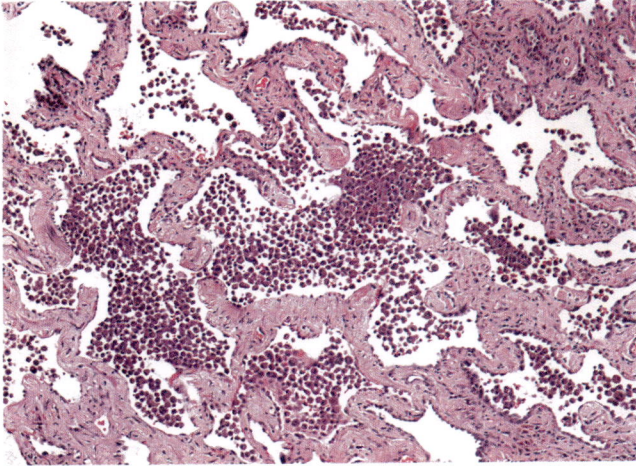

**Fig. 3.9** Intermediate-magnification photomicrograph showing the features that historically defined DIP: an interstitial pneumonia characterized by mild fibrosis and inflammation resulting in uniform thickening of alveolar septa lined by reactive type II pneumocytes and prominent pigmented macrophages within alveolar spaces (hematoxylin and eosin stain; original magnification ×100). Increasingly, patients historically assigned to the category of DIP are more likely to be classified as either RBILD (with *smoking-related interstitial fibrosis*—SRIF) or NSIP depending on the characteristics and extent of the interstitial changes

**Significance of Pathologic Diagnoses of DIP or RBILD**

Neither RBILD nor DIP should be viewed as free-standing histopathologic entities, because areas resembling both commonly occur as incidental findings in cigarette smokers with other lung diseases including UIP [29, 46]. In addition, there are no histologic changes that reliably separate patients with DIP/RBILD from those with other lung diseases in whom RB and "DIP-like reactions" represent incidental findings [46]. For that reason, DIP/RBILD should be diagnosed only when other forms of interstitial lung disease have been vigorously excluded by carefully examining all aspects of the microscopic slides and by correlating the surgical lung biopsy diagnosis with clinical and radiological features to establish the presence of physiologically meaningful restrictive lung disease [47]. While incidental RB can be recognized on TBB, this technique cannot be used to diagnose DIP/RBILD.

## *Nonspecific Interstitial Pneumonia*

Nonspecific interstitial pneumonia/fibrosis (NSIP) was proposed in 1994 as a form of chronic interstitial pneumonia characterized by relatively uniform expansion of alveolar septa by inflammation and/or fibrosis without the geographic and temporal heterogeneity of UIP [48]. As the term implies, the histologic findings in NSIP are not specific. Findings indistinguishable from NSIP can occur focally in other conditions, most importantly in UIP. The findings are also nonspecific from a clinical perspective, given that identical changes can occur in surgical lung biopsies from patients with a variety of underlying causes or associations including hypersensitivity pneumonia and various systemic connective tissue diseases [40, 48, 49]. Recognizing idiopathic NSIP as a distinct entity is, therefore, a process of exclusion that, like DIP/RBILD, requires careful correlation with clinical and radiological information. While the previously referenced 2002 consensus classification suggested that NSIP should be considered "a *provisional diagnosis* until there is further clarity on the nature of the corresponding clinical condition," the revised document [6] and other authorities recognize NSIP as a distinct entity that should be separated from UIP due to important differences in natural history, treatment, and outcome [28, 30, 40, 49].

## Clinical Features

NSIP is the second most common idiopathic interstitial pneumonia, accounting for as many as a third of patients undergoing surgical lung biopsy in retrospective series [8–12, 40]. NSIP fails to show the gender predilection for men seen in UIP, and in some series NSIP is more common in women [48]. NSIP also differs from UIP in that it tends to affect younger patients with an average age at diagnosis of around 50 years [40, 49]. Shortness of breath and dry cough are the most common complaints, which often develop in an insidious fashion that is indistinguishable from that described for UIP. Pulmonary function studies show restricted lung volumes and abnormalities of oxygenation, although the degree of abnormality tends to be less severe compared to patients with UIP. CT scans show a nonspecific but characteristic combination of ground-glass opacities, irregular lines, and traction bronchiectasis, occasionally with subpleural sparing.

Multiple studies have now confirmed the survival advantage associated with a diagnosis of NSIP compared to UIP [40, 49]. Median survival for all NSIP cases is over 9 years with the best prognosis occurring in patients with minimal fibrosis (i.e., "cellular NSIP"). Most patients with cellular NSIP survive, but about half have persistent stable disease. Patients in whom fibrosis predominates in surgical lung biopsies do worse than those with more cellular lesions (although survival is still better than UIP) [11, 48, 50–53]. Mortality rates for patients with fibrotic NSIP vary widely, ranging from 11 % to 68 % in various studies (mean ± STD, 30.4 % ± 18.9 %) [10, 11, 48–51, 54]. Reported 5-year survivals of such patients are about 76 % compared to about 45 % for UIP [38, 53]. Survivors typically have persistent lung disease, and to some extent variation in mortality rates reported for patients with fibrotic NSIP reflects differences in histologic definitions and the difficulty in separating fibrotic NSIP from UIP. Corticosteroids have not been prospectively evaluated in a randomized fashion but may be effective in a subset of patients, especially those with minimal associated fibrosis [50].

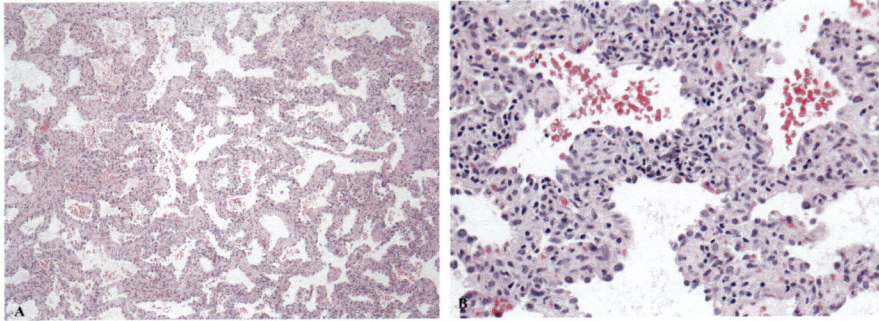

**Fig. 3.10** (**a**) Intermediate-magnification photomicrograph of cellular NSIP (hematoxylin and eosin stain; original magnification ×100). Alveolar septa are uniformly thickened by an infiltrate of mononuclear inflammatory cells with minimal fibrosis and preservation of lung architecture. (**b**) High-magnification photomicrograph showing expansion of alveolar septa by an interstitial infiltrate of predominantly lymphocytes and occasional plasma cells in the same patient with cellular NSIP (hematoxylin and eosin stain; original magnification ×400)

## Pathologic Features

A diagnosis of NSIP in surgical lung biopsies requires the presence of a chronic interstitial pneumonia without findings to prompt diagnosis of a more specific pathologic process. Unlike UIP, NSIP is in many respects a diagnosis of exclusion. Defined in this way, NSIP spans a range of histologic abnormalities ranging from a predominantly cellular process (i.e., cellular NSIP) to paucicellular lung fibrosis (i.e., fibrotic NSIP). The most cellular forms are characterized by an alveolar septal infiltrate of mononuclear cells that may be patchy or diffuse (Fig. 3.10). Whether patchy or diffuse, the qualitative features of the interstitial abnormalities remain constant without the geographic and temporal heterogeneity associated with UIP. The inflammatory infiltrate consists of lymphocytes and variable numbers of admixed plasma cells. Neutrophils, eosinophils, and histiocytes are relatively inconspicuous. Granulomas are rare in NSIP and, if present, should raise other considerations such as infection or hypersensitivity pneumonia.

The relative frequency of fibrosis in NSIP is variable. Patients with fibrotic NSIP outnumber patients with cellular NSIP by a ratio of nearly 4–1 in published studies, but this may reflect selection bias in that most reports are from tertiary referral centers where patients with fibrotic interstitial lung disease may be overrepresented. In addition, there are no clearly articulated criteria for separating cellular from fibrotic NSIP. The term, fibrotic NSIP, should be limited to those cases in which paucicellular fibrosis with minimal or mild inflammation is the predominant feature. If fibrotic NSIP is defined in this way, the extent of interstitial fibrosis is variable. Fibrosis takes the form of uniform collagen accumulation resulting in expansion of alveolar septa and peribronchiolar interstitium (Fig. 3.11) without the patchwork distribution characteristic of UIP. Pathology reports should comment on the presence and extent of interstitial fibrosis, since it is associated with significantly increased

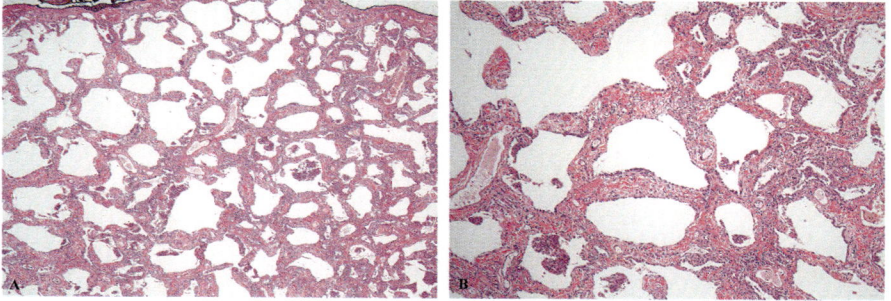

**Fig. 3.11** (**a**) Low-magnification photomicrograph illustrating fibrotic NSIP (hematoxylin and eosin stain; original magnification ×40). Alveolar septa are uniformly expanded by collagen deposition with mild inflammation. There is no associated scarring or honeycomb change. (**b**) Intermediate-magnification photomicrograph from same patient with fibrotic NSIP illustrating expansion of alveolar septa by eosinophilic collagen with a mild and patchy associated infiltrate of mononuclear inflammatory cells (hematoxylin and eosin stain; original magnification ×100). Thickened alveolar septa are lined by reactive pneumocytes, a nonspecific but common manifestation of interstitial injury

risk for disease-specific mortality [1, 2, 40, 48, 49]. Associated smooth muscle hyperplasia tends to be less extensive than that seen in UIP. Fibroblast foci should be absent or, at most, rare and inconspicuous, and honeycomb change and broad zones of scarring should be absent. Absence of honeycomb change is perhaps the single most important feature in distinguishing fibrotic NSIP from UIP. Patchy intraluminal fibrosis resembling organizing pneumonia is common, but this should be a focal and relatively inconspicuous finding.

## The Role of Surgical Lung Biopsy in Classification and Diagnosis of Idiopathic Interstitial Pneumonias

### *"Pattern" Versus "Diagnosis" for Reporting the Results of Surgical Lung Biopsy*

The authors of the 2002 consensus classification advocated use of the term "pattern" when reporting lung biopsy findings in order to distinguish the pathologic diagnosis from a final "clinical-radiologic-pathologic diagnosis." This emphasizes the value of an iterative, dynamic, multidisciplinary process that correlates histologic findings with other relevant data, as reviewed in greater detail in Chap. 5, but this may be unnecessary and, in some cases, potentially dangerous [30]. Indeed, many pathologic diagnoses are not isolated events but rather essential components of an iterative process in which final interpretation is dynamic and framed by ongoing data collection. For example, a lung biopsy diagnosis of adenocarcinoma may be reinterpreted as metastatic adenocarcinoma after discovery of a previously occult primary malignancy outside the lung. This possibility should not drive an argument for substituting the term "adenocarcinoma pattern," terminology that may interfere with the end user's recognition that the diagnosis of malignancy is certain. Use of the term "pattern" may result in confusion regarding the circumstances in which the specificity of the histopathologic findings is, in fact, the primary driver of a final diagnosis.

UIP stands alone among the idiopathic interstitial pneumonias in being a specific histopathologic entity. Several studies have demonstrated the primary role of a lung biopsy diagnosis of UIP in establishing a clinical diagnosis of IPF [23, 24, 27, 55, 56]. This is especially important given that patients are increasingly selected for lung biopsy because there is some level of doubt regarding the likelihood of IPF, which is usually based on an atypical radiological pattern of disease. It is precisely in this context that a biopsy diagnosis of UIP establishes the clinical diagnosis with certainty, and in this context the biopsy result remains the single most powerful predictor of disease-specific mortality at the time of diagnosis [10, 23]. The histopathologic findings are less specific in all other forms of idiopathic interstitial pneumonia, and perhaps for these non-UIP entities a stronger argument can be made for using the term "pattern." In the biased view of this author, however, this diminishes the role of the pathologist to that of technician rather than a diagnostician engaged in proactively integrating histologic observations with clinical information. This proactive approach is common in other areas of medicine in which the pathology report serves as a platform for integrating relevant clinical, laboratory, and radiological information that facilitates accurate interpretation of microscopic findings.

The second argument for using the term "pattern" in reporting diagnoses of UIP is that it occurs in patients for whom the term "IPF" is deemed inappropriate. The implication is that sorting patients with UIP into different clinical groups impacts therapeutic options and outcome. The preponderance of evidence suggests that patients with a biopsy diagnosis of UIP have a form of fibrotic lung disease that is relatively insensitive to conventional immunosuppressive therapy and likely to be associated with a progressive course regardless of the underlying or associated condition. Although a number of studies have indicated a better prognosis for UIP associated with connective tissue diseases, others have failed to demonstrate the same survival advantage [17, 57–59]. The differences observed in some studies may be related to confounding factors such as younger age, greater prevalence of women, and lower smoking rates in patients with connective tissue diseases, factors that themselves are associated with a better prognosis in patients with UIP/IPF. In addition, the survival advantage does not apply to patients with rheumatoid arthritis, the largest subset of patients with connective tissue disease-associated UIP [59]. Similarly, asbestos can be viewed as a potential cause of UIP that carries significant legal ramifications, but there are few, if any, meaningful differences between asbestosis and IPF in terms of signs and symptoms, morphology, treatment response, or natural history [60, 61]. Even in patients with an exposure history suggesting chronic hypersensitivity pneumonias as an alternative, a biopsy diagnosis of UIP predicts a natural history indistinguishable from IPF [62–66].

## Distinguishing Fibrotic NSIP from UIP

Separating fibrotic NSIP from UIP is perhaps the greatest challenge when it comes to making meaningful distinctions among the idiopathic interstitial pneumonias [28]. Separating fibrotic NSIP from UIP hinges on recognition of the patchwork distribution, fibroblast foci, and honeycomb change typical of UIP. Recognition of any one of these features in a biopsy for which a diagnosis of fibrotic NSIP is being contemplated is reason for caution. In this circumstance, correlation with other clinical data (especially HRCT findings) may be helpful.

The primary problem is that areas typical of NSIP can occur as a focal phenomenon in other conditions, which makes sampling bias a potential barrier to accurate diagnosis. In a review of 20 explanted lungs with UIP, for example, all but three showed isolated areas that were indistinguishable from NSIP ("NSIP-like areas") [29]. Other studies have shown that when surgical lung biopsies taken from more than one site demonstrated both UIP and NSIP ("discordant UIP"), the presence of UIP in even a single piece of tissue defined a survival curve typical of IPF in patients [67, 68]. For these reasons, establishing a diagnosis of idiopathic NSIP requires the absence of clinical, radiological, or pathologic findings to suggest an alternative. For example, a biopsy diagnosis of fibrotic NSIP in a patient with bibasilar honeycomb change on HRCT is almost certainly a sampling error in a patient with UIP. While the 2002 consensus classification would suggest that this issue could be resolved by producing a pathology report with a diagnosis of *fibrotic NSIP pattern*, it may be more prudent to instead offer a descriptive diagnosis in the pathology report that synthesizes histopathologic, clinical, and radiological data (e.g., *chronic interstitial pneumonia with fibrosis most consistent with UIP*) with a comment acknowledging that the biopsy is not by itself diagnostic, but that correlation with imaging studies indicates UIP as the correct diagnosis. This approach avoids the risk that others engaged in a patient's care will have to reconcile seemingly discordant information when comparing pathology reports with other clinical or radiological data.

## Role of Transbronchial Biopsies

Transbronchial biopsies may be useful in managing selected patients suspected of having idiopathic interstitial pneumonias, but its role in establishing a diagnosis of UIP remains controversial [69, 70]. The 2011 ATS/ERS/JRS/ALAT statement on IPF recommends that, "Transbronchial biopsy should not be used in the evaluation of IPF in the majority of patients, but may be appropriate in a minority (weak recommendation, low-quality evidence)" [14]. In a retrospective case study limited to patients with UIP, about a third of transbronchial biopsies showed some combination of fibrosis distributed in a patchwork pattern, fibroblast foci, and honeycomb change considered diagnostic or at least suggestive of UIP [69]. Additional studies are necessary to more fully understand the diagnostic sensitivity and specificity of transbronchial lung biopsy in this setting, but in the author's anecdotal experience, there is a small selected subset of patients in whom UIP can be diagnosed with confidence on transbronchial biopsies if carefully correlated with clinical and radiological findings.

## Summary

Surgical lung biopsy diagnosis is an essential component of the diagnostic algorithm for the majority of patients with idiopathic interstitial pneumonia. Differentiating these entities is important because of significant differences in therapeutic options and outcome. As HRCT gains widespread acceptance as a primary diagnostic modality for a subset of patients with UIP, lung biopsies will be increasingly limited to patients with atypical and nondiagnostic radiological findings. It is in this subset of patients that surgical lung biopsy plays a key role in diagnosis and management.

## References

 1. Myers J. Idiopathic interstitial pneumonias. In: Churg A, Myers J, Tazelaar HD, Wright JL, editors. Thurlbeck's pathology of the lung. New York, NY: Thieme; 2004. p. 563–600.
 2. Katzenstein AL. Katzenstein and askin's surgical pathology of non-neoplastic lung disease. 4th ed. Philadelphia, PA: Saunders Elsevier; 2006.
 3. Katzenstein AL, Myers JL. Idiopathic pulmonary fibrosis: clinical relevance of pathologic classification. Am J Respir Crit Care Med. 1998;157(4 Pt 1):1301–15.
 4. Liebow AA, Steer A, Billingsley JG. Desquamative interstitial pneumonia. Am J Med. 1965;39:369–404.
 5. American Thoracic Society/European Respiratory Society. American Thoracic Society/ European Respiratory Society International Multidisciplinary Consensus Classification of the Idiopathic Interstitial Pneumonias. Am J Respir Crit Care Med. 2002;165(2):277–304.
 6. Travis W, Gostabel U, Hensell D, et al. An official American Thoracic Society/European Respiratory Society Statement: Update of the international multidisciplinary classification of the Idiopathic interstitional pneumonias. Am J Respir Crit Care Med. 2013 (in press).
 7. Hamman BL, Rich AR. Acute diffuse interstitial fibrosis of the lung. Bull Johns Hopkins Hosp. 1944;74:177–212.
 8. Katzenstein AL, Myers JL, Mazur MT. Acute interstitial pneumonia. A clinicopathologic, ultrastructural, and cell kinetic study. Am J Surg Pathol. 1986;10(4):256–67.
 9. Bjoraker JA, Ryu JH, Edwin MK, Myers JL, Tazelaar HD, Schroeder DR, et al. Prognostic significance of histopathologic subsets in idiopathic pulmonary fibrosis. Am J Respir Crit Care Med. 1998;157(1):199–203.
10. Flaherty KR, Toews GB, Travis WD, Colby TV, Kazerooni EA, Gross BH, et al. Clinical significance of histological classification of idiopathic interstitial pneumonia. Eur Respir J. 2002;19(2):275–83.
11. Nicholson AG, Colby TV, du Bois RM, Hansell DM, Wells AU. The prognostic significance of the histologic pattern of interstitial pneumonia in patients presenting with the clinical entity of cryptogenic fibrosing alveolitis. Am J Respir Crit Care Med. 2000;162(6):2213–7.
12. Riha RL, Duhig EE, Clarke BE, Steele RH, Slaughter RE, Zimmerman PV. Survival of patients with biopsy-proven usual interstitial pneumonia and nonspecific interstitial pneumonia. Eur Respir J. 2002;19(6):1114–8.

13. Idiopathic Pulmonary Fibrosis: diagnosis and treatment. Am J Respir Crit Care Med. 2000;161(2):646–64.
14. Raghu G, Collard HR, Egan JJ, Martinez FJ, Behr J, Brown KK, et al. An official ATS/ERS/ JRS/ALAT statement: idiopathic pulmonary fibrosis: evidence-based guidelines for diagnosis and management. Am J Respir Crit Care Med. 2011;183(6):788–824.
15. Lee HL, Ryu JH, Wittmer MH, Hartman TE, Lymp JF, Tazelaar HD, et al. Familial idiopathic pulmonary fibrosis: clinical features and outcome. Chest. 2005;127(6):2034–41.
16. Steele MP, Speer MC, Loyd JE, Brown KK, Herron A, Slifer SH, et al. Clinical and pathologic features of familial interstitial pneumonia. Am J Respir Crit Care Med. 2005;172(9): 1146–52.
17. Flaherty KR, Colby TV, Travis WD, Toews GB, Mumford J, Murray S, et al. Fibroblastic foci in usual interstitial pneumonia: idiopathic versus collagen vascular disease. Am J Respir Crit Care Med. 2003;167(10):1410–5.
18. Collard HR, Moore BB, Flaherty KR, Brown KK, Kaner RJ, King Jr TE, et al. Acute exacerbations of idiopathic pulmonary fibrosis. Am J Respir Crit Care Med. 2007;176(7):636–43.
19. Parambil JG, Myers JL, Ryu JH. Histopathologic features and outcome of patients with acute exacerbation of idiopathic pulmonary fibrosis undergoing surgical lung biopsy. Chest. 2005;128(5):3310–5.
20. Azuma A, Nukiwa T, Tsuboi E, Suga M, Abe S, Nakata K, et al. Double-blind, placebo-controlled trial of pirfenidone in patients with idiopathic pulmonary fibrosis. Am J Respir Crit Care Med. 2005;171(9):1040–7.
21. Martinez FJ, Safrin S, Weycker D, Starko KM, Bradford WZ, King Jr TE, et al. The clinical course of patients with idiopathic pulmonary fibrosis. Ann Intern Med. 2005;142(12 Pt 1):963–7.
22. Daniels C, Yi E, Ryu JH. Autopsy findings in 42 consecutive patients with idiopathic pulmonary fibrosis. Eur Respir J. 2008;32:170–4.
23. Flaherty KR, Thwaite EL, Kazerooni EA, Gross BH, Toews GB, Colby TV, et al. Radiological versus histological diagnosis in UIP and NSIP: survival implications. Thorax. 2003;58(2):143–8.
24. Hunninghake GW, Zimmerman MB, Schwartz DA, King Jr TE, Lynch J, Hegele R, et al. Utility of a lung biopsy for the diagnosis of idiopathic pulmonary fibrosis. Am J Respir Crit Care Med. 2001;164(2):193–6.
25. Johkoh T, Muller NL, Cartier Y, Kavanagh PV, Hartman TE, Akira M, et al. Idiopathic interstitial pneumonias: diagnostic accuracy of thin-section CT in 129 patients. Radiology. 1999;211(2):555–60.
26. Sumikawa H, Johkoh T, Ichikado K, Taniguchi H, Kondoh Y, Fujimoto K, et al. Usual interstitial pneumonia and chronic idiopathic interstitial pneumonia: analysis of CT appearance in 92 patients. Radiology. 2006;241(1):258–66.
27. Sumikawa H, Johkoh T, Colby TV, Ichikado K, Suga M, Taniguchi H, et al. Computed tomography findings in pathological usual interstitial pneumonia: relationship to survival. Am J Respir Crit Care Med. 2008;177(4):433–9.
28. Katzenstein AL, Mukhopadhyay S, Myers JL. Diagnosis of usual interstitial pneumonia and distinction from other fibrosing interstitial lung diseases. Hum Pathol. 2008;39(9):1275–94.
29. Katzenstein AL, Zisman DA, Litzky LA, Nguyen BT, Kotloff RM. Usual interstitial pneumonia: histologic study of biopsy and explant specimens. Am J Surg Pathol. 2002;26(12):1567–77.
30. Myers JL, Katzenstein AL. Beyond a consensus classification for idiopathic interstitial pneumonias: progress and controversies. Histopathology. 2009;54(1):90–103.
31. Myers JL, Katzenstein AL. Fibroblasts in focus. Am J Respir Crit Care Med. 2006;174(6):623–4.
32. Atkins SR, Turesson C, Myers JL, Tazelaar HD, Ryu JH, Matteson EL, et al. Morphologic and quantitative assessment of CD20+ B cell infiltrates in rheumatoid arthritis-associated nonspecific interstitial pneumonia and usual interstitial pneumonia. Arthritis Rheum. 2006;54(2):635–41.

33. Enomoto N, Suda T, Kato M, Kaida Y, Nakamura Y, Imokawa S, et al. Quantitative analysis of fibroblastic foci in usual interstitial pneumonia. Chest. 2006;130(1):22–9.
34. King Jr TE, Schwarz MI, Brown K, Tooze JA, Colby TV, Waldron Jr JA, et al. Idiopathic pulmonary fibrosis: relationship between histopathologic features and mortality. Am J Respir Crit Care Med. 2001;164(6):1025–32.
35. Nicholson AG, Fulford LG, Colby TV, du Bois RM, Hansell DM, Wells AU. The relationship between individual histologic features and disease progression in idiopathic pulmonary fibrosis. Am J Respir Crit Care Med. 2002;166(2):173–7.
36. Tiitto L, Bloigu R, Heiskanen U, Paakko P, Kinnula VL, Kaarteenaho-Wiik R. Relationship between histopathological features and the course of idiopathic pulmonary fibrosis/usual interstitial pneumonia. Thorax. 2006;61(12):1091–5.
37. Hanak V, Ryu JH, de Carvalho E, Limper A, Hartman TE, Decker PA, et al. Profusion of fibroblast foci in patients with idiopathic pulmonary fibrosis does not predict outcome. Respir Med. 2008;102:852–6.
38. Myers JL, Veal Jr CF, Shin MS, Katzenstein AL. Respiratory bronchiolitis causing interstitial lung disease. A clinicopathologic study of six cases. Am Rev Respir Dis. 1987;135(4):880–4.
39. Ryu JH, Myers JL, Capizzi SA, Douglas WW, Vassallo R, Decker PA. Desquamative interstitial pneumonia and respiratory bronchiolitis-associated interstitial lung disease. Chest. 2005;127(1):178–84.
40. Myers JL. Nonspecific interstitial pneumonia: pathologic features and clinical implications. Semin Diagn Pathol. 2007;24(3):183–7.
41. Portnoy J, Veraldi KL, Schwarz MI, Cool CD, Curran-Everett D, Cherniack RM, et al. Respiratory bronchiolitis-interstitial lung disease: long-term outcome. Chest. 2007; 131(3):664–71.
42. Craig PJ, Wells AU, Doffman S, Rassl D, Colby TV, Hansell DM, et al. Desquamative interstitial pneumonia, respiratory bronchiolitis and their relationship to smoking. Histopathology. 2004;45(3):275–82.
43. Yousem SA. Respiratory bronchiolitis-associated interstitial lung disease with fibrosis is a lesion distinct from fibrotic nonspecific interstitial pneumonia: a proposal. Mod Pathol. 2006;19(11):1474–9.
44. Katzenstein AL. Smoking-related interstitial fibrosis (SRIF), pathogenesis and treatment of usual interstitial pneumonia (UIP), and transbronchial biopsy in UIP. Mod Pathol. 2012;25 Suppl 1:S68–78.
45. Gaensler EA, Goff AM, Prowse CM. Desquamative interstitial pneumonia. N Engl J Med. 1966;274(3):113–28.
46. Fraig M, Shreesha U, Savici D, Katzenstein AL. Respiratory bronchiolitis: a clinicopathologic study in current smokers, ex-smokers, and never-smokers. Am J Surg Pathol. 2002; 26(5):647–53.
47. Wells AU, Nicholson AG, Hansell DM. Challenges in pulmonary fibrosis. 4: smoking-induced diffuse interstitial lung diseases. Thorax. 2007;62(10):904–10.
48. Katzenstein AL, Fiorelli RF. Nonspecific interstitial pneumonia/fibrosis. Histologic features and clinical significance. Am J Surg Pathol. 1994;18(2):136–47.
49. Travis WD, Hunninghake G, King Jr TE, Lynch DA, Colby TV, Galvin JR, et al. Idiopathic nonspecific interstitial pneumonia: report of an American Thoracic Society project. Am J Respir Crit Care Med. 2008;177(12):1338–47.
50. Nagai S, Kitaichi M, Itoh H, Nishimura K, Izumi T, Colby TV. Idiopathic nonspecific interstitial pneumonia/fibrosis: comparison with idiopathic pulmonary fibrosis and BOOP. Eur Respir J. 1998;12(5):1010–9 [erratum appears in Eur Respir J 1999 Mar;13(3):711].
51. Travis WD, Matsui K, Moss J, Ferrans VJ. Idiopathic nonspecific interstitial pneumonia: prognostic significance of cellular and fibrosing patterns: survival comparison with usual interstitial pneumonia and desquamative interstitial pneumonia. Am J Surg Pathol. 2000;24(1):19–33.
52. Latsi PI, du Bois RM, Nicholson AG, Colby TV, Bisirtzoglou D, Nikolakopoulou A, et al. Fibrotic idiopathic interstitial pneumonia: the prognostic value of longitudinal functional trends. Am J Respir Crit Care Med. 2003;168(5):531–7.

53. Shin KM, Lee KS, Chung MP, Han J, Bae YA, Kim TS, et al. Prognostic determinants among clinical, thin-section CT, and histopathologic findings for fibrotic idiopathic interstitial pneumonia: tertiary hospital study. Radiology. 2008;249(1):328–37.
54. Jegal Y, Kim DS, Shim TS, Lim CM, Do Lee S, Koh Y, et al. Physiology is a stronger predictor of survival than pathology in fibrotic interstitial pneumonia. Am J Respir Crit Care Med. 2005;171(6):639–44.
55. Flaherty KR, Andrei AC, King Jr TE, Raghu G, Colby TV, Wells A, et al. Idiopathic interstitial pneumonia: do community and academic physicians agree on diagnosis? Am J Respir Crit Care Med. 2007;175(10):1054–60.
56. Flaherty KR, King Jr TE, Raghu G, Lynch 3rd JP, Colby TV, Travis WD, et al. Idiopathic interstitial pneumonia: what is the effect of a multidisciplinary approach to diagnosis? Am J Respir Crit Care Med. 2004;170(8):904–10.
57. Hubbard R, Venn A. The impact of coexisting connective tissue disease on survival in patients with fibrosing alveolitis. Rheumatology. 2002;41(6):676–9.
58. Kocheril SV, Appleton BE, Somers EC, Kazerooni EA, Flaherty KR, Martinez FJ, et al. Comparison of disease progression and mortality of connective tissue disease-related interstitial lung disease and idiopathic interstitial pneumonia. Arthritis Rheum. 2005;53(4):549–57.
59. Park JH, Kim DS, Park IN, Jang SJ, Kitaichi M, Nicholson AG, et al. Prognosis of fibrotic interstitial pneumonia: idiopathic versus collagen vascular disease-related subtypes. Am J Respir Crit Care Med. 2007;175(7):705–11.
60. Copley SJ, Wells AU, Sivakumaran P, Rubens MB, Lee YC, Desai SR, et al. Asbestosis and idiopathic pulmonary fibrosis: comparison of thin-section CT features. Radiology. 2003;229(3):731–6.
61. Gaensler EA, Jederlinic PJ, Churg A. Idiopathic pulmonary fibrosis in asbestos-exposed workers. Am Rev Respir Dis. 1991;144(3 Pt 1):689–96.
62. Perez-Padilla R, Salas J, Chapela R, Sanchez M, Carrillo G, Perez R, et al. Mortality in Mexican patients with chronic pigeon breeder's lung compared with those with usual interstitial pneumonia. Am Rev Respir Dis. 1993;148(1):49–53.
63. Churg A, Sin DD, Everett D, Brown K, Cool C. Pathologic patterns and survival in chronic hypersensitivity pneumonitis. Am J Surg Pathol. 2009;33(12):1765–70.
64. Hayakawa H, Shirai M, Sato A, Yoshizawa Y, Todate A, Imokawa S, et al. Clinicopathological features of chronic hypersensitivity pneumonitis. Respirology. 2002;7(4):359–64.
65. Ohtani Y, Saiki S, Kitaichi M, Usui Y, Inase N, Costabel U, et al. Chronic bird fancier's lung: histopathological and clinical correlation. An application of the 2002 ATS/ERS consensus classification of the idiopathic interstitial pneumonias. Thorax. 2005;60(8):665–71.
66. Trahan S, Hanak V, Ryu JH, Myers JL. Role of surgical lung biopsy in separating chronic hypersensitivity pneumonia from usual interstitial pneumonia/idiopathic pulmonary fibrosis: analysis of 31 biopsies from 15 patients. Chest. 2008;134(1):126–32.
67. Flaherty KR, Travis WD, Colby TV, Toews GB, Kazerooni EA, Gross BH, et al. Histopathologic variability in usual and nonspecific interstitial pneumonias. Am J Respir Crit Care Med. 2001;164(9):1722–7.
68. Monaghan H, Wells AU, Colby TV, du Bois RM, Hansell DM, Nicholson AG. Prognostic implications of histologic patterns in multiple surgical lung biopsies from patients with idiopathic interstitial pneumonias. Chest. 2004;125(2):522–6.
69. Berbescu EA, Katzenstein AL, Snow JL, Zisman DA. Transbronchial biopsy in usual interstitial pneumonia. Chest. 2006;129(5):1126–31.
70. Ensminger SA, Prakash UB. Is bronchoscopic lung biopsy helpful in the management of patients with diffuse lung disease? Eur Respir J. 2006;28(6):1081–4.

# Chapter 4
# Imaging of Idiopathic Pulmonary Fibrosis

Jonathan H. Chung and Jeffrey P. Kanne

**Abstract** Imaging is an essential part of establishing a confident diagnosis in the setting of suspected idiopathic pulmonary fibrosis (IPF), and usual interstitial pneumonia (UIP) represents the imaging and histopathologic correlate of IPF. Although chest radiographs often show abnormalities in patients with UIP, the findings are typically nonspecific. High-resolution computed tomography (HRCT) allows for accurate characterization of many types of pulmonary fibrosis and can be used to establish a confident diagnosis of UIP. When a confident diagnosis of UIP can be made on HRCT, the high accuracy of a high-confidence diagnosis obviates the need to perform a surgical lung biopsy. However, due to significant overlap in the imaging appearance of UIP with other causes of pulmonary fibrosis, caution is necessary in making a diagnosis of IPF when low-confidence patterns of pulmonary fibrosis are present.

**Keywords** Idiopathic pulmonary fibrosis • IPF • Usual interstitial pneumonia • UIP • HRCT

## Introduction

Idiopathic pulmonary fibrosis (IPF) is the most common cause of fibrotic lung disease. Approximately, 1–2/10,000 people are diagnosed with IPF, with an increased prevalence in elderly patients. Men are affected nearly twice as often as women [1]. There is a strong association between IPF and cigarette smoking, especially in

J.H. Chung, M.D. (✉)
Department of Radiology, National Jewish Health, 1400 Jackson Street, Denver,
CO 80206, USA
e-mail: chungj@njhealth.org

J.P. Kanne, M.D.
Department of Radiology, University of Wisconsin School of Medicine
and Public Health, Madison, WI, USA

K.C. Meyer and S.D. Nathan (eds.), *Idiopathic Pulmonary Fibrosis: A Comprehensive Clinical Guide*, Respiratory Medicine 9, DOI 10.1007/978-1-62703-682-5_4, © Springer Science+Business Media New York 2014

patients with a >20 pack-year smoking history [2]. Additionally, gastroesophageal reflux disease (GERD) is also very common in patients with IPF; 90 % of patients with IPF have GERD, and treatment for GERD has been associated with increased survival [3]. The prognosis of patients with IPF is poor (approaching levels similar to non-small cell lung cancer), with a median survival of approximately 3 years [4]. The clinical presentation is nonspecific and includes progressive dyspnea (especially upon exertion), dry cough, early inspiratory crackles on chest auscultation, and digital clubbing. Usual interstitial pneumonia (UIP) is the most common imaging correlate in patients with IPF [5, 6]. Based on imaging, a confident diagnosis of UIP can often be made, obviating the need for biopsy.

# Radiography

Given its poor contrast resolution compared to computerized tomography (CT), routine use of radiography in the work-up of patients with known or suspected IPF has markedly decreased with the widespread availability of multidetector CT. However, because imaging findings of UIP may be detected before patients become symptomatic, recognition of the radiographic pattern of UIP remains important, because the radiologist may be the first to suggest underlying pulmonary fibrosis. The main pattern on chest radiography is that of bilateral symmetric reticulation and irregular linear opacities [7]. Superimposition of reticulation on radiography may lead to apparent reticulonodular opacities, though no nodules are actually present. Traction bronchiectasis may also be evident. UIP favors the subpleural and basal lung regions (Fig. 4.1). In typical cases, pulmonary fibrosis will lead to basilar-predominant volume loss. In cases of concomitant upper lobe-predominant emphysema from smoking, total lung volume may be normal. In more advanced cases, subpleural honeycombing, which manifests as basilar-predominant cystic spaces, may be apparent [8]. Honeycombing implies local areas of end-stage pulmonary fibrosis and is highly specific for the diagnosis of UIP [9]. In a study of 16 patients with UIP, 15 had interstitial opacities on the chest radiograph; 10 patients had reticular opacities, 2 had reticulonodular opacities, 3 had frank honeycombing, and 1 patient had mixed alveolar and interstitial opacities. Lung volumes were decreased in the majority of patients (12/16 = 75 %). No patients had increased lung volumes in keeping with the restrictive nature of pulmonary fibrosis [10]. If pulmonary fibrosis is suspected on radiography, the next step is further evaluation with high-resolution CT (HRCT).

# Technical Aspects of HRCT

The introduction of CT in the late 1970s and the explosion in CT utilization in the late 1990s have revolutionized the manner in which the lungs are imaged. Because images are acquired in cross-section with CT, contrast resolution is superior to radiography (where overlapping structures complicate an accurate assessment of the

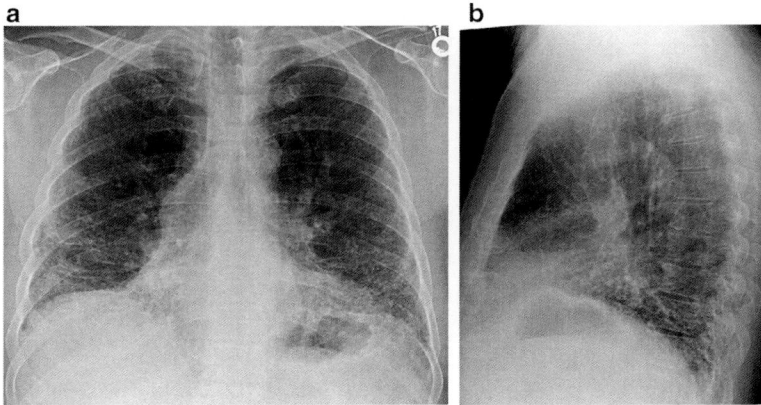

**Fig. 4.1** PA (**a**) and lateral (**b**) chest radiographs show low lung volumes and basilar-predominant reticulation highly suggestive of pulmonary fibrosis. Further evaluation with HRCT would be necessary to more accurately characterize the fibrotic lung disease

lung parenchyma) [11]. CT scans can be acquired to maximize spatial resolution or contrast resolution. Given the inherent high contrast within the lungs, CT of the chest is most often tailored to optimize spatial resolution, which results in HRCT [12]. HRCT is the reference standard for imaging the lungs in the setting of diffuse lung disease, and with current multidetector scanners, images can be reconstructed in any plane given the near-isovolumetric acquisition.

Unfortunately, there is no standard HRCT protocol. CT scans can be acquired in a helical manner (most common) or in a sequential or "step-and-shoot" fashion. Helical CT acquisition allows for more diverse reconstruction parameters and images the entire chest as opposed to the step-and-shoot strategy. However, the step-and-shoot method allows for gapped imaging such that significant portions of the chest are not scanned, leading to substantial reduction in radiation dose. This is most advantageous in the setting of diffuse lung diseases where complete imaging of the thorax is not usually necessary [7]. However, given the short life spans of most patients with pulmonary fibrosis and the long lead time for the development of radiation-induced malignancy, volumetric HRCT is preferred, as it can detect subtle fibrosis and honeycombing, which may alter management. Different centers use different acquisition parameters [CT scanner make and model, tube peak kilovoltage (kVp), tube current (mA), tube rotation time, table speed] as well as different image reconstruction parameters (slice thickness, slice interval, reconstruction kernel and method, field of view). Typically, the kVp should be 80–120, depending on patient size, and the mA should be less than 250. Tube current modulation, available on most modern scanners, has become the standard of care because it significantly reduces patient radiation exposure [13–15]. Field of view should include both lungs, while the inclusion of an excess amount of overlying air should be avoided. Prone and expiratory imaging can be helpful in distinguishing mild pulmonary fibrosis from peripheral atelectasis (particularly in the dependent aspect of the lungs) and to assess for air trapping, respectively. A dynamic expiratory scan can also be included to assess for tracheobronchomalacia. Although there are many variations, any HRCT scan should include a number of mandatory requirements that include (1) thin-section reconstruction (0.5–1.5 mm), (2) high spatial frequency (edge-enhancing) reconstruction kernel, (3) full inspiration, and (4) absence of motion artifact.

## Typical HRCT Pulmonary Findings

The vast majority of patients with UIP have reticulation in a subpleural and basilar-predominant distribution. A small percentage of patients have upper lobe-predominant fibrosis, although this pattern is more suggestive of non-UIP conditions such as sarcoidosis [16]. Associated architectural distortion with traction bronchiectasis and bronchiolectasis are the rule. Honeycombing occurs in the subpleural lung and typically manifests as "clustered cystic air spaces, typically of comparable diameters on the order of 3–10 mm" [17]. Honeycombing, in addition to upper lobe, subpleural linear lines, is the most specific finding of UIP on HRCT and is quite common, occurring in up to 90 % of UIP cases [9, 18]. A small amount of ground-glass opacity is not uncommon [19] (Fig. 4.2). When there are other findings of frank fibrosis (traction bronchiectasis and bronchiolectasis, reticulation, and honey-combing), ground-glass opacity almost assuredly represents microscopic pulmonary fibrosis. In cases in which ground-glass opacity is isolated, it may alternatively represent active inflammation [20, 21].

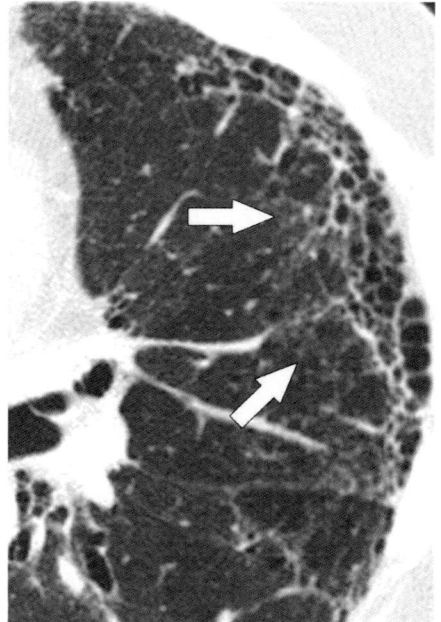

**Fig. 4.2** Axial HRCT image shows a small amount of ground-glass opacity (*arrow*) in the left upper lobe. Given the large degree of adjacent pulmonary fibrosis, ground-glass opacity likely represents microscopic pulmonary fibrosis rather than inflammation

**Fig. 4.3** Axial CT image
shows mild mediastinal
lymphadenopathy (*arrows*) in
this patient with UIP

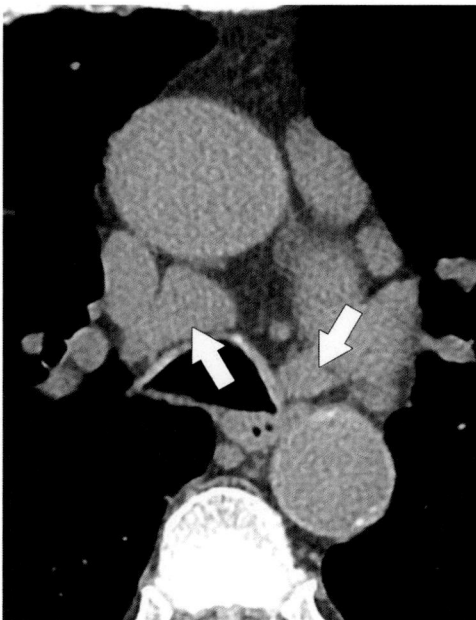

Mild mediastinal and hilar lymphadenopathy is present on HRCT in up to 70–86 % of patients with UIP [22–24] (Fig. 4.3). Lymph node size usually does not exceed 1.5 cm in short axis and is typically isolated to one or two lymph node stations, most commonly levels 4 (lower paratracheal), 5 (aortopulmonary window), 7 (subcarinal), and 10R (right hilar) [22]. In one study of 30 patients with pulmonary fibrosis (25 of whom had IPF), patients with more ground-glass opacity tended to have larger individual lymph nodes, while those with more fibrosis had an overall greater number of enlarged lymph nodes [24]. However, a larger study with similar design showed that the presence of lymph node enlargement did not correlate to any specific pattern or to the extent of disease on HRCT [23].

The syndrome of combined pulmonary fibrosis and emphysema (CPFE) has recently gained increased recognition. Approximately one-third of patients with IPF also have emphysema [25]. This association is not surprising, considering that smoking is a common risk factor for both emphysema and IPF (Fig. 4.4). As is typical for smoking-related emphysema, emphysema predominates in the upper lobes and has a centrilobular distribution. Fibrosis is peripheral and basilar predominant and has typical findings of UIP. Pulmonary function testing in patients with combined IPF and emphysema usually shows little or modest decreases in forced vital capacity and forced expiratory volume in 1 s, but a marked decrease in the diffusion capacity is typically present [26]. Interestingly, there is a strong association with combined disease and pulmonary hypertension; in one series, 47 % of patients with combined emphysema and IPF had pulmonary hypertension on initial diagnosis, which increased to 55 % on follow-up [26]. Patients with CPFE tend to have a poor

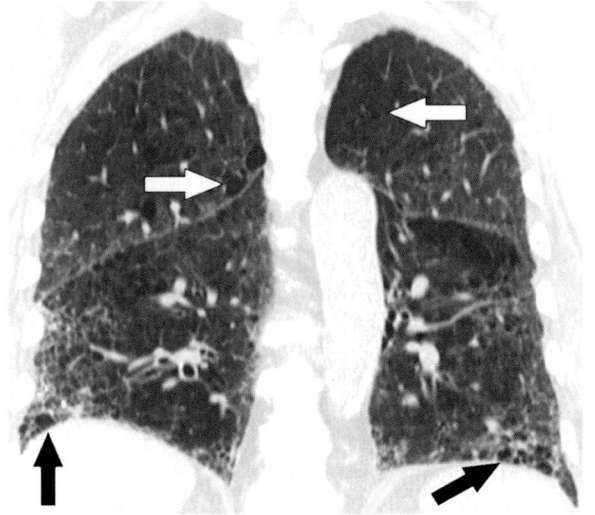

**Fig. 4.4** Coronal reformatted HRCT image shows basilar-predominant pulmonary fibrosis (*black arrows*) with upper lung zone emphysema (*white arrows*) consistent with combined pulmonary fibrosis and emphysema

prognosis. This is especially true if there is concomitant pulmonary hypertension; one study showed that patients with CPFE and pulmonary hypertension have a 1-year survival of only 60 % [26].

## Accuracy of HRCT

The accuracy of HRCT in the setting of UIP is approximately 80–90 % [9, 27–30] when UIP is the first-choice diagnosis. However, when a confident diagnosis of UIP can be made on HRCT, the accuracy increases to 90–100 %. Unfortunately, HRCT is not a perfect tool for the diagnosis of pulmonary fibrosis because different conditions may manifest with similar imaging findings. A confident diagnosis of UIP cannot be established by HRCT in approximately 50 % of patients who are ultimately diagnosed with IPF [31, 32].

A recent consensus statement from the American Thoracic Society, European Respiratory Society, Japanese Respiratory Society, and Latin American Thoracic Association on Idiopathic Pulmonary Fibrosis suggested guidelines for radiologists when interpreting and reporting cases in which UIP is being considered [33]. In the setting of fibrotic interstitial lung diseases, the three classes of UIP diagnoses on HRCT are (definite) UIP pattern, possible UIP pattern, and inconsistent with UIP pattern. A confident diagnosis of UIP can be made on HRCT if the following four imaging parameters are met: (1) basilar and subpleural predominance, (2) reticulation, (3) honeycombing (with or without traction bronchiectasis), and (4) absence of features to suggest another diagnosis (inconsistent with UIP pattern) (Fig. 4.5). When there is a definite UIP pattern, the diagnosis will almost always be IPF,

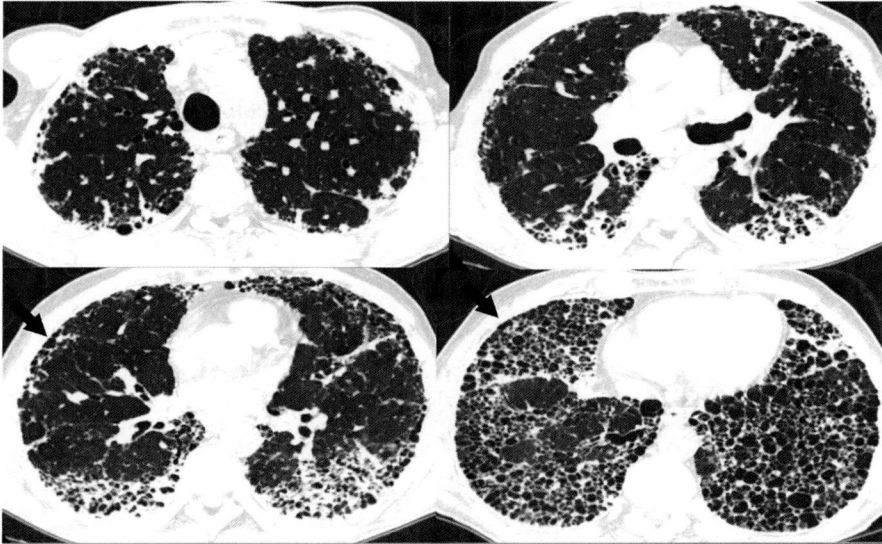

**Fig. 4.5** Multiple axial HRCT images show basilar- and peripheral-predominant pulmonary fibrosis characterized by reticulation, traction bronchiolectasis, and subpleural honeycombing (*arrows*), diagnostic of UIP

although a definite UIP pattern can occasionally be seen with collagen vascular disease, asbestosis, familial fibrosis, chronic hypersensitivity pneumonitis, or drug-related pulmonary fibrosis. The possible UIP pattern on HRCT includes all the imaging parameters of the definite UIP pattern with the exception of honeycombing, which is absent (Fig. 4.6). The distinction between a confident UIP diagnosis and possible UIP diagnosis can be challenging, given that the main distinction between these two groups is the presence or absence of honeycombing, which may be difficult to identify when honeycombing is subtle or when HRCT images are noncontiguous. This is highlighted by the finding that only fair-to-moderate agreement exists among expert readers for the identification of honeycombing (mean kappa of 0.45 in one study) [34]. The pattern should be considered as inconsistent with UIP if any one of the following imaging parameters are present: (1) upper or mid-lung predominance (Fig. 4.7), (2) peribronchovascular predominance (Fig. 4.8), (3) extensive ground-glass opacity (more extensive than reticulation) (see Fig. 4.8), (4) profuse micronodules (Fig. 4.9), (5) discrete cysts (multiple, not consistent with honeycombing) (Fig. 4.10), (6) diffuse mosaic attenuation or air trapping (involving three or more lobes and bilateral) (Fig. 4.11), or (7) consolidation (Fig. 4.12). The presence of any of these findings is much more suggestive of an alternative diagnosis to UIP (Table 4.1). Patients with a HRCT pattern of possible UIP or inconsistent with UIP need further work-up and will often require biopsy to establish a confident diagnosis.

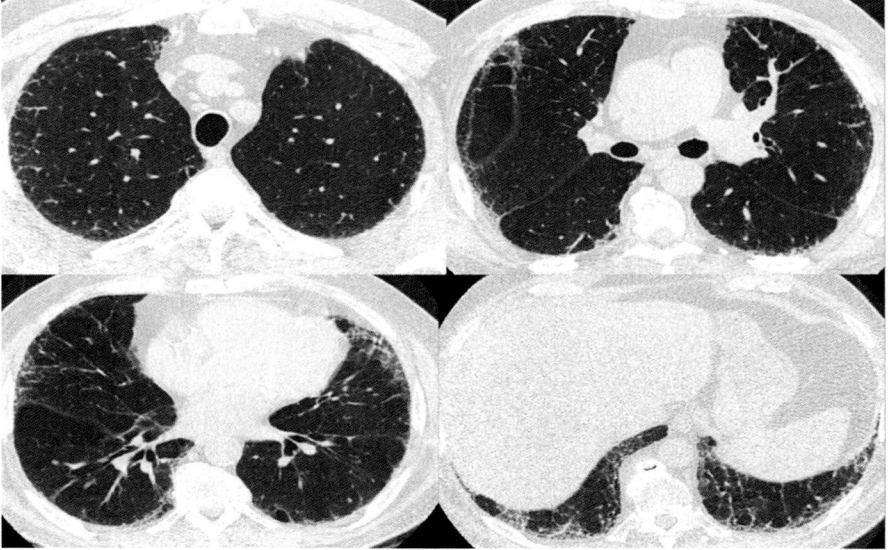

**Fig. 4.6** Multiple axial HRCT images show basilar and peripheral-predominant pulmonary fibrosis characterized by reticulation, mild ground-glass opacity, and traction bronchiolectasis, meeting criteria for possible usual interstitial pneumonia. The main distinction between an HRCT diagnosis of definite UIP and possible UIP is the presence or absence of honeycombing

**Fig. 4.7** Coronal reformatted HRCT image shows peripheral-predominant pulmonary fibrosis. However, as opposed to typical cases of UIP, fibrosis in this case predominates in the upper lungs. This patient was shown to have sarcoidosis-related pulmonary fibrosis

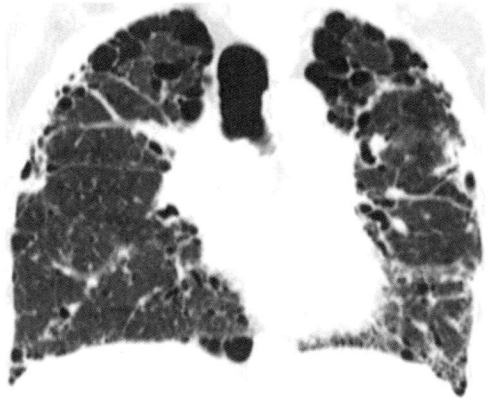

# Prognosis

Unfortunately, a diagnosis of UIP carries a poor prognosis. In a study in patients with various interstitial lung diseases, UIP histopathology was shown to have the worst prognosis [35]. Interestingly, imaging findings, which may be discordant with histopathologic findings, correlate with survival, even in patients with known histopathology; patients with a nonspecific interstitial pneumonia (NSIP) pattern on

a                                          b

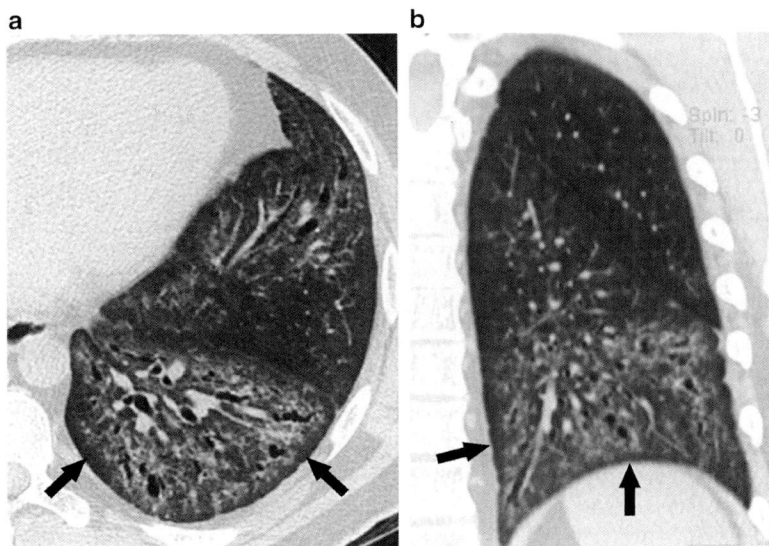

**Fig. 4.8** Axial (**a**) and coronal (**b**) HRCT images show basilar and bronchovascular-predominant pulmonary fibrosis characterized by ground-glass opacity, mild reticulation, and traction bronchiectasis. There is relative sparing of the subpleural lung (*arrows*). These findings strongly favor NSIP over UIP

**Fig. 4.9** Coronal reformatted HRCT image shows multiple nodules (*arrows*) in the mid- and upper lungs in a perilymphatic distribution along bronchovascular structures, interlobular septa, and subpleural lung in this patient with sarcoidosis

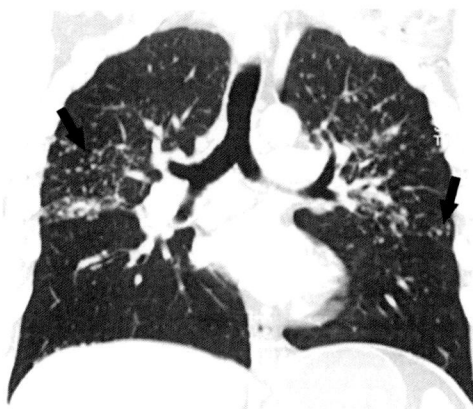

HRCT but UIP on histopathology have survival rates that are more similar to patients with NSIP. Patients with indeterminate HRCT patterns with UIP on histopathology also have 3.68 years of increased median survival relative to patients with a UIP HRCT pattern and histopathologic UIP [27]. The extent of honeycombing and pulmonary fibrosis has been shown to be associated with prognosis in the setting of pulmonary fibrosis [18, 36–39]. Lead time bias may play a role in the longer survival of patients with milder fibrosis, because honeycombing and more extensive fibrosis suggest that the fibrosis has likely been present for a longer duration.

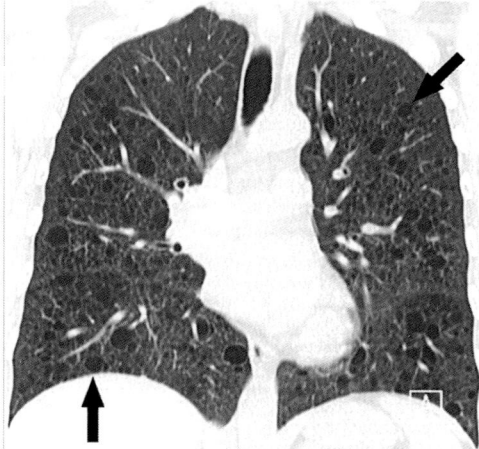

**Fig. 4.10** Coronal reformatted HRCT image shows multiple uniform thin-walled lung cysts (*arrows*), which are more profuse in the mid- and lower lungs in this patient with lymphangioleiomyomatosis

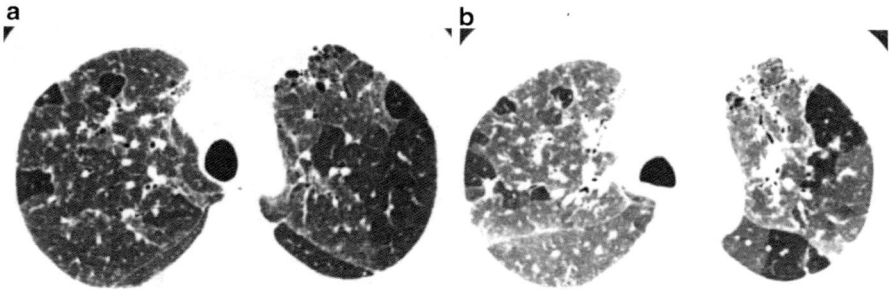

**Fig. 4.11** Axial HRCT images taken during inspiration (**a**) and end-expiration (**b**) show lobular areas of air trapping with adjacent pulmonary fibrosis, typical of hypersensitivity pneumonitis. The combination of fibrosis and air trapping represents a combination of the subacute and chronic phases of hypersensitivity pneumonitis

**Fig. 4.12** Axial HRCT image shows subpleural consolidation (*arrow*) and ground-glass opacity in the right lower lobe in this patient with organizing pneumonia

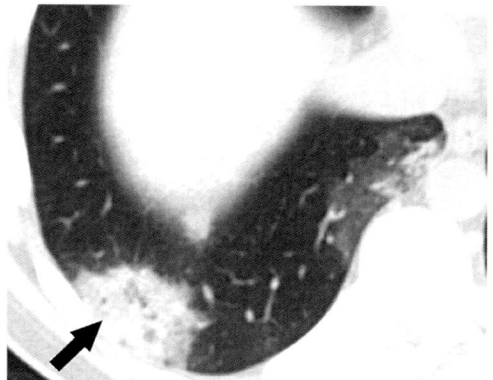

**Table 4.1** Differential diagnosis of imaging features that are considered to be inconsistent with a diagnosis of UIP

| Imaging finding | Differential diagnosis (diffuse lung diseases) |
| --- | --- |
| Upper or mid-lung predominance | Sarcoidosis, HP, familial pulmonary fibrosis, pleuroparenchymal fibroelastosis |
| Peribronchovascular predominance | NSIP |
| Extensive ground-glass abnormality | NSIP, HP, DIP, PAP |
| Profuse micronodules (predominantly in upper lobes) | Ground-glass: HP, RB<br>Solid: sarcoidosis, silicosis/CWP |
| Discrete cysts (not consistent with honeycombing) | Cystic lung disease (LAM, LCH, LIP) |
| Diffuse mosaic attenuation/air trapping | HP, OB |
| Consolidation | COP, CEP |

*CEP* chronic eosinophilic pneumonia, *COP* cryptogenic organizing pneumonia, *CWP* coal workers' pneumoconiosis, *DIP* desquamative pneumonitis, *HP* hypersensitivity pneumonia, *LAM* lymphangioleiomyomatosis, *LCH* Langerhans cell histiocytosis, *LIP* lymphocytic interstitial pneumonitis, *NSIP* nonspecific interstitial pneumonia, *PAP* pulmonary alveolar proteinosis, *RB* respiratory bronchiolitis, *OB* obliterative bronchiolitis

Nonetheless, the ability to predict survival from the time of CT scanning still has importance. Therefore, either qualitative or quantitative assessment of the degree of pulmonary fibrosis and of honeycombing is mandatory. It is intuitive that the rate of progression of fibrosis and honeycombing would be associated with survival in the setting of fibrosing interstitial pneumonitis; a recent study demonstrated that progression of honeycombing on follow-up CT is an important determinant of survival in patients with fibrosing interstitial pneumonia [40].

# Thoracic Complications of IPF

An acute exacerbation of IPF carries a poor prognosis, with most patients eventually dying within weeks to months after the initial onset of acute respiratory worsening [41–43]. The most common histological correlate is diffuse alveolar damage, with organizing pneumonia occurring less commonly [44]. The HRCT manifestations reflect the underlying histology; ground-glass opacity, consolidation, or both are superimposed on underlying pulmonary fibrosis [45, 46] (Fig. 4.13). Given the somewhat nonspecific pattern of HRCT abnormalities, pneumonia and pulmonary edema must first be excluded. The distribution of lung disease may be peripheral, patchy, or diffuse. Based on limited data, it appears that a peripheral pattern of disease is less often fatal than multifocal or diffuse patterns [45, 46]. Patients with an organizing pneumonia have a better prognosis than those with diffuse alveolar damage. Therefore, one would expect patients with more consolidation, which is a pattern that is more typical of organizing pneumonia (peripheral and bronchovascular), to have a better prognosis than those patients with ground-glass opacities that are more typical for diffuse alveolar damage (Fig. 4.14). However, this has not been shown conclusively.

a                                          b

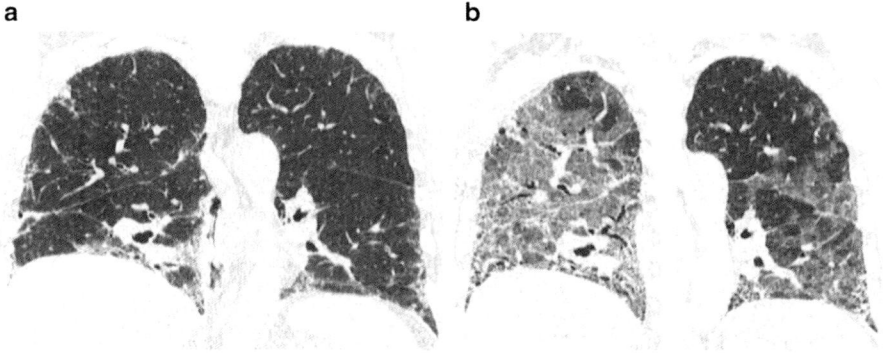

**Fig. 4.13** Coronal reformatted HRCT image (**a**) shows typical findings of basilar and peripheral-predominant pulmonary fibrosis in UIP. Coronal reformatted HRCT image obtained approximately 18 months later (**b**) shows diffuse ground-glass opacity in this patient with acute exacerbation of IPF. Ground-glass opacity in this case is consistent with diffuse alveolar damage histopathology

a                                          b

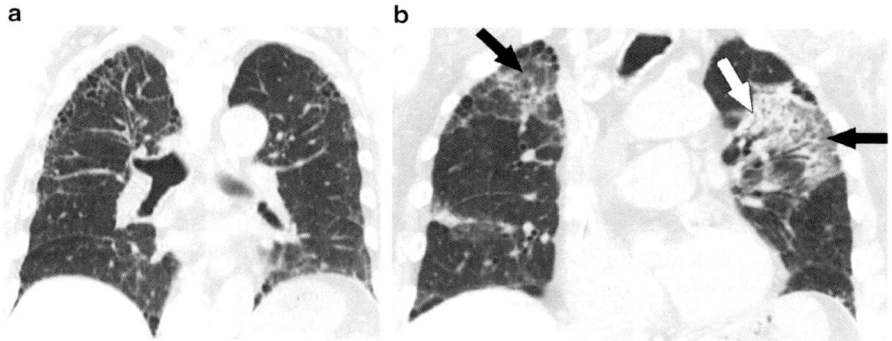

**Fig. 4.14** Coronal reformatted HRCT image (**a**) shows pulmonary fibrosis in this patient with UIP. Coronal reformatted HRCT image obtained approximately 2 years later (**b**) shows bronchovascular-predominant ground-glass opacity (*black arrows*) and consolidation (*white arrow*) in this patient with acute exacerbation of IPF. The pattern of bronchovascular ground-glass opacity and consolidation is consistent with organizing pneumonia histopathology

Patients with IPF are at fivefold increased risk of developing lung cancer than the general population [47], and older men with a history of smoking are most often affected. Synchronous cancers are not uncommon and occur in up to 15 % of patients [48]. Lung cancers in these patients arise most frequently in the peripheral lung in areas of more severe fibrosis or at the junction of fibrosis and normal lung [49–52] (Fig. 4.15). With regard to lobar distribution, lung cancers in patients with IPF have been reported to occur more often in the lower lobes [53, 54], but other studies report a more balanced distribution of cancer between the upper and lower lobes [49, 55]. The most common types of primary lung cancer in IPF are adenocarcinoma and squamous cell carcinoma [49]. On HRCT, the most common

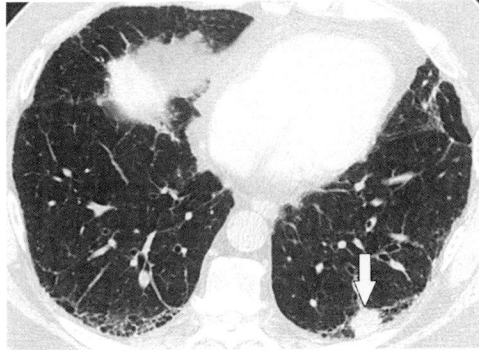

**Fig. 4.15** Axial HRCT image shows typical findings of UIP (peripheral-predominant reticulation and honeycombing). The nodule (*arrow*) in the peripheral left lower lobe was new. Transcutaneous needle biopsy showed primary lung adenocarcinoma

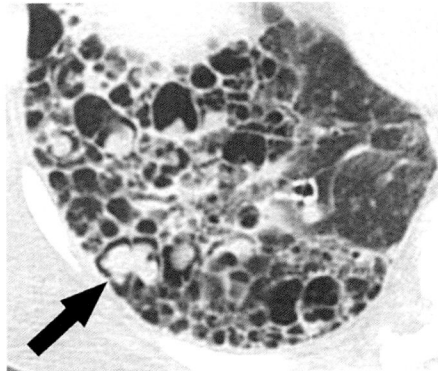

**Fig. 4.16** Axial HRCT image shows nodular filling defects (*arrow*) in cystic areas of bronchiectasis and honeycombing shown to represent aspergillomas

manifestation of lung cancer in association with IPF is an ill- or well-defined nodule or mass. At times, lung cancer can present as air-space consolidation, which usually represents a mucinous adenocarcinoma. Given that lung cancer tends to arise in or adjacent to areas of fibrosis, the early detection of lung cancer in IPF can be challenging. Therefore, comparison of current images to previous studies to assess for any new focal nodular or consolidative opacity is, therefore, paramount. In one retrospective study, the authors found that there was a 409-day median delay in lung cancer diagnosis in patients with pulmonary fibrosis, indicating the subtle nature of early lung cancer in this setting [52].

Patients with pulmonary fibrosis are also predisposed to pneumonia, especially from mycobacterial and *Aspergillus* species as well as *Pneumocystis jirovecii* pneumonia (PJP). These tend to develop during periods of immunosuppression in patients with worsening fibrosis and clinical disease progression [56]. *Aspergillus* infection in patients with IPF usually manifests as an aspergilloma in areas of pre-existing fibrocavitary disease or as chronic necrotizing aspergillosis [57, 58]. Aspergillomas represent a saprophytic infection in which the fungus ball can shift freely within a lung cavity or dilated bronchus (Fig. 4.16). Because the associated

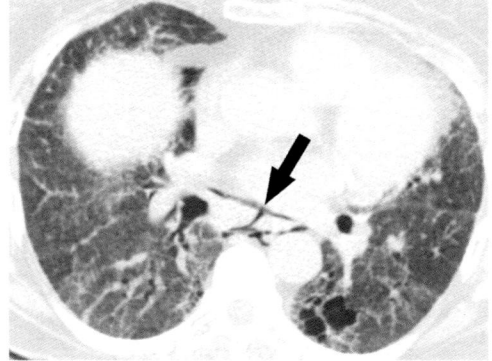

inflammatory response leads to friable and hypervascular cavity walls, patients can develop hemoptysis, which may be life-threatening. Chronic necrotizing aspergillosis presents as focal consolidation, usually within the upper lobes, that eventually cavitates [57]. Patients with secondary pulmonary tuberculosis in the setting of IPF may present with an atypical imaging pattern. Rather than classic upper lobe-predominant cavitary disease with tree-in-bud opacities and centrilobular nodules, subpleural nodules, masses, coalescent consolidation, or a combination of these findings may be seen [59]. Although patients with IPF are unlikely to be at significantly increased risk for PJP if not immunosuppressed, individuals on even mild corticosteroid therapy are more susceptible to PJP. Unfortunately, the HRCT manifestations of PJP in IPF may mimic the findings of an acute exacerbation, with bilateral, diffuse ground-glass opacities, reticulation, and mild consolidation all possible on HRCT imaging. Patients with IPF (especially those on immunosuppression) who present with acute to subacute dyspnea in the context of one of the latter HRCT patterns should be evaluated for infection (including PJP) before the initiation or augmentation of immunosuppression is considered.

Spontaneous pneumomediastinum and pneumothorax develop in up to 11.5 % of patients with IPF [60–62] (Fig. 4.17). Pneumothoraces are likely caused by rupture of honeycomb cysts into the pleural space. Pneumomediastinum may be caused by the Macklin effect, in which increased intrathoracic pressure results in alveolar rupture with subsequent dissection of gas along the peribronchial sheaths centrally into the mediastinum. Accurate estimates of the incidence of events where gas gains access to extra-alveolar spaces are difficult to make, because in many cases, patients may be only mildly symptomatic or even asymptomatic. The clinical significance of pneumomediastinum and pneumothorax in asymptomatic patients is unclear. However, when patients present with cough, dyspnea, or chest pain, extra-alveolar gas may portend a poor prognosis, although the evidence for this is weak [61].

Pulmonary hypertension (PH) is present in up to 46 % of patients with IPF referred for lung transplantation [63, 64]. In addition, patients with concomitant IPF and PH have a worse prognosis compared to patients with IPF without PH [65]. In one study, the 1-year mortality rate was 28.0 % for patients with IPF and PH compared to 5.5 % for patients with IPF but without PH [66]. In another study, IPF patients with mean systolic pulmonary artery pressure above 50 mmHg had a mean survival of only 0.7 years compared to 4.8 years for IPF patients with mean systolic pulmonary artery pressure below 35 mmHg [67]. The pathophysiological relationship between IPF and PH is complex and likely includes fibrotic destruction of the vasculature and chronic hypoxic vasoconstriction of small pulmonary vessels. However, these factors in isolation may not explain the relationship between IPF and PH. There are a significant number of cases in which there is discordance between the degree of IPF or oxygen saturation and PH, which implies that other underlying factors may be present that have not yet been fully identified [68]. Although a correlation between pulmonary arterial diameter and mean pulmonary artery pressure has been shown in the general population, it appears that this relationship may not be extrapolated to patients with IPF. One study showed that the diameter of the main pulmonary artery and the pulmonary artery to aorta diameter ratio did not differ between those with and without PH, and no significant correlation was found between the mean pulmonary artery pressure and pulmonary arterial diameter [69]. Another study also showed that pulmonary artery diameters or ratios were unreliable in predicting mean pulmonary artery pressure. In fact, pulmonary artery dilation may occur in the absence of significant pulmonary hypertension [70].

## Atypical UIP on HRCT and How to Distinguish It from Other Common Fibrotic Lung Diseases

In addition to indeterminate HRCT patterns in patients with UIP, the pattern of lung disease on HRCT in UIP may mimic other interstitial lung diseases, most commonly NSIP or chronic hypersensitivity pneumonitis (HP), and less commonly sarcoidosis (Figs. 4.18 and 4.19). In one study of 55 patients with biopsy-proven UIP, UIP was considered low probability (<30 %) by at least two out of three observers on HRCT for 34 of the 55 patients, and NSIP (18/34 = 53 %), chronic HP (4/34 = 12 %), and sarcoidosis (3/34 = 9 %) were scored as the most likely (high degree of probability) first-choice diagnoses. Additionally, NSIP, chronic HP, and sarcoidosis were also most often included in the differential diagnosis, even when these were not scored as the first-choice diagnosis [71]. Silva et al. also compared HRCT appearances of patients with IPF, NSIP, and chronic HP and found that in 23 cases of histopathologically proven UIP, observers chose NSIP or chronic HP as a first-choice diagnosis 25.7 % of the time (exclusive of cases in which the first-choice diagnosis was "indeterminate") [30].

Findings suggestive of NSIP include ground-glass opacity (the salient feature, which is present in all cases), fine reticulation, traction bronchiectasis, and lower lobe volume loss [72–76]. Basilar and peribronchovascular predominance is the rule, and upper lobe-predominant disease favors an alternative diagnosis such as sarcoidosis, HP, or familial pulmonary fibrosis. Because UIP is also nearly always basilar preponderant, the cranio-caudad distribution of disease is not helpful

**Fig. 4.18** Axial HRCT image during expiration shows lobular areas of air trapping (*arrows*) as well as mild pulmonary fibrosis, consistent with chronic hypersensitivity pneumonitis; however, open lung biopsy showed UIP. Based on clinical work-up, the patient was diagnosed with IPF

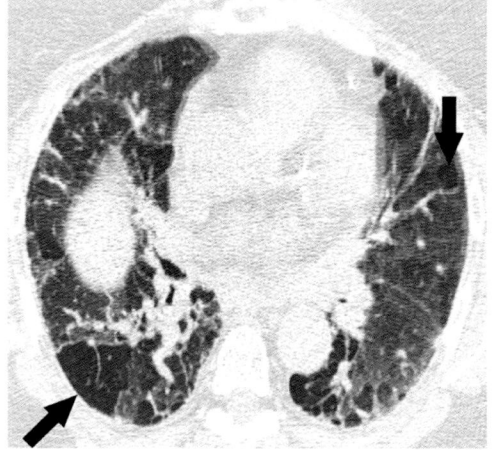

**Fig. 4.19** Axial HRCT image shows basilar ground-glass opacity, reticulation, and traction bronchiectasis, most consistent with NSIP. However, open lung biopsy showed UIP. Based on clinical work-up, the patient was diagnosed with IPF

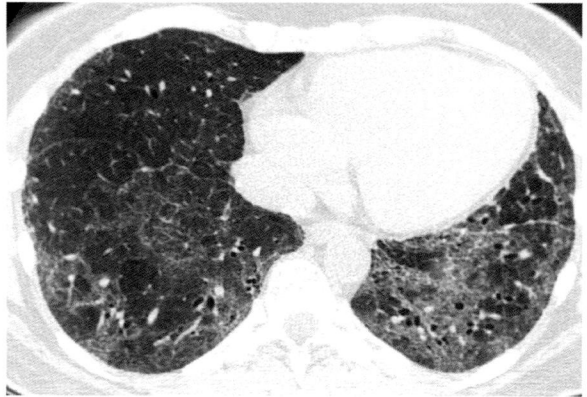

in distinguishing NSIP from UIP. However, the axial distribution of disease can be quite helpful in distinguishing NSIP from IPF. Specifically, although the axial distribution of fibrosis in NSIP can be peripheral, diffuse, or peribronchovascular, the latter pattern combined with relative sparing of the subpleural lung is much more suggestive of NSIP rather than UIP [30] (see Fig. 4.8).

Chronic HP may have findings on HRCT that are identical to those of UIP [77]. However, a confident diagnosis of chronic HP can be made if certain imaging parameters are present. The most specific findings for chronic HP include centrilobular ground-glass nodules, mosaic attenuation (reflecting air trapping), and mid- to upper lobe-predominant pulmonary fibrosis [30, 78, 79]. This combination of findings actually represents overlap of the subacute and chronic phases of HP [80] (see Fig. 4.11). In more advanced cases of chronic HP, honeycombing is quite common, and the HRCT pattern may mimic that of UIP [30, 81].

In the absence of a high-confidence diagnosis of UIP on HRCT, no single test or set of tests has proven to be adequately sensitive and specific in the diagnosis of UIP. In fact, because of the difficulty in establishing a firm diagnosis of UIP (as well as other diffuse lung diseases), a multidisciplinary review of cases by pulmonologists, radiologists, and pathologists is essential in establishing the most accurate diagnosis. One study of 58 patients with suspected interstitial lung disease showed that after consensus review of the clinical, radiological, and pathological data, radiologists changed their initial diagnosis in 50 % of cases, pulmonologists in 30 % of cases, and pathologists in 20 % of cases [82]. Radiologists most commonly changed their initial diagnoses of NSIP to UIP as well as respiratory bronchiolitis or desquamative interstitial pneumonia, and HP was often changed to NSIP. In a study of patients with IPF diagnosed locally by international consensus criteria, the diagnosis of IPF was rejected by an expert panel in 12.8 % of cases based on their review of the HRCT and histopathologic findings [83]. Interestingly, the mean kappa value for three expert thoracic radiologists' HRCT evaluations was 0.40, and the kappa value was even lower at 0.30 for two expert pulmonary pathologists' histopathologic evaluations. This further supports the importance of a multidisciplinary diagnostic approach, as disagreements clearly occur even among experts. By increasing the opportunities for the pulmonologist, radiologist, or pathologist to make a confident diagnosis of a specific diagnosis (often UIP), a more accurate diagnosis can be established in a greater percentage of patients with diffuse lung disease.

## Summary

UIP is the imaging and histopathologic correlate of IPF. If the typical pattern of UIP is present on HRCT, a confident and accurate diagnosis of UIP can be made, obviating the need for lung biopsy. However, in up to half of patients, who ultimately are proven to have UIP on biopsy, a confident diagnosis of UIP cannot be made by HRCT; these patients often require further work-up with a surgical lung biopsy. The most common diseases that mimic UIP are NSIP and chronic HP. Although there is often overlap in radiographic appearance among these conditions, HRCT can often distinguish UIP from NSIP or chronic HP if certain imaging patterns are present.

## References

1. Coultas DB, Zumwalt RE, Black WC, Sobonya RE. The epidemiology of interstitial lung diseases. Am J Respir Crit Care Med. 1994;150:967–72.
2. Baumgartner KB, Samet JM, Stidley CA, Colby TV, Waldron JA. Cigarette smoking: a risk factor for idiopathic pulmonary fibrosis. Am J Respir Crit Care Med. 1997;155:242–8.
3. Raghu G, Freudenberger TD, Yang S, Curtis JR, Spada C, Hayes J, et al. High prevalence of abnormal acid gastro-oesophageal reflux in idiopathic pulmonary fibrosis. Eur Respir J. 2006;27:136–42.

4. Collard HR, King Jr TE, Bartelson BB, Vourlekis JS, Schwarz MI, Brown KK. Changes in clinical and physiologic variables predict survival in idiopathic pulmonary fibrosis. Am J Respir Crit Care Med. 2003;168:538–42.
5. Katzenstein AL, Myers JL. Idiopathic pulmonary fibrosis: clinical relevance of pathologic classification. Am J Respir Crit Care Med. 1998;157:1301–15.
6. Bjoraker JA, Ryu JH, Edwin MK, Myers JL, Tazelaar HD, Schroeder DR, et al. Prognostic significance of histopathologic subsets in idiopathic pulmonary fibrosis. Am J Respir Crit Care Med. 1998;157:199–203.
7. Mathieson JR, Mayo JR, Staples CA, Muller NL. Chronic diffuse infiltrative lung disease: comparison of diagnostic accuracy of CT and chest radiography. Radiology. 1989;171:111–6.
8. Johnson Jr TH. Radiology and honeycomb lung disease. Am J Roentgenol Radium Ther Nucl Med. 1968;104:810–21.
9. Hunninghake GW, Lynch DA, Galvin JR, Gross BH, Müller N, Schwartz DA, et al. Radiologic findings are strongly associated with a pathologic diagnosis of usual interstitial pneumonia. Chest. 2003;124:1215–23.
10. Chandler PW, Shin MS, Friedman SE, Myers JL, Katzenstein AL. Radiographic manifestations of bronchiolitis obliterans with organizing pneumonia vs usual interstitial pneumonia. AJR Am J Roentgenol. 1986;147:899–906.
11. Staples CA, Muller NL, Vedal S, Abboud R, Ostrow D, Miller RR. Usual interstitial pneumonia: correlation of CT with clinical, functional, and radiologic findings. Radiology. 1987;162:377–81.
12. Mayo JR. CT evaluation of diffuse infiltrative lung disease: dose considerations and optimal technique. J Thorac Imaging. 2009;24:252–9.
13. Papadakis AE, Perisinakis K, Damilakis J. Automatic exposure control in pediatric and adult multidetector CT examinations: a phantom study on dose reduction and image quality. Med Phys. 2008;35:4567–76.
14. Tack D, De Maertelaer V, Gevenois PA. Dose reduction in multidetector CT using attenuation-based online tube current modulation. AJR Am J Roentgenol. 2003;181:331–4.
15. Kalra MK, Rizzo S, Maher MM, Halpern EF, Toth TL, Shepard JA, et al. Chest CT performed with z-axis modulation: scanning protocol and radiation dose. Radiology. 2005;237:303–8.
16. Sumikawa H, Johkoh T, Ichikado K, Taniguchi H, Kondoh Y, Fujimoto K, et al. Usual interstitial pneumonia and chronic idiopathic interstitial pneumonia: analysis of CT appearance in 92 patients. Radiology. 2006;241:258–66.
17. Hansell DM, Bankier AA, MacMahon H, McLoud TC, Muller NL, Remy J. Fleischner Society: glossary of terms for thoracic imaging. Radiology. 2008;246:697–722.
18. Lynch DA, Godwin JD, Safrin S, Starko KM, Hormel P, Brown KK, et al. High-resolution computed tomography in idiopathic pulmonary fibrosis: diagnosis and prognosis. Am J Respir Crit Care Med. 2005;172:488–93.
19. Remy-Jardin M, Giraud F, Remy J, Copin MC, Gosselin B, Duhamel A. Importance of ground-glass attenuation in chronic diffuse infiltrative lung disease: pathologic-CT correlation. Radiology. 1993;189:693–8.
20. Nishimura K, Kitaichi M, Izumi T, Nagai S, Kanaoka M, Itoh H. Usual interstitial pneumonia: histologic correlation with high-resolution CT. Radiology. 1992;182:337–42.
21. Leung AN, Miller RR, Muller NL. Parenchymal opacification in chronic infiltrative lung diseases: CT-pathologic correlation. Radiology. 1993;188:209–14.
22. Niimi H, Kang EY, Kwong JS, Carignan S, Muller NL. CT of chronic infiltrative lung disease: prevalence of mediastinal lymphadenopathy. J Comput Assist Tomogr. 1996;20:305–8.
23. Souza CA, Muller NL, Lee KS, Johkoh T, Mitsuhiro H, Chong S. Idiopathic interstitial pneumonias: prevalence of mediastinal lymph node enlargement in 206 patients. AJR Am J Roentgenol. 2006;186:995–9.
24. Jung JI, Kim HH, Jung YJ, Park SH, Lee JM, Hahn ST. Mediastinal lymphadenopathy in pulmonary fibrosis: correlation with disease severity. J Comput Assist Tomogr. 2000;24:706–10.
25. Wells AU, Desai SR, Rubens MB, Goh NS, Cramer D, Nicholson AG, et al. Idiopathic pulmonary fibrosis: a composite physiologic index derived from disease extent observed by computed tomography. Am J Respir Crit Care Med. 2003;167:962–9.

26. Cottin V, Nunes H, Brillet PY, Delaval P, Devouassoux G, Tillie-Leblond I, et al. Combined pulmonary fibrosis and emphysema: a distinct underrecognised entity. Eur Respir J. 2005;26:586–93.
27. Flaherty KR, Thwaite EL, Kazerooni EA, Gross BH, Toews GB, Colby TV, et al. Radiological versus histological diagnosis in UIP and NSIP: survival implications. Thorax. 2003;58:143–8.
28. Tsubamoto M, Muller NL, Johkoh T, Ichikado K, Taniguchi H, Kondoh Y, et al. Pathologic subgroups of nonspecific interstitial pneumonia: differential diagnosis from other idiopathic interstitial pneumonias on high-resolution computed tomography. J Comput Assist Tomogr. 2005;29:793–800.
29. Johkoh T, Muller NL, Cartier Y, Kavanagh PV, Hartman TE, Akira M, et al. Idiopathic interstitial pneumonias: diagnostic accuracy of thin-section CT in 129 patients. Radiology. 1999;211:555–60.
30. Silva CI, Muller NL, Lynch DA, Curran-Everett D, Brown KK, Lee KS, et al. Chronic hypersensitivity pneumonitis: differentiation from idiopathic pulmonary fibrosis and nonspecific interstitial pneumonia by using thin-section CT. Radiology. 2008;246:288–97.
31. Hunninghake GW, Zimmerman MB, Schwartz DA, King Jr TE, Lynch J, Hegele R, et al. Utility of a lung biopsy for the diagnosis of idiopathic pulmonary fibrosis. Am J Respir Crit Care Med. 2001;164:193–6.
32. Swensen SJ, Aughenbaugh GL, Myers JL. Diffuse lung disease: diagnostic accuracy of CT in patients undergoing surgical biopsy of the lung. Radiology. 1997;205:229–34.
33. Raghu G, Collard HR, Egan JJ, Martinez FJ, Behr J, Brown KK, et al. An official ATS/ERS/JRS/ALAT statement: idiopathic pulmonary fibrosis: evidence-based guidelines for diagnosis and management. Am J Respir Crit Care Med. 2011;183:788–824.
34. Sundaram B, Gross BH, Martinez FJ, Oh E, Müller NL, Schipper M, et al. Accuracy of high-resolution CT in the diagnosis of diffuse lung disease: effect of predominance and distribution of findings. AJR Am J Roentgenol. 2008;191:1032–9.
35. Flaherty KR, Toews GB, Travis WD, Colby TV, Kazerooni EA, Gross BH, et al. Clinical significance of histological classification of idiopathic interstitial pneumonia. Eur Respir J. 2002;19:275–83.
36. Gay SE, Kazerooni EA, Toews GB, Lynch 3rd JP, Gross BH, Cascade PN, et al. Idiopathic pulmonary fibrosis: predicting response to therapy and survival. Am J Respir Crit Care Med. 1998;157:1063–72.
37. Nagao T, Nagai S, Hiramoto Y, Hamada K, Shigematsu M, Hayashi M, et al. Serial evaluation of high-resolution computed tomography findings in patients with idiopathic pulmonary fibrosis in usual interstitial pneumonia. Respiration. 2002;69:413–9.
38. Sumikawa H, Johkoh T, Colby TV, Ichikado K, Suga M, Taniguchi H, et al. Computed tomography findings in pathological usual interstitial pneumonia: relationship to survival. Am J Respir Crit Care Med. 2008;177:433–9.
39. Shin KM, Lee KS, Chung MP, Han J, Bae YA, Kim TS, et al. Prognostic determinants among clinical, thin-section CT, and histopathologic findings for fibrotic idiopathic interstitial pneumonias: tertiary hospital study. Radiology. 2008;249:328–37.
40. Hwang JH, Misumi S, Curran-Everett D, Brown KK, Sahin H, Lynch DA. Longitudinal follow-up of fibrosing interstitial pneumonia: relationship between physiologic testing, computed tomography changes, and survival rate. J Thorac Imaging. 2011;26:209–17.
41. Parambil JG, Myers JL, Ryu JH. Histopathologic features and outcome of patients with acute exacerbation of idiopathic pulmonary fibrosis undergoing surgical lung biopsy. Chest. 2005;128:3310–5.
42. Kim DS, Park JH, Park BK, Lee JS, Nicholson AG, Colby T. Acute exacerbation of idiopathic pulmonary fibrosis: frequency and clinical features. Eur Respir J. 2006;27:143–50.
43. Collard HR, Moore BB, Flaherty KR, Brown KK, Kaner RJ, King Jr TE, et al. Acute exacerbations of idiopathic pulmonary fibrosis. Am J Respir Crit Care Med. 2007;176:636–43.
44. Churg A, Muller NL, Silva CI, Wright JL. Acute exacerbation (acute lung injury of unknown cause) in UIP and other forms of fibrotic interstitial pneumonias. Am J Surg Pathol. 2007;31:277–84.

45. Akira M, Hamada H, Sakatani M, Kobayashi C, Nishioka M, Yamamoto S. CT findings during phase of accelerated deterioration in patients with idiopathic pulmonary fibrosis. AJR Am J Roentgenol. 1997;168:79–83.
46. Silva CI, Muller NL, Fujimoto K, Kato S, Ichikado K, Taniguchi H, et al. Acute exacerbation of chronic interstitial pneumonia: high-resolution computed tomography and pathologic findings. J Thorac Imaging. 2007;22:221–9.
47. Hubbard R, Venn A, Lewis S, Britton J. Lung cancer and cryptogenic fibrosing alveolitis. A population-based cohort study. Am J Respir Crit Care Med. 2000;161:5–8.
48. Mizushima Y, Kobayashi M. Clinical characteristics of synchronous multiple lung cancer associated with idiopathic pulmonary fibrosis. A review of Japanese cases. Chest. 1995;108:1272–7.
49. Kishi K, Homma S, Kurosaki A, Motoi N, Yoshimura K. High-resolution computed tomography findings of lung cancer associated with idiopathic pulmonary fibrosis. J Comput Assist Tomogr. 2006;30:95–9.
50. Matsushita H, Tanaka S, Saiki Y, Hara M, Nakata K, Tanimura S, et al. Lung cancer associated with usual interstitial pneumonia. Pathol Int. 1995;45:925–32.
51. Aubry MC, Myers JL, Douglas WW, Tazelaar HD, Washington Stephens TL, Hartman TE, et al. Primary pulmonary carcinoma in patients with idiopathic pulmonary fibrosis. Mayo Clin Proc. 2002;77:763–70.
52. Yoshida R, Arakawa H, Kaji Y. Lung cancer in chronic interstitial pneumonia: early manifestation from serial CT observations. AJR Am J Roentgenol. 2012;199:85–90.
53. Lee HJ, Im JG, Ahn JM, Yeon KM. Lung cancer in patients with idiopathic pulmonary fibrosis: CT findings. J Comput Assist Tomogr. 1996;20:979–82.
54. Sakai S, Ono M, Nishio T, Kawarada Y, Nagashima A, Toyoshima S. Lung cancer associated with diffuse pulmonary fibrosis: CT-pathologic correlation. J Thorac Imaging. 2003;18:67–71.
55. Park J, Kim DS, Shim TS, Lim CM, Koh Y, Lee SD, et al. Lung cancer in patients with idiopathic pulmonary fibrosis. Eur Respir J. 2001;17:1216–9.
56. Lloyd CR, Walsh SL, Hansell DM. High-resolution CT of complications of idiopathic fibrotic lung disease. Br J Radiol. 2011;84:581–92.
57. Saraceno JL, Phelps DT, Ferro TJ, Futerfas R, Schwartz DB. Chronic necrotizing pulmonary aspergillosis: approach to management. Chest. 1997;112:541–8.
58. Roberts CM, Citron KM, Strickland B. Intrathoracic aspergilloma: role of CT in diagnosis and treatment. Radiology. 1987;165:123–8.
59. Chung MJ, Goo JM, Im JG. Pulmonary tuberculosis in patients with idiopathic pulmonary fibrosis. Eur J Radiol. 2004;52:175–9.
60. Picado C, Gomez de Almeida R, Xaubet A, Montserrat J, Letang E, Sanchez-Lloret J. Spontaneous pneumothorax in cryptogenic fibrosing alveolitis. Respiration. 1985;48:77–80.
61. Fujiwara T. Pneumomediastinum in pulmonary fibrosis. Detection by computed tomography. Chest. 1993;104:44–6.
62. Franquet T, Gimenez A, Torrubia S, Sabate JM, Rodriguez-Arias JM. Spontaneous pneumothorax and pneumomediastinum in IPF. Eur Radiol. 2000;10:108–13.
63. Shorr AF, Wainright JL, Cors CS, Lettieri CJ, Nathan SD. Pulmonary hypertension in patients with pulmonary fibrosis awaiting lung transplant. Eur Respir J. 2007;30:715–21.
64. King Jr TE, Tooze JA, Schwarz MI, Brown KR, Cherniack RM. Predicting survival in idiopathic pulmonary fibrosis: scoring system and survival model. Am J Respir Crit Care Med. 2001;164:1171–81.
65. Hamada K, Nagai S, Tanaka S, Handa T, Shigematsu M, Nagao T, et al. Significance of pulmonary arterial pressure and diffusion capacity of the lung as prognosticator in patients with idiopathic pulmonary fibrosis. Chest. 2007;131:650–6.
66. Lettieri CJ, Nathan SD, Barnett SD, Ahmad S, Shorr AF. Prevalence and outcomes of pulmonary arterial hypertension in advanced idiopathic pulmonary fibrosis. Chest. 2006;129:746–52.

67. Nadrous HF, Pellikka PA, Krowka MJ, Swanson KL, Chaowalit N, Decker PA, et al. Pulmonary hypertension in patients with idiopathic pulmonary fibrosis. Chest. 2005;128:2393–9.
68. Corte TJ, Wort SJ, Wells AU. Pulmonary hypertension in idiopathic pulmonary fibrosis: a review. Sarcoidosis Vasc Diffuse Lung Dis. 2009;26:7–19.
69. Zisman DA, Karlamangla AS, Ross DJ, Keane MP, Belperio JA, Saggar R, et al. High-resolution chest CT findings do not predict the presence of pulmonary hypertension in advanced idiopathic pulmonary fibrosis. Chest. 2007;132:773–9.
70. Devaraj A, Wells AU, Meister MG, Corte TJ, Hansell DM. The effect of diffuse pulmonary fibrosis on the reliability of CT signs of pulmonary hypertension. Radiology. 2008;249:1042–9.
71. Sverzellati N, Wells AU, Tomassetti S, Desai SR, Copley SJ, Aziz ZA, et al. Biopsy-proved idiopathic pulmonary fibrosis: spectrum of nondiagnostic thin-section CT diagnoses. Radiology. 2010;254:957–64.
72. Elliot TL, Lynch DA, Newell Jr JD, Cool C, Tuder R, Markopoulou K, et al. High-resolution computed tomography features of nonspecific interstitial pneumonia and usual interstitial pneumonia. J Comput Assist Tomogr. 2005;29:339–45.
73. Johkoh T, Muller NL, Colby TV, Ichikado K, Taniguchi H, Kondoh Y, et al. Nonspecific interstitial pneumonia: correlation between thin-section CT findings and pathologic subgroups in 55 patients. Radiology. 2002;225:199–204.
74. Hartman TE, Swensen SJ, Hansell DM, Colby TV, Myers JL, Tazelaar HD, et al. Nonspecific interstitial pneumonia: variable appearance at high-resolution chest CT. Radiology. 2000;217:701–5.
75. MacDonald SL, Rubens MB, Hansell DM, Copley SJ, Desai SR, du Bois RM, et al. Nonspecific interstitial pneumonia and usual interstitial pneumonia: comparative appearances at and diagnostic accuracy of thin-section CT. Radiology. 2001;221:600–5.
76. Kligerman SJ, Groshong S, Brown KK, Lynch DA. Nonspecific interstitial pneumonia: radiologic, clinical, and pathologic considerations. Radiographics. 2009;29:73–87.
77. Lynch DA, Newell JD, Logan PM, King Jr TE, Muller NL. Can CT distinguish hypersensitivity pneumonitis from idiopathic pulmonary fibrosis? AJR Am J Roentgenol. 1995;165:807–11.
78. Hansell DM, Wells AU, Padley SP, Muller NL. Hypersensitivity pneumonitis: correlation of individual CT patterns with functional abnormalities. Radiology. 1996;199:123–8.
79. Small JH, Flower CD, Traill ZC, Gleeson FV. Air-trapping in extrinsic allergic alveolitis on computed tomography. Clin Radiol. 1996;51:684–8.
80. Silva CI, Churg A, Muller NL. Hypersensitivity pneumonitis: spectrum of high-resolution CT and pathologic findings. AJR Am J Roentgenol. 2007;188:334–44.
81. Remy-Jardin M, Remy J, Wallaert B, Muller NL. Subacute and chronic bird breeder hypersensitivity pneumonitis: sequential evaluation with CT and correlation with lung function tests and bronchoalveolar lavage. Radiology. 1993;189:111–8.
82. Flaherty KR, King Jr TE, Raghu G, Lynch 3rd JP, Colby TV, Travis WD, et al. Idiopathic interstitial pneumonia: what is the effect of a multidisciplinary approach to diagnosis? Am J Respir Crit Care Med. 2004;170:904–10.
83. Thomeer M, Demedts M, Behr J, Buhl R, Costabel U, Flower CD, et al. Multidisciplinary interobserver agreement in the diagnosis of idiopathic pulmonary fibrosis. Eur Respir J. 2008;31:585–91.

# Chapter 5
# The Keys to Making a Confident Diagnosis of IPF

**Anish Wadhwa and Kevin R. Flaherty**

**Abstract** Diffuse parenchymal lung diseases (DPLDs) are characterized by injury primarily to the interstitium of the lung, but may involve alveolar spaces, airways, and vessels (American Thoracic Society/European Respiratory Society. Am J Respir Crit Care Med 165(2):277–304, 2002). Many DPLDs are idiopathic (referred to as idiopathic interstitial pneumonias, or IIPs), but DPLD can develop secondary to other factors, including connective tissue disease (CTD), environmental exposures, and drugs/toxins (American Thoracic Society/European Respiratory Society. Am J Respir Crit Care Med 165(2):277–304, 2002). The IIPs include idiopathic pulmonary fibrosis (IPF), nonspecific interstitial pneumonia (NSIP), cryptogenic organizing pneumonia (COP), respiratory bronchiolitis interstitial lung disease (RB-ILD), acute interstitial pneumonia (AIP), lymphocytic interstitial pneumonia (LIP), and desquamative interstitial pneumonia (DIP) (American Thoracic Society/European Respiratory Society. Am J Respir Crit Care Med 165(2):277–304, 2002). There is significant overlap in the clinical features of the IIPs, including chronic dyspnea, interstitial changes on imaging studies, reduction in lung volumes, and impairment in diffusion capacity (DLCO) (American Thoracic Society/European Respiratory Society. Am J Respir Crit Care Med 165(2):277–304, 2002). Distinct radiographic and histopathological features can distinguish between the clinical entities, and establishing an accurate diagnosis is critical to determining treatment and understanding prognosis (Flaherty et al. Eur Respir J 19(2):275–83, 2002; Bjoraker et al. Am J Respir Crit Care Med 157(1):199–203, 1998).

A. Wadhwa, M.D.
Division of Pulmonary and Critical Care Medicine, University of Michigan Health System, Ann Arbor, MI, USA

K.R. Flaherty, M.D., M.S. (✉)
Department of Internal Medicine, Division of Pulmonary and Critical Care Medicine, University of Michigan Health System, 3916 Taubman Center, Ann Arbor, MI 49109, USA
e-mail: flaherty@umich.edu

K.C. Meyer and S.D. Nathan (eds.), *Idiopathic Pulmonary Fibrosis: A Comprehensive Clinical Guide*, Respiratory Medicine 9, DOI 10.1007/978-1-62703-682-5_5,
© Springer Science+Business Media New York 2014

Of the over 150 recognized types of DPLDs, IPF is the most common and has the worst prognosis (Flaherty et al. Eur Respir J 19(2):275–83, 2002; Bjoraker et al. Am J Respir Crit Care Med 157(1):199–203, 1998). IPF is defined as a specific form of chronic, progressive fibrosing interstitial pneumonia of unknown etiology that occurs primarily in older adults, is limited to the lungs, and is associated with a histopathological and/or radiologic pattern of usual interstitial pneumonia (UIP) (Raghu et al. Am J Respir Crit Care Med 183(6):788–824, 2011). As outlined in the ATS/ERS 2011 consensus statement, the diagnosis requires the exclusion of known causes of DPLD and the presence of a UIP pattern on high-resolution computed tomography (HRCT) or surgical lung biopsy (SLB) (Raghu et al. Am J Respir Crit Care Med 174(7):810–6, 2006). The incidence and prevalence of IPF increase with age, and the diagnosis should be considered in older adult patients who present with nonproductive cough, dyspnea, and bibasilar crackles (Raghu et al. Am J Respir Crit Care Med 174(7):810–6, 2006; Douglas et al. Am J Respir Crit Care Med 161 (4 Pt 1):1172–8, 2000; Fell et al. Am J Respir Crit Care Med 181(8):832–7, 2010).

This chapter reviews the key historical, physiologic, radiographic, and histopathological features that are key to establishing a confident diagnosis of IPF.

**Keywords** Pulmonary fibrosis • Phenotype • Mimics • Multidisciplinary • Confidence

# Introduction

Diffuse parenchymal lung diseases (DPLDs) are characterized by injury primarily to the interstitium of the lung, but may involve alveolar spaces, airways, and vessels [1]. Many DPLDs are idiopathic (referred to as idiopathic interstitial pneumonias, or IIPs), but DPLD can develop secondary to other factors, including connective tissue disease (CTD), environmental exposures, and drugs/toxins [1]. The IIPs include idiopathic pulmonary fibrosis (IPF), nonspecific interstitial pneumonia (NSIP), cryptogenic organizing pneumonia (COP), respiratory bronchiolitis interstitial lung disease (RB-ILD), acute interstitial pneumonia (AIP), lymphocytic interstitial pneumonia (LIP), and desquamative interstitial pneumonia (DIP) [1]. There is significant overlap in the clinical features of the IIPs, including chronic dyspnea, interstitial changes on imaging studies, reduction in lung volumes, and impairment in diffusion capacity (DLCO) [1]. Distinct radiographic and histopathological features can distinguish between the clinical entities, and establishing an accurate diagnosis is critical to determining treatment and understanding prognosis [2, 3].

Of the over 150 recognized types of DPLDs, IPF is the most common and has the worst prognosis [2, 3]. IPF is defined as a specific form of chronic, progressive fibrosing interstitial pneumonia of unknown etiology that occurs primarily in older adults, is limited to the lungs, and is associated with a histopathological and/or radiologic pattern of usual interstitial pneumonia (UIP) [4]. As outlined in the ATS/ERS 2011 consensus statement, the diagnosis requires the exclusion of known causes of DPLD and the presence of a UIP pattern on high-resolution computed tomography (HRCT) or surgical lung biopsy (SLB) [5]. The incidence and prevalence of IPF increase with age, and the diagnosis should be considered in older adult patients who present with nonproductive cough, dyspnea, and bibasilar crackles [5–7].

This chapter reviews the key historical, physiologic, radiographic, and histopathological features that are key to establishing a confident diagnosis of IPF.

# Clinical Presentation, Disease Course, and Phenotypes

## *Signs and Symptoms*

The clinical features of IPF are nonspecific. Most patients complain of a dry cough and dyspnea. These symptoms are sometimes attributed to comorbid conditions such as cardiac disease, infections, normal aging, or deconditioning, which can lead to a delay in diagnosis. A high index of suspicion is required to avoid missing a diagnosis of DPLD, including IPF. The most characteristic physical exam finding of IPF is bibasilar crackles, and clubbing may be present but is nonspecific.

The duration of symptoms prior to presentation may offer insight in a patient without an obvious proximate cause for dyspnea. The classical chronic and insidious presentation of ILDs contrasts with the acute/subacute development and progression of particular diagnoses, including AIP, acute eosinophilic pneumonia, COP, drug-induced lung diseases, and CTD-related ILD (CTD-ILD). Sarcoidosis and hypersensitivity pneumonitis (HP) may present in an acute, subacute, or chronic fashion. Chronic HP has overlapping radiologic features with IPF and must always be considered if the HRCT is not definitive for IPF. Evaluation for chronic HP is discussed later.

Age and gender may also help to distinguish among DPLDs, as certain diagnoses may be more common in particular age groups or have a male or female predominance. The prevalence of IPF is estimated to range from 0.8 (age, 18–34) to 64.7 (age ≥75) per 100,000, and it is generally higher among men than women [5]. The index of suspicion for a diagnosis of CTD-ILD should be higher in younger patients (<50), especially in women. In contrast to other IIPs, most patients with IPF are older than 50 at the time of diagnosis [8]. Increasing age has been shown to be a powerful predictor of IPF, particularly in patients with mild radiographic disease, as shown in Table 5.1 [7].

Although IPF is by definition idiopathic, there are several risk factors that seem to be associated with it. Gastroesophageal reflux disease (GERD) is frequent in patients with IPF [9, 10], as is pulmonary fibrosis associated with scleroderma [11]. Tobacco use is associated with the development of both sporadic and familial IPF [12–14], and smoking cessation may be the most modifiable risk factor [15]. Occupations such as hair dressing and farm working are also associated with the development of IPF [16]. The clinical evaluation is critical to look for exam findings or historical features that may suggest an exposure or systemic illness leading to the DPLD.

**Table 5.1** Positive predictive value, specificity, sensitivity, and negative predictive value when classifying patients with IPF who are at least as old as the age specified[a,b]

| Age | PPV | Specificity | Sensitivity | NPV |
|---|---|---|---|---|
| 30 | 72 | 0 | 100 | N/A |
| 40 | 74 | 11 | 98 | 67 |
| 50 | 78 | 34 | 92 | 62 |
| 60 | 87 | 89 | 61 | 43 |
| 70 | 95 | 97 | 21 | 32 |
| 80 | 100 | 100 | 1 | 28 |

[a]Adapted from [7]
[b]Classification of patients with IPF based on age, positive predictive value (PPV), specificity, sensitivity, and negative predictive value (NPV). PPV and specificity increase in older patients. Data expressed as percentages

Genetic factors, particularly in familial and sporadic forms of IPF, must also be evaluated, especially when considering the likelihood of disease progression. These factors are discussed elsewhere in this review. Genetic analyses evaluating differential expression of genes have identified unique patterns that suggest there are different phenotypes of IPF and hold promise in identifying subgroups of patients who are likely to have differing clinical courses. For example, data suggest that predominantly male smokers with <6 months of symptoms before first presentation may be "rapid" progressors and show an upregulation of genes involved in cell motility, myofibroblast differentiation, coagulation, oxidative stress, and development [17]. These patients differ from those with greater than 24 months of symptoms prior to presentation, as "slow" progressors [17].

## Clinical Course

The importance of a diagnosis of IPF as related to disease progression and poor prognosis is well established [2]. IPF is characterized by a progressive decline in pulmonary function until death. Data suggest that 40–60 % of patients will die from a respiratory cause, with comorbid coronary artery disease or infections comprising the most common other proximate causes of mortality [18, 19]. The time and path of progression from asymptomatic to symptomatic IPF are variable. Patients may demonstrate a slow progression over years, a rapid progression over a few months, or episodes of sudden deterioration in their condition during a period of relative stability, often called "exacerbations."

The potential clinical courses in IPF are depicted in Fig. 5.1 [20]. The rate of decline and progression to death may present in several clinical forms: subclinical IPF, where disease precedes symptoms; slowly progressive IPF, where there is a gradual physiologic decline and increasing exertional dyspnea; and rapidly progressive IPF, characterized by an acute decline from the time of presentation. This is frequently accompanied by progression to death or may be characterized by periods

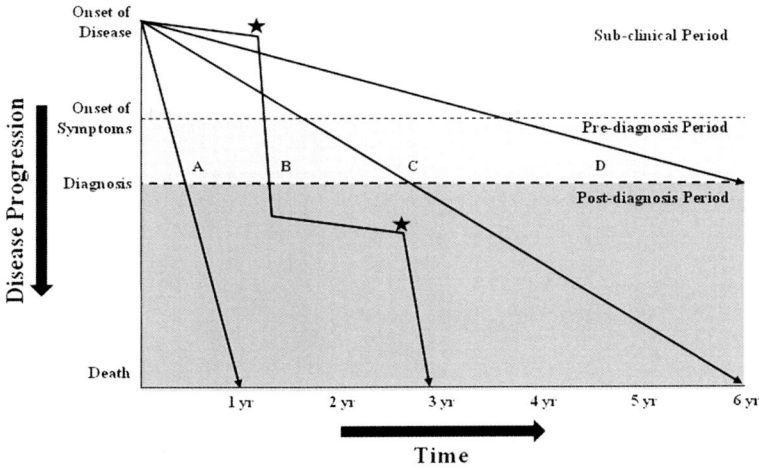

**Fig. 5.1** Potential clinical courses of idiopathic pulmonary fibrosis (IPF). During the subclinical period, only radiographic findings of disease may be present. The rate of decline may be accelerated in some (*line A*), although the majority of patients experience a gradual progressive worsening of their disease (*lines C and D*). The rate of decline may have periods of relative stability interposed with periods of rapid progression of disease (*line B, stars*). Reprinted with permission from Ley B, Collard HR, King TE Jr. Clinical course and prediction of survival in idiopathic pulmonary fibrosis. Am J Respir Crit Care Med. 2011;183(4):431–40

of stability alternating with periods of acute decline (so-called acute exacerbations of IPF [AE-IPF]) that are often associated with hospitalizations for respiratory failure [20].

Accelerated worsening of IPF may occur at any time during the disease course and may be the initial manifestation of disease in some patients. The etiology of decompensation may be related to pulmonary embolism, infection, congestive heart failure, pneumothorax, or drugs. When a cause cannot be determined, the worsening is typically characterized as an episode of AE-IPF. Although Epstein-Barr virus has been identified with a high prevalence in the lung tissue of patients with IPF and the general population [21], definitive conclusions about the contribution of acute infection in disease causation/progression cannot be made. Moreover, recent studies evaluating gene expression profiles in explanted tissue samples from patients with AE-IPF suggest that a marked inflammatory response, secondary to infection or otherwise, is less likely to contribute to the phenotype of AE-IPF [22]. The true incidence of AE-IPF is not known, but two retrospective studies suggest a 1-year incidence of 14.2 % and 8.6 %, respectively, with a 3-year incidence of 20.7 % and 23.9 %, respectively, in two separate studies of 461 and 74 patients [23, 24]. Subclinical IPF may be a risk factor for the development of an acute exacerbation, especially after surgery or invasive procedures [25]. Thoracic surgery, including lung resection or SLB, can precipitate an AE-IPF, often in the non-biopsied side and perhaps secondary to barotrauma incurred during the single-lung ventilation process [23, 26]. The risk for exacerbation is not likely related to the level of pulmonary function abnormality, although patients with lower FVC have more total and frequent respiratory hospitalizations during subsequent follow-up [27, 28]. Although the numbers of fibroblastic foci in lung samples before death are associated with poor survival [29–32], they cannot predict the development of acute exacerbations of IPF/UIP [31].

## Combined Pulmonary Fibrosis and Emphysema

Smoking increases the risk of developing IPF [14]. Patients with combined emphysema and pulmonary fibrosis are recognized as a unique clinical entity [33]. Patients with both emphysema and interstitial disease often present with severe dyspnea, preserved lung volumes, and marked reduction in DLCO and have radiographic evidence of lower lobe-predominant pulmonary fibrosis and upper lobe-predominant emphysema [34, 35]. In a series of 110 cases with IPF, 28 % of patients were found to have at least 10 % of the lung affected with emphysema and were thus considered to have combined pulmonary fibrosis and emphysema (CPFE) [35]. The risk of development of pulmonary hypertension (PH) is notably higher in patients with IPF and concomitant emphysema, as demonstrated by echocardiographic estimates of systolic pulmonary artery pressures (sPAP) [35]. Survival is worse for patients with CPFE versus those with IPF alone [35], and survival is even worse if these patients develop PH; 5-year survival may be as low as 25 % for patients with PH on echocardiogram versus 75 % for patients without PH [36].

Since lung volumes are relatively preserved in patients with CPFE [36] (unlike in IPF patients without emphysema), serial measurement of lung volumes may not be relevant in these patients. Instead, changes in $FEV_1$ or echocardiographic evidence for PH could be more appropriate surrogates for progression of disease and prediction of mortality [36, 37]. On the other hand, DLCO may not reliably predict mortality [37]. Of note, clinical prediction tools like the clinical-radiographic-physiologic (CRP) score do not consider the presence and severity of emphysema and thus have limited utility in the assessment of patients with CPFE [38]. A separate clinical tool, the composite physiologic index (CPI), predicts mortality more accurately than individual pulmonary function tests (PFTs) alone in patients with CPFE, although this composite is not helpful in establishing a diagnosis and is less useful than forced expiratory volume in 1 s ($FEV_1$) in predicting mortality when the disease progresses [37, 39].

## Pulmonary Fibrosis with Pulmonary Hypertension

Patients with IPF may present with PH that is disproportionate to the severity of underlying lung disease [40]. The prevalence of PH in a series of patients with

DPLD may range from 14 % to 41 % [41], and most studies have used the NIH definition of pulmonary artery hypertension as a mean pulmonary artery pressure (PAP) of >25 mmHg at rest with normal pulmonary capillary wedge pressure [42, 43]. Estimates of severity and decisions regarding treatment of PH should not be based on echocardiography, as this modality may overestimate the degree of PH when compared to right heart catheterization [44]. The incidence and severity of PH tend to correlate with the need for supplemental oxygen and decrements in DLCO [43, 45], while the presence of PH is associated with an increased risk of subsequent mortality [45–47]. Of note, a prospective analysis of IPF patients undergoing initial workup with RHC and PFTs identified a mean PAP of 17 mmHg as an appropriate value to discriminate 5-year mortality [48].

The subset of patients with IPF who develop PH at earlier stages of disease may have disproportionate PH due to molecular mediators that are common to PH and IPF. There may be increases in 5-lipoxygenase (LO), transforming growth factor-$\beta$ (beta) (TGF-$\beta$), and endothelin-1 (ET-1), but decreases in prostaglandin-$E_2$ (PGE$_2$) [49–51]. An altered balance between angiogenesis and angiostasis, as well as intermittent hypoxia (especially during sleep and exercise), may also contribute [40]. Pulmonary vascular remodeling, associated with chronic alveolar hypoxia, may be a consequence of "desensitization" to hypoxia (as seen in patients with nocturnal hypoventilation syndromes [52]) and thus makes patients more vulnerable to daytime and exercise-induced hypoxia [40].

## Physiologic Evaluation

Reduced lung volumes and impairment in DLCO are common to all the IIPs, although normal PFTs cannot exclude a diagnosis of IPF [53]. Specifically, the discrimination of IPF from other IIPs by scrutiny of PFTs alone is limited by a lack of specificity. Typical physiologic changes include an increase in elastic recoil and decrease in lung compliance that lead to reductions in the vital capacity (VC) and total lung capacity (TLC) [54], while the functional residual capacity remains either normal or only mildly reduced [55]. Preserved residual volume (RV) may be secondary to honeycombing or cystic air spaces that contribute to the TLC, or it may represent an increase in dead space ventilation [54, 55]. Both the FEV$_1$ and FVC may be reduced if lung volumes are reduced, but usually the FEV$_1$/FVC ratio is normal or elevated [54, 55]. As noted previously, concomitant emphysema and IPF can render measurements of lung volumes less reliable, as hyperinflation and increased compliance can lead to pseudonormalization of the VC and TLC [34, 36].

Hypoxemia is thought to be secondary to various mechanisms, including ventilation-perfusion mismatch, impaired diffusion secondary to abnormality of the alveolar-capillary membrane, and right-to-left shunting (from intracardiac/intrapulmonary shunting or elevated PAPs) [54]. Increased dead space ventilation likely accounts for the characteristic changes noted during exercise assessment, including increased minute ventilation ($V_E$) at rest and increased $V_E$ as oxygen consumption ($VO_2$) increases [54]. A reduction in DLCO may manifest with resting or exercise-induced hypoxemia, a reduced partial pressure of oxygen in arterial blood ($PaO_2$), or an elevated alveolar–arterial gradient ($P(A-a)O_2$) [55]. A decreased DLCO below 40 % predicts a subsequent risk of increased mortality [56]. Similarly, desaturation to <88 % during a 6-min hallwalk test [57, 58], low thresholds of maximal oxygen uptake during exercise [59], and declines in lung function over time also correlate with an increased risk of mortality [57, 58, 60–62].

The classical phenotype of IPF, where there is progressive decline in lung function and increasing dyspnea, demonstrates a mean rate of decline in forced vital capacity (FVC) of 150–200 mL/year [20]. However, there is typically great variability in the rate of progression of IPF, and identification of baseline and short-term serial predictors of survival is therefore critical to the accurate characterization of disease progression and consideration of appropriate interventions. In addition to providing evidence that a restrictive and probable interstitial pulmonary process is present, physiologic studies can aid in establishing baseline and longitudinal prognoses [56, 60, 63, 64].

## Radiographic Evaluation

Utilization of HRCT has become a key aspect in the evaluation of patients with a suspected IIP. Although typical radiographic changes are usually noted in established disease, normal radiology does not exclude the presence of IPF [65]. The recent ATS/ERS consensus statement clearly outlines the HRCT characteristics associated with a diagnosis of IPF: specifically, the disease is characterized by subpleural reticulation with a basal predominance and honeycombing without associated extensive ground-glass abnormality, micronodules, discrete cysts, mosaic attenuation/air trapping, or consolidation [4]. Honeycombing on HRCT, which is critical for establishing a definitive HRCT diagnosis of IPF, manifests as clustered cystic spaces varying between 3 and 25 mm in diameter, usually with well-defined walls [66]. The appearance of honeycomb lung with serial imaging over time may be preceded by the presence of patchy ground-glass opacities and reticulations within a secondary lobule [67]. Importantly, HRCT features of ground glass, fibrosis, and honeycombing correlate with measurements of FVC and DLCO and pathological fibrosis [68, 69]. Although HRCT can be used to make a definitive diagnosis with a pattern of UIP, it cannot do the same for NSIP. In current practice, the presence of honeycombing is considered specific for UIP. Thus, per recent Fleischner society recommendations, the term should be used with caution, given the potential impact on care [66].

HRCT findings of UIP with other associated abnormalities (e.g., plaques, calcifications, and pleural effusions) should prompt consideration of alternative etiologies for the UIP pattern [4]. The list of alternative diagnoses to consider includes CTD-ILD, chronic HP, and certain pneumoconioses, particularly asbestosis [4]. With the exception of honeycomb changes, many of the characteristic features of UIP overlap with HRCT features of NSIP, as listed in Table 5.2 [70]. Examples of HRCT images showing NSIP, UIP, and CPFE patterns are shown in Fig. 5.2. Patients

**Table 5.2** Characteristic
radiographic findings in NSIP
overlap with typical findings
in UIP[a,b]

| Radiologic finding | Number (%) |
|---|---|
| Lower lobe distribution | 56 (92) |
| Diffuse (axial) distribution | 29 (47) |
| Peripheral (axial) distribution | 28 (46) |
| Reticulation | 53 (87) |
| Traction bronchiectasis | 50 (82) |
| Lobar volume loss | 47 (77) |
| Ground-glass attenuation | 27 (44) |
| Subpleural sparing | 13 (21) |
| Substantial micronodules | 2 (3) |
| Honeycombing | 3 (5) |

[a]Adapted from [70]
[b]Diffuse bilateral reticular opacities that are mostly lower lobe predominant, associated traction bronchiectasis and lobar volume loss, and relative sparing of the subpleural space in approximately 20 % of patients are common findings. Data expressed as percentages in a series of 61 cases

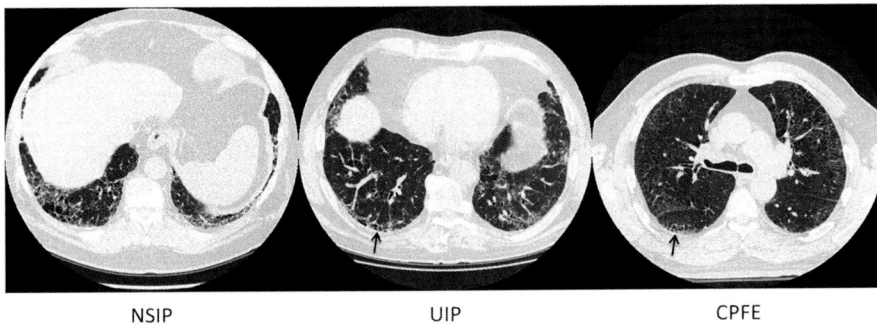

NSIP                    UIP                    CPFE

**Fig. 5.2** HRCT images from three different patients with ILD. Areas of honeycombing are indicated by *black arrows*. *Left*: Peripheral and lower lung-predominant interstitial disease without honeycombing in a patient with radiographic diagnosis of NSIP, although surgical lung biopsy was consistent with UIP. *Middle*: There are areas of lower lobe-predominant septal thickening, traction bronchiectasis, and honeycombing that are consistent with UIP. *Right*: Upper lobe emphysema changes and lower lobe interstitial changes compatible with UIP in a patient with CPFE. Figures courtesy of Kevin R. Flaherty, MD, MS, University of Michigan

with suspected NSIP by HRCT require a SLB for confirmation, since many of these patients will have a histopathological pattern of UIP [71].

Concurrence between radiologists regarding the presence of honeycomb lung may be inconsistent, as demonstrated in a study of 314 patients where interobserver agreement for the presence of honeycomb lung ranged from 0.21 to 0.31 [69]. The presence of emphysema and cystic spaces can make the diagnostic process more challenging, especially in the presence of overlapping ground-glass opacities [72], which may possibly lead to misdiagnoses. The development of chronic interstitial pneumonia in emphysematous lung or patterns of NSIP and DIP that demonstrate predominantly ground-glass opacities and have a honeycomb appearance (especially if involving areas of emphysematous lung) may also be misdiagnosed as UIP [67]. Emphysema and interstitial fibrosis can develop and progress simultaneously in the same lung area and lead to honeycomb changes, which may also contribute to misdiagnoses [73]. Paraseptal emphysema, which has definite walls and is located subpleurally (and often in clusters), may be accompanied by fibrosis. When such changes occur in the upper and middle lobes, and coexist with typical honeycomb changes in the lower lobes, distinguishing the disease entities via imaging could conceivably be more difficult.

# Bronchoscopy, Surgical Lung Biopsy, and Histopathology

## Bronchoscopy

The 2000 ATS/ERS consensus statement regarding the diagnosis and treatment of IPF included the use of transbronchial lung biopsy or BAL, to identify any features that could support an alternative to IPF, as a criterion for diagnosis in patients who did not undergo SLB [74]. These criteria were not included in the 2011 statement, although bronchoscopy should still be considered when non-IPF diagnoses are in the differential [4]. Bronchoscopy is useful for the diagnosis of sarcoidosis, infections, malignancy, and potentially HP; specifically, a cell count of more than 30 % lymphocytes has been suggested as predictive of HP [4, 75].

Conventional wisdom suggests that the amount of tissue obtained by transbronchial biopsy is inadequate to make a diagnosis of UIP, although in a recent series of 22 patients with UIP, 7 of 18 adequate specimens contained features diagnostic of UIP, and an additional two cases were considered consistent with UIP [76]. A second study of 32 patients found changes consistent with UIP in only 9.4 % of patients, although the authors did suggest the approach could be helpful in patients unable to undergo SLB [77]. As the sensitivity and specificity of this approach for the diagnosis of UIP is unknown, the most recent ATS/ERS statement suggests transbronchial biopsy should not be used in the evaluation of IPF, but should be considered in the evaluation of selected conditions (e.g., granulomatous disorders such as sarcoidosis) for which there is a reasonable expectation of establishing a diagnosis [4].

## Surgical Lung Biopsy

Enabling an accurate diagnosis of an IIP often requires obtaining a SLB, as histopathology may serve as the only distinguishing feature between similar clinical and radiographic presentations [78]. As many patients with advanced lung disease are of older age, have impaired lung function, require oxygen, have pulmonary hypertension, and demonstrate impaired functional capacity at the time of evaluation, decision making regarding biopsy is complex [26, 79, 80]. In patients with nondiagnostic HRCT findings, SLB should be considered, although 30-day mortality has been described in as many as 17 % of patients following the procedure [26]. The possibility of complication, including bleeding, prolonged mechanical ventilation, or prolonged air leak, should always be considered. Acute respiratory failure following surgery carries a high mortality [26, 27]. Risk factors for increased morbidity and mortality following SLB include prior treatment with immunosuppression, mechanical ventilation at the time of biopsy, pulmonary hypertension, lower levels of lung function (specifically regarding lung volumes or DLCO <40 % predicted), and the need for supplemental oxygen [1, 79, 81–83]. Although HRCT features of UIP in the presence of honeycombing have a diagnostic accuracy of greater than 90 % [2, 71, 84, 85], other diseases with specific historical and radiographic findings may also be diagnosed without biopsy. For example, asbestosis should be considered in patients with extensive exposure history, pleural plaques, and classical CT findings.

The recent ATS/ERS consensus statement reiterates that findings on transbronchial biopsy and BAL fluid are not reliable for establishing a diagnosis [4]. With improvements in minimally invasive techniques, including video-assisted thoracoscopic surgery (VATS), complication rates have declined. Thirty-day mortality is estimated at 4 %, but this decreases to 1.5–3 % when those already on mechanical ventilation, patients with an acute exacerbation, or individuals on immunosuppression are excluded from the analysis [79, 86]. Moreover, VATS lung biopsy has a diagnostic yield that is comparable to open lung biopsy for both diffuse and focal pathology [87]. Biopsy is ideally performed early in the disease course, since histologic distinctions can be more difficult as disease progresses. Obtaining biopsies from multiple lobes is recommended; in two single-center analyses, patterns of both UIP and NSIP were identified in 12–26 % of patients with biopsies from multiple lobes [88, 89]. In addition, the diagnostic yield is improved when diseased (but not end-stage) areas are targeted, reducing the risk of finding nonspecific changes [90]. Biopsies from areas of severe fibrosis are likely to show end-stage lung and not the histopathological patterns required to differentiate UIP from other IIPs (see "Histopathology" below). HRCT may be helpful in guiding surgeons to areas that show intermediate or relatively preserved lung, as a pathological identification of fibrotic lung next to normal lung aids in confirmation of a UIP pattern [88].

## Histopathology

Prior to the 1960s, the term "honeycomb lung" had been used to describe the macroscopic appearance of lung diseases comprising various histopathological processes and causes, but in 1965 the definition was limited to include chronic interstitial pneumonia (pulmonary fibrosis) regardless of etiology [73, 91]. The presence of honeycomb lung should not be considered specific as to cause, and disease entities apart from IPF should be included in a list of differential diagnoses, including other IIPs, sarcoidosis, chronic hypersensitivity pneumonia, and Langerhans cell histiocytosis [92, 93]. One of the IIPs, respiratory bronchiolitis associated ILD (RB-ILD), which is also referred to as smoking-related interstitial fibrosis (SRIF), may have fibroblastic foci present, but rarely demonstrates honeycomb changes, and is accompanied by respiratory bronchiolitis in all cases [94]. Studies of honeycomb lung found in diseases other than IPF (scleroderma, dermatomyositis, Langerhans cell histiocytosis, tuberculosis, lipoid pneumonia, and sarcoidosis) suggest that the pathophysiologic changes may be independent of the original disease [95].

The most important criteria for the pathological diagnosis of UIP are temporal and spatial heterogeneity in the distribution of normal lung, interstitial inflammation, fibroblastic foci, and honeycomb changes. Scattered fibroblastic foci are usually found between areas of normal lung and older fibrosis, and the majority of changes are often in a lower lobe-predominant distribution. A prospective cohort study of 87 patients with biopsy-proven UIP showed that the degree of granulation/connective tissue deposition, which is characteristic of fibroblastic foci, could predict lower survival [29]. The importance of the number of foci to the clinical phenotype was also demonstrated by a separate study of 108 patients with UIP, where the nine patients with collagen vascular disease-associated UIP had fewer foci and improved survival [96]. At low magnification, the pattern has a heterogeneous appearance, and identification of normal parenchyma interspersed with areas of fibrosis and honeycomb cysts can help to distinguish UIP from NSIP, where temporal and spatial uniformity are common, honeycomb changes are rare, interstitial inflammation is more likely, and fewer fibroblastic foci may be found [72]. A UIP pattern may be found in non-UIP diagnoses, although the possibility of other diagnoses does not necessarily confer a survival advantage, as in a series of 168 patients including various different IIPs (i.e., not just IPF), the risk ratio of histologic classification of UIP for mortality was 11.46 (95 % confidence interval 4.13–31.83; $p < 0.0001$) [2].

A summary of contrasting histologic features of SRIF, UIP, and NSIP is listed in Table 5.3, and representative images for these diagnoses are shown in Fig. 5.3.

Interobserver variation in the pathological diagnosis of DPLDs parallels the variation that has been described with radiologic diagnoses. One study of 133 biopsy specimens identified a 100 % confidence level for a single diagnosis in only 39 % of biopsy specimens reviewed by ten pulmonary pathologists ($\kappa = 0.38$) [97]. The level of agreement increased when multiple biopsy specimens were taken and when diagnostic confidence was higher ($\kappa = 0.43$ and $\kappa = 0.50$, respectively). Agreement improved only marginally for a diagnosis of UIP, even with multiple biopsy specimens and high diagnostic confidence ($\kappa = 0.42$, $\kappa = 0.49$ and $\kappa = 0.58$, respectively) [97]. Agreement was significantly improved for sarcoidosis ($\kappa = 0.76$, $\kappa = 0.82$ and $\kappa = 0.86$, respectively) [97]. Not surprisingly, significant variability was seen for a diagnosis of NSIP ($\kappa = 0.29$, $\kappa = 0.32$ and $\kappa = 0.31$, respectively), while the distinction of NSIP from UIP was noted to be particularly problematic [97]. The degree of

**Table 5.3**  Characteristic histologic findings in UIP, NSIP, and SRIF[a,b]

|                          | UIP            | NSIP           | SRIF         |
|--------------------------|----------------|----------------|--------------|
| Distribution             | Heterogeneous  | Uniform        | Uniform      |
| Emphysema                | Usually absent | Usually absent | Often severe |
| Respiratory bronchiolitis| Possible       | Possible       | Present      |
| Honeycombing             | Present        | None/minimal   | None/minimal |
| Fibroblastic foci        | Present        | None/rare      | None/rare    |

[a]Adapted from [98]
[b]UIP is distinguished by the heterogeneous distribution of areas of active fibrosis with collagen deposition, parenchymal distortion, and honeycomb changes. In contrast, the fibrosis in SRIF and NSIP is more uniform and less patchy, and it lacks the characteristic honeycomb changes seen in UIP

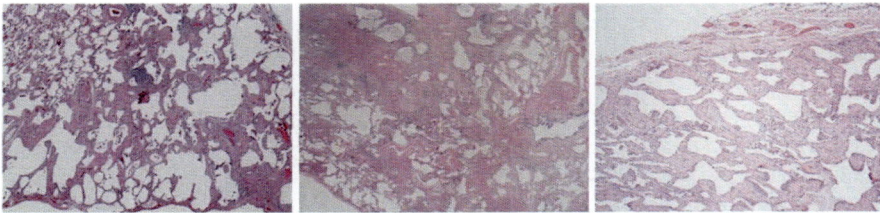

**Fig. 5.3**  Histologic images of SRIF, UIP, and NSIP. Original magnification ×40, hematoxylin, and eosin staining. *Left*: A typical SRIF has more emphysema changes with collagen deposition around airways and evidence of macrophages in airways (consistent with respiratory bronchiolitis). *Middle*: A pathological diagnosis of UIP requires identification of normal areas of lung interspersed with fibroblastic foci and honeycomb changes. *Right*: A NSIP pattern has interstitial inflammation that is diffuse without evidence of honeycombing and scant evidence of fibroblastic foci. Images courtesy of Lindsay Schmidt, MD, University of Michigan

uncertainty in differentiating histologic patterns of DPLDs, particularly NSIP versus UIP, supports the use of a multidisciplinary approach to confirm a diagnosis. This paradigm is discussed later in this chapter.

## Close Mimics of IPF

In patients with a suspected IIP, a histologic diagnosis of UIP confers a nearly 30-fold increased risk of mortality when compared to an alternative histologic diagnosis. Similarly, the relative risk of mortality for a histologic diagnosis of UIP is more than ten times higher than that associated with only the presence of honeycomb changes on HRCT [2]. Evaluation of patients with presentations similar to UIP should include consideration of differences in history, exposures, and HRCT patterns. Exclusion of other known causes of ILD is important given differences in clinical course, management, and outcomes.

## Chronic HP and NSIP

A thorough review of history and physical examination, medications, environmental exposures, and family history can be useful to distinguish certain causes of ILD, particularly chronic HP [4]. In HP, type III hypersensitivity reactions related to precipitin-antibody deposition in alveolar walls may be considered pathological, although 20–30 % of patients may not have an inciting antigen identified by exposure history or serologic testing [99–101]. Histologic findings of lymphocytic interstitial infiltrates with granuloma formation and BAL findings of lymphocytosis are typical [99]. Patients with chronic HP and a fibrotic histopathology demonstrate a predominant $T_H2$ response in comparison to patients with OP or NSIP-like histopathology [102]. With chronic exposure, the typical histopathological findings in subacute HP (cellular NSIP and bronchiolitis, granulomatous inflammation, involvement of central regions of secondary lobules) can progress to fibrotic changes with honeycombing [103]. A review of 13 cases of chronic HP (all with presence of granulomas and/or giant cells) suggested that patterns of fibrosis may be in a typical UIP distribution (peripheral, patchy, with fibroblastic foci), UIP-like (irregular, predominantly peribronchiolar), or similar to fibrotic NSIP (homogeneous linear fibrosis) [104].

The HRCT distribution of changes in HP may be more prominent in the upper lobes, but can occur in the lower lobes, although subpleural involvement is less likely [105]. The presence of poorly defined centrilobular micronodules is often suggestive of the diagnosis [99]. A study evaluating the role of HRCT in distinguishing chronic HP from UIP and NSIP found that the presence of lobular areas with decreased attenuation, centrilobular nodules, and a lack of lower lung predominance of changes to be most consistent with chronic HP; basal predominance of honeycombing and absence of pleural sparing and centrilobular nodules are particularly useful to distinguish UIP versus HP, although up to 64 % of patients with chronic HP may have honeycomb changes as well [106].

Idiopathic NSIP is a distinct clinical entity with features that distinguish it from the other IIPs. Symptoms of breathlessness and cough are often present. Patients are usually nonsmokers, are more often women, are usually in the sixth decade of life, and may have serologic testing that is positive for collagen vascular disease [70]. Characteristic HRCT features include reticular opacities with lower lung zone predominance, traction bronchiectasis with lobar volume loss, and a diffuse or subpleural distribution [70]. The most common finding may be symmetric ground-glass opacities [92, 107]. Key histopathological features differ between predominantly cellular patterns and fibrosing patterns. The former are characterized by mild to moderate interstitial chronic inflammation and type II pneumocyte hyperplasia in areas of inflammation, while fibrosing NSIP usually demonstrates areas of interstitial fibrosis with a uniform appearance, lung architecture that is frequently preserved, and mild to moderate interstitial chronic inflammation [70]. Studies suggest that the distinction between cellular and fibrosing patterns is important, as a more favorable prognosis is seen with the cellular variant [108].

## Connective Tissue Disease-Related ILD

Pulmonary disease may manifest in several CTDs, including rheumatoid arthritis (RA), systemic sclerosis/scleroderma (SSc), polymyositis(PM)/dermatomyositis (DM), Sjögren syndrome, and systemic lupus erythematosus (SLE). Patients often present with nonspecific complaints of cough, dyspnea, and fatigue. Approximately 15 % of patients with UIP have an underlying CTD as well [4], and the incidence of IPF diagnosis in younger women may be overstated due to the misdiagnosis of these patients [109]. Within the CTDs, a pattern of UIP is most common in RA [110]; interestingly, both the disease course and prognosis for UIP-RA are similar to that of IPF [111]. Although ILD associated with RA is often secondary to long-standing disease and progression of disease is usually slow, it may be an early manifestation of disease in up to 20 % of patients and can occur prior to classical exam findings of synovitis [112, 113]. Risk factors for RA-associated ILD include older age, male sex, and history of tobacco use.

The most recent ATS/ERS consensus statement provides a weak positive recommendation (given low quality evidence) for CTD serologic testing in the evaluation for IPF, even in the absence of signs or symptoms of disease [4]. Rheumatoid factor, anti-citrullinated peptide, and antinuclear antibody titer and pattern should be considered first, while the use of other serologic tests may only be helpful in select cases. Regarding bronchoscopy, BAL neutrophilia correlates with poor lung function but has not been shown to consistently correlate with prognosis and/or response to therapy [114–117]. In select cases, there might be utility in evaluating for possible drug reactions (for evidence of eosinophilia), diffuse alveolar hemorrhage (DAH), and opportunistic infection [118–120].

A typical pattern of bibasilar subpleural reticulations and honeycombing likely predicts a pathological finding of UIP [110, 121], while a ground-glass predominance may confer a better prognosis [122]. In addition to ground-glass opacities, common HRCT features of CTD-ILD include reticulation, bronchiectasis, and micronodules [123]. Abnormalities are found predominantly at the periphery of the lung and are usually associated with architectural distortion, traction bronchiectasis, and honeycombing. Therefore, these abnormalities can make the distinction from other IIPs difficult [124]. The correlation that exists between radiographic UIP and pathological UIP is thought to exist in patients with CTD-ILD as well [121], whereas the correlations between radiographic and histologic patterns of NSIP are not reliable [125]. Serial HRCT manifestations may include progressive reticular and honeycomb changes [122] with progressive fibrosis being associated with a worse prognosis [124].

A number of histopathological patterns, including NSIP and UIP, may exist simultaneously in a single specimen in patients with CTD-ILD [126]. Overall, the prognosis of patterns of NSIP and UIP in CTD-ILD is felt to be better than in idiopathic disease [88, 109, 124, 127, 128]. This may relate in part to a higher profusion of fibroblastic foci noted on histopathology in idiopathic ILD compared to CTD-ILD [96]. It is unclear whether a different fibroblast phenotype exists in idiopathic UIP versus CTD-ILD, or if there is an effect of age on fibroblast function, as studies of fibroblasts undergoing replicative senescence suggest that the senescent state mimics inflammatory wound repair processes [129].

## The Elderly Patient

As stated previously, the incidence of IPF is increased in older patients [5]. Mechanisms of disease pathogenesis suggest that the aging process itself may contribute to clinical progression through the effects of cellular and molecular factors such as mutations in surfactant protein C and mutations in telomerase. Additional factors that might affect the disease course include environmental factors such as tobacco use and viral infections, as well as comorbid conditions, including GERD and PH [130]. Improvements in radiographic studies facilitate the diagnosis of some DPLDs without the need for SLB, although histopathological evaluation is often required to establish diagnosis and determine appropriate prognosis and treatment. However, the use and need for a SLB must be carefully weighed in the context of the patient's overall clinical condition, as age itself is a known risk factor for complications and mortality from SLB [26]. There may be a risk for an acute exacerbation even for patients undergoing BAL [131], and the role of transbronchial biopsy specimens is not yet established as a reliable way to make a diagnosis of IPF [4]. One retrospective series identified age as a reliable sole predictor for the diagnosis of IPF. A cutoff of 75 years provided a 100 % predictive value of confirming UIP/IPF by SLB, and a cutoff of 70 years was nearly as good. The predictive value increased when interstitial changes were also present on HRCT [7]. These data afford the clinician some measure of confidence when considering this diagnosis, thereby further raising the bar to obtain surgical confirmation in elderly higher-risk patients. However, this single series was limited by a high proportion of IPF in the cohort as well as possible referral bias, thus further data are needed to verify these findings.

## The Multidisciplinary Approach

Establishing the correct diagnosis in a patient with a suspected IIP can be challenging. The ATS/ERS consensus recommends a collaborative process involving clinicians, radiologists, and pathologists working together to improve the diagnostic confidence for patients with suspected IPF. This is predicated on the knowledge that the combination of HRCT and histologic features is more robust in predicting prognosis versus either modality alone [71]. Previous data suggested that a histologic diagnosis of IPF as a standard by itself was limited by interobserver variation, as the ability of experienced pathologists to discriminate between NSIP and UIP produced agreement only 50 % of the time [97]. Radiologists' assessment of ILD was also

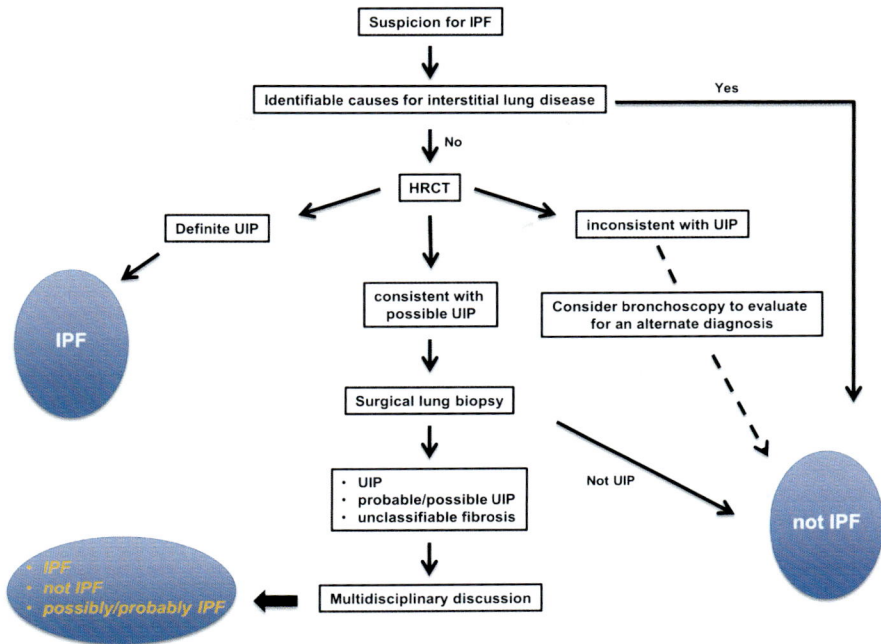

**Fig. 5.4** Algorithm for evaluation of suspected IPF. HRCT may establish a diagnosis if there is a pattern consistent with UIP. Absent a pattern of UIP, a bronchoscopy should be considered to further evaluate for alternate diagnoses. A surgical lung biopsy should be considered if HRCT suggests possible UIP, but is not diagnostic for UIP. The accuracy of diagnosis of IPF increases with collaboration among a multidisciplinary team of specialists. Adapted from [4]

found to be limited by nonspecific findings and interobserver variations, with disagreement being highest for the diagnosis of NSIP, especially pertaining to its distinction from UIP [132]. The creation of an interdisciplinary algorithm for clinicians, radiologists, and pathologists determined that SLB can be deferred if the clinical/radiographic impression is consistent with IPF [133]. On the other hand, the diagnosis of non-IPF IIPs does usually require a biopsy [133]. A comparison of academic-based clinicians and community-based physicians found significant disagreement in the diagnosis of IIPs and identified a tendency for community-based physicians to be more likely to make a diagnosis of IPF. The inference from this is that overall clinical experience likely has a profound effect on diagnostic confidence [134]. In summary, pathologists should consider additional data (clinical, radiologic) when making diagnoses, and patients should be referred to tertiary centers with expertise in DPLDs in order to better clarify diagnoses and provide suggestions regarding treatment options. Figure 5.4 demonstrates a diagnostic algorithm for the evaluation of suspected IPF.

## Future Directions

Long-term follow-up data will continue to provide insights regarding the natural history of IPF, while the identification of biomarkers that have prognostic significance will further improve upon established multivariate predictive models. As more insight is gained, this will hopefully aid in the stratification of unique subpopulations to facilitate the goal of targeting therapies more efficiently. Specifically, the use of molecular and genetic techniques to establish diagnoses and distinguish among subtypes of IPF will be paramount. As suggested above, relatively specific gene expression profiles exist for "rapid" versus "slow" progressors [17]. Recent gene expression studies comparing patients with HP and IPF suggest a phenotype that is particular for IPF [135]. Other work has identified Toll-like receptor 9 (TLR9) as a possible biomarker for patients with the rapidly progressive form of IPF [136]. Future investigation to elucidate other mechanisms as part of a broader collaboration between basic and clinical scientists will help to achieve goals of facilitating detection, improving quality of life, and prolonging survival.

## References

1. American Thoracic Society/European Respiratory Society. American Thoracic Society/ European Respiratory Society International Multidisciplinary Consensus Classification of the Idiopathic Interstitial Pneumonias. This joint statement of the American Thoracic Society (ATS), and the European Respiratory Society (ERS) was adopted by the ATS board of directors, June 2001 and by the ERS Executive Committee, June 2001. Am J Respir Crit Care Med. 2002;165(2):277–304.
2. Flaherty KR, Toews GB, Travis WD, Colby TV, Kazerooni EA, Gross BH, et al. Clinical significance of histological classification of idiopathic interstitial pneumonia. Eur Respir J. 2002;19(2):275–83.
3. Bjoraker JA, Ryu JH, Edwin MK, Myers JL, Tazelaar HD, Schroeder DR, et al. Prognostic significance of histopathologic subsets in idiopathic pulmonary fibrosis. Am J Respir Crit Care Med. 1998;157(1):199–203.
4. Raghu G, Collard HR, Egan JJ, Martinez FJ, Behr J, Brown KK, et al. An official ATS/ERS/ JRS/ALAT statement: idiopathic pulmonary fibrosis: evidence-based guidelines for diagnosis and management. Am J Respir Crit Care Med. 2011;183(6):788–824.
5. Raghu G, Weycker D, Edelsberg J, Bradford WZ, Oster G. Incidence and prevalence of idiopathic pulmonary fibrosis. Am J Respir Crit Care Med. 2006;174(7):810–6.
6. Douglas WW, Ryu JH, Schroeder DR. Idiopathic pulmonary fibrosis: impact of oxygen and colchicine, prednisone, or no therapy on survival. Am J Respir Crit Care Med. 2000;161 (4 Pt 1):1172–8.
7. Fell CD, Martinez FJ, Liu LX, Murray S, Han MK, Kazerooni EA, et al. Clinical predictors of a diagnosis of idiopathic pulmonary fibrosis. Am J Respir Crit Care Med. 2010; 181(8):832–7.
8. Wade 3rd JF, King Jr TE. Infiltrative and interstitial lung disease in the elderly patient. Clin Chest Med. 1993;14(3):501–21.
9. Lee JS, Ryu JH, Elicker BM, Lydell CP, Jones KD, Wolters PJ, et al. Gastroesophageal reflux therapy is associated with longer survival in patients with idiopathic pulmonary fibrosis. Am J Respir Crit Care Med. 2011;184(12):1390–4.

10. Raghu G, Freudenberger TD, Yang S, Curtis JR, Spada C, Hayes J, et al. High prevalence of abnormal acid gastro-oesophageal reflux in idiopathic pulmonary fibrosis. Eur Respir J. 2006;27(1):136–42.
11. D'Ovidio F, Singer LG, Hadjiliadis D, Pierre A, Waddell TK, de Perrot M, et al. Prevalence of gastroesophageal reflux in end-stage lung disease candidates for lung transplant. Ann Thorac Surg. 2005;80(4):1254–60.
12. Steele MP, Speer MC, Loyd JE, Brown KK, Herron A, Slifer SH, et al. Clinical and pathologic features of familial interstitial pneumonia. Am J Respir Crit Care Med. 2005;172(9):1146–52.
13. Schwartz DA, Merchant RK, Helmers RA, Gilbert SR, Dayton CS, Hunninghake GW. The influence of cigarette smoking on lung function in patients with idiopathic pulmonary fibrosis. Am Rev Respir Dis. 1991;144(3 Pt 1):504–6.
14. Baumgartner KB, Samet JM, Stidley CA, Colby TV, Waldron JA. Cigarette smoking: a risk factor for idiopathic pulmonary fibrosis. Am J Respir Crit Care Med. 1997;155(1):242–8.
15. Schwartz DA, Van Fossen DS, Davis CS, Helmers RA, Dayton CS, Burmeister LF, et al. Determinants of progression in idiopathic pulmonary fibrosis. Am J Respir Crit Care Med. 1994;149(2 Pt 1):444–9.
16. Baumgartner KB, Samet JM, Coultas DB, Stidley CA, Hunt WC, Colby TV, et al. Occupational and environmental risk factors for idiopathic pulmonary fibrosis: a multicenter case–control study. Collaborating Centers. Am J Epidemiol. 2000;152(4):307–15.
17. Selman M, Carrillo G, Estrada A, Mejia M, Becerril C, Cisneros J, et al. Accelerated variant of idiopathic pulmonary fibrosis: clinical behavior and gene expression pattern. PLoS One. 2007;30:2(5).
18. Daniels CE, Yi ES, Ryu JH. Autopsy findings in 42 consecutive patients with idiopathic pulmonary fibrosis. Eur Respir J. 2008;32(1):170–4.
19. Panos RJ, Mortenson RL, Niccoli SA, King TE. Clinical deterioration in patients with idiopathic pulmonary fibrosis - causes and assessment. Am J Med. 1990;88(4):396–404.
20. Ley B, Collard HR, King Jr TE. Clinical course and prediction of survival in idiopathic pulmonary fibrosis. Am J Respir Crit Care Med. 2011;183(4):431–40.
21. Stewart JP, Egan JJ, Ross AJ, Kelly BG, Lok SS, Hasleton PS, et al. The detection of Epstein-Barr virus DNA in lung tissue from patients with idiopathic pulmonary fibrosis. Am J Respir Crit Care Med. 1999;159(4 Pt 1):1336–41.
22. Konishi K, Gibson KF, Lindell KO, Richards TJ, Zhang Y, Dhir R, et al. Gene expression profiles of acute exacerbations of idiopathic pulmonary fibrosis. Am J Respir Crit Care Med. 2009;180(2):167–75.
23. Kondoh Y, Taniguchi H, Katsuta T, Kataoka K, Kimura T, Nishiyama O, et al. Risk factors of acute exacerbation of idiopathic pulmonary fibrosis. Sarcoidosis Vasc Diffuse Lung Dis. 2010;27(2):103–10.
24. Song JW, Hong SB, Lim CM, Koh Y, Kim DS. Acute exacerbation of idiopathic pulmonary fibrosis: incidence, risk factors and outcome. Eur Respir J. 2011;37(2):356–63.
25. Chida M, Ono S, Hoshikawa Y, Kondo T. Subclinical idiopathic pulmonary fibrosis is also a risk factor of postoperative acute respiratory distress syndrome following thoracic surgery. Eur J Cardiothorac Surg. 2008;34(4):878–81.
26. Utz JP, Ryu JH, Douglas WW, Hartman TE, Tazelaar HD, Myers JL, et al. High short-term mortality following lung biopsy for usual interstitial pneumonia. Eur Respir J. 2001; 17(2):175–9.
27. Kim DS, Park JH, Park BK, Lee JS, Nicholson AG, Colby T. Acute exacerbation of idiopathic pulmonary fibrosis: frequency and clinical features. Eur Respir J. 2006;27(1):143–50.
28. Martinez FJ, Safrin S, Weycker D, Starko KM, Bradford WZ, King Jr TE, et al. The clinical course of patients with idiopathic pulmonary fibrosis. Ann Intern Med. 2005;142(12 Pt 1):963–7.
29. King Jr TE, Schwarz MI, Brown K, Tooze JA, Colby TV, Waldron Jr JA, et al. Idiopathic pulmonary fibrosis: relationship between histopathologic features and mortality. Am J Respir Crit Care Med. 2001;164(6):1025–32.

30. Nicholson AG, Fulford LG, Colby TV, du Bois RM, Hansell DM, Wells AU. The relationship between individual histologic features and disease progression in idiopathic pulmonary fibrosis. Am J Respir Crit Care Med. 2002;166(2):173–7.
31. Tiitto L, Bloigu R, Heiskanen U, Paakkc P, Kinnula VL, Kaarteenaho-Wiik R. Relationship between histopathological features and the course of idiopathic pulmonary fibrosis/usual interstitial pneumonia. Thorax. 2006;61(12):1091–5.
32. King Jr TE, Tooze JA, Schwarz MI, Brown KR, Cherniack RM. Predicting survival in idiopathic pulmonary fibrosis: scoring system and survival model. Am J Respir Crit Care Med. 2001;164(7):1171–81.
33. Cottin V, Cordier JF. The syndrome of combined pulmonary fibrosis and emphysema. Chest. 2009;136(1):1–2.
34. Doherty MJ, Pearson MG, O'Grady EA, Pellegrini V, Calverley PM. Cryptogenic fibrosing alveolitis with preserved lung volumes. Thorax. 1997;52(11):998–1002.
35. Mejia M, Carrillo G, Rojas-Serrano J, Estrada A, Suarez T, Alonso D, et al. Idiopathic pulmonary fibrosis and emphysema: decreased survival associated with severe pulmonary arterial hypertension. Chest. 2009;136(1):10–5.
36. Cottin V, Nunes H, Brillet PY, Delaval P, Devouassoux G, Tillie-Leblond I, et al. Combined pulmonary fibrosis and emphysema: a distinct underrecognised entity. Eur Respir J. 2005;26(4):586–93.
37. Schmidt SL, Nambiar AM, Tayob N, Sundaram B, Han MK, Gross BH, et al. Pulmonary function measures predict mortality differently in IPF versus combined pulmonary fibrosis and emphysema. Eur Respir J. 2011;38(1):176–83.
38. Watters LC, King TE, Schwarz MI, Waldron JA, Stanford RE, Cherniack RM. A clinical, radiographic, and physiologic scoring system for the longitudinal assessment of patients with idiopathic pulmonary fibrosis. Am Rev Respir Dis. 1986;133(1):97–103.
39. Wells AU, Desai SR, Rubens MB, Goh NS, Cramer D, Nicholson AG, et al. Idiopathic pulmonary fibrosis: a composite physiologic index derived from disease extent observed by computed tomography. Am J Respir Crit Care Med. 2003;167(7):962–9.
40. Corte TJ, Wort SJ, Wells AU. Pulmonary hypertension in idiopathic pulmonary fibrosis: a review. Sarcoidosis Vasc Diffuse Lung Dis. 2009;26(1):7–19.
41. Andersen CU, Mellemkjaer S, Hilberg O, Nielsen-Kudsk JE, Simonsen U, Bendstrup E. Pulmonary hypertension in interstitial lung disease: prevalence, prognosis and 6 min walk test. Respir Med. 2012;106(6):875–82.
42. D'Alonzo GE, Barst RJ, Ayres SM, Bergofsky EH, Brundage BH, Detre KM, et al. Survival in patients with primary pulmonary hypertension. Results from a national prospective registry. Ann Intern Med. 1991;115(5):343–9.
43. Patel NM, Lederer DJ, Borczuk AC, Kawut SM. Pulmonary hypertension in idiopathic pulmonary fibrosis. Chest. 2007;132(3):998–1006.
44. Arcasoy SM, Christie JD, Ferrari VA, Sutton MS, Zisman DA, Blumenthal NP, et al. Echocardiographic assessment of pulmonary hypertension in patients with advanced lung disease. Am J Respir Crit Care Med. 2003;167(5):735–40.
45. Nathan SD, Shlobin OA, Ahmad S, Koch J, Barnett SD, Ad N, et al. Serial development of pulmonary hypertension in patients with idiopathic pulmonary fibrosis. Respiration. 2008;76(3):288–94.
46. Lettieri CJ, Nathan SD, Barnett SD, Ahmad S, Shorr AF. Prevalence and outcomes of pulmonary arterial hypertension in advanced idiopathic pulmonary fibrosis. Chest. 2006;129(3):746–52.
47. Nathan SD, Noble PW, Tuder RM. Idiopathic pulmonary fibrosis and pulmonary hypertension: connecting the dots. Am J Respir Crit Care Med. 2007;175(9):875–80.
48. Hamada K, Nagai S, Tanaka S, Handa T, Shigematsu M, Nagao T, et al. Significance of pulmonary arterial pressure and diffusion capacity of the lung as prognosticator in patients with idiopathic pulmonary fibrosis. Chest. 2007;131(3):650–6.
49. Charbeneau RP, Peters-Golden M. Eicosanoids: mediators and therapeutic targets in fibrotic lung disease. Clin Sci (Lond). 2005;108(6):479–91.

50. Richter A, Yeager ME, Zaiman A, Cool CD, Voelkel NF, Tuder RM. Impaired transforming growth factor-beta signaling in idiopathic pulmonary arterial hypertension. Am J Respir Crit Care Med. 2004;170(12):1340–8.
51. Wright L, Tuder RM, Wang J, Cool CD, Lepley RA, Voelkel NF. 5-Lipoxygenase and 5-lipoxygenase activating protein (FLAP) immunoreactivity in lungs from patients with primary pulmonary hypertension. Am J Respir Crit Care Med. 1998;157(1):219–29.
52. Weitzenblum E, Chaouat A. Sleep and chronic obstructive pulmonary disease. Sleep Med Rev. 2004;8(4):281–94.
53. Risk C, Epler GR, Gaensler EA. Exercise alveolar-arterial oxygen pressure difference in interstitial lung disease. Chest. 1984;85(1):69–74.
54. O'Donnell D. Physiology of interstitial lung disease. In: Schwarz MI, King TE, editors. Interstitial lung disease. Hamilton, ON: Marcel Dekker; 1998. p. 51–70.
55. Gottlieb D, Snider G. Lung function in pulmonary fibrosis. In: Phan S, Thrall R, editors. Lung biology in health and disease: pulmonary fibrosis. New York, NY: Marcel Dekker; 1995. p. 85–135.
56. Collard HR, King Jr TE, Bartelson BB, Vourlekis JS, Schwarz MI, Brown KK. Changes in clinical and physiologic variables predict survival in idiopathic pulmonary fibrosis. Am J Respir Crit Care Med. 2003;168(5):538–42.
57. Flaherty KR, Andrei AC, Murray S, Fraley C, Colby TV, Travis WD, et al. Idiopathic pulmonary fibrosis: prognostic value of changes in physiology and six-minute-walk test. Am J Respir Crit Care Med. 2006;174(7):803–9.
58. Lama VN, Flaherty KR, Toews GB, Colby TV, Travis WD, Long Q, et al. Prognostic value of desaturation during a 6-minute walk test in idiopathic interstitial pneumonia. Am J Respir Crit Care Med. 2003;168(9):1084–90.
59. Fell CD, Liu LX, Motika C, Kazerooni EA, Gross BH, Travis WD, et al. The prognostic value of cardiopulmonary exercise testing in idiopathic pulmonary fibrosis. Am J Respir Crit Care Med. 2009;179(5):402–7.
60. Latsi PI, du Bois RM, Nicholson AG, Colby TV, Bisirtzoglou D, Nikolakopoulou A, et al. Fibrotic idiopathic interstitial pneumonia: the prognostic value of longitudinal functional trends. Am J Respir Crit Care Med. 2003;168(5):531–7.
61. du Bois RM, Weycker D, Albera C, Bradford WZ, Costabel U, Kartashov A, et al. Six-minute-walk test in idiopathic pulmonary fibrosis: test validation and minimal clinically important difference. Am J Respir Crit Care Med. 2011;183(9):1231–7.
62. du Bois RM, Weycker D, Albera C, Bradford WZ, Costabel U, Kartashov A, et al. Ascertainment of individual risk of mortality for patients with idiopathic pulmonary fibrosis. Am J Respir Crit Care Med. 2011;184(4):459–66.
63. Flaherty KR, Mumford JA, Murray S, Kazerooni EA, Gross BH, Colby TV, et al. Prognostic implications of physiologic and radiographic changes in idiopathic interstitial pneumonia. Am J Respir Crit Care Med. 2003;168(5):543–8.
64. Jegal Y, Kim DS, Shim TS, Lim CM, Do Lee S, Koh Y, et al. Physiology is a stronger predictor of survival than pathology in fibrotic interstitial pneumonia. Am J Respir Crit Care Med. 2005;171(6):639–44.
65. Orens JB, Kazerooni EA, Martinez FJ, Curtis JL, Gross BH, Flint A, et al. The sensitivity of high-resolution CT in detecting idiopathic pulmonary fibrosis proved by open lung biopsy. A prospective study. Chest. 1995;108(1):109–15.
66. Hansell DM, Bankier AA, MacMahon H, McLoud TC, Muller NL, Remy J. Fleischner Society: glossary of terms for thoracic imaging. Radiology. 2008;246(3):697–722.
67. Akira M, Sakatani M, Ueda E. Idiopathic pulmonary fibrosis: progression of honeycombing at thin-section CT. Radiology. 1993;189(3):687–91.
68. Kazerooni EA, Martinez FJ, Flint A, Jamadar DA, Gross BH, Spizarny DL, et al. Thin-section CT obtained at 10-mm increments versus limited three-level thin-section CT for idiopathic pulmonary fibrosis: correlation with pathologic scoring. AJR Am J Roentgenol. 1997;169(4):977–83.

69. Lynch DA, Godwin JD, Safrin S, Starko KM, Hormel P, Brown KK, et al. High-resolution computed tomography in idiopathic pulmonary fibrosis: diagnosis and prognosis. Am J Respir Crit Care Med. 2005;172(4):488–93.
70. Travis WD, Hunninghake G, King Jr TE, Lynch DA, Colby TV, Galvin JR, et al. Idiopathic nonspecific interstitial pneumonia: report of an American Thoracic Society project. Am J Respir Crit Care Med. 2008;177(12):1338–47.
71. Flaherty KR, Thwaite EL, Kazerooni EA, Gross BH, Toews GB, Colby TV, et al. Radiological versus histological diagnosis in UIP and NSIP: survival implications. Thorax. 2003;58(2):143–8.
72. du Bois R, King Jr TE. Challenges in pulmonary fibrosis x 5: the NSIP/UIP debate. Thorax. 2007;62(11):1008–12.
73. Arakawa H, Honma K. Honeycomb lung: history and current concepts. AJR Am J Roentgenol. 2011;196(4):773–82.
74. American Thoracic Society. Idiopathic pulmonary fibrosis: diagnosis and treatment. International consensus statement. American Thoracic Society (ATS), and the European Respiratory Society (ERS). Am J Respir Crit Care Med. 2000;161(2 Pt 1):646–64.
75. Ohshimo S, Bonella F, Cui A, Beume M, Kohno N, Guzman J, et al. Significance of bronchoalveolar lavage for the diagnosis of idiopathic pulmonary fibrosis. Am J Respir Crit Care Med. 2009;179(11):1043–7.
76. Berbescu EA, Katzenstein AL, Snow JL, Zisman DA. Transbronchial biopsy in usual interstitial pneumonia. Chest. 2006;129(5):1126–31.
77. Shim HS, Park MS, Park IK. Histopathologic findings of transbronchial biopsy in usual interstitial pneumonia. Pathol Int. 2010;60(5):373–7.
78. Hunninghake GW, Zimmerman MB, Schwartz DA, King Jr TE, Lynch J, Hegele R, et al. Utility of a lung biopsy for the diagnosis of idiopathic pulmonary fibrosis. Am J Respir Crit Care Med. 2001;164(2):193–6.
79. Lettieri CJ, Veerappan GR, Helman DL, Mulligan CR, Shorr AF. Outcomes and safety of surgical lung biopsy for interstitial lung disease. Chest. 2005;127(5):1600–5.
80. Kreider ME, Hansen-Flaschen J, Ahmad NN, Rossman MD, Kaiser LR, Kucharczuk JC, et al. Complications of video-assisted thoracoscopic lung biopsy in patients with interstitial lung disease. Ann Thorac Surg. 2007;83(3):1140–4.
81. Canver CC, Mentzer Jr RM. The role of open lung biopsy in early and late survival of ventilator-dependent patients with diffuse idiopathic lung disease. J Cardiovasc Surg (Torino). 1994;35(2):151–5.
82. Hazelrigg SR, Nunchuck SK, LoCicero 3rd J. Video assisted thoracic surgery study group data. Ann Thorac Surg. 1993;56(5):1039–43 [discussion 43–4].
83. Nicod P, Moser KM. Primary pulmonary hypertension. The risk and benefit of lung biopsy. Circulation. 1989;80(5):1486–8.
84. Hunninghake GW, Lynch DA, Galvin JR, Gross BH, Muller N, Schwartz DA, et al. Radiologic findings are strongly associated with a pathologic diagnosis of usual interstitial pneumonia. Chest. 2003;124(4):1215–23.
85. Raghu G, Mageto YN, Lockhart D, Schmidt RA, Wood DE, Godwin JD. The accuracy of the clinical diagnosis of new-onset idiopathic pulmonary fibrosis and other interstitial lung disease: a prospective study. Chest. 1999;116(5):1168–74.
86. Park JH, Kim DK, Kim DS, Koh Y, Lee SD, Kim WS, et al. Mortality and risk factors for surgical lung biopsy in patients with idiopathic interstitial pneumonia. Eur J Cardiothorac Surg. 2007;31(6):1115–9.
87. Kadokura M, Colby TV, Myers JL, Allen MS, Deschamps C, Trastek VF, et al. Pathologic comparison of video-assisted thoracic surgical lung biopsy with traditional open lung biopsy. J Thorac Cardiovasc Surg. 1995;109(3):494–8.
88. Park JH, Kim DS, Park IN, Jang SJ, Kitaichi M, Nicholson AG, et al. Prognosis of fibrotic interstitial pneumonia: idiopathic versus collagen vascular disease-related subtypes. Am J Respir Crit Care Med. 2007;175(7):705–11.

89. Monaghan H, Wells AU, Colby TV, du Bois RM, Hansell DM, Nicholson AG. Prognostic implications of histologic patterns in multiple surgical lung biopsies from patients with idiopathic interstitial pneumonias. Chest. 2004;125(2):522–6.
90. Qureshi RA, Ahmed TA, Grayson AD, Soorae AS, Drakeley MJ, Page RD. Does lung biopsy help patients with interstitial lung disease? Eur J Cardiothorac Surg. 2002;21(4):621–6 [discussion 6].
91. Meyer EC, Liebow AA. Relationship of interstitial pneumonia honeycombing and atypical epithelial proliferation to cancer of the lung. Cancer. 1965;18:322–51.
92. Johkoh T, Muller NL, Colby TV, Ichikado K, Taniguchi H, Kondoh Y, et al. Nonspecific interstitial pneumonia: correlation between thin-section CT findings and pathologic subgroups in 55 patients. Radiology. 2002;225(1):199–204.
93. Katzenstein AL, Mukhopadhyay S, Zanardi C, Dexter E. Clinically occult interstitial fibrosis in smokers: classification and significance of a surprisingly common finding in lobectomy specimens. Hum Pathol. 2010;41(3):316–25.
94. Fraig M, Shreesha U, Savici D, Katzenstein AL. Respiratory bronchiolitis: a clinicopathologic study in current smokers, ex-smokers, and never-smokers. Am J Surg Pathol. 2002;26(5):647–53.
95. Pimentel JC. Tridimensional photographic reconstruction in a study of the pathogenesis of honeycomb lung. Thorax. 1967;22(5):444–52.
96. Flaherty KR, Colby TV, Travis WD, Toews GB, Mumford J, Murray S, et al. Fibroblastic foci in usual interstitial pneumonia: idiopathic versus collagen vascular disease. Am J Respir Crit Care Med. 2003;167(10):1410–5.
97. Nicholson AG, Addis BJ, Bharucha H, Clelland CA, Corrin B, Gibbs AR, et al. Inter-observer variation between pathologists in diffuse parenchymal lung disease. Thorax. 2004;59(6):500–5.
98. Katzenstein, AL, et al. Smoking-related interstitial fibrosis (SRIF), pathogenesis and treatment of usual interstitial pneumonia (UIP), and transbronchial biology in UIP. Mod Pathol. 2012;25 Suppl 1:S68–78.
99. Costabel U, Bonella F, Guzman J. Chronic hypersensitivity pneumonitis. Clin Chest Med. 2012;33(1):151–63.
100. Hanak V, Golbin JM, Hartman TE, Ryu JH. High-resolution CT findings of parenchymal fibrosis correlate with prognosis in hypersensitivity pneumonitis. Chest. 2008;134(1):133–8.
101. Sahin H, Brown KK, Curran-Everett D, Hale V, Cool CD, Vourlekis JS, et al. Chronic hypersensitivity pneumonitis: CT features comparison with pathologic evidence of fibrosis and survival. Radiology. 2007;244(2):591–8.
102. Kishi M, Miyazaki Y, Jinta T, Furusawa H, Ohtani Y, Inase N, et al. Pathogenesis of cBFL in common with IPF? Correlation of IP-10/TARC ratio with histological patterns. Thorax. 2008;63(9):810–6.
103. Coleman A, Colby TV. Histologic diagnosis of extrinsic allergic alveolitis. Am J Surg Pathol. 1988;12(7):514–8.
104. Churg A, Muller NL, Flint J, Wright JL. Chronic hypersensitivity pneumonitis. Am J Surg Pathol. 2006;30(2):201–8.
105. Lynch DA, Newell JD, Logan PM, King Jr TE, Muller NL. Can CT distinguish hypersensitivity pneumonitis from idiopathic pulmonary fibrosis? AJR Am J Roentgenol. 1995;165(4):807–11.
106. Silva CI, Muller NL, Lynch DA, Curran-Everett D, Brown KK, Lee KS, et al. Chronic hypersensitivity pneumonitis: differentiation from idiopathic pulmonary fibrosis and nonspecific interstitial pneumonia by using thin-section CT. Radiology. 2008;246(1):288–97.
107. Park JS, Lee KS, Kim JS, Park CS, Suh YL, Choi DL, et al. Nonspecific interstitial pneumonia with fibrosis: radiographic and CT findings in seven patients. Radiology. 1995;195(3):645–8.

108. Travis WD, Matsui K, Moss J, Ferrans VJ. Idiopathic nonspecific interstitial pneumonia: prognostic significance of cellular and fibrosing patterns: survival comparison with usual interstitial pneumonia and desquamative interstitial pneumonia. Am J Surg Pathol. 2000;24(1):19–33.

109. Kim DS, Yoo B, Lee JS, Kim EK, Lim CM, Lee SD, et al. The major histopathologic pattern of pulmonary fibrosis in scleroderma is nonspecific interstitial pneumonia. Sarcoidosis Vasc Diffuse Lung Dis. 2002;19(2):121–7.

110. Lee HK, Kim DS, Yoo B, Seo JB, Rho JY, Colby TV, et al. Histopathologic pattern and clinical features of rheumatoid arthritis-associated interstitial lung disease. Chest. 2005;127(6): 2019–27.

111. Kim EJ, Elicker BM, Maldonado F, Webb WR, Ryu JH, Van Uden JH, et al. Usual interstitial pneumonia in rheumatoid arthritis-associated interstitial lung disease. Eur Respir J. 2010;35(6):1322–8.

112. Gochuico BR, Avila NA, Chow CK, Novero LJ, Wu HP, Ren P, et al. Progressive preclinical interstitial lung disease in rheumatoid arthritis. Arch Intern Med. 2008;168(2):159–66.

113. Mori S, Cho I, Koga Y, Sugimoto M. A simultaneous onset of organizing pneumonia and rheumatoid arthritis, along with a review of the literature. Mod Rheumatol. 2008; 18(1):60–6.

114. Biederer J, Schnabel A, Muhle C, Gross WL, Heller M, Reuter M. Correlation between HRCT findings, pulmonary function tests and bronchoalveolar lavage cytology in interstitial lung disease associated with rheumatoid arthritis. Eur Radiol. 2004;14(2):272–80.

115. Garcia JG, James HL, Zinkgraf S, Perlman MB, Keogh BA. Lower respiratory tract abnormalities in rheumatoid interstitial lung disease. Potential role of neutrophils in lung injury. Am Rev Respir Dis. 1987;136(4):811–7.

116. Komocsi A, Kumanovics G, Zibotics H, Czirjak L. Alveolitis may persist during treatment that sufficiently controls muscle inflammation in myositis. Rheumatol Int. 2001;20(3): 113–8.

117. Nagasawa Y, Takada T, Shimizu T, Narita J, Moriyama H, Terada M, et al. Inflammatory cells in lung disease associated with rheumatoid arthritis. Intern Med. 2009;48(14):1209–17.

118. Costabel U, Guzman J, Bonella F, Oshimo S. Bronchoalveolar lavage in other interstitial lung diseases. Semin Respir Crit Care Med. 2007;28(5):514–24.

119. Ramirez P, Valencia M, Torres A. Bronchoalveolar lavage to diagnose respiratory infections. Semin Respir Crit Care Med. 2007;28(5):525–33.

120. Schnabel A, Richter C, Bauerfeind S, Gross WL. Bronchoalveolar lavage cell profile in methotrexate induced pneumonitis. Thorax. 1997;52(4):377–9.

121. Kim EJ, Collard HR, King Jr TE. Rheumatoid arthritis-associated interstitial lung disease: the relevance of histopathologic and radiographic pattern. Chest. 2009;136(5):1397–405.

122. Dawson JK, Fewins HE, Desmond J, Lynch MP, Graham DR. Predictors of progression of HRCT diagnosed fibrosing alveolitis in patients with rheumatoid arthritis. Ann Rheum Dis. 2002;61(6):517–21.

123. Stack BH, Grant IW. Rheumatoid interstitial lung disease. Br J Dis Chest. 1965;59(4): 202–11.

124. Kocheril SV, Appleton BE, Somers EC, Kazerooni EA, Flaherty KR, Martinez FJ, et al. Comparison of disease progression and mortality of connective tissue disease-related interstitial lung disease and idiopathic interstitial pneumonia. Arthritis Rheum. 2005;53(4):549–57.

125. Kligerman SJ, Groshong S, Brown KK, Lynch DA. Nonspecific interstitial pneumonia: radiologic, clinical, and pathologic considerations. Radiographics. 2009;29(1):73–87.

126. Leslie KO, Trahan S, Gruden J. Pulmonary pathology of the rheumatic diseases. Semin Respir Crit Care Med. 2007;28(4):369–78.

127. Douglas WW, Tazelaar HD, Hartman TE, Hartman RP, Decker PA, Schroeder DR, et al. Polymyositis-dermatomyositis-associated interstitial lung disease. Am J Respir Crit Care Med. 2001;164(7):1182–5.

128. Tansey D, Wells AU, Colby TV, Ip S, Nikolakoupolou A, du Bois RM, et al. Variations in histological patterns of interstitial pneumonia between connective tissue disorders and their relationship to prognosis. Histopathology. 2004;44(6):585–96.

129. Shelton DN, Chang E, Whittier PS, Choi D, Funk WD. Microarray analysis of replicative senescence. Curr Biol. 1999;9(17):939–45.
130. Castriotta RJ, Eldadah BA, Foster WM, Halter JB, Hazzard WR, Kiley JP, et al. Workshop on idiopathic pulmonary fibrosis in older adults. Chest. 2010;138(3):693–703.
131. Sakamoto K, Taniguchi H, Kondoh Y, Wakai K, Kimura T, Kataoka K, et al. Acute exacerbation of IPF following diagnostic bronchoalveolar lavage procedures. Respir Med. 2012;106(3):436–42.
132. Aziz ZA, Wells AU, Hansell DM, Bain GA, Copley SJ, Desai SR, et al. HRCT diagnosis of diffuse parenchymal lung disease: inter-observer variation. Thorax. 2004;59(6):506–11.
133. Flaherty KR, King Jr TE, Raghu G, Lynch 3rd JP, Colby TV, Travis WD, et al. Idiopathic interstitial pneumonia: what is the effect of a multidisciplinary approach to diagnosis? Am J Respir Crit Care Med. 2004;170(8):904–10.
134. Flaherty KR, Andrei AC, King Jr TE, Raghu G, Colby TV, Wells A, et al. Idiopathic interstitial pneumonia: do community and academic physicians agree on diagnosis? Am J Respir Crit Care Med. 2007;175(10):1054–60.
135. Selman M, Pardo A, Barrera L, Estrada A, Watson SR, Wilson K, et al. Gene expression profiles distinguish idiopathic pulmonary fibrosis from hypersensitivity pneumonitis. Am J Respir Crit Care Med. 2006;173(2):188–98.
136. Trujillo G, Meneghin A, Flaherty KR, Sholl LM, Myers JL, Kazerooni EA, et al. TLR9 differentiates rapidly from slowly progressing forms of idiopathic pulmonary fibrosis. Sci Transl Med. 2010;2(57):57ra82.

# Chapter 6
# Pulmonary Function Tests in Idiopathic Pulmonary Fibrosis

**Athol U. Wells and Simon Ward**

**Abstract** It is generally acknowledged that in interstitial lung disease (ILD), pulmonary function tests (PFTs) reflect the histologic severity of disease more closely than plain chest radiography or symptoms [1]. It is not known whether PFTs are more accurate than high-resolution computed tomography (HRCT) in this regard, but the exact quantification of the morphologic extent of disease on HRCT is not practicable in routine practice. Thus, the measurement of PFT has been central to the evaluation of disease severity in ILD in general and in idiopathic pulmonary fibrosis (IPF) in particular.

The primary roles of PFT estimation in IPF have been to quantify disease at baseline (both as continuous variables and in disease staging) and to detect changes in disease severity during follow-up. Also covered in this chapter are the ancillary uses of PFT to detect the presence of disease and the range of patterns of functional impairment in IPF (including the deconstruction of complex PFT impairment due to coexistent disease processes). Exercise testing, quality assurance, and the performance of fitness-to-fly tests are also reviewed.

**Keywords** Pulmonary function tests • Lung restriction • Severity • Progression • Pulmonary hypertension • Quality assurance • Fitness to fly

A.U. Wells, M.D. (✉)
Interstitial Lung Disease Unit, Royal Brompton Hospital, Emmanuel Kaye Building, Manresa Rd., Chelsea, London, SW3 6LR, UK
e-mail: Athol.Wells@rbht.nhs.uk

S. Ward, B.Sc., Hons.
Lung Function Unit, Royal Brompton and Harefield NHS Trust, London, UK

K.C. Meyer and S.D. Nathan (eds.), *Idiopathic Pulmonary Fibrosis: A Comprehensive Clinical Guide*, Respiratory Medicine 9, DOI 10.1007/978-1-62703-682-5_6, © Springer Science+Business Media New York 2014

# Introduction

It is generally acknowledged that in ILD, PFTs reflect the histologic severity of disease more closely than plain chest radiography or symptoms [1]. It is not known whether PFTs are more accurate than HRCT in this regard, but the exact quantification of the morphologic extent of disease on HRCT is difficult to incorporate into routine practice. Thus, the measurement of PFT has been central to the evaluation of disease severity in ILD in general and in IPF in particular.

In the last century, attempts were made to link the level of impairment of individual PFT (including exercise variables) to the histological severity of inflammation in surgical biopsy specimens. At that time, the term "idiopathic pulmonary fibrosis" was an umbrella term that included IPF, nonspecific interstitial pneumonia (NSIP), and other disorders mimicking IPF in non-biopsied patients. In this context, best management was hampered by the absence of a reliable, noninvasive marker for reversible disease. In historical reports, correlations of lung function with histopathology were examined in small patient series containing a variety of diffuse lung disorders, which lead to conflicting findings that included the identification of a significant relationship between the severity of inflammation at biopsy and maximum exercise data in one report [2]. This finding led some experts to argue for routine maximal exercise testing in the evaluation of ILD. However, it was eventually shown in a large study of IPF (which at that time must also have included patients with NSIP) that PFT provided no useful link to the histologic severity of inflammation [3]. In contrast, significant relationships were observed between PFT and the overall morphologic severity of disease with carbon monoxide diffusing capacity (DLCO) levels being most accurate in this regard.

Since these early studies, the primary roles of PFT estimation in IPF have been to quantify disease at baseline (both as continuous variables and in disease staging) and to detect changes in disease severity during follow-up. Also covered in this chapter are the ancillary uses of PFT to detect the presence of disease and the range of patterns of functional impairment in IPF (including the deconstruction of complex PFT impairment due to coexistent disease processes). Exercise testing, quality assurance, and the performance of fitness-to-fly tests are also reviewed. A glossary of abbreviations for PFT is provided in Table 6.1.

Table 6.1 A glossary of abbreviations for routine pulmonary function variables

| | |
|---|---|
| $FEV_1$ | Forced expiratory volume in 1 s |
| FVC | Forced vital capacity |
| TLC | Total lung capacity |
| RV | Residual volume |
| VA | Alveolar volume |
| DLCO | Carbon monoxide diffusing capacity |
| KCO | Carbon monoxide transfer coefficient |
| MEF25 | Maximum expiratory flow at 25 % forced vital capacity |

# PFT in "Early" IPF

In cases of IPFs that are sufficiently advanced to cause major exercise limitation, HRCT and PFT abnormalities are almost always evident. The earlier detection of "preclinical" IPF, by screening with PFT, is not a realistic goal, in view of the low prevalence of IPF in the community. However, in occasional patients with smoking-related chronic obstructive pulmonary disease (COPD), coexistent ILD can result in concurrent obstruction and restriction. Thus, in the setting of otherwise typical COPD, the presence of an unexplained mixed ventilatory defect is an indication for the performance of HRCT (as limited IPF is not always evident on chest radiography).

A more frequent clinical scenario occurs when patients with minor exercise limitation (which may also be ascribable to cardiac disease or loss of fitness) are evaluated in the context of normal or subtle chest radiographic abnormalities. Spirometric volumes are often used as a screening test in such situations to determine whether further investigation, including the performance of HRCT, is warranted. However, this algorithm is sometimes misleading for two reasons. First, expected PFT values in health, calculated from age, gender, and height, are expressed as a normal range (80–120 % of predicted values). It follows logically that in an individual patient, an FVC level of 80 % of predicted might equally represent a normal lung function value or a striking reduction in FVC from a premorbid value of 120 % of predicted. A second important consideration is the fact that when emphysema coexists with IPF, spirometric volumes may be preserved, even when IPF is more advanced (as discussed in more detail later in this chapter).

Thus, the detection of early IPF should not be based on the performance of spirometry to obtain lung volumes but requires more detailed evaluation that includes the measurement of DLCO levels and the performance of HRCT. It should be stressed that the greater sensitivity of DLCO (compared to spirometric volumes) can sometimes lead to difficulties. While normal DLCO levels effectively exclude the presence of clinically significant IPF, reductions in this parameter are not necessarily indicative of the presence of ILD [4]. Reductions in the DLCO tend to be highly nonspecific and may be influenced by interstitial processes, pulmonary vasculopathies, and smoking-related damage alike. Thus, PFTs are useful in the exclusion of an occult ILD when spirometric volumes and DLCO levels are well within normal limits, but HRCT is warranted if PFT values lie at the lower limit of normal and no alternative cause of exercise limitation is apparent.

# Typical Patterns of Pulmonary Function Impairment

Variations in the pattern of pulmonary function impairment in patients with IPF reflect the presence or absence of concurrent disorders including pulmonary hypertension (PH) and smoking-related emphysema. Commonly encountered PFT patterns include a classical restrictive defect, a mixed (restriction plus airflow obstruction) ventilatory defect, and an isolated or disproportionate reduction in measures of gas transfer.

A *restrictive ventilatory defect* (reduced TLC and FVC, increased $FEV_1$/FVC ratio) is the most prevalent PFT pattern in IPF (and other idiopathic interstitial pneumonias), in association with a reduction in the DLCO [5], which is usually significantly more impaired than the fall in lung volumes. Arterial hypoxemia in IPF tends to be a feature of advanced disease (as judged by the extent of disease on HRCT) [6]. In earlier stages of the disease, arterial blood gases typically show preservation of $pO_2$ levels with $pCO_2$ levels in the lower end of the normal range, indicating an increase in alveolar ventilation that may initially mask any impairment in gas exchange. Hypoxemia in the setting of less advanced IPF suggests the presence of coexisting PH or emphysema. The alveolar-arterial oxygen gradient, which removes the confounding effect of changes in the level of alveolar ventilation, widens earlier in the course of disease.

The typical restrictive ventilatory defect of IPF is indistinguishable from that of extra-pulmonic restriction [7], although in pleural disease, relative preservation of RV (as judged by an increased RV/TLC ratio) is often present [8]. However, in isolated extra-pulmonic restriction, DLCO levels are reduced minimally and the DLCO/VA ratio (KCO) increases, often manifesting with supranormal values [9]. This is due to the relatively small change in blood volume within ventilated lung, even when extra-pulmonic restriction is severe.

An *isolated reduction in DLCO* is also a prevalent PFT pattern in IPF, reflecting the presence of coexistent emphysema, which is frequently evident on HRCT and was found to be present in nearly 40 % of patients in one large series [6]. The presence of interstitial fibrosis increases traction on airways, which counters the collapse of small airways that is the hallmark of emphysema (without parenchymal fibrosis) and leads to preserved ventilation of emphysematous lung. Thus, the coexistence of emphysema and IPF results in a sparing effect on spirometric and plethysmographic volumes [10, 11], which, in many cases, lie within the normal range, even when both processes are advanced. By contrast, the additive effect on measures of gas transfer and $pO_2$ levels (which are influenced by both processes) results in disproportionate reductions that may be devastatingly severe, even when lung volumes are misleadingly normal. It has been argued that the high prevalence of PH in this setting justifies the designation of a separate "combined pulmonary fibrosis and emphysema" syndrome, although it is currently unclear whether the excess of PH merely reflects the combined total impact of two separate disease processes. This smoking-related PFT phenotype [10] may result in either an isolated or a disproportionate reduction in DLCO, which can be quantified by a reduction in KCO or a rise in the FVC/DLCO ratio. In one series, the presence of emphysema on HRCT was associated with a 35 % reduction in KCO after matching for the extent of fibrosis on HRCT [10].

A disproportionate reduction in DLCO is not solely due to the combination of emphysema and fibrosis but can also be found in IPF patients with PH (with or without emphysema on CT). Thus, a low KCO level or a high FVC/DLCO ratio should be interpreted with caution, and the HRCT should be carefully reviewed for the presence of emphysema. In the absence of emphysema, this PFT profile should prompt the clinician to exclude PH. The role of PFT as an aid to the detection of PH in IPF is discussed in greater detail later in this chapter.

Patterns of pulmonary function impairment are seldom diagnostically useful in suspected IPF. The exception to this rule is the presence of a mixed ventilatory defect in a nonsmoker or a smoker with no evidence of emphysema on HRCT, as this may be seen in some patients with hypersensitivity pneumonitis or rheumatoid lung. In both disorders, HRCT appearances may mimic IPF, and a histologic pattern of usual interstitial pneumonia is sometimes present. Thus, the presence of unexplained coexistent airflow obstruction and restriction should prompt a review of the diagnosis of IPF.

## Baseline PFT: Disease Severity and Prognostic Evaluation

Key conclusions with regard to the quantification of disease severity and prognostic evaluation are shown in Table 6.2.

In ILD in general, and in IPF in particular, the measurement of pulmonary function has a central role in the initial evaluation and serves to quantify the severity of disease. Indeed, many PFT variables are routinely measurable, including spirometric volumes ($FEV_1$, FVC, the $FEV_1$/FVC ratio), plethysmographic volumes (RV, TLC, the RV/TLC ratio), measures of gas transfer (DLCO, KCO), measures of gas exchange ($pO_2$, the alveolar-arterial oxygen gradient), the 6-minute walk test (6MWT; 6-minute walk distance [6MWD] and maximal desaturation during the 6-minute walk test), and maximal exercise variables. The multiplicity of PFT has stimulated attempts to identify variables that most accurately capture disease severity and predict mortality.

Historical attempts to identify the pulmonary function variable that correlates best with the histological severity of disease at surgical biopsy were hampered by "sampling error," since the severity of disease in biopsy specimens is not necessarily indicative of disease severity throughout the lung. Given this fact, it is not surprising that even in the relatively large series of Cherniack [3], functional-histologic relationships were weak. In that study, DLCO levels (which best reflect histologic findings) accounted for only 15 % of the variation in histologic severity. However, the advent of HRCT provided, for the first time, a means of quantifying the global morphologic severity of IPF, against which individual pulmonary function variables could be evaluated. It should be stressed that in the absence of an alternative measure of overall morphologic severity, the extent of disease on HRCT has not been validated as a reference standard. Methods of measuring disease extent on HRCT have varied, and the subjective estimation of disease extent is prone to observer variation, which is of the same order of magnitude as the measurement of DLCO. The advantage of PFT–HRCT correlations is that *independent* measures of global extent and global severity are reconciled. Those working in this field have argued that despite flaws in the quantification of both disease severity and extent, the PFT variable most accurately capturing disease severity should best correlate

**Table 6.2** Key points in the use of PFT to stage disease severity

1. DLCO levels best reflect CT morphologic severity
2. Lung volumes and arterial oxygen levels correlate poorly with CT morphologic severity
3. DLCO is the resting PFT variable that best predicts mortality
4. Oxygen desaturation to <88 % during a 6-minute walk test is associated with increased mortality
5. Maximal exercise testing has no role in routine prognostic evaluation

with HRCT as the only sensitive means of quantifying global morphologic extent of disease.

PFT–HRCT correlations have largely been explored in the context of the historical entity of "IPF" [10, 12, 13] before the idiopathic interstitial pneumonias were reclassified in 2002. However, the findings in earlier series have been reproduced in a large cohort of patients with IPF who were diagnosed using the 2002 diagnostic criteria [4]. PFT–HRCT correlations were virtually identical when patients with IPF were compared with systemic sclerosis patients with ILD (predominantly NSIP) [14], suggesting that these observations are likely to hold true across the fibrotic idiopathic interstitial pneumonias.

Based on published series, DLCO levels have a stronger correlation with the extent of disease on HRCT than other resting PFT variables. Lung volumes, including FVC and TLC, are an inaccurate reflection of the morphologic extent of disease. It is clear from these observations that the morphologic severity of disease in IPF is not captured by spirometric volumes but requires the measurement of DLCO. However, spirometric volumes and DLCO levels are independently linked to the extent of disease on HRCT [4], with the clear implication being that these variables should be integrated when disease severity is evaluated. The reconciliation of spirometric volumes and DLCO is particularly important in patients with coexistent emphysema and IPF, a context in which the severity of IPF is seriously understated by spirometric measures but is overstated by DLCO levels.

Arterial hypoxemia at rest is an expected finding in IPF patients with extensive disease on HRCT [4]. However, there is a poor correlation between arterial oxygen levels and disease extent when less extensive disease is present, and the presence of hypoxemia is unpredictable in less advanced disease. This finding may reflect the fact that the presence of PH as a potent cause of impaired gas exchange is not closely linked to other PFT and HRCT findings in IPF.

Many clinicians strongly advocated maximal exercise testing as a means of evaluating the severity of pulmonary fibrosis prior to our current era. However, the level of desaturation during exercise has a weaker correlation with disease extent on HRCT than DLCO levels in patients with IPF, even with adjustment for maximum oxygen consumption [10]. The relationships between HRCT disease extent and submaximal exercise variables, including 6MWT data, have not been compared with those between HRCT and maximal exercise testing.

Taken together, histologic and HRCT data indicate that DLCO levels best reflect the morphologic severity of IPF, but it should again be stressed that the optimal

level of 35 %), a 6MWD of <72 % of predicted, and a Medical Research Council dyspnea score of >3 units [29]. This modification of severity staging with the use of exercise data represents an innovative approach that may help to overcome inaccuracies resulting from variations in premorbid values. However, further validation is required before such a staging system can be advocated in routine evaluation.

## PFT in the Monitoring of Change over Time

Key points in the use of PFT to monitor change in disease severity in IPF are presented in Table 6.3.

The fact that the most accurate discriminatory variables are not always the most desirable evaluative tests is a universally acknowledged truism. The PFT variables that are most helpful in quantifying disease severity at a single point in time are not necessarily the most accurate variables in detecting serial change. As discussed earlier, FVC levels have a poor correlation with the extent of disease on HRCT in IPF and are confounded by the presence of concurrent emphysema. However, changes in disease severity are more accurately captured by FVC trends than by serial DLCO data (although no comparison has been made between FVC and other lung volumes including slow VC). This conclusion has been distilled from a large number of IPF studies in which PFT trends at 6 months or 1 year have been examined against survival [25, 27, 28, 30–38]. In all these series, subsequent mortality has been substantially higher in patients with a "significant" decline in FVC values (although FVC thresholds for significant change have varied between studies). In all but one series, serial FVC trends have provided more accurate prognostic information than serial DLCO trends. The advantage of FVC over DLCO in this regard is due, in part, to the inherently greater variability in the measurement of the DLCO. As discussed later, the minimization of "drift" in DLCO estimation requires the calibration of lung function equipment daily against normal biological controls, but this level of quality assurance is seldom achievable in busy pulmonary function laboratories.

The optimal threshold that should be regarded as a "significant" change in FVC remains uncertain. Both in clinical practice and in some published studies, there is often a lack of clarity on whether a 10 % change in FVC denotes a 10 % change from baseline values (e.g., a fall in FVC from 2.0 to 1.8 L) or a 10 % change in predicted normal values (e.g., a fall from 60 to 50 % of predicted). The latter is often referred to as an "absolute change" because the threshold for change is independent of baseline values. Confusingly, the term "absolute change" has also been used to indicate a change in absolute baseline values (e.g., a 10 % reduction in FVC from 2.0 to 1.8 L, as opposed to a fall from 40 to 36 % of predicted) [17].

Relative change from baseline values [25, 30, 32–36] has historically been used most often rather than absolute change [27, 28, 31]. In a recent study, it was established that the two approaches provide equivalent prognostic significance, although relative change is substantially more sensitive [37]. It is important to recognize that thresholds for "significant" PFT change (a 10 % change from baseline FVC, a 15 %

**Table 6.3** Key points in the use of PFT to monitor change in disease severity in idiopathic pulmonary fibrosis

| |
|---|
| 1.  Serial FVC trends predict mortality better than trends in other PFT |
| 2.  "Significant" change is defined as a 10 % change in FVC or a 15 % change in DLCO, from *baseline* values |
| 3.  FVC and DLCO levels should both be measured, to improve the accuracy of monitoring |
| 4.  Serial DLCO trends are more sensitive to change than serial FVC trends in patients who desaturate below 88 % during a 6-minute walk test and when emphysema is admixed with interstitial fibrosis |
| 5.  6-minute walk testing may have a role in monitoring for the need for supplemental oxygen, as a predictor of complicating PH, as well as the timing for referral for lung transplant consideration |

change from baseline DLCO) are based on reproducibility data. Short-term changes in PFT values from baseline should be calculated from absolute measured values rather than percentage predicted levels (which are modified depending upon whether the timing of patient birthdays lies within or outside the monitored time period). The use of a 10 % FVC threshold for change is based on the fact that when FVC measurements are repeated at a short time interval, whether in health or disease, FVC values differ by less than 10 % between measurements in 95 % of subjects (i.e., the 10 % threshold corresponds to two standard deviations of change). This statement captures variability at both initial and follow-up measurements. The greater inherent variability in DLCO estimation demands a higher DLCO threshold for "significant" change of 15 % from baseline values. With rigorous quality assurance in the PFT laboratory, albeit at a level that is seldom realistic, measurement variation can be reduced. However, in routine practice as well as in large multicenter pharmaceutical trials, these thresholds remain appropriate.

Further confusion has arisen from the term "significant," which is used to define thresholds for PFT change. Measurement variation can equally result in an overstatement or an understatement of change. A measured change in FVC of 10 % from baseline in an individual represents, in reality, a true change of between 1 and 19 %, which represents a change that ranges from the trivial to the substantial. Thus, a change of this magnitude is not necessarily indicative of a clinically significant alteration in disease severity in a given individual but merely establishes that such change is almost certainly real and is unlikely to be ascribable to measurement variation.

Unfortunately, thresholds for change to deal with the problem of PFT measurement variation have been erroneously applied to the evaluation of average serial PFT change in a patient cohort. For example, it has been argued that for a treatment to be regarded as clinically beneficial, an average FVC benefit of 10 % is required and corresponds to significant change [38]. However, average PFT change in a patient cohort is not influenced by measurement variation (as the overstatement and understatement of change in individual patients is equally prevalent). In this context, the use of thresholds for change (that were initially promulgated to exclude measurement variation in individual patients) is misdirected and, therefore, may be erroneous.

Thus, traditional thresholds for "significant" PFT change in individual patients serve only to establish that change is real. Lesser change (e.g., a 5–10 % change in FVC) is moderately likely to denote real change and has also been shown to predict a worse average outcome in several studies [27, 36, 37]. However, measurement variation cannot be excluded with the same confidence as an explanation for a change of this amplitude in an individual patient. It is partly for this reason that it has been recommended that serial measurements of both FVC and DLCO should be made during routine monitoring [17]. By evaluating PFT change using separate measurement techniques, the clinician is often able to conclude that a trend common to both FVC and DLCO, perhaps associated with concordant symptomatic change, is unlikely to be spurious, even when such changes are marginal (e.g., a 9 % decline in FVC and a 13 % change in DLCO). Furthermore, the understatement of FVC change due to measurement variation can be recognized when there is a more striking change in DLCO (e.g., a 7 % decline in FVC and a 17 % decline in DLCO). When a "significant" decline is evident in both FVC and DLCO, progression of disease can be identified with confidence, even when symptoms are stable.

In IPF, it is not useful to repeat pulmonary function tests more frequently than every 3 months in the absence of a clinical indication such as increasing dyspnea, as there is insufficient time for pulmonary function trends to reach thresholds for change. In clinical practice, the FVC and DLCO should be monitored every 3–6 months, with the exact time interval dependent on the likelihood that observation of a decline will lead to a change in management (such as referral for lung transplantation). The exception to this recommendation is the scenario in which significant decline may be ascribable to a cause other than disease progression (usually lower respiratory tract infection), and early demonstration of a return to baseline values is clinically important.

As discussed earlier, the coexistence of emphysema and IPF results in a paradoxical preservation of lung volumes and a disproportionate reduction in the DLCO. Therefore, serial FVC trends may sometimes be insensitive to major disease progression due to the unpredictable confounding effects of emphysema on serial spirometric volumes. In a recent study, it was shown that when emphysema coexists with IPF, serial $FEV_1$ trends are more closely related than serial FVC trends to subsequent mortality [35], while in some patients, serial reductions in DLCO may be more sensitive. However, in many patients with advanced IPF, the extent of fibrosis greatly exceeds that of emphysema, and FVC levels can be used to monitor progression. On the other end of the spectrum, when spirometric volumes are minimally reduced or lie within the normal range, serial DLCO trends should probably be given more weight. Based on these foregoing considerations, it can be concluded that trends in $FEV_1$, FVC, and DLCO should all be considered and reconciled in the monitoring of IPF patients with concurrent emphysema.

Despite its widespread use in the last century, there is no evidence that serial maximal exercise testing provides useful prognostic information in IPF, perhaps because of the associated poor reproducibility of this test. The 6MWD is highly reproducible in the short term in fibrotic idiopathic interstitial pneumonia [18] and in pulmonary fibrosis in patients with systemic sclerosis [39]. However, in the longer term, major changes in the 6MWD may occur due to other factors, such as deconditioning or musculoskeletal factors, as well as the salutary effects of pulmonary rehabilitation. In IPF treatment trials, striking changes in both directions are apparent at 1 year in the absence of change in PFT or other specific measures of the severity of pulmonary fibrosis [40, 41]. It is not clear whether large declines in the 6MWD, which have been shown to have prognostic significance [42, 43], add utility to the information obtained from routine monitoring that reflects progression of fibrosis [17]. However, using serial 6MWTs may be useful in decision making with regard to referral for lung transplantation or increasing the index of suspicion for underlying PH (oxygen desaturation, reduced pulse rate recovery), and the 6MWT can provide guidance with regard to the need for ambulatory oxygen therapy.

## Pulmonary Function Tests in the Detection of Pulmonary Hypertension

The detection of PH in patients with IPF causes particular clinical difficulty, as the echocardiogram often significantly overstates the pulmonary artery systolic pressure value. The pattern of PFT impairment provides ancillary information that, although it is not definitive, may heighten the suspicion for the presence of PH and thus reduce the threshold for performing a diagnostic right heart catheterization study. The severity of pulmonary fibrosis, as judged by spirometric and plethysmographic lung volumes, differs little between IPF patients with or without PH [44]. However, as in PAH [45], a reduction in the DLCO that is disproportionate to lung volumes should prompt suspicion that PH is present, although no consistently reliable diagnostic threshold has been identified. Historically, disproportionate reductions in DLCO have been quantified as reductions in KCO levels (the DLCO/VA ratio). More recently, an increase in the FVC/DLCO ratio [46, 47] has been preferred, but the logic of this change can be questioned. Disproportionate hypoxemia at rest or on exercise is another feature of PH in IPF. Both the DLCO and $pO_2$ levels are lower in IPF patients with PH [44], and the presence of PH can be predicted with reasonable accuracy by a formula containing the FVC, DLCO, and room air oxygen saturation [48].

However, a prevailing difficulty in the detection of evolving PH is that PFT measurements may be suggestive of pulmonary vascular limitation long before there is sufficient loss of pulmonary vascular reserve to give rise to clinically evident PH. Evidence of increasing pulmonary vasculopathy on serial PFT is of major prognostic significance in IPF. In patients with desaturation to 88 % during a 6MWT, serial DLCO decline predicts mortality more strongly than reductions in FVC levels [42]. Similarly, serial reductions in KCO (which occur too rapidly to be ascribable to emphysema) have been associated with striking increases in mortality [33, 34]. A "pulmonary vascular index" has been constructed based on these observations, although it should be stressed that this provides evidence of declining pulmonary vascular reserve and is not specific to PH per se [34].

## PFT Quality Control and Quality Assurance

Quality control and quality assurance protocols in lung function laboratories are essential to minimize measurement variability and guarantee technical accuracy [49, 50]. Rigor in this regard is central to the accurate use of PFT threshold values to designate "significant" change. The ATS/ERS standards provide guidance on quality control and quality procedures relevant to the performance of routine PFT and include recommendations on the calibration and verification of equipment.

The acquisition of biological control data is essential [51–54]. Trends in PFT performed by "normal" staff members should be analyzed frequently. Equipment malfunction, which may not be disclosed by routine calibration, is readily detected by this means. In some PFT laboratories (including our own institution), PFT are measured by staff members at the start of every working day with the recalibration of equipment as necessary. The value of this approach is reinforced by our own experience, especially in the estimation of gas transfer variables, which is notoriously more variable than the measurement of lung volumes. In reality, this demanding requirement cannot always be satisfied in routine practice, but, at the least, the weekly acquisition of biological control data is highly desirable. This recommendation is more stringent than recommendations made in some guideline statements. However, the requirement in some IPF pharmaceutical trials for the monthly evaluation of biological control data is, in our view, insufficiently rigorous given that FVC and DLCO trends, which are often designated as primary or co-primary end points, are measured across many PFT laboratories in multicenter studies.

A coefficient of variation ([standard deviation/mean] $\times$ 100) of more than 4–8 % is unacceptable [52]. In well-managed PFT laboratories, the rigorous monitoring of performance, quality assurance, quality control, and test results allows a coefficient of variation of 2–4 % to be achieved for spirometric volumes, total lung capacity, and measures of gas transfer. The variability of maximum expiratory flow at 25 % of FVC ($MEF_{25}$) and RV is significantly higher than that of other routine variables. $MEF_{25}$ values are generally low (less than 2 L/s), which increases relative measurement "noise" and the corresponding coefficient of variation. The RV is calculated from two measured variables (functional residual capacity and expiratory reserve volume), which also results in an increased coefficient of variation. Neither variable is suited to the detection of PFT change in treatment trials or in routine clinical practice.

Variability between laboratories is often overlooked when PFTs are compared to those previously performed elsewhere. When rigorous quality assurance is performed at both laboratory facilities, discrepancies in FVC values will be minimized. By contrast, DLCO values are notoriously inconsistent (even when quality assurance is impeccable) due to the many technical variations that exist in gas transfer measurement. When spirometric volumes are stable, the accuracy of major gas transfer trends between laboratories should be viewed with suspicion (although it must also be remembered that isolated reductions in gas transfer changes may denote worsening pulmonary vasculopathy).

## Fitness-to-Fly Tests

A hypoxic inhalation test should be performed in patients with minor hypoxemia who wish to travel by air. The impact of the inverse relationship between oxygen partial pressure and altitude can be evaluated by measuring hypobaric hypoxemia at sea level, which captures the effect of decreases in ambient pressure in a pressurized aircraft cabin. Due to engineering and financial constraints, sea-level pressurization cannot be maintained: the pressurization of an aircraft cabin to an equivalent maximum altitude of 2,500 m equates to breathing 15 % oxygen at sea level [55]. In normal individuals, falls of 8–10 kPa ($SpO_2$ 90–94 %) can be expected at this altitude, but the partial pressure of oxygen in arterial blood ($PaO_2$) is surprisingly variable and only partially explained by variations in age and minute ventilation [56, 57]. In patients with respiratory disease, a low threshold for performing preflight assessments is appropriate, especially in those with severe lung function impairment and major exercise intolerance [58, 59].

Data acquired in hypobaric chambers, the referred standard for preflight assessment, are seldom practicable due to the associated expense. Predictive equations based on PFT at sea level will often considerably overestimate the need for in-flight oxygen [60]. Furthermore, these have not been validated in IPF and may be confounded by the presence of coexisting PH. The hypoxic inhalation test is the preferred alternative procedure. Cabin pressure at altitude is simulated by the inhalation of a gas mixture containing 15 % oxygen in nitrogen for 20 min, and ECG and oxygen saturation should be monitored throughout and the arterial gases measured at the end of the test. The flow rate of supplemental oxygen required to restore oxygen saturation to an adequate level is then established. An important caveat is that hypoxemia may be masked by short-term hyperventilation during the test; thus, a decline in $PaCO_2$ levels should be taken into account, especially in patients wishing to undertake prolonged flights.

## References

1. Keogh BA, Crystal RG. Pulmonary function testing in interstitial pulmonary disease. What does it tell us? Chest. 1980;78:856–964.
2. Fulmer JD, Roberts WC, Von Gal ER, Crystal RG. Morphologic-physiologic correlates of the severity of fibrosis and degree of cellularity in idiopathic pulmonary fibrosis. J Clin Invest. 1979;63:665–76.
3. Cherniack RM, Colby TV, Flint A, Thurlbeck WM, Waldron Jr JA, Ackerson L, et al. Correlation of structure and function in idiopathic pulmonary fibrosis. Am J Respir Crit Care Med. 1995;151:1180–8.
4. Wells AU. Pulmonary function tests in connective tissue disease. Semin Respir Crit Care Med. 2007;28:379–88.
5. Gibson GJ. Clinical tests of respiratory function. London: Chappell and Hall; 1996. p. 223–4.
6. Wells AU, Desai SR, Rubens MB, Goh NS, Cramer D, Nicholson AG, et al. Idiopathic pulmonary fibrosis: a composite physiologic index derived from disease extent observed on computed tomography. Am J Respir Crit Care Med. 2003;167:962–9.

7. Broderich A, Fuortes LJ, Merchant JA, Galvin JR, Shwartz DA. Pleural determinants of restrictive lung function and respiratory symptoms in an asbestos-exposed population. Chest. 1992;101:684–91.
8. Colp C, Reichel J, Park SS. Severe pleural restriction: the maximum static pulmonary recoil pressure as an aide in diagnosis. Chest. 1975;67:658–64.
9. Wright PH, Hansen A, Kreel L, Capel LH. Respiratory function changes after asbestos pleurisy. Thorax. 1980;35:31–6.
10. Wells AU, King AD, Rubens MB, Cramer D, du Bois RM, Hansell DM. Lone CFA: a functional-morphological correlation based on extent of disease on thin-section computed tomography. Am J Respir Crit Care Med. 1997;155:1367–75.
11. Mura M, Zompatori M, Pacilli AM, Fasano L, Schiavina M, Fabbri M. The presence of emphysema further impairs physiologic function in patients with idiopathic pulmonary fibrosis. Respir Care. 2006;51:257–65.
12. Staples CA, Muller NL, Vedal S, Abboud R, Ostrow DN, Miller RR. Usual interstitial pneumonia: correlation of CT with clinical, functional and radiologic findings. Radiology. 1987;162:377–81.
13. Xaubet Am Agusti C, Luburich P, Roca J, Montón C, Ayuso MC, et al. Pulmonary function tests and CT scan in the management of idiopathic pulmonary fibrosis. Am J Respir Crit Care Med. 1998;168:431–6.
14. Wells AU, Hansell DM, Rubens MB, King AD, Cramer D, Black CM, et al. Fibrosing alveolitis in systemic sclerosis: indices of lung function in relation to extent of disease on computed tomography. Arthritis Rheum. 1997;40:1229–36.
15. Watters LC, King TE, Schwarz MI, Waldron JA, Stanford RE, Cherniack RM. A clinical, radiographic and physiologic scoring system for the longitudinal assessment of patients with idiopathic pulmonary fibrosis. Am Rev Respir Dis. 1986;133:97–103.
16. King TE, Tooze JA, Schwarz MI, Brown KR, Cherniack RM. Predicting survival in idiopathic pulmonary fibrosis: scoring system and survival model. Am J Respir Crit Care Med. 2001;164:1171–81.
17. Raghu G, Collard HR, Egan JJ, Martinez FJ, Behr J, Brown KK, et al. An official ATS/ERS/JRS/ALAT statement: idiopathic pulmonary fibrosis: evidence-based guidelines for diagnosis and management. Am J Respir Crit Care Med. 2011;183:788–824.
18. Eaton T, Young P, Milne D, Wells AU. Six-minute walk, maximal exercise tests: reproducibility in fibrotic interstitial pneumonia. Am J Respir Crit Care Med. 2005;171:1150–7.
19. Idiopathic Pulmonary Fibrosis Clinical Research Network, Zisman DA, Schwarz M, Angstgrom KJ, Collard HR, Flaherty KR, Hunninghake GW. A controlled trial of sildenafil in advanced idiopathic pulmonary fibrosis. N Engl J Med. 2010;363:620–8.
20. Lama VN, Flaherty KR, Toews GB, Colby TV, Travis WD, Long Q, et al. Prognostic value of desaturation during a six-minute walk test in idiopathic interstitial pneumonia. Am J Respir Crit Care Med. 2003;168:1084–90.
21. Hallstrand TS, Boitano LJ, Johnson WC, Spada CA, Hayes JG, Raghu G. The timed walk test as a measure of severity and survival in idiopathic pulmonary fibrosis. Eur Respir J. 2006;25:96–103.
22. Lederer DJ, Arcasoy SM, Wilt JS, D'Ovidio F, Sonett JR, Kawut SM. Six minute walk distance predicts waiting list survival in idiopathic pulmonary fibrosis. Am J Respir Crit Care Med. 2006;174:659–64.
23. Martinez FJ, Safrin S, Weycker D, Starko KM, Bradford WZ, King Jr TE, et al. The clinical course of patients with idiopathic pulmonary fibrosis. Ann Intern Med. 2006;142:963–7.
24. Egan JJ, Martinez FJ, Wells AU, Williams T. Lung function estimates in idiopathic pulmonary fibrosis: the potential for a simple classification. Thorax. 2005;60:270–3.
25. Latsi PI, du Bois RM, Nicholson AG, Colby TV, Bisirtzoglou D, Nikolakopoulou A, et al. Fibrotic idiopathic interstitial pneumonia: the prognostic value of longitudinal functional trends. Am J Respir Crit Care Med. 2003;168:531–7.
26. Ley B, Ryerson CJ, Vittinghoff E, Ryu JH, Tomassetti S, Lee JS, et al. A multidimensional index and staging system for idiopathic pulmonary fibrosis. Ann Intern Med. 2012;156:684–91.

27. du Bois RM, Weycker D, Albera C, Bradford WZ, Costabel U, Kartashov A, et al. Ascertainment of individual risk of mortality for patients with idiopathic pulmonary fibrosis. Am J Respir Crit Care Med. 2011;184:459–66.
28. Collard HR, King Jr TE, Bartelson BB, Vourlekis JS, Schwarz MI, Brown KK. Changes in clinical and physiologic variables predict survival in idiopathic pulmonary fibrosis. Am J Respir Crit Care Med. 2003;168:538–42.
29. Mura M, Porretta MA, Bargagli E, Sergiacomi G, Zompatori M, Sverzellati N, et al. Predicting survival in newly diagnosed idiopathic pulmonary fibrosis: a 3-year prospective study. Eur Respir J. 2012;040:101–9.
30. Flaherty KR, Mumford JA, Murray S, Kazerooni EA, Gross BH, Colby TV, et al. Prognostic implications of physiologic and radiographic changes in idiopathic interstitial pneumonia. Am J Respir Crit Care Med. 2003;168:543–8.
31. King Jr TE, Safrin S, Starko KM, Brown KK, Noble PW, Raghu G, et al. Analyses of efficacy end points in a controlled trial of interferon-gamma1b for idiopathic pulmonary fibrosis. Chest. 2005;127:171–7.
32. Jegal Y, Kim DS, Shim TS, Lim CM, Do Lee S, Koh Y, et al. Physiology is a stronger predictor of survival than pathology in fibrotic interstitial pneumonia. Am J Respir Crit Care Med. 2005;171:639–44.
33. Peelen L, Wells AU, Prijs M, Blumenthal JP, van Steenwijk RP, Jonkers RE, et al. Fibrotic idiopathic interstitial pneumonias: mortality is linked to a decline in gas transfer. Respirology. 2010;15:1233–43.
34. Corte TJ, Wort SJ, Macdonald PS, Edey A, Hansell DM, Renzoni E, et al. Pulmonary function vascular index predicts prognosis in idiopathic interstitial pneumonia. Respirology. 2012;17:674–80.
35. Schmidt SL, Nambiar AM, Tayob N, Sundaram B, Han MK, Gross BH, et al. Pulmonary function measures predict mortality differently in idiopathic pulmonary fibrosis versus combined pulmonary fibrosis and emphysema. Eur Respir J. 2011;38:176–83.
36. Zappala CJ, Latsi PI, Nicholson AG, Colby TV, Cramer D, Renzoni EA, et al. Marginal decline in forced vital capacity is associated with a poor outcome in idiopathic pulmonary fibrosis. Eur Respir J. 2010;35:830–6.
37. Richeldi L, Ryerson CJ, Lee JS, Wolters PJ, Koth LL, Ley B, et al. Relative versus absolute change in forced vital capacity in idiopathic pulmonary fibrosis. Thorax. 2012;67:407–11.
38. Hunninghake GW. Antioxidant therapy for idiopathic pulmonary fibrosis. N Engl J Med. 2005;353:2285–7.
39. Buech MH, Denton CP, Furst DE, Guillevin L, Rubin LJ, Wells AU, et al. Submaximal exercise testing in the assessment of interstitial lung disease secondary to systemic sclerosis: reproducibility and correlations of the 6-min walk test. Ann Rheum Dis. 2007;66:169–73.
40. King Jr TE, Behr J, Brown KK, du Bois RM, Lancaster L, de Andrade JA, et al. BUILD-1: a randomized placebo-controlled trial of bosentan in idiopathic pulmonary fibrosis. Am J Respir Crit Care Med. 2008;177:75–81.
41. Raghu G, Brown KK, Costabel U, Cottin V, du Bois RM, Lasky JA, et al. Treatment of idiopathic pulmonary fibrosis with etanercept: an exploratory, placebo-controlled trial. Am J Respir Crit Care Med. 2008;178:948–55.
42. Flaherty KR, Andrei AC, Murray S, Fraley C, Colby TV, Travis WD, et al. Idiopathic pulmonary fibrosis: prognostic value of changes in physiology and six-minute-walk test. Am J Respir Crit Care Med. 2006;174:803–9.
43. du Bois RM, Weycker D, Albera C, Bradford WZ, Costabel U, Kartashov A, et al. Six-minute-walk test in idiopathic pulmonary fibrosis: test validation and minimal clinically important difference. Am J Respir Crit Care Med. 2011;183:1231–7.
44. Lettieri CJ, Nathan SD, Barnett SD, Ahmad S, Shorr AF. Prevalence and outcomes of pulmonary arterial hypertension in advanced idiopathic pulmonary fibrosis. Chest. 2006;129(3):746–52.
45. Burke CM, Glanville AR, Morris AJR, Rubin D, Harvey JA, Theodore J, et al. Pulmonary function in advanced pulmonary hypertension. Thorax. 1987;42:151–5.

46. Nathan SD, Shlobin OA, Ahmad S, Urbanek S, Barnett SD. Pulmonary hypertension and pulmonary function testing in idiopathic pulmonary fibrosis. Chest. 2007;131:657–63.
47. Steen VD, Graham G, Conte C, Owens G, Medsger TAJR. Isolated diffusing capacity reduction in systemic sclerosis. Arthritis Rheum. 1992;35:765–70.
48. Zisman DA, Karlamangla AS, Kawut SM, Shlobin OA, Saggar R, Ross DJ, et al. Validation of a method to screen for pulmonary hypertension in advanced idiopathic pulmonary fibrosis. Chest. 2008;133:640–5.
49. ATS/ERS Task Force, Brusasco V, Crapo R, Viegi G, et al. General considerations for lung function. Eur Respir J. 2005;26:153–61.
50. ATS/ERS Task Force, Brusasco V, Crapo R, Viegi G, et al. Standardisation of the single breath determination of carbon monoxide uptake in the lung. Eur Respir J. 2005;26:720–35.
51. ARTP Working Groups on Standards of Care and Recommendations for Lung Function Departments. 2006. Quality assurance for lung function laboratories. Available from: http://www.ARTP.org.uk/
52. Cotes JE, Chinn DJ, Miller MR. Lung function. 6th ed. Oxford: Blackwell; 2006. p. 79. ISBN 13:978-0-6320-6493-9.
53. ERS Task Force on Standardization of Clinical Exercise Testing, Roca J, Whipp BJ, et al. Clinical exercise testing with reference to lung diseases: indications, standardization and interpretation strategies. Eur Respir J. 1997;10:2662–89.
54. Reville SM, Morgan M. Biological quality control for exercise testing. Thorax. 2000;55:63–6.
55. Seccombe LM, Kelly PT, Wong CK, Rogers PG, Lim S, Peters MJ. Effect of simulated commercial flight on oxygenation in patients with interstitial lung disease and chronic obstructive pulmonary disease. Thorax. 2004;59:966–70.
56. Cramer D, Ward S, Geddes D. Assessment of oxygen supplementation during air travel. Thorax. 1996;51:202–3.
57. Ernsting J, Nicholson AN, Rainford DJ, editors. Aviation medicine. 3rd ed. Oxford: Butterworth-Heinmann; 2000.
58. British Thoracic Society Standards of Care Committee. Managing passengers with respiratory disease planning air travel: British Thoracic Society recommendations. Thorax. 2002;57:289–304.
59. British Thoracic Society Standards of Care Committee. Managing passengers with respiratory disease planning air travel: summary for primary care. 2004. Available from: http://www.britthoracic.org.uk/c2/uploads/FlightPCsummary04.pdf
60. Martin SE, Bradley JM, Buick JB, Bradbury I, Elborn JS. Flight assessment in patients with respiratory disease: hypoxic challenge testing vs. predictive equations. Q J Med. 2007;100:361–7.

# Chapter 7
# The Role of Adaptive Immunity in Idiopathic Pulmonary Fibrosis: Hiding in Plain Sight

**Steven R. Duncan**

**Abstract**  Deleterious actions of antigen-activated T and B lymphocytes, the major cellular effectors of adaptive immune host defenses, underlie the pathogenesis of nearly every human fibroproliferative disease. Misdirected or especially intense and persistent adaptive immune responses can cause recurrent cellular injury and dys-regulated tissue repair in other organs that are comparable to the lung abnormalities found in patients with idiopathic pulmonary fibrosis (IPF). This chapter includes a brief discussion of some relevant basic immunobiology to facilitate a better under-standing of the mechanisms and typifying features of pathological adaptive immune responses. Subsequent sections then review findings of the numerous translational studies that implicate adaptive immunity in the development and progression of IPF. Many diseases caused by adaptive immune responses are, like IPF, refractory to treatment with nonspecific glucocorticoid regimens. However, patients with these other immunological disorders often benefit from treatment regimens that specifi-cally target the causal inflammatory mechanism(s). The author believes that appre-ciation of the abnormal immune processes associated with IPF would justify trials of novel, mechanistically focused therapies that have the potential to benefit patients with this morbid and heretofore intractable lung disease.

**Keywords**  T cells • B cells • HLA molecules • Autoimmunity • Autoantibodies • Anti-B cell therapies • Biomarkers

S.R. Duncan, M.D. (✉)
Department of Pulmonary, Allergy, and Critical Care Medicine, University of Pittsburgh
Medical Center, 628 NW MUH, 3459 Fifth Ave, Pittsburgh, PA 15213, USA
e-mail: duncsr@upmc.edu

K.C. Meyer and S.D. Nathan (eds.), *Idiopathic Pulmonary Fibrosis: A Comprehensive Clinical Guide*, Respiratory Medicine 9, DOI 10.1007/978-1-62703-682-5_7, © Springer Science+Business Media New York 2014

# Background

Idiopathic pulmonary fibrosis (IPF) was widely regarded to be an immunological disease until relatively recently. In part, those beliefs were due to considerations that adaptive immune responses play a central causal role in nearly every other human fibroproliferative disease [1]. Moreover, a series of studies had shown that overtly abnormal adaptive immune responses were prevalent in IPF patients [2–56]. Within the last decade or so, however, contrary opinions have been widely promoted [57, 58]. Accordingly, immunology is no longer generally regarded as relevant to IPF. The foundations of this paradigm shift were fueled in large part by frustration with the therapeutic ineffectiveness of nonspecific immunosuppressive regimens (largely glucocorticoid based) to alter the natural history of IPF [59]. However, many immune disorders are also often refractory to steroid treatments, particularly when they are severe, far-advanced (e.g., fibrotic), or rapidly progressive [60–70]. Indeed, arguments that IPF cannot have an immunological basis because it is steroid resistant ignore a wealth of data to the contrary.

IPF pathogenesis is now most often attributed to recurrent injuries of alveolar epithelium in conjunction with dysregulated epithelial–fibroblast interactions [57, 58, 71]. Aside from the assertions these processes cannot be immunological, the etiology of the underlying injury remains enigmatic despite long and intense study. However, analogous chronic fibrotic disorders that are completely devoid of an immunological component are not common in other organs (or organisms) [1, 72]. Hence, the pathogenesis of IPF seemingly has to involve a biological process that is unique to the lungs of older humans.

Notwithstanding contemporary opinions to the contrary, at least some investigators believe the evidence that adaptive immune responses are critically involved in IPF is overwhelming and irrefutable. Numerous recent studies have corroborated and extended earlier investigations by showing that myriad, highly pathogenic immunological responses are common, if not ubiquitous, among IPF patients (as will be detailed in subsequent sections of this chapter). Moreover, these immune abnormalities are also known to cause analogous chronic tissue injuries and fibroproliferation in other human diseases [1, 72] and are, thus, biologically plausible causes for the lung pathology that typifies IPF [59]. Furthermore, many of the immunologic abnormalities found in individual IPF patients are also highly associated with their clinical manifestations and disease prognoses, again paralleling findings in populations afflicted by other recognized immune disorders.

Observations made in a variety of animal models are often raised during discussions of IPF pathogenesis, even though animal models do not accurately replicate human IPF [73, 74]. Accordingly, the use of imperfect animal models to extrapolate the causal mechanisms of IPF has limited rationale. It is clear from animal modeling that many mediators promote fibrosis [75, 76]. These and other similar basic investigations illuminate the importance of particular cytokines amid the complex, interactive, and redundant mediator cascades that result in pathological fibroproliferation [1, 72]. However, isolated, de novo, primary overproduction of a profibrotic cytokine or other mediator has not been identified among human patients, and this seems very unlikely to be a frequent cause of IPF. Conversely, adaptive immune responses are characteristically accompanied by increased productions of a wide variety of potent mediators and effectors that cause or promote injury and fibroproliferation (including TNF-α and TGF-β) as will be subsequently described. Furthermore, several other animal models also show that aberrations of immunological host defenses per se readily cause chronic, progressive pulmonary fibrosis [77–79].

Rather than add further obfuscation with arguments based on studies of animal models that likely have tenuous direct applicability to understanding human IPF, the following discussions in this chapter are largely focused on translational investigations of actual IPF patients and their clinical specimens. The author believes the number, quality, and rigor of these observations are more than adequate to support the theme and contention of this chapter.

To follow is a brief overview of key adaptive immune elements. The remainder of this chapter will then focus on the evidence that immune responses play a central role in the development and/or progression of IPF.

## Basics of the Adaptive Immune System

### *General*

A comprehensive review of immunology is beyond the scope and purpose of this chapter, and interested readers are directed to more detailed and elegant presentations elsewhere, including several outstanding general texts [80–82]. Appreciation and critical interpretation of the relevant research findings in IPF patients, however, requires at least some familiarity with fundamental aspects of the adaptive immune system.

Adaptive immunity is an essential component of our defenses against microbes, noxious environmental agents, and malignancies, and it is usually highly efficient, focused, and self-limited. Nonetheless, for a variety of reasons, only some of which are known, an inflammatory cascade that is initially and appropriately targeted at an appropriate antigen (e.g., a microbial protein) can itself cause disease if unchecked or if misdirected against an autologous protein (i.e., autoimmunity) [83–86].

Adaptive immunity exhibits two hallmark features that distinguish it from other host defense processes (e.g., the innate immune system), namely, the exquisite antigen specificity of individual immune effector cells (i.e., lymphocytes) and amplification of these immune responses by sometimes prodigious proliferations of the antigen-activated lymphocyte(s). These unique characteristics are conferred by the immunobiology of the three major components of the adaptive immune system: (1) human leukocyte antigen (HLA) molecules, (2) T cells, and (3) B cells. Interrelated abnormalities of all three elements have been described in IPF patients.

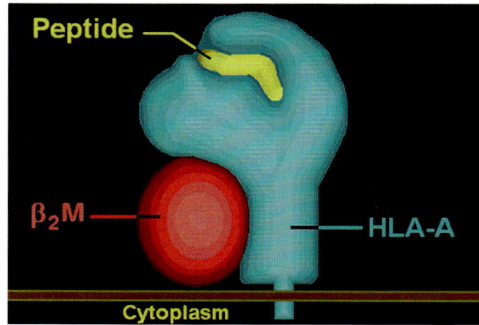

**Fig. 7.1** HLA molecules present peptides to T cells. Schematically depicted here is a small peptide fragment presented in the cleft of a HLA Class I molecule (HLA-A) on the surface of an antigen-presenting cell (APC). Dendritic cells, B cells, macrophages and, in some circumstances, other parenchymal and mesenchymal cells can effectively function as APC. The clefts of each HLA allele are distinctive, and only a finite number of specific, defined peptide motifs will bind in any particular HLA. Most peptide-HLA complexes are ignored by T-cell surveillance, but those HLA-bound peptides that trigger T-cell responses are "antigens." The invariant $\beta_2$ microglobulin ($\beta_2M$) depicted here is a unique feature of HLA Class I molecules. HLA Class II molecule structures consist of heterodimeric $\alpha$ and $\beta$ chains (from Wikipedia.com)

## HLA Alleles

HLA molecules (the human version of the major histocompatability complex) are highly specialized glycoproteins that present short peptides on the surfaces of antigen-presenting cells (APC) to adjacent T cells [87]. HLA-bound peptides, particularly those that are fragments of self-proteins (and these are often fragments of the HLA themselves), are usually ignored by T cells, whereas those that evoke a lymphocyte response (whether appropriately or inappropriately) are denoted as "antigens."

HLA molecules are the most polymorphic proteins of humans, being encoded by a series of gene loci clustered on chromosome 6, and there are dozens or even hundreds of distinct alleles that can occupy each of these loci [88, 89]. The major HLA loci can be subdivided into two classes. Although there are some notable exceptions, HLA Class I alleles (-A, -B, -Cw) primarily present peptides that are synthesized endogenously within the APC per se (including viral proteins) and are recognized by CD8 T cells. HLA Class II alleles (-DR, -DQ, -DP) typically bind peptides that were synthesized exogenously to the APC, which are then engulfed, processed, and usually presented to CD4 T lymphocytes [87].

Due to the unique physicochemical effects and interactions rendered by their respective, highly varied protein structures, each polymorphic HLA molecule is capable of efficiently binding and presenting only a restricted set (motif) of peptides [87] (Fig. 7.1). Hence, HLA haplotype inheritance determines the finite repertoire of antigens that can evoke adaptive immune responses in an individual. The evolution of HLA polymorphisms are the result of a fascinating interplay of environmental and sexual selective pressures [90, 91]. The net result is the presence of an incalculable range of potential antigen-binding motifs within the population, even if these are limited in any particular individual. This extreme diversity increases the probability that at least some individuals will be able to present the unique antigen sequences of newly encountered pathogens. Those who have fortunately inherited these particular HLA alleles will thus be more likely to mount an effective immune response and survive what could otherwise be an extinction event.

A classic feature of adaptive immune disorders, especially autoimmune syndromes, is the presence of one or more HLA allele frequency abnormalities within the disease population [89, 92–98]. Although critical for host defense, the presentation of peptides to T cells may instead be injurious if a particular antigen triggers an especially intense or prolonged immune response that escapes normal homeostatic controls, is a self-protein to which immunological tolerance has been lost (or was never established), or is sufficiently similar in structure to evoke a cross-response to a self-protein (i.e., epitope mimicry) [83–86, 99, 100]. Individuals with a HLA polymorphism that efficiently presents the disease-associated antigen(s) are more likely to have these deleterious immune responses, and the prevalence of that allele is thus overrepresented among the disease cohort [89, 92–98]. In contrast, individuals lacking these specific "predisposing" HLA allele(s) are less prone to develop that disease. Other HLA alleles may also more effectively induce immunologic tolerance to the disease-associated antigen/autoantigen or present different, relatively benign epitopes of the antigen and, thus, appear to be "protective" for this particular disease [83–86, 101].

Alternatively, the presence of abnormal HLA allele frequencies in a disease population may in some cases be unrelated to the unique peptide binding motifs of that HLA per se, but are instead a genetic "marker" denoting the presence of a pathogenic immunomodulatory gene(s) that is/are in linkage disequilibrium (LD) with the HLA allele. Many important immune-related genes are located within or in proximity to the HLA region and are often in LD with particular HLA alleles [89, 98].

## T Cells

Thymus-dependent lymphocytes (T cells) function as the "sharp end of the immunologic spear," in that they initiate and sustain the complex inflammatory cascades that occur after encounters and activation by appropriate or "inappropriate" (i.e., disease-causing) antigens [84, 85, 102–106].

The antigen specificity of T cells is a result of the extreme individual variability of cell surface antigen receptors (TCR) present on each of these lymphocytes [87]. In effect, T cells are like snowflakes in that, at least for practical purposes, every newly emergent lymphocyte bears completely distinct TCR (Fig. 7.2).

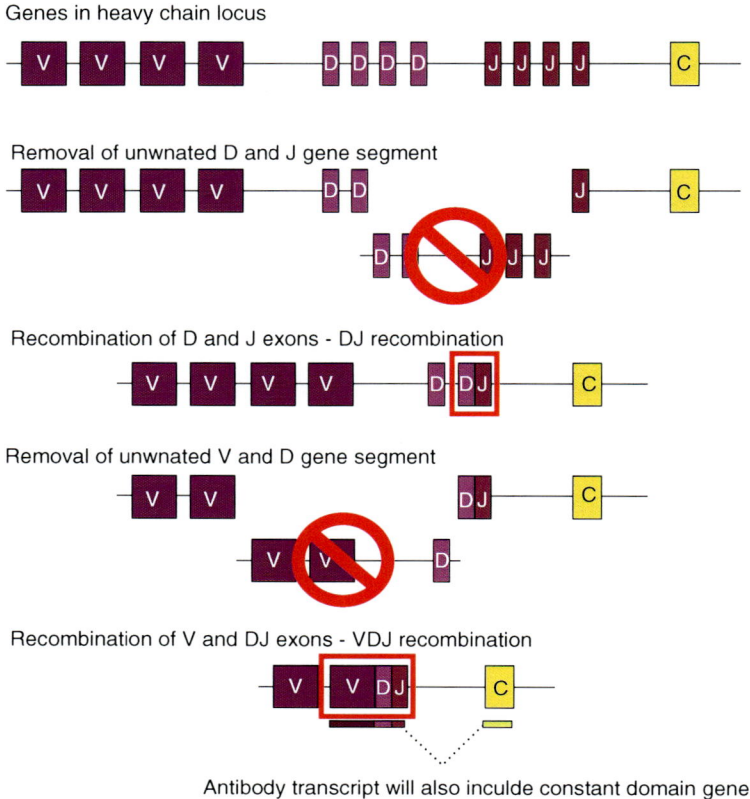

Fig. 7.2 Combinatorial rearrangements of lymphocyte antigen receptor genes. Each developing lymphocyte randomly (or near randomly) rearranges the numerous genes that encode their singular antigen receptors. One variable (V) gene recombines with one (each) diversity (D), joining (J) and constant region (C) genes. In addition, various numbers of nucleotides may be added or deleted, which results in frame shifts. The net effect is that each newly emergent lymphocyte has a unique antigen receptor nucleotide sequence that encodes their correspondingly highly variable antigen receptor proteins. In turn, this uniqueness imparts the distinctive avidities of these receptors for particular peptide antigens (B cells) or antigen-HLA complexes (T cells) (see Fig. 7.3). The immunoglobulin (antibody) gene rearrangements of B cells are depicted here, but the processes involved in the development of distinctive T-cell antigen receptors (TCR) are very analogous [107, 108] (from Wikipedia.com)

This individuality is a function of near-random recombinations of the multiple adjacent genes that encode the TCR proteins that occur during intrathymic maturation [107, 108]. The resulting primary sequence of the TCR proteins on a particular lymphocyte affects the configurations (i.e., secondary and tertiary protein structures) of these receptors and, consequently, determines the physicochemical binding strengths (avidities) of their interactions with HLA–peptide complexes on the surfaces of APC (Fig. 7.3).

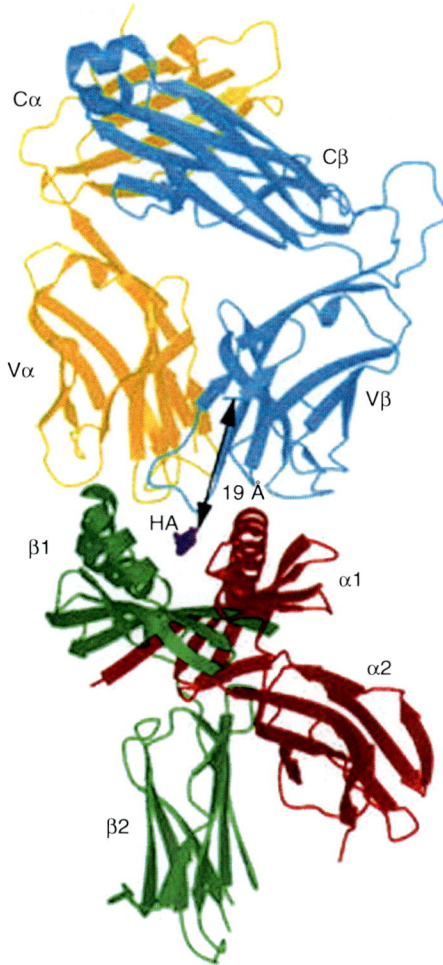

**Fig. 7.3** Schematic of the trimolecular complex that initiates adaptive immune responses. The heterodimeric T-cell antigen receptor (TCR) is depicted at *top* (*yellow* and *blue*). HLA Class II structures (*bottom*) are depicted in *red* and *green*. The antigen is located centrally (which is a hemagglutinin (HA) peptide fragment in this example). *C* denotes the TCR constant region; *V* denotes the TCR variable region; α and β depict respective alpha and beta chains of the TCR and HLA. The *blue double-headed arrow* is a distance scale. The avidity of TCR for antigen-HLA complexes is determined by the complex configurations of the respective molecules and the strengths of interactive forces (e.g., electrostatic, van der Waals) between them. The intricacies and distinctiveness of these complexes imparts the antigen specificity of the adaptive immune system (reprinted by permission from Macmillan Publishers Ltd: The EMBO Journal, Jens Hennecke, Andrea Carfi, Don C. Wiley, Structure of a covalently stabilized complex of a human αβ T-cell receptor, influenza HA peptide and MHC class II molecule, HLA-DR1, Nov;19(21):5611–5624, copyright 2000)

Nascent T cells are highly selected during their intrathymic maturations to eliminate those bearing TCR that cannot efficiently interact with self-HLA, as well as those with unduly high avidity for self-peptide–HLA complexes [108]. Additional lymphocyte selection processes occur in the periphery after their export from the thymus [109]. These serial selections ultimately result in individuals having repertoires of T cells that bear potentially useful, but not (usually) self-damaging, avidities for autologous HLA–peptide complexes. Obviously, however, this intricate system is imperfect, given that some unlucky individuals are unable to mount an effective immune response to certain microbes or tumor antigens, whereas others are prone to develop autoimmune disorders [83–86].

The uniqueness and finite specificity of TCR result in only a very small proportion of the naive T cells in an individual that can avidly bind to and initiate responses to any given antigen. As an example, viral capsid peptides are typically recognized by only 1 out of 10,000 to100,000 circulating T cells [110]. Thus, in order to mount an effective immune response to a particular antigen, activated T cells undergo repetitive cycles of proliferation that can result in extraordinarily large numbers of lymphocytes (clones) with identically rearranged TCR genes and identical antigen specificities [111, 112]. In especially prolonged and intense responses, as many as half or more of the circulating T cells in a diseased individual may be comprised of daughter progeny from a single or a very small number of antigen-stimulated progenitors [111–113]. Although the ability to marshal a huge number of T cells with common specificity for an important antigen(s) is highly adaptive for host defenses against virulent organisms, these exponential clonal amplifications can have deleterious consequences when the provocative stimuli are persistent/recurrent extrinsic antigens or self-peptides.

Expanded lymphocyte clones can be easily detected in clinical specimens by various laboratory techniques [113, 114]. The probability of finding even two T cells that share identical TCR purely by chance in a specimen has been conservatively estimated as <1 in $1 \times 10^7$ [115]. Although some CD8 T cell clonality can be seen among apparently healthy aged subjects, circulating CD4 T cell clones are highly abnormal. Hence, findings of CD4 T cell clonality are unmistakable evidence of an adaptive immune response and most often represent a pathogenic process, especially when these expansions are numerous and/or extreme [111–113, 116, 117]. In distinction, immune responses to nonspecific mitogens or microbial superantigens are not mediated by engagements with distinct, specific individual TCR, and such responses are thus characterized by promiscuous (polyclonal) T-cell proliferations.

Under appropriate circumstances, TCR cross-linking by engagements with antigen-HLA complexes on the surfaces of APC mediate a series of intracellular signaling events that result in activation of the lymphocyte(s). Antigen-activated T cells begin transcription (and later translation) of a succession of intercellular mediators (e.g., IL-2 followed by other cytokines and chemokines, enzymes, etc.). Activation also triggers DNA replication as a prelude to subsequent mitosis of that T cell [102–106]. Activated T cells have pleiotropic effector capabilities to effectively counter microbes and tumors, but these same processes can cause or contribute to tissue injuries when they become dysregulated, misdirected, or inordinately intense and prolonged [1, 72, 83–86, 102–106].

## B Cells

Antibody-producing lymphocytes were first discovered in the bursa of birds (hence the "B-cell" designation) and are the third major element of the human adaptive immune system [118]. B cells share many features and general characteristics of T cells and were almost certainly the evolutionary progenitors of T cells. Like T cells, B lymphocytes also express individual cell surface antigen receptors (i.e., immunoglobulins [antibodies]) such that each has a limited number of specificities. B cells are also selected during maturation in the bone marrow, and later in the periphery, to remove (albeit imperfectly) those lymphocytes that have enhanced potential for autoreactivity [119]. Much like TCR on T cells, the highly variable sequences of individual B cell antibodies are conferred by near-random rearrangements of the genes that encode these immunoglobulins [120] (see Fig. 7.2). The antibodies of each particular B cell have finite, restricted antigen specificity. However, the huge number of these unique B lymphocytes in an individual, each with their respective, distinctive cell surface antibody, ensures that effective host responses can be mounted to a wide range of potential antigens.

B-cell activation is also triggered by antigen binding and cross-linking of the corresponding avidly bound cell surface antibodies, which are typically IgD or IgM isotypes on early/naïve lymphocytes. This antigen cross-linking initiates a series of transcriptional and translational events that result in an ordered series of cell maturations and divisions that can result in huge numbers of genetically identical, antigen-specific (clonal) B-cell progeny. Among other consequences of this cascade of cell proliferation, the increasingly differentiated B cells, which eventually culminate in plasmablasts and plasma cells, are the most efficient producers and secretors of antibodies [118, 121].

Interactions of B cells and T cells are important in the development of fully functional adaptive immune responses [121]. Activated B cells act as APC by internalizing antigens bound to their surface antibodies, and the intracellular antigens are then processed, packaged, and eventually presented in the clefts of the B cell HLA on the cell surface to proximate T cells (see Figs. 7.1 and 7.3). In turn, activated T cells (especially among the CD4 subpopulation) that share antigen specificity with the B cell(s) provide "help" to the latter, a process that is mediated by specialized receptor–ligand interactions and soluble cytokines. This T-cell help further promotes B-cell differentiation and is an absolute requisite for B cells to undergo isotype switching and produce IgG antibodies that are directed against and avidly bind protein antigens [121, 122]. Hence, finding antigen-specific IgG isotype antibodies (or autoantibodies) against peptide epitopes is de facto evidence of concomitant T-cell reactivity to those same antigens.

The antigen specificity of B cells appears to be more plastic than that of T cells. Later generations of the B-cell progeny produced during repetitive, antigen-driven cell divisions can begin to incrementally alter their immunoglobulin gene rearrangements, resulting in productions of differently configured antibodies with potentially greater avidity for the antigen(s) (i.e., affinity maturation) [123]. In some cases, especially in the context of intense or protracted immune responses, some of these antibodies might also recognize irrelevant proteins (including otherwise inert self-antigens). This generalization of immune responses (epitope spread) has been implicated in the development of many autoimmune syndromes that are associated with infections and malignancies [83–86, 99, 100].

B cells can cause disease by a variety of mechanisms (Fig. 7.4). Antigen–antibody (immune) complexes that are deposited in tissues can activate complement cascades. In turn, the activated complement components are cytotoxic to proximate cells and can serve as potent chemoattractants for neutrophils [125]. Additionally, immunoglobulins bound to cellular targets can trigger NK cell-mediated cytotoxicity [126]. These B-cell- and immune complex-mediated phenomena are of particular interest, as intrapulmonary cell apoptosis and neutrophil infiltration also happen to be characteristic histological findings in IPF lungs, especially during acute exacerbations [59, 130, 131]. Antibodies can also have function-altering effects by cross-linking antigens bound to cell surface receptors (which can transduce cell signaling) or after gaining access to intracellular antigens [20, 124, 132–135]. While often overlooked, activated B cells also directly produce numerous cytokines and other mediators that have vasoactive, proinflammatory, and profibrotic actions [118].

## Adaptive Immune Abnormalities in IPF Patients

### HLA Biases

As described earlier, HLA allele frequency biases are a characteristic of adaptive immune diseases (and especially autoimmune disorders) [84, 85, 89, 92–98].

A series of early studies examined HLA allele frequencies in IPF patients prior to the paradigm shift that discounted adaptive immune processes in this disease [136–141]. HLA expressions were defined by using reference antibodies that have avidity to particular HLA alleles. This (now obsolete) method suffers both from poor specificity (frequent antibody cross-reactivity to two or more distinct HLA alleles) and lack of sensitivity (antibodies are not available for all HLA alleles). Moreover, the full extent of HLA polymorphisms was not yet appreciated during that time period, and a number of alleles that are now known to be prevalent in humans (especially Class II alleles) were not even assayed. Other limitations of these earlier reports include what now seem to be very small numbers of subject's (hence limited study power) absence of replication cohorts, and uncertain case definitions such that subjects with other interstitial lung diseases were enrolled and

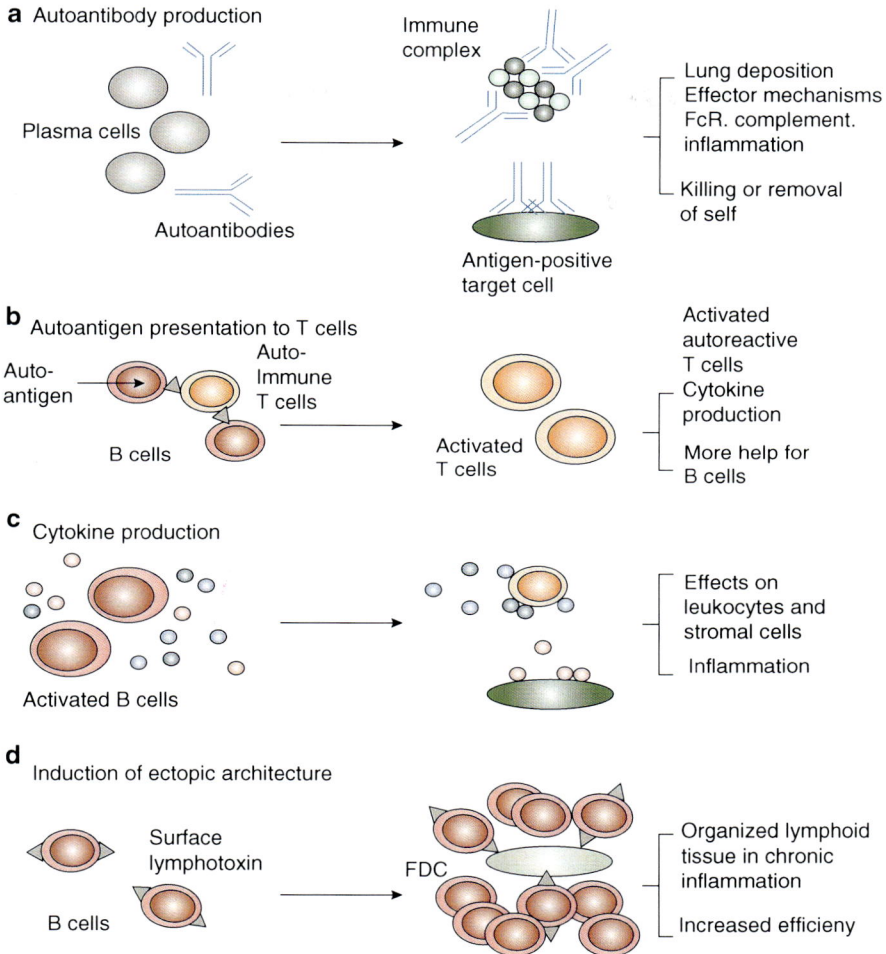

**Fig. 7.4** Pathogenic effects of B cells. (**a**) Autoantibodies produced by B cells can form immune complexes in tissues (see also Fig. 7.15) that engage and activate Fc-receptor bearing cells. The latter include NK cells (which can then kill antibody-bound cells [126]) and macrophages (which elaborate proinflammatory mediators [124] as well as activate the cytotoxic and neutrophil-attracting complement system [125]). (**b**) B cells can also effectively present antigen and provide costimulatory signals to T cells, which can lead to T-cell activation. (**c**) B cells also release potent proinflammatory and vasoactive cytokines (similar to T cells). (**d**) B-cell aggregates in disease tissue enhance immune responses (see also Fig. 7.14) (reprinted by permission from Macmillan Publishers Ltd: Nature Rev Drug Discovery, Jeffrey L. Browning, B cells move to center stage: novel opportunities for autoimmune disease treatment, Jul;5(7):564–575, copyright 2006)

admixed with IPF patients. Nevertheless, the findings in all but two of these previous studies [137, 138] suggested that HLA allele frequency perturbations are present in IPF.

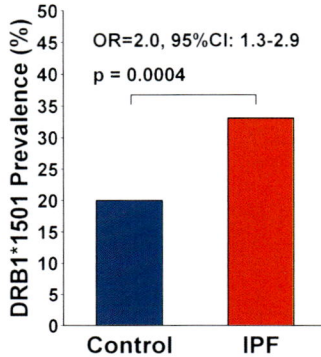

**Fig. 7.5** DRB1*1501 is over-represented in IPF patients. DRB1*1501 was significantly more prevalent in the cumulative IPF population ($n = 275$) compared to demographically and geographically matched healthy controls ($n = 285$). *OR* odds ratio, *CI* confidence interval. HLA allele biases are a characteristic feature of immunological disorders, and autoimmune diseases in particular [85, 89, 92–98] (reprinted from [142])

To our knowledge, there has been only one study of HLA allele prevalence in IPF patients that used contemporary molecular methodologies and disease criteria and prospectively replicated findings in distinct cohorts (a current standard of genomic research) [142]. HLA Class II alleles were characterized in this study, which evaluated 275 heterogeneous IPF patients from five major US medical centers, by sequence-specific primers in polymerase chain reactions (SSP-PCR) and/or specific oligonucleotide probe assays. HLA DRβ1*15 was shown to be consistently overrepresented in the IPF cohorts compared to demographically matched healthy controls (Fig. 7.5). Those IPF patients who were positive for DRβ1*15 also had greater decrements of diffusing capacity for carbon monoxide (DLCO) when compared to the subjects lacking this allele, and this finding appeared to be independent of pulmonary artery pressures or lung volumes.

Overrepresentation of HLA DRβ1*15 is the most frequently reported immunogenetic finding in patients with diverse immunologic diseases, including Goodpasture's syndrome and systemic lupus erythematosus (SLE), both of which are autoantibody-mediated illnesses, as well as multiple sclerosis, sarcoidosis, various other autoimmune syndromes, and interstitial lung disease associated with rheumatoid arthritis (RA) [89, 92–98]. This particular allele has been implicated as conferring a genetic predilection for increased production of autoantibodies [143], and it was also recently linked to autoantibody production in IPF patients [124].

## T Cells in IPF

Numerous reports show that many T-cell processes are manifestly abnormal in IPF patients [2–5, 7, 23–39, 45, 48–50, 52–55, 124, 130, 131, 144–150].

The usual interstitial pneumonia (UIP) or end-stage fibrosis that typifies IPF lung histopathology is often (if somewhat glibly) described as lacking the inflammatory cell influx that would seemingly be necessary to account for an immunological disease [57, 58]. However, it is by no means evident that lung biopsies of individuals with established fibrotic disease, which in all probability has been present (and progressive) over many years, can be extrapolated to accurately deduce the pathological process(es) that occurred early in disease development. IPF is characteristically an insidious disease of older, more sedentary individuals, in whom the extent of lung dysfunction is often severe by the time of initial diagnosis [39, 151].

With the exception of a very few focused research studies, isolated asymptomatic and functionally benign (and presumably early) interstitial lung diseases are often not detected, and even when they are, the patients with these disorders typically do not have lung biopsies [152–154]. As shown by some studies and other anecdotal reports, however, the development of UIP precedes the onset of symptoms and physiological abnormalities of IPF, and it often does so by several years [152]. Abnormal intrapulmonary influxes of activated T cells and characteristic chest CT infiltrates were found to be present among much younger (by ~20 years) asymptomatic first-order relatives of patients with familial IPF, implying that overt disease takes decades to fully manifest itself [153]. Matrix metalloproteinase-7 (MMP-7) was also abnormally increased in the sera of these younger subjects with early, asymptomatic lung disease [154]. MMP7 catalyzes the breakdown of extracellular matrix proteins during wound remodeling, and has been implicated as a pathological mediator as well as a biomarker of interstitial lung diseases [155]. Moreover, serial histological assessments of injuries mediated by adaptive immune processes in other diseases and animal models follow a predictable pattern of initial T-cell infiltration with subsequent reduction in the relative number of these lymphocytes as they are succeeded by the influxes of other immune effector cells (e.g., activated macrophages). The extensive fibrosis that eventually ensues after a prolonged adaptive immune response is, like IPF, typically pauci-cellular and may sometimes even be acellular [79, 156, 157].

Furthermore, despite some suggestions to the contrary, infiltrating T cells are much more numerous in IPF lungs than in normal lung specimens [26–54, 130, 131, 141, 147–150, 158, 159]. The T cells in IPF lungs are heterogeneously distributed, but are especially prominent in proximity to active fibroproliferative foci [149, 150] (Fig. 7.6) as well as among specimens from patients with rapidly progressive disease [131]. The magnitude of intrapulmonary T-cell infiltration in IPF is also correlated with the disease severity and prognosis of afflicted patients [148, 149]. These findings would, in and of themselves, be curiously coincidental if immunological processes were irrelevant to the disease pathogenesis.

Circulating T cells in IPF patients are also abnormally activated [145], deficient in homeostatic, immune-dampening regulatory T-cell ($T_{reg}$) numbers and functions [146], and are characterized by the increased production of numerous intercellular mediators (Fig. 7.7). Several T cell-mediated processes injure or kill proximate bystander epithelium (e.g., FasL, perforin, granzyme B), and epithelial

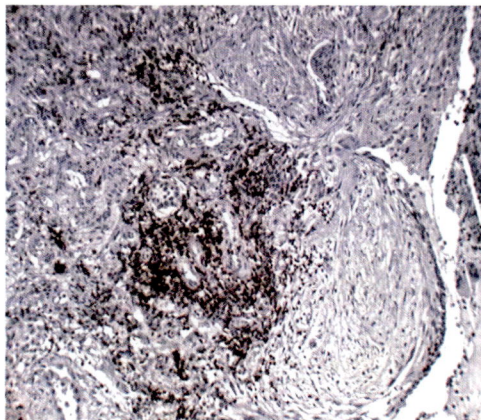

**Fig. 7.6** T cells in IPF lungs. Immunohistochemical staining shows that abnormal CD3+ T cell infiltrates (*black cells* near *arrow*) in lungs of IPF patients are distributed heterogeneously, and are often especially prominent in proximity to fibroproliferative foci (*star*), in the UIP lung. These infiltrates include both CD4+ and CD8+ T cells (not shown). Similar associations between infiltrating T cells and fibroproliferation are present in other chronic human lung diseases (×10) (image courtesy of G. Rosen)

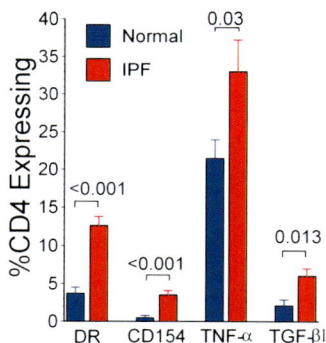

**Fig. 7.7** T-cell activation and mediator production in IPF. Circulating T cells of IPF patients exhibit several abnormalities that show their participation in ongoing adaptive immune responses. Among many other alterations, CD4 T cells from patients with IPF are more activated than those of demographically matched healthy controls, which is illustrated here by their expressions of HLA Class II DR and CD154 (CD40L), and these T cells more frequently produce proinflammatory and/or profibrotic cytokines (including TNF-α and TGF-β). (Reprinted with permission from The Journal of Immunology 2007 Aug;179(4):2592–9. Copyright 2007. American Association of Immunologists, Inc)

cell apoptosis is a frequent finding in IPF lungs [59, 130]. Additional T-cell products associated with IPF can activate, recruit, and/or alter functions of other immune effector cells including macrophages, neutrophils, and B cells (e.g., IL-1, IL-4, IL-6, TNF-α) [145–148].

**Fig. 7.8** T-cell clonality in IPF patients. Partial characterizations of circulating CD4 T-cell repertoires in IPF patients show the universal presence of clonal expansions. This is a pathognomonic finding of adaptive immune responses to repetitive specific antigen encounters [111–113] (reprinted with permission from The Journal of Immunology 2007 Aug;179(4):2592–9. Copyright 2007. American Association of Immunologists, Inc)

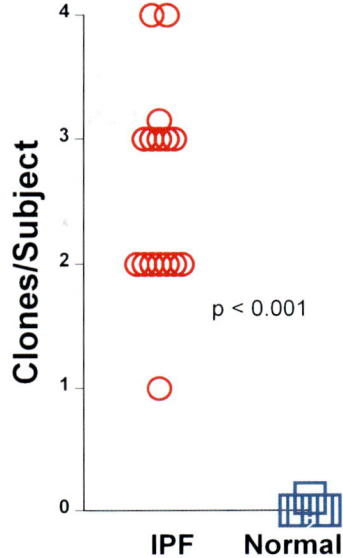

As described in an earlier section of this chapter, clonal proliferation of CD4 T cells is a pathognomonic finding that establishes the existence of an antigen-driven, adaptive immune response [111–113]. Lymphocyte clonality assessments have been used for decades to identify and confirm the immunological basis of many diseases in other organ systems [111–113, 160–162]. Independent corroborative investigations have shown that T-cell populations in IPF patients consistently show the presence of numerous clonal proliferations [4, 5], including the striking observation that highly abnormal CD4 T-cell clonality was evident in every IPF subject tested, in striking distinction to age-matched, healthy individuals [145] (Fig. 7.8).

With few exceptions, the identities of the antigen(s) that are driving T-cell activation and proliferation in IPF patients remain unknown. The IPF-associated antigen(s) could be a viral or another microbial product [163], an environmental agent [164], a chemically modified self-protein [165], or an autologous protein to which immunological tolerance has been lost or never developed [11, 13–23, 145, 166, 167]. Identifying the inciting agent(s) has considerable potential importance for possibly illuminating remedial or preventive strategies for IPF. As examples, if particular microbes triggered these pathogenic immune responses, eradication therapies could be beneficial, as could minimizing or avoiding exposures to particular disease-associated environmental agents. Since adaptive immune inflammatory cascades triggered by diverse antigens are typically indistinguishable when disease is far advanced or fulminant [1, 102–105], it is not inconceivable that numerous, distinctly different antigens can cause or contribute to the pathological immune responses that are common among IPF patients.

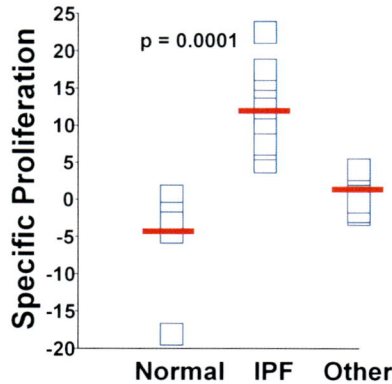

**Fig. 7.9** Intrapulmonary antigens in IPF lungs. Boiled (denatured) water-soluble protein extracts of IPF lungs cause proliferation of autologous CD4 T cells, unlike the preparations from normal controls or patients with other lung diseases (most of which were COPD). Specific proliferation = proliferation in extract supplemented cultures minus media control proliferation. This is an extremely abnormal finding, and specific evidence of an ongoing immunological process. T cells do not normally react to proteins in tissues (because if they do so, they cause disease), and this is an upstream inciting event in many serious human disorders [1, 84, 85, 102–105]. The responses to IPF lung antigens here are not attributable to nonspecific mitogens (which have been denatured) or intrapulmonary microbes (none were found in the IPF specimens), whereas all of the COPD lungs had microbial colonization. One (of possibly many) intrapulmonary antigens of IPF patients is heat shock protein 70 [124] (reprinted with permission from The Journal of Immunology 2007 Aug;179(4):2592–9. Copyright 2007. American Association of Immunologists, Inc)

One or more protein antigens within IPF lungs have been shown to induce autologous CD4 T-cell proliferations, unlike analogous preparations from lungs of normal subjects or other disease controls [124, 145] (Fig. 7.9). This is a very abnormal and specific ("gold standard") pathological finding, because T cells in healthy individuals are normally inert to anatomically accessible self-proteins [84, 85, 102]. T cells of some IPF patients were also recently shown to proliferate and produce IL-4 when co-cultured with heat shock protein 70 (HSP70) [124]. Expression of HSP70 is increased in IPF lungs [124], and the magnitude of this production is correlated with patient outcomes [168]. Given the important role of antigen-activated CD4 T cells in initiating and sustaining inflammatory lesions that can result in severe organ injury [1, 72, 102], lymphocyte reactivity and profibrotic mediator production triggered by a protein that is abundantly expressed in diseased lungs (e.g., HSP70) are very unlikely to have benign consequences [124].

The T-cell clonal expansions in IPF specimens (see Fig. 7.8) [4, 5, 145] also have additional pathological implications. Daughter progeny of T cells that have undergone multiple cell divisions in response to repetitive antigen stimulation (i.e., clonally expanded T cells) develop profound phenotypic and functional changes. Among many other alterations, end-differentiated CD4 T lymphocytes permanently lose their cell surface CD28, whereas almost all circulating CD4 T cells in healthy

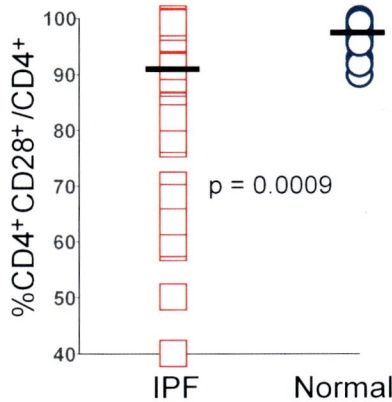

**Fig. 7.10** CD4 T-cell differentiation in IPF patients. In comparison to demographically matched normal controls, circulating CD4 T cells of many IPF subjects are highly differentiated, as evidenced (among other characteristics) by their downregulation of cell surface CD28. This T-cell differentiation is a consequence of prior repetitive antigen stimulation and multiple cell divisions, and it is a specific biomarker for the presence of a chronic adaptive immune responses [169–180] (reprinted from [147])

normal subjects express this costimulatory molecule [169]. Another unusual feature and facile marker of end-differentiated CD4 T cells is their production of granzyme b and perforin [147, 170, 171]. In contrast, "normal" (naïve or less repetitively stimulated) CD4 T cells do not produce these potent cytotoxic mediators (Fig. 7.10). Granzyme b and perforin are especially useful specific markers for end-differentiation among the CD4 T cells localized in tissues, since many parenchymal infiltrating lymphocytes transiently downregulate CD28 with their initial, acute activation in situ (for a few hours). However, these particular T cells do not exhibit the numerous other phenotypic and functional characteristics of end-differentiated lymphocytes (unpublished observations).

Thus, the presence of increased proportions of circulating CD4 T cells that lack CD28 or tissue-infiltrating CD4 T cells that express cytotoxic mediators are surrogate markers that identify clonal, antigen-differentiated effector memory lymphocytes, and this is pathognomonic for the presence of a chronic adaptive immune response [169–174]. The circulating peripheral blood of many IPF patients contains significantly increased proportions of end-differentiated CD4 T cells (Fig. 7.11), and these highly altered, disease-associated lymphocytes are also present and easily identified in the lungs of these patients (Fig. 7.12). Moreover, and as often described in many other immune-mediated disease populations [169, 170, 172, 174], the magnitude of this T cell differentiation in individual IPF patients is also correlated with their disease manifestations and outcomes (Fig. 7.13) [147].

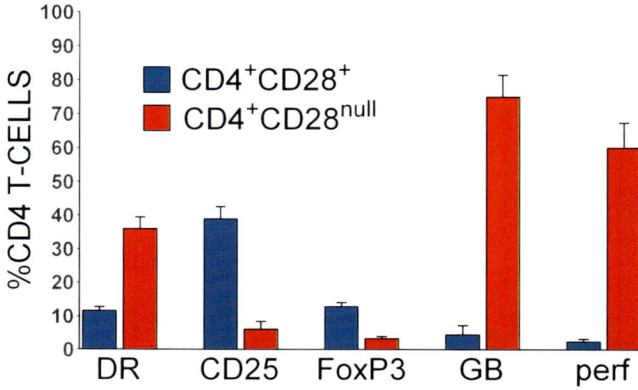

**Fig. 7.11** Altered characteristics of T cells in IPF patients. Among many other phenotypic and functional alterations not shown here, end-differentiated effector memory CD4 T cells (CD28$^{null}$) in IPF patients have discordant expression of activation markers (HLA Class II DR$\beta$1 and CD25), diminished production of FoxP3 (a transcription factor associated with regulatory T cell functions), and enhanced production of cytotoxic mediators (e.g., granzyme b and perforin). All comparisons here to autologous "normal" (naïve or less differentiated CD28$^+$ CD4 T cells) were highly significant. Analogous end-differentiation and essentially identically altered lymphocyte functions are seen in patients with numerous other chronic immune disorders [169–180] (reprinted from [147])

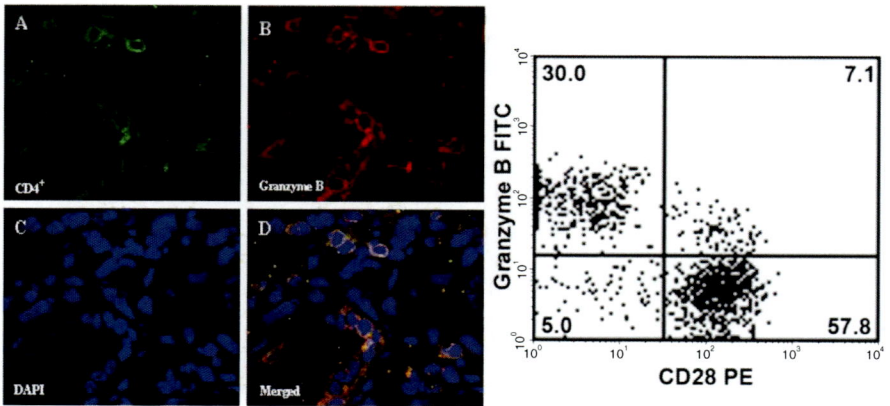

**Fig. 7.12** End-differentiated T cells in IPF lungs. (**a**) Confocal images show granzyme b$^+$ CD4$^+$ cells in IPF lung specimens. Other images (not shown here) confirm that these cells co-express CD3 and are thus CD4 T cells. Effector memory CD4 T cells that have become highly differentiated by repeated, antigen-driven proliferation produce cytotoxic mediators, including granzyme b, whereas "normal" (undifferentiated or minimally differentiated) CD4 T cells do not (see Fig. 7.10). (**b**) Flow cytometric analyses of cells isolated from IPF lungs by enzymatic digestion confirm that end-differentiated granzyme b$^+$CD28$^{null}$ cells comprise a large proportion of the CD4 T lymphocytes in these specimens. These analyses were performed by gating on CD4$^+$CD3$^+$ CD56$^{null}$ cells in the digests. In contrast, end-differentiated CD4 T cells are rare in normal lung specimens (reprinted from [147])

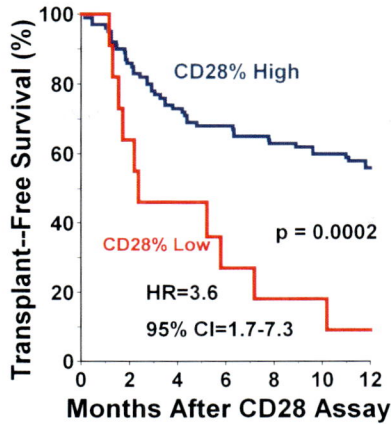

**Fig. 7.13** The extent of CD4 T cell end-differentiation is associated with IPF outcomes. Chronic antigen encounters result in repeated divisions of T cells that bear identical antigen receptors and specificity (clones). The daughter progeny of these T-cell expansions have numerous functional and phenotypic alterations compared to normal (naïve or less differentiated) CD4 T cells, including downregulated cell surface expression of CD28 (see Figs. 7.10, 7.11, and 7.12). CD28 is a costimulatory molecule for naïve T lymphocytes, but end-differentiated, CD28$^{null}$ effector memory CD4 T cells do not require costimulation. The magnitude of this process, easily ascertained by flow cytometric assays of circulating T cells, is highly associated with the manifestations and prognoses of patients with a variety of chronic immunological diseases [169, 170, 172, 174]. IPF patients with greater proportions of circulating, end-differentiated CD4 T cells (CD28 % Low) similarly have much worse prognoses than the patient cohort with more normal CD28 expression (CD28 % High). *HR* hazard ratio; *CI* confidence interval (reprinted from [147])

In addition to their enhanced production of cytotoxic mediators such as granzyme b and perforin, end-differentiated lymphocytes display autonomous and facultatively increased elaboration of multiple cytokines and chemokines that are implicated in IPF pathogenesis (including IL-4, IL-6, IL-13, TNF-α, TGF-β), diminished FoxP3 expression and $T_{reg}$ function, and resistance to apoptosis and the effects of multiple immunosuppressant medications [147, 170, 175–180]. CD4$^+$CD28$^{null}$ T cells isolated from clinical specimens are able to replicate [147, 170, 175, 178], but these have a finite, limited replication potential ex vivo due to their shortened telomeres, which is, in turn, a consequence of their having undergone multiple prior cell divisions. This feature is likely to confound assays of telomere lengths based on the study of peripheral blood leukocytes among patients with IPF as well as non-IPF chronic immune diseases [181].

Analogous T-cell differentiation does not occur in rodents, rendering study of these immunological processes dependent on the procurement of (typically) limited human specimens. The enhanced cytotoxic, proinflammatory, and profibrotic functions of these CD4$^+$CD28$^{null}$ T cells are remarkably similar among the lymphocytes found in patient populations afflicted with very different clinical syndromes [147, 169–180]. Thus, it appears that this lymphocyte differentiation process is an important, biologically conserved adaptation to chronic/repetitive antigen exposures.

Generation of CD4$^+$CD28$^{null}$ T cells has been hypothesized to augment the effectiveness of defenses against difficult-to-eradicate infections (especially intracellular pathogens) that undoubtedly were scourges of early humans (and proto-humans) [169]. Nonetheless, this vestigial mechanism has been implicated as a dysfunctional contributor to many modern afflictions, including various autoimmune syndromes, coronary artery disease, and IPF [147, 170–180].

Many abnormalities of IPF T cells can cause or contribute to the recurrent injuries and disordered repair processes that typify this lung disease. The deleterious cytotoxic actions of activated T cells on proximate tissues (including epithelia and endothelium) have long been recognized as critical steps in the genesis of diverse chronic diseases by investigators of gastrointestinal, renal, cardiac, dermatologic, and rheumatologic disorders [1, 72, 84, 85, 102, 104, 179]. Activated T cells also have many other direct effects on mesenchymal cells that promote the development of fibrosis [1, 84, 182–201]. IPF T cells have increased surface expression of CD40L (CD154) [145], which has the potential to stimulate fibroblasts bearing CD40 and thereby enhance their production of collagen and proinflammatory mediators [185–188]. TGF-β plays a singularly important role in IPF through multiple profibrotic effects [1, 76] that include stimulation of fibroblast chemotaxis and the augmentation of extracellular matrix production [79, 198]. The TGF-β in diseased lungs has largely been attributed to production by epithelial cells or macrophages [1, 57], but activated CD4 T cells of IPF patients are also sources of this cytokine (see Fig. 7.7) [145, 147]. T cells from RA patients with phenotypes indistinguishable from those of IPF subjects [169, 173–178] were recently also shown to promote fibroproliferation mediated by CX$_3$CR1 and TNF-α [197]. The fibroproliferative effects of T cells that have been specifically isolated from IPF patients have been less extensively studied, but these particular lymphocytes have, nonetheless, been shown to similarly stimulate fibroblast proliferation and extracellular matrix production [55, 144, 200]. CD4$^+$CD28$^{null}$ T cells of RA patients are especially potent stimulators of fibroproliferation [197] and, although not yet directly tested, the otherwise identical end-differentiated T cells of IPF patients [147] almost certainly have similarly enhanced effects on fibroblasts.

## B Cells in IPF

Numerous striking B-cell abnormalities are also found in IPF patients. The presence of focal B-cell aggregates in diseased tissues is a pathognomonic feature of an ongoing, abnormal, adaptive immune response [129], and these aggregates are prevalent in IPF lungs [7, 8, 127, 128] (Fig. 7.14). In addition to being a nidus for the production of antibodies (and/or autoantibodies), B cells in these aggregates produce a variety of pathogenic cytokines, chemokines, and vasoactive mediators [118, 129, 202–204]. Lymphoid aggregates in proximity to pulmonary blood vessels are associated with anatomic and functional vascular abnormalities in other disease populations [204]. Identical lesions in IPF lungs seem likely to play an analogous

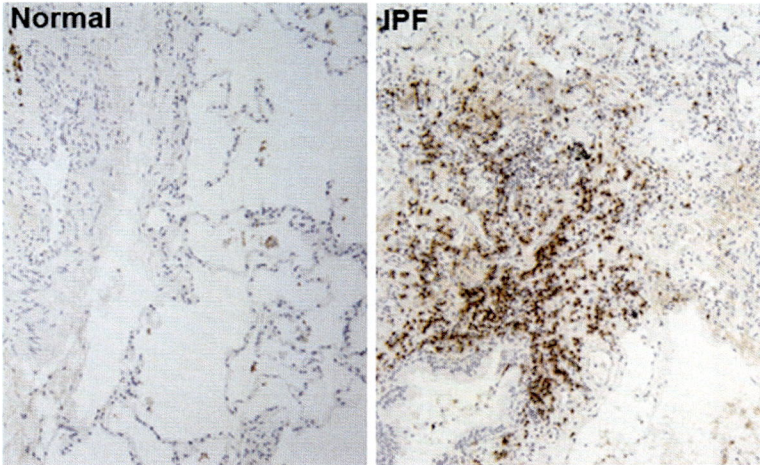

**Fig. 7.14** B-cell aggregates in IPF lungs. Focal CD19+ B-cell aggregates are prevalent in IPF lungs [7, 8, 127, 128]. These findings are pathognomonic for the presence of chronic immune responses [129] and are associated with numerous disease-promoting effects [118]

role in the dysfunctional pulmonary circulation and/or gas exchange abnormalities that are common among these patients [59, 128, 205].

A considerable body of compelling evidence implicates a role for autoantibodies in the progression of IPF. The immunoglobulin genes that encode antibodies are abnormally overexpressed in IPF lungs [6]. Additionally, pathogenic antibody–antigen (immune) complexes [125] are abundant in the sera, bronchoalveolar lavage fluid, and lung parenchyma of IPF patients [9–13, 124] (Fig. 7.15). Diverse autoantibodies against a variety of autologous proteins are found in IPF subjects [11, 13–23, 56, 124, 166, 167], and, by using sensitive methods, autoantibodies can be detected in >80 % of these subjects [124, 145] (Fig. 7.16). In addition to having direct cytotoxic effects [21], autoantibodies isolated from IPF patients have been shown to increase alveolar epithelial cell production of TGF-β [20], and such autoantibodies can also activate monocytes, which then increase their production of IL-8 [124], a potent neutrophil chemotactic and activating chemokine that has been implicated in the pathogenesis of IPF [206]. Other autoantibodies isolated from IPF patients have direct cytotoxic effects [21], and immunoglobulins with specific binding avidity for IL-1α [21], periplakin [166], annexin 1 [167], and HSP70 [124] are significantly associated with IPF progression (Fig. 7.17). The presence of anti-HSP70 autoantibodies in IPF patients are also linked to HLA Class II allele frequency perturbations (Fig. 7.18).

B-lymphocyte stimulating factor (BLyS), also known as B-cell activating factor (BAFF), is a specific, obligate, and nonredundant cytokine product of diverse cell types; BLyS has been demonstrated to be critical for B-cell survival, differentiation, and antibody production [207, 208]. Circulating concentrations of BLyS are increased

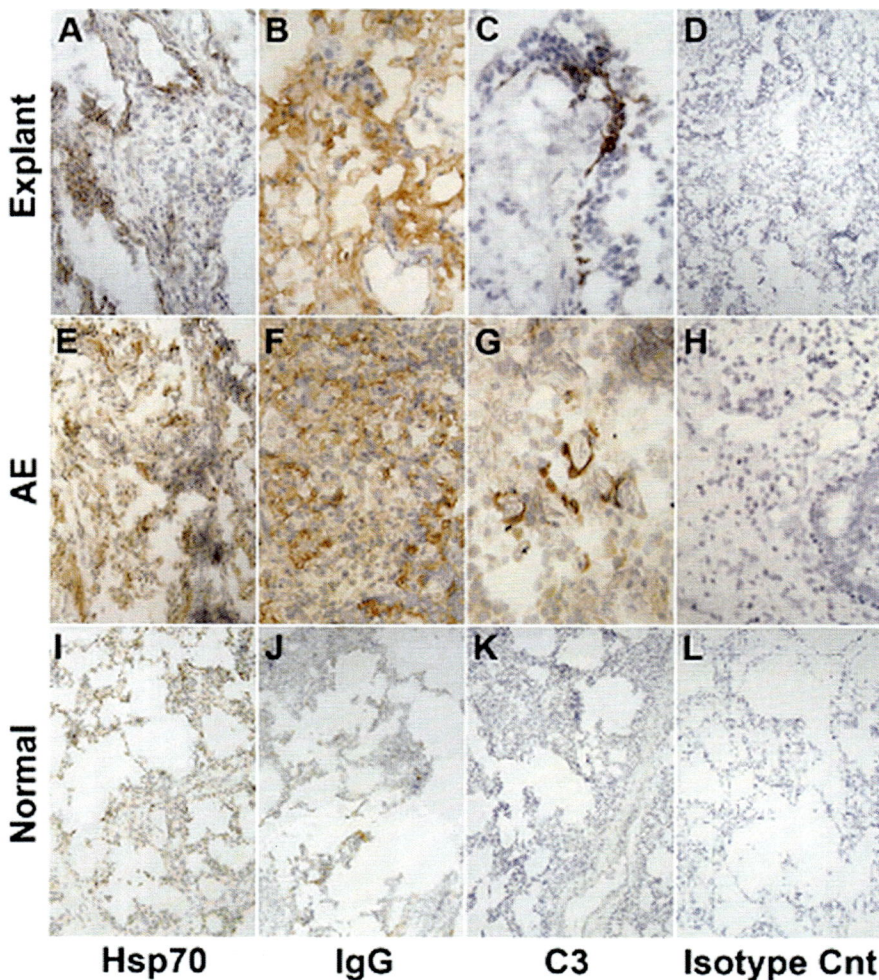

**Fig. 7.15** Antibody-mediated processes in IPF lungs. Columns from *left* to *right* depict expression of heat shock protein 70 (HSP70), IgG, fixed complement (C3), and isotype controls. Rows, from *top* to *bottom* depict lungs explanted during therapeutic transplantation from clinically stable IPF patients (Explant), warm autopsy specimens from IPF patients who died due to acute exacerbations (AE), and normal lungs. IPF lungs invariably show over-expression of HSP70, which has also been identified as an autoantigen in some IPF patients [124], and nearly all of these specimens also have deposits of IgG immune complexes and complement. Findings of immune complexes and complement in tissue indicate the presence of highly abnormal, antibody-mediated pathogenic processes [125], and these were not present in sections normal lungs. These abnormalities are even more prominent in the lungs of IPF patients dying with AE (*middle row*) (modified and reprinted with permission of the American Thoracic Society. Copyright © 2013 American Thoracic Society. Kahloon RA, Xue J, Bhargava A, Csizmadia E, Otterbein L, Kass DJ, et al. idiopathic pulmonary fibrosis patients with antibodies to heat shock protein 70 have poor prognoses. Am J Respir Crit Care Med. 2013 Apr;187(7):768–75. Official journal of the American Thoracic Society)

in conventional autoantibody-mediated disease syndromes (e.g., RA, SLE, Sjögren syndrome), and levels of this cytokine also correlate with clinical progression among the afflicted individuals [207–209]. BLyS levels are similarly elevated in IPF, and are also highly correlated with pulmonary artery pressures and mortality of these patients [128]. A specific anti-BLyS monoclonal antibody that inhibits the function of this cytokine (belimumab) was recently approved for use in SLE patients with pathological autoantibody disease manifestations, and the agent appears to have clinical efficacy and minimal toxicity [66, 207]. If initial indications that BLyS is increased in IPF and strongly associated with clinical manifestations of individual patients are corroborated [128], it may provide the rationale for experimental treatment of this disease cohort with belimumab and/or other analogous agents that are currently in development [207]. Circulating B cells in IPF patients were also described in this report to have greater proportions of antigen-differentiated, antibody-producing lymphocytes [128], which is also consistent with near-identical findings in patients with other autoantibody-mediated diseases [210–212].

Acute exacerbations of classic autoantibody-mediated pulmonary syndromes are characterized by histological findings of diffuse alveolar damage with immune complex and complement deposition, and such exacerbations, which are often associated with rapidly progressive lung function deterioration, are almost always refractory to treatments with steroids and other nonspecific medications [60–70]. However, these otherwise unremitting and lethal disorders may be amenable to directed, specific therapies that remove autoantibodies (e.g., plasma exchange) [61, 63, 213–215], decrease autoantibody production by depleting B cells (e.g., rituximab) [62–65, 67–70, 212], interfere with B-cell maturation (e.g., belimubab) [207–209], and/or inhibit B-cell antibody production (e.g., intravenous immunoglobulin) [63, 213, 215].

Acute exacerbations also occur in a sizeable proportion of IPF patients (see Chap. 16) and are associated with rapid (and often lethal) clinical progression, and such exacerbations are singularly refractory to treatment with corticosteroids and the conventional medical regimens that have been used to date [131, 216]. Also, like many other recognized autoimmune disorders, acute IPF exacerbations are characterized by diffuse alveolar damage [17] and the presence of autoantibodies with defined specificities [21, 124, 167]. Indeed, autopsy specimens from IPF patients who die during acute exacerbations show especially prominent intrapulmonary immune complex and complement deposition (see Fig. 7.15).

If the pathogenesis of acute exacerbations of IPF is autoantibody-mediated, mechanistically based therapies that are analogous to those used in conventional autoimmune disorders could benefit patients with this rapidly progressive syndrome. Preliminary results of a pilot clinical trial to test this hypothesis will be presented soon [217].

## Summary

The many interrelated and overlapping adaptive immune abnormalities among IPF patients more than fulfill criteria that have established the immunological basis of numerous, non-IPF diseases in various other organ systems. No other process, aside

**A**

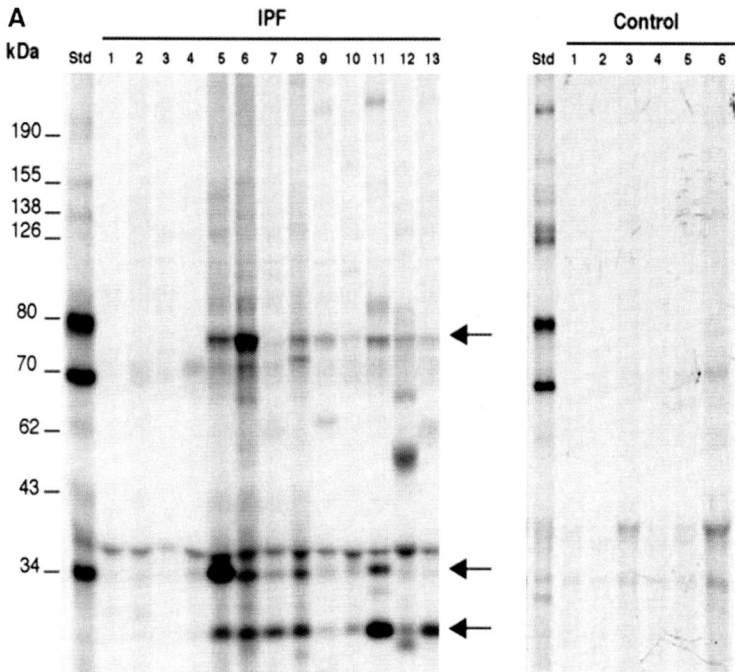

**B**

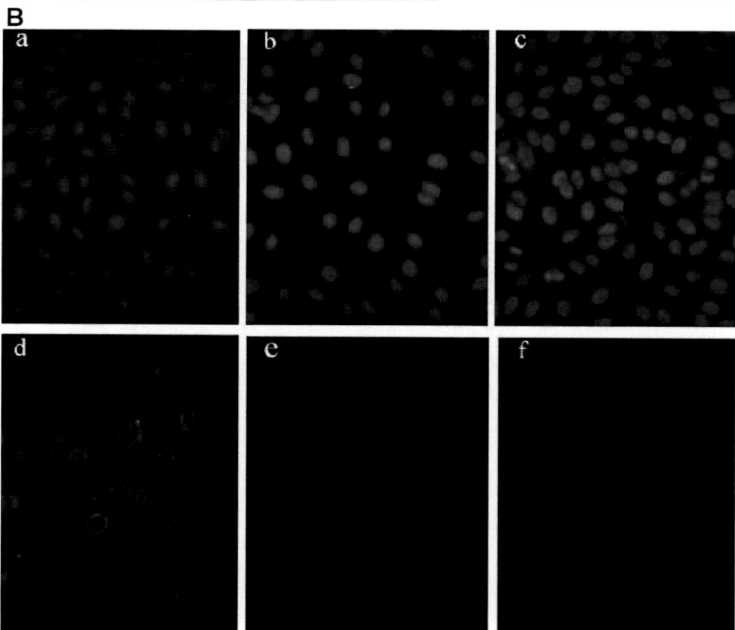

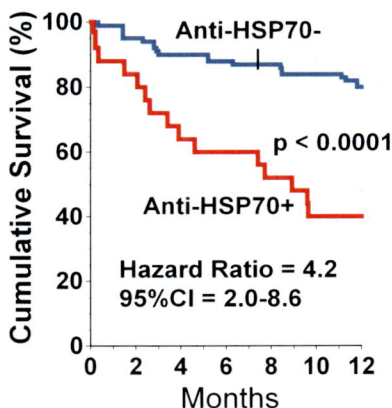

**Fig. 7.17** Association of autoreactivity with outcome in IPF patients. Although there were no intergroup demographic or clinical differences at the time of specimen acquisitions, IPF patients with circulating autoantibodies against heat shock protein 70 (HSP70) had much greater 1-year mortality than anti-HSP70 negative subjects (reprinted with permission of the American Thoracic Society. Copyright © 2013 American Thoracic Society. Kahloon RA, Xue J, Bhargava A, Csizmadia E, Otterbein L, Kass DJ, et al. idiopathic pulmonary fibrosis patients with antibodies to heat shock protein 70 have poor prognoses. Am J Respir Crit Care Med. 2013 Apr;187(7):768–75. Official Journal of the American Thoracic Society)

from the presence of an active, ongoing immune response(s), can readily account for the concurrent HLA allele frequency biases, intrapulmonary lymphocyte infiltrates, and activated, mediator-producing, autoreactive, clonally expanded, and end-differentiated T and B cells seen in IPF. Indeed, many IPF immunological abnormalities are also highly correlated with the observed disease manifestations

**Fig. 7.16** Autoantibodies in IPF patients. (**a**) Plasma autoantibodies of IPF patients cause immunoprecipitation of a variety of cell proteins (i.e., autoantigens). Each lane depicts an immunoprecipitant (IP) of a plasma sample from an individual with IPF or that from a demographically matched, healthy control. Molecular weight standards (kDa) are also shown, and defined, conventional, autoimmune disease antigen standards (Std) (which were not autoantigens of these IPF patients) are also depicted. *Arrows* denote frequently seen ~75, 34, and 25 kDa autoantigens in IPF patients. One or more IP autoantibodies were present in >80 % of IPF specimens (reprinted with permission from The Journal of Immunology 2007 Aug;179(4):2592–9. Copyright 2007. American Association of Immunologists, Inc.). (**b**) Indirect immunofluorescence assays (IFA) corroborate >80 % of IPF plasma specimens (from different subjects than those in *left panel* IP) are positive for anti-epithelial cell autoantibodies, compared to specimens from normal subjects. All specimens from IPF patients with acute exacerbations tested (*n* = 12) were similarly positive. Different patterns of immunofluorescence, as seen here (**a–d**), are consistent with the presence of numerous autoantibodies with specificities for diverse autoantigens located in varied cell compartments. Normal plasma specimens are depicted in panels **e** and **f** (reprinted with permission from the American Thoracic Society. Copyright © 2013 American Thoracic Society. Kahloon RA, Xue J, Bhargava A, Csizmadia E, Otterbein L, Kass DJ, et al. idiopathic pulmonary fibrosis patients with antibodies to heat shock protein 70 have poor prognoses. Am J Respir Crit Care Med. 2013 Apr;187(7):768–75. Official Journal of the American Thoracic Society)

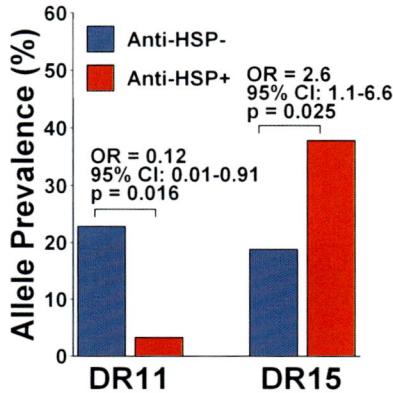

**Fig. 7.18** HLA allele biases of IPF autoimmunity. HLA-DRβ*11*15 is over-represented among IPF patients with circulating autoantibodies to HSP70, whereas HLA-DRβ1*11 appeared to be "protective" (see also Fig. 7.5). HLA allele biases are considered to be a hallmark characteristic of antigen-specific autoimmune responses [85, 89, 92–98] (Reprinted with permission of the American Thoracic Society. Copyright © 2013 American Thoracic Society. Kahloon RA, Xue J, Bhargava A, Csizmadia E, Otterbein L, Kass DJ, et al. idiopathic pulmonary fibrosis patients with antibodies to heat shock protein 70 have poor prognoses. Am J Respir Crit Care Med. 2013 Apr;187(7):768–75. Official Journal of the American Thoracic Society)

and outcomes among individual patients. Analogous adaptive immune processes have been directly linked to the pathogenesis of most (if not all) other fibrotic disorders in humans, and one need not evoke speculation of a heretofore unidentified, unprecedented disease mechanism to account for the pathogenesis of IPF. The cumulative data strongly suggest that T-cell responses to an antigen, or perhaps a series of antigens, occur early in IPF, and such T-cell responses cause and/or promote lung injury. Additional studies have shown that these immune responses can subsequently generalize to also include autoreactivity, which almost certainly contributes to disease progression among many IPF patients.

In light of the many positive and unequivocal findings of biologically plausible, pathogenic immune responses in IPF patients, the current tendency for many leaders in the field to dismiss considerations that immunologic processes are involved in the genesis or progression of IPF seems unjustified. This oversight may, in some instances, reflect an incomplete understanding of fundamental immunobiological processes (e.g., not appreciating the importance and implications of finding lymphocyte clonal proliferations and autoreactivity). Another argument that is often heard is that "because IPF does not respond to steroids, it cannot be immunological." As detailed in this chapter, however, repetitively antigen-stimulated, end-differentiated, and highly pathological T cells found in IPF subjects are especially resistant to the effects of corticosteroids. Moreover, patients with any one of a variety of severe, rapidly progressive autoimmune syndromes, especially autoantibody-mediated lung diseases, typically progress and often die when treated merely with corticosteroids, but some patients can and do respond to specific, mechanistically focused regimens.

Current notions that the chronic lung injury that characterizes IPF are devoid of a significant adaptive immune component have not led to an encompassing, cogent mechanism that explains the development or progression of IPF, nor have they resulted in practical treatments for this disease. New (or resurrected) paradigms, especially those with obvious novel treatment implications, should be entertained on the basis of scientific merit, and then scrupulously tested and advanced as appropriate.

A better understanding of the underlying pathogenic processes that cause or promote IPF could have tangible benefits for patients afflicted with this morbid disease. Valid, scientifically based insights into the pathological processes of IPF will enable us to rationally select and test specific, mechanistically targeted biological response modifiers that have the potential to be uniquely beneficial for these otherwise doomed patients.

**Acknowledgments**  Supported in part by NIH grant: HL107172.

# References

1. Wynn TA. Fibrotic disease and the TH1/TH2 paradigm. Nat Rev Immunol. 2004;4(8):583–94.
2. Kravis TC, Ahmed A, Brown TE, Fulmer JD, Crystal RG. Pathogenic mechanisms in pulmonary fibrosis. Collagen-induced migration inhibition factor production and cytotoxicity mediated by lymphocytes. J Clin Invest. 1976;58(5):1223–32.
3. Bitterman PB, Rennard SI, Keogh BA, Wewers MD, Adelberg S, Crystal RG. Familial idiopathic pulmonary fibrosis. Evidence of lung inflammation in unaffected family members. N Engl J Med. 1986;314(21):1343–7.
4. Lympany PA, Southcott AM, Welsh KI, Black CM, Boylston AW, du Bois RM. T cell receptor gene usage in patients with fibrosing alveolitis and control subjects. Eur J Clin Invest. 1999;29(2):173–81.
5. Shimizudani N, Murata H, Keino H, Kogo S, Nakamura H, Morishima Y, et al. Conserved CDR 3 region of T cell receptor BV gene in lymphocytes from bronchoalveolar lavage fluid of patients with idiopathic pulmonary fibrosis. Clin Exp Immunol. 2002;129(1):140–9.
6. Zuo F, Kaminski N, Eugui E, Allard J, Yakhini Z, Ben-Dor A, et al. Gene expression analysis reveals matrilysin as a key regulator of pulmonary fibrosis in mice and humans. Proc Natl Acad Sci USA. 2002;99(9):6292–7.
7. Campbell DA, Poulter LW, Janossy G, du Bois RM. Immunohistological analysis of lung tissue from patients with cryptogenic fibrosing alveolitis suggesting local expression of immune hypersensitivity. Thorax. 1985;40(6):405–11.
8. Wallace WA, Howie SEM, Krajewski AS, Lamb D. The immunologic architecture of B-lymphocyte aggregates in cryptogenic fibrosing alveolitis. J Pathol. 1996;178(3):323–9.
9. Dreisin RB, Schwarz MI, Theofilopoulos AN, Stanford RE. Circulating immune complexes in the idiopathic interstitial pneumonias. N Engl J Med. 1978;298(7):353–7.
10. Dall'Aglio PP, Pesci A, Bertorelli G, Brianti E, Scarpa S. Study of immune complexes in broncholaveolar lavage fluids. Respiration. 1988;54 Suppl 1:36–41.
11. Dobashi N, Fujita J, Ohtsuki Y, Yamadori I, Yoshinouchi T, Kamei T, et al. Circulating cytokeratin 8: anti-cytokeratin 8 antibody complexes in sera of patients with pulmonary fibrosis. Respiration. 1999;67(4):397–401.
12. Haslam PL, Thompson B, Mohammed I, Townsend PJ, Hodson ME, Holborow EJ, et al. Circulating immune complexes in patients with cryptogenic fibrosing alveolitis. Clin Exp Immunol. 1979;37(3):381–90.

13. Dobashi N, Fujita J, Murota M, Ohtsuki Y, Yamadori I, Yoshinouchi T, et al. Elevation of anti-cytokeratin 18 antibody and circulating cytokeratin 18: anti-cytokeratin 18 antibody immune complexes in sera of patients with idiopathic pulmonary fibrosis. Lung. 2000;178(3):171–9.
14. Chapman JR, Charles PJ, Venables PJ, Thompson PJ, Haslam PL, Maini RN, et al. Definition and clinical relevance of antibodies to nuclear ribonucleoprotein and other nuclear antigens in patients with cryptogenic fibrosing alveolitis. Am Rev Respir Dis. 1984;130(3):439–43.
15. Grigolo B, Mazzetti I, Borzi RM, Hickson ID, Fabbri M, Fasano L, Meliconi R, et al. Mapping of topoisomerase II alpha epitopes recognized by autoantibodies in idiopathic pulmonary fibrosis. Clin Exp Immunol. 1998;114(3):339–46.
16. Meliconi R, Negri C, Borzi RM, Facchini A, Sturani C, Fasano L, et al. Antibodies to topoisomerase II in idiopathic pulmonary fibrosis. Clin Rheumatol. 1993;12(3):311–5.
17. Yang Y, Fujita J, Bandho S, Ohtsuki Y, Yamadori I, Yoshinouchi T, et al. Detection of antivimentin antibody in sera of patients with idiopathic pulmonary fibrosis and non-specific interstitial pneumonia. Clin Exp Immunol. 2002;128(1):169–74.
18. Fujita J, Dobashi N, Ohtsuki Y. Elevation of anti-cytokeratin 19 antibody in sera of the patients with idiopathic pulmonary fibrosis and pulmonary fibrosis associated with collagen vascular disorders. Lung. 1999;177(11):311–9.
19. Wallace WA, Schofield JA, Lamb D, Howie SE. Localization of a pulmonary autoantigen in cryptogenic fibrosing alveolitis. Thorax. 1994;49(11):1139–45.
20. Wallace WA, Howie SE. Upregulation of tenascin and TGF-β production in a type II alveolar epithelial cell line by antibody against a pulmonary auto-antigen. J Pathol. 2001;195(2):251–6.
21. Ogushi F, Tani K, Endo T, Tada H, Kawano T, Asano T, et al. Autoantibodies to IL-1α in sera from rapidly progressive idiopathic pulmonary fibrosis. J Med Invest. 2001;48(3–4):181–9.
22. Wallace WA, Roberts SN, Caldwell H, Thornton E, Greening PA, Lamb D, et al. Circulating antibodies to lung proteins in patients with cryptogenic fibrosing alveolitis. Thorax. 1993; 49(3):218–24.
23. Nakos G, Adams A, Andriopoulos N. Antibodies to collagen in patients with idiopathic pulmonary fibrosis. Chest. 1993;103(4):1051–8.
24. Homolka J, Ziegenhagen MW, Gaede KI, Entzian P, Zissel G, Muller-Quernheim J. Systemic immune cell activation in a subgroup of patients with idiopathic pulmonary fibrosis. Respiration. 2003;70(3):262–9.
25. Stewart GA, Hoyne GF, Ahmad SA, Jarman E, Wallace WA, Harrison DJ, et al. Expression of the developmental Sonic hedgehog (Shh) signaling pathway is upregulated in chronic lung fibrosis and the Shh receptor patched 1 is present in circulating T lymphocytes. J Pathol. 2003;199(4):488–9.
26. Suzuki E, Tsukada H, Ishida T, Ishizuka O, Hasegawa T, Gejyo F. Correlation between the numbers of gamma delta T cells and CD4+ HLA-DR+ T cells in broncho-alveolar lavage fluid from patients with diffuse lung disease. Tohoku J Exp Med. 2002;196(4):231–40.
27. Ma W, Cui W, Lin Q. Improved immnunophenotyping of lymphocytes in bronchoalveolar lavage fluid (BALF) by flow cytometry. Clin Chim Acta. 2001;313(1–2):133–8.
28. Kaneko Y, Kuwano K, Kunitake R, Kawasaki M, Hagimoto N, Hara N. B7-1, B7-2 and class II MHC molecules in idiopathic pulmonary fibrosis and bronchiolitis obliterans-organizing pneumonia. Eur Respir J. 2000;15(1):49–55.
29. Nagai S, Fujimura N, Hirata T, Izumi T. Differentiation between idiopathic pulmonary fibrosis and interstitial pneumonia associated with collagen vascular diseases by comparison of the ratio of OKT4+ cells and OKT8+ cells in BALF T lymphocytes. Eur J Respir Dis. 1985;67(1):1–9.
30. Garcia JG, Wolven RG, Garcia PL, Keogh BA. Assessment of interlobar variation of bronchoalveolar lavage cellular differentials in interstitial lung diseases. Am Rev Respir Dis. 1986;133(3):444–9.
31. Fireman E, Vardinon N, Burke M, Spizer S, Levin S, Endler A, et al. Predictive value of response to treatment of T-lymphocyte subpopulations in idiopathic pulmonary fibrosis. Eur Respir J. 1998;11(3):706–11.

32. Agostini C, Siviero M, Semenzato G. Immune effector cells in idiopathic pulmonary fibrosis. Curr Opin Pulm Med. 1997;3(5):348–55.
33. Emura M, Nagai S, Takeuchi M, Kitaichi M, Izumi T. In vitro production of B cell growth factor and B cell differentiation factor by peripheral blood mononuclear cells and bronchoalveolar lavage T lymphocytes from patients with idiopathic pulmonary fibrosis. Clin Exp Immunol. 1990;82(1):133–9.
34. Rihs S, Walker C, Virchow Jr JC, Boer C, Kroegel C, Giri SN, et al. Differential expression of alpha E beta 7 integrins on bronchoalveolar lavage T lymphocyte subsets: regulation by alpha 4 beta 1-integrin crosslinking and TGF-beta. Am J Respir Cell Mol Biol. 1996;15(5):600–10.
35. Gruber R, Pforte A, Beer B, Riethmuller G. Determination of gamma/delta and other T-lymphocyte subsets in bronchoalveolar lavage fluid and peripheral blood from patients with sarcoidosis and idiopathic fibrosis of the lung. APMIS. 1996;104(3):199–205.
36. Utsumi K, Kawanishi K, Kuriyama Y, Nakano M, Ichinose Y, Toyama K. Gamma delta T cells in peripheral blood and in bronchoalveolar lavage fluid from patients with sarcoidosis and idiopathic pulmonary fibrosis. Nihon Kyobu Shikkan Gakkai Zasshi. 1995;33(11): 1186–90.
37. Nakao A, Hasegawa Y, Tsuchiya Y, Shimokata K. Expression of cell adhesion molecules in the lungs of patients with idiopathic pulmonary fibrosis. Chest. 1995;108(1):233–9.
38. Walker C, Bauer W, Braun RK, Menz G, Braun P, Schwarz F, et al. Activated T cells and cytokines in bronchoalveolar lavages from patients with various lung diseases associated with eosinophilia. Am J Respir Crit Care Med. 1994;150(4):1038–48.
39. Groen H, Hamstra M, Aalbers R, van der Mark TW, Koeter GH, Postma DS. Clinical evaluation of lymphocyte sub-populations and oxygen radical production in sarcoidosis and idiopathic pulmonary fibrosis. Respir Med. 1994;88(1):55–64.
40. Striz I, Wang YM, Svarcova I, Trnka L, Sorg C, Costabel U. The phenotype of alveolar macrophages and its correlation with immune cells in bronchoalveolar lavage. Eur Respir J. 1993;6(9):1287–94.
41. van Dinther-Janssen AC, van Maarsseveen TC, Eckert H, Newman W, Meijer CJ. Identical expression of ELAM-1, VCAM-1, and ICAM-1 in sarcoidosis and usual interstitial pneumonitis. J Pathol. 1993;170(2):157–64.
42. Costabel U, Guzman J. Bronchoalveolar lavage in interstitial lung disease. Curr Opin Pulm Med. 2001;7(5):255–61.
43. Robinson BW, Rose AH. Pulmonary gamma interferon production in patients with fibrosing alveolitis. Thorax. 1990;45(2):105–8.
44. Meliconi R, Lalli E, Borzi RM, Sturani C, Galavotti V, Gunell G, et al. Idiopathic pulmonary fibrosis: can cell mediated immunity markers predict clinical outcome? Thorax. 1990;45(7): 536–40.
45. Karpel JP, Norin AJ. Association of activated cytolytic lung lymphocytes with response to prednisone therapy in patients with idiopathic pulmonary fibrosis. Chest. 1989;96(4):794–8.
46. Reynolds SP, Jones KP, Edwards JH, Davies BH. Immunoregulatory proteins in bronchoalveolar lavage fluid. A comparative analysis of pigeon breeders' disease, sarcoidosis and idiopathic pulmonary fibrosis. Sarcoidosis. 1989;6(2):125–34.
47. Kallenberg CG, Schilizzi BM, Beaumont F, De Leij L, Poppema S, The TH. Expression of class II major histocompatibility complex antigens on alveolar epithelium in interstitial lung disease: relevance to pathogenesis of idiopathic pulmonary fibrosis. J Clin Pathol. 1987;40(7):725–33.
48. Watters LC, Schwarz MI, Cherniack RM, Waldron JA, Dunn TL, Stanford RE, et al. Idiopathic pulmonary fibrosis. Pretreatment bronchoalveolar lavage cellular constituents and their relationship with lung histopathology and clinical response to therapy. Am Rev Respir Dis. 1987;135(3):696–704.
49. Turner-Warwick M, Haslam PL. The value of serial bronchoalveolar lavages in assessing the clinical progress of patients with cryptogenic fibrosing alveolitis. Am Rev Respir Dis. 1987;135(1):26–34.

50. Kallenberg CG, Schilizzi BM, Beaumont F, Poppema S, De Leij L. The expression of class II MHC antigens on alveolar epithelium in fibrosing alveolitis. Clin Exp Immunol. 1987;67(1):182–90.
51. Kradin RL, Divertie MB, Colvin RB, Ramirez J, Ryu J, Carpenter HA, et al. Usual interstitial pneumonitis is a T cell alveolitis. Clin Immunol Immunopathol. 1986;40(2):224–35.
52. Paradis IL, Dauber JH, Rabin BS. Lymphocyte phenotypes in bronchoalveolar lavage and lung tissue in sarcoidosis and idiopathic pulmonary fibrosis. Am Rev Respir Dis. 1986;133(5):855–60.
53. Norin A, Karpel J, Fleitman J, Kamholz S, Pinsker K. Concanavalin A dependent cell-mediated cytotoxicity (CDCMC) in bronchoalveolar lavage (BAL) fluid of patients with interstitial lung diseases (ILD). Evidence of cytolytic T-lymphocyte (CTL) activity. Chest. 1986;89(3 Suppl):144S–5.
54. Pesci A, Bertorelli G, Manganelli P. Differentiation between idiopathic pulmonary fibrosis and interstitial pneumonia associated with collagen vascular diseases by comparison of the ratio of OKT4+ cells and OKT8+ in BALF T-lymphocytes. Eur J Respir Dis. 1986;68(2):155–6.
55. Cathcart MK, Emdur LI, Ahtiala-Stewart K, Ahmad M. Excessive helper T cell function in patients with idiopathic pulmonary fibrosis: correlation with disease activity. Clin Immunol Immunopathol. 1987;43(3):382–94.
56. Crystal RG, Fulmer JD, Roberts WC, Moss ML, Line BR, Reynolds HY. Idiopathic pulmonary fibrosis. Clinical, histologic, radiographic, physiologic, scintigraphic, cytologic, and biochemical aspects. Ann Intern Med. 1976;85(6):769–887.
57. Selman M, Thannickal VJ, Pardo A, Zisman DA, Martinez FJ, Lynch III JP. Idiopathic pulmonary fibrosis: pathogenesis and therapeutic approaches. Drugs. 2004;64(4):406–30.
58. Gauldie J. Inflammatory mechanisms are a minor component of the pathogenesis of idiopathic pulmonary fibrosis. Am J Respir Crit Care Med. 2002;165(9):1205–6.
59. Raghu G, Collard HR, Egan JJ, Martinez FJ, Behr J, Brown KK, et al. An official ATS/ERS/JRS/ALAT statement: idiopathic pulmonary fibrosis: evidence-based guidelines for diagnosis and management. Am J Respir Crit Care Med. 2011;183(6):788–824.
60. Arzoo K, Sadeghi S, Liebman HA. Treatment of refractory antibody mediated autoimmune disorders with an anti-CD20 monoclonal antibody (rituximab). Ann Rheum Dis. 2002;61(10):922–4.
61. Erickson SB, Kurtz SB, Donadio JV, Holley KE, Wilson CB, Pineda AA. Use of combined plasmapharesis and immunosuppression in the treatment of Goodpasture's syndrome. Mayo Clin Proc. 1979;54(11):714–20.
62. Sem M, Molberg O, Lund MB, Gran JT. Rituximab treatment of the anti-synthetase syndrome: a retrospective case series. Rheumatology (Oxford). 2009;48(8):968–71.
63. Martinu T, Howell DN, Palmer SM. Acute cellular rejection and humoral sensitization in lung transplant recipients. Semin Respir Crit Care Med. 2010;31(2):179–88.
64. Borie R, Debray MP, Laine C, Aubier M, Crestani B. Rituximab therapy in autoimmune pulmonary alveolar proteinosis. Eur Respir J. 2009;33(6):1503–6.
65. Keir GJ, Maher TM, Hansell DM, Denton CP, Ong VH, Singh S, et al. Severe interstitial lung disease in connective tissue disease: rituximab as rescue therapy. Eur Respir J. 2012;40(3):641–8.
66. Furie R, Petri M, Zamani O, Cervera R, Wallace DJ, Tegzová D, et al. A phase III, randomized, placebo-controlled study of belimumab, a monoclonal antibody that inhibits B lymphocyte stimulator, in patients with systemic lupus erythematosus. Arthritis Rheum. 2011;63(12):3918–30.
67. Stone JH, Merkel PA, Spiera R, Seo P, Langford CA, Hoffman GS, et al. Rituximab versus cyclophosphamide for ANCA-associated vasculitis. N Engl J Med. 2010;363(3):221–32.
68. Shah Y, Mohiuddin A, Sluman C, Daryanani I, Ledson T, Banerjee A, et al. Rituximab in anti-glomerular basement membrane disease. QJM. 2011;105(2):195–7.
69. Perosa F, Prete M, Racanelli V, Dammacco F. CD20-depleting therapy in autoimmune diseases: from basic research to the clinic. J Intern Med. 2010;267(3):260–77.

70. Daoussis D, Liossis SN, Tsamandas AC, Kalogeropoulou C, Paliogianni F, Sirinian C, et al. Effect of long-term treatment with rituximab on pulmonary function and skin fibrosis in patients with diffuse systemic sclerosis. Clin Exp Rheumatol. 2012;30(2 Sup 71):S17–22.
71. Coward WR, Saini G, Jenkins G. The pathogenesis of idiopathic pulmonary fibrosis. Ther Adv Respir Dis. 2010;4(6):316–88.
72. Barron L, Wynn TA. Fibrosis is regulated by Th2 and Th17 responses and by dynamic interactions between fibroblasts and macrophages. Am J Physiol Gastrointest Liver Physiol. 2011;300(5):G723–8.
73. Moore BB, Hogaboam CM. Murine models of pulmonary fibrosis. Am J Physiol Lung Cell Mol Physiol. 2008;294(2):L152–60.
74. Gauldie J, Kolb M. Animal models of pulmonary fibrosis: how far from effective reality? Am J Physiol Lung Cell Mol Physiol. 2008;294(2):L151.
75. Lundblad LK, Thompson-Figueroa J, Leclair T, Sullivan MJ, Poynter ME, Irvin CG, et al. Tumor necrosis factor-alpha overexpression in lung disease: a single cause behind a complex phenotype. Am J Respir Crit Care Med. 2005;171(12):1363–70.
76. Sime PJ, Xing Z, Graham FL, Csaky KG, Gauldie J. Adenovector-mediated gene transfer of active transforming growth factor-beta1 induces prolonged severe fibrosis in rat lung. J Clin Invest. 1997;100(4):768–76.
77. Hao Z, Hampel B, Yagita H, Rajewsky K. T cell-specific ablation of Fas leads to Fas ligand-mediated lymphocyte depletion and inflammatory pulmonary fibrosis. J Exp Med. 2004;199(10):1355–65.
78. Shum AK, DeVoss J, Tan CL, Hou Y, Johannes K, O'Gorman CS, et al. Identification of an autoantigen demonstrates a link between interstitial lung disease and a defect in central tolerance. Sci Transl Med. 2009;1(9):9ra20. doi: 10.1126/scitranslmed.3000284.
79. Xue J, Tomai L, Leme A, Schneider F, Duncan SR. A humanized mouse model replicates the pathologic CD4 T cell differentiation of patients with chronic immunologic lung diseases. Am J Respir Crit Care Med. 2011;183(7), A16325 (Abstract).
80. Murphy K. Janeway's Immunobiology. 8th ed. New York: Garland Science; 2011.
81. Abbas AK, Lichtman AHH, Pillal S. Cellular and molecular immunology. 7th ed. Philadelphia: Elsevier; 2011.
82. Delves PJ, Martin SJ, Burton DR, Roitt IM. Roitt's Essential immunology. 12th ed. Hoboken, NJ: John Wiley and Sons; 2011.
83. Ermann J, Fathman CG. Autoimmune diseases: genes, bugs, and failed regulation. Nat Immunol. 2001;2(9):759–61.
84. Marrack P, Kappler J, Kotzin BL. Autoimmune disease: why and where it occurs. Nat Immunol. 2001;7(8):899–905.
85. Fu SM, Deshmukh US, Gaskin F. Pathogenesis of systemic lupus erythematosus revisited 2011: end organ resistance to damage, autoantibody initiation and diversification, and HLA-DR. J Autoimmun. 2011;37(2):104–12.
86. Pordeus V, Szyper-Kravitz M, Levy RA, Vaz NM, Shoenfeld Y. Infections and autoimmunity: a panorama. Clin Rev Allergy Immunol. 2008;34(3):283–99.
87. Rudolph MG, Stanfield RL, Wilson IA. How TCRs bind MHCs, peptides, and coreceptors. Annu Rev Immunol. 2006;24:419–66.
88. Marsh SG, Albert ED, Bodmer WF, Bontrop RE, Dupont B, Erlich HA, et al. Nomenclature for factors of the HLA System, 2010. Tissue Antigens. 2010;75(4):291–455.
89. de Bakker PI, McVean G, Sabeti PC, Miretti MM, Green T, Marchini J, et al. A high-resolution HLA and SNP haplotype map for disease association studies in the extended human MHC. Nat Genet. 2006;38(10):1166–72.
90. Apanius V, Penn D, Slev PR, Ruff LR, Potts WK. The nature of selection on the major histocompatibility complex. Crit Rev Immunol. 1997;17(2):179–224.
91. Wedekind C, Seebeck T, Bettens F, Paepke AJ. MHC-dependent mate preferences in humans. Proc Biol Sci. 1995;260(1359):245–9.
92. Hall FC, Bowness P. HLA and disease: from molecular function to disease association? In: Browning MJ, McMichael AJ, editors. HLA and MHC: genes, molecules, and function. Oxford: BIOS Scientific Publishers Ltd; 1996. p. 353–81.

93. Furukawa H, Oka S, Shimada K, Sugii S, Ohashi J, Matsui T, et al. Association of humal leukocyte antigen with interstitial lung disease in rheumatoid arthritis: a protective role for shared epitope. PLoS One. 2012;7(5):e33133.
94. Schmidt H, Williamson D, Ashley-Koch A. HLA-DR15 haplotype and multiple sclerosis: a huge review. Am J Epidemiol. 2007;165(10):1097–109.
95. Takeuchi F, Nakano K, Nabeta H, Hong GH, Kawasugi K, Mori M, et al. Genetic contribution of the tumor necrosis factor (TNF) B+252*2/2 genotype, but not the TNFa, b microsatellite alleles, to system lupus erythematosis in Japanese patients. Int J Immunogenet. 2005;32(3):173–8.
96. Voorter CEM, Drent M, van den Berg-Loonen EM. Severe pulmonary sarcoidosis is strongly associated with the haplotype HLA-DQB1*0602-DRB1*1501. Hum Immunol. 2005;66(7):826–35.
97. Stewart CA, Horton R, Allcock RJN, Ashurst JL, Atrazhev AM, Coggill P, et al. Complete MHC haplotype sequencing for common disease gene mapping. Genome Res. 2004;14(6):1176–87.
98. Shiina T, Hosomichi K, Inoko H, Kulski JK. The HLA genomic loci map: expression, interaction, diversity and disease. J Hum Genet. 2009;54(1):15–39.
99. Oldstone MB. Molecular mimicry, microbial infection and autoimmune disease: evolution of the concept. Curr Top Microbiol Immunol. 2005;296:1–17.
100. Vanderlugt CL, Miller SD. Epitope spreading in immune mediated diseases: implications for immunotherapy. Nat Rev Immunol. 2002;109(2):85–94.
101. Day EB, Charlton KL, La Gruta NL, Doherty PC, Turner SJ. Effect of MHC class I diversification on influenza epitope-specific CD8+ T cell precursor frequency and subsequent effector function. J Immunol. 2011;186(11):6319–28.
102. Monaco C, Andreakos E, Kiriakidis S, Feldman M, Paleolog E. T cell-mediated signaling in immune, inflammatory and angiogenic processes: the cascade of events leading to inflammatory diseases. Curr Drug Targets Inflamm Allergy. 2004;3(1):35–42.
103. Crane IJ, Forrester JV. Th1 and Th2 lymphoyctes in autoimmune disease. Crit Rev Immunol. 2005;25(2):75–102.
104. Skapenko A, Leipe J, Libsky PE, Schulze-Koops H. The role of the T cell in autoimmune inflammation. Arthritis Res Ther. 2005;7 Suppl 2:S4–14.
105. Fabbri M, Smart C, Pardi R. T lymphocytes. Int J Biochem Cell Biol. 2003;35(7):1004–8.
106. Bevan MJ. Helping the CD8+ T cell response. Nat Rev Immunol. 2004;4(8):595–602.
107. Thomas LR, Cobb RM, Oltz EM. Dynamic regulation of antigen receptor gene assembly. Adv Exp Med Biol. 2009;650:103–15.
108. Goldrath AW, Bevan MJ. Selecting and maintaining a diverse T cell repertoire. Nature. 1999;402(6759):255–62.
109. Xing Y, Hogquist KA. T cell tolerance: central and peripheral. Cold Spring Harb Perspect Biol. 2012;4(6). doi: 10.1101/cshperspect.a006957.
110. Doherty PC, Christensen JP. Accessing complexity: the dynamics of virus-specific T cell responses. Annu Rev Immunol. 2000;18:561–92.
111. Maini MK, Casorati G, Dellabona P, Wack A, Beverely PC. T cell clonality in immune responses. Immunol Today. 1999;20(6):161–6.
112. Turner SJ, Doherty PC, McCluskey J, Rossjohn J. Structural determinants of T cell receptor bias in immunity. Nat Rev Immunol. 2006;6(12):883–94.
113. Duncan SR, Leonard C, Theodore J, Lega M, Girgis RE, Rosen GD, et al. Oligoclonal CD4+ T cell expansions in lung transplant recipients with obliterative bronchioloitis. Am J Respir Crit Care Med. 2002;165(10):1439–46.
114. Long SA, Khalili J, Ashe J, Berenson R, Ferrand C, Bonyhadi M. Standardized analysis for the quantitation of Vbeta CDR3 T cell receptor diversity. J Immunol Methods. 2006;317(1–2):100–13.
115. Ogle BM, Cascalho M, Joao C, Taylor W, West LJ, Platt JL. Direct measurement of lymphocyte receptor diversity. Nucleic Acids Res. 2003;31(22):e139.

116. Posnett DN, Sinha R, Kabak S, Russo C. Clonal populations of T cells in normal elderly humans: the T cell equivalent to "benign monoclonal gammapathy.". J Exp Med. 1994;179(2):609–18.

117. Hingorani R, Choi I-H, Akolhar P, Gulwani-Akollar B, Pergolizzi R, Silver J, et al. Clonal predominance of T cell receptors within the CD8+ CD45RO+ subset in normal human subjects. J Immunol. 1993;151(10):5762–9.

118. Browning JL. B cells move to center stage: novel opportunities for autoimmune disease treatment. Nat Rev Drug Discov. 2006;5(7):564–75.

119. Goodnow CC, Fazekas de St. Groth B, Goodnow CC, Vinuesa CG. Cellular and genetic mechanisms of self tolerance and autoimmunity. Nature. 2005;435(7042):590–7.

120. Tonegawa S. Somatic generation of antibody diversity. Nature. 1983;302(5909):575–81.

121. McHeyzer-Williams M, Okitsu S, Wang N, McHeyzer-Williams L. Molecular programming of B cell memory. Nat Rev Immunol. 2011;12(1):24–34.

122. Shapiro-Shelef M, Calame K. Regulation of plasma-cell development. Nat Rev Immunol. 2005;5(3):230–42.

123. Detanico T, St Clair JB, Aviszus K, Kirchenbaum G, Guo W, Wysocki LJ. Somatic mutagenesis in autoimmunity. Autoimmunity. 2013;46(2):102–14.

124. Kahloon RA, Xue J, Bhargava A, Csizmadia E, Otterbein L, Kass DJ. Idiopathic pulmonary fibrosis patients with antibodies to heat shock protein 70 have poor prognoses. Am J Respir Crit Care Med. 2013;187(7):768–75.

125. Mayadas TN, Tsokos GC, Tsuboi N. Mechanisms of immune complex-mediated neutrophil recruitment and tissue injury. Circulation. 2009;120(20):2012–24.

126. Feghali-Bostwick CA, Gadgil AS, Otterbein LE, Pilewski JM, Stoner MW, Csizmadia E, et al. Autoantibodies in patients with chronic obstructive pulmonary disease. Am J Respir Crit Care Med. 2008;177(2):156–63.

127. Marchal-Somme J, Uzunhan Y, Marchand-Adam S, Valeyre D, Soumelis V, Crestani B, et al. Cutting edge: non-proliferating mature immune cells form a novel type of organizing lymphoid structure in idiopathic pulmonary fibrosis. J Immunol. 2006;176(10):5735–9.

128. Xue J, Kass DJ, Bon J, Vuga L, Tan J, Czimadia E, et al. Plasma B-lymphocyte stimulator (BLyS) and B-cell differentiation in patients with in idiopathic pulmonary fibrosis J Immunol. 2013;191(5):2089–95.

129. Aloisi F, Pujol-Borrell R. Lymphoid neogenesis in chronic inflammatory disease. Nat Rev Immunol. 2006;6(3):205–11.

130. Katzenstein A-L, Myers JL. Idiopathic pulmonary fibrosis. Clinical relevance of pathologic classification. Am J Respir Crit Care Med. 1998;157(4 part 1):1301–15.

131. Collard HR, Moore BB, Flaherty KR, Brown KK, Kaner RJ, King TE, et al. Acute exacerbations of idiopathic pulmonary fibrosis. Am J Respir Crit Care Med. 2007;176(7):636–43.

132. Yokota S, Chiba S, Furuyama H, Fujii N. Cerebrospinal fluids containing anti-HSP70 autoantibodies from multiple sclerosis patients augment HSP70-induced proinflammatory cytokine production in monocytic cells. J Neuroimmunol. 2010;218(1–2):129–33.

133. Yokota S, Seiji Minota S, Fujii N. Anti-HSP auto-antibodies enhance HSP-induced proinflammatory cytokine production in human monocytic cells via Toll-like receptors. Int Immunol. 2006;18(4):573–80.

134. Lu MC, Lai NS, Yu HC, Huang HB, Hsieh SC, Yu CL. Anti-citrullinated protein antibodies bind surface-expressed citrullinated Grp78 on monocyte/macrophages and stimulate tumor necrosis factor alpha production. Arthritis Rheum. 2010;62(5):1213–23.

135. Racanelli V, Prete M, Musaraj G, Dammacco F, Perosa F. Autoantibodies to intracellular antigens: generation and pathogenetic role. Autoimmun Rev. 2011;10(8):503–8.

136. Evans C. HLA antigens in diffuse fibrosing alveolitis. Thorax. 1976;31(4):483.

137. Strimlan CV, Taswell HF, DeRemee RA, Kuepper F. HLA antigens and fibrosing alveolitis. Am Rev Respir Dis. 1977;116(6):1120–1.

138. Fulmer JD, Sposovska MS, von Gal ER, Crystal RG, Mittal KK. Distribution of HLA antigens in idiopathic pulmonary fibrosis. Am Rev Respir Dis. 1978;118(1):141–7.

139. Turton CWG, Morris LM, Lawler SD, Turner-Warwick M. HLA in cryptogenic fibrosing alveolitis. Lancet. 1978;1(8062):507–8.

140. Varpela E, Tiililkainen A, Varpela M, Tukiainen P. High prevalences of HLA-B15 and HLA-Dw6 in patients with cryptogenic fibrosing alveolitis. Tissue Antigens. 1979;14(1): 68–71.
141. Libby DM, Gibofsky A, Fotino M, Waters SJ, Smith JP. Immunogenetic and clinical findings in idiopathic pulmonary fibrosis. Am Rev Respir Dis. 1983;127(5):618–22.
142. Xue J, Gochuico BR, Alawad AS, Feghali-Bostwick CA, Noth I, Nathan SD, et al. The HLA Class II allele DRB1*1501 is over-represented in patients with idiopathic pulmonary fibrosis. PLoS One. 2011;6(2):e14715.
143. Pozsonyi E, György B, Berki T, Bánlaki Z, Buzás E, Rajczy K, et al. HLA-association of serum levels of natural antibodies. Mol Immunol. 2009;46(7):1416–23.
144. Reilkoff RA, Peng H, Murray LA, Peng X, Russell T, Montgomery R, et al. Semaphorin 7a+ regulatory T cells are associated with progressive IPF and are implicated in TGF-β1-induced pulmonary fibrosisAm J Respir. Crit Care Med. 2013;187(2):180–8.
145. Feghali-Bostwick CA, Tsai CG, Valentine VG, Kantrow S, Stoner MW, Pilewski JM, et al. Cellular and humoral autoreactivity in idiopathic pulmonary fibrosis. J Immunol. 2007; 179(4):2592–9.
146. Kotslanidis I, Nakou E, Bouchliou I, Tzouvelekis A, Spanoudakis E, Steiropoulos P, et al. Global impairment of CD4+CD25+FoxP3+ regulatory T cells in idiopathic pulmonary fibrosis. Am J Respir Crit Care Med. 2009;179(12):1121–30.
147. Gilani SR, Vuga LJ, Lindell KO, Gibson KF, Xue J, Kaminski N, et al. CD28 down-regulation on circulating CD4 T cells is associated with poor prognoses of patients with idiopathic pulmonary fibrosis. PLoS One. 2010;5(1):e8959.
148. Daniil Z, Kitsanta P, Kapotsis G, Mathioudaki M, Kollintza A, Karatza M, et al. CD8+ T lymphocytes in lung tissue from patients with idiopathic pulmonary fibrosis. Respir Res. 2005;6:81.
149. Parra ER, Kairalla RA, Ribeiro de Carvalho CR, Eher E, Capelozzi VL. Inflammatory cell phenotyping of the pulmonary interstitium in idiopathic interstitial pneumonia. Respiration. 2007;74(2):159–69.
150. Nuovo GJ, Hagood JS, Magro CM, Chin N, Kapil R, Davis L, et al. The distribution of immunomodulatory cells in the lungs of patients with idiopathic pulmonary fibrosis. Mod Pathol. 2012;25(3):416–33.
151. Nathan SD, Shlobin OA, Weir N, Ahmad S, Kaldjob JM, Battle E, et al. Long-term course and prognosis of idiopathic pulmonary fibrosis in the new millenium. Chest. 2011;140(1): 221–9.
152. Tabuena RP, Nagai S, Tsutsumi T, Handa T, Minoru T, Mikuniya T, et al. Cell profiles of bronchoalveolar lavage fluid as prognosticators of idiopathic pulmonary fibrosis/usual interstitial pneumonia among Japanese Patients. Respiration. 2005;72(5):490–8.
153. Rosas IO, Ren P, Avila NA, Chow CK, Franks TJ, Travis WD, McCoy Jr JP, et al. Early interstitial lung disease in familial pulmonary fibrosis. Am J Respir Crit Care Med. 2007;176(7):698–705.
154. Rosas IO, Richards TJ, Konishi K, Zhang Y, Gibson K, Lokshin AE, et al. MMP1 and MMP7 as potential peripheral blood biomarkers in idiopathic pulmonary fibrosis. PLoS Med. 2008;5(4):e93.
155. Vuorinen K, Myllarniemi M, Lammi L, Piirla P, Salmenkivi K, et al. Elevated matrilysin levels in bronchoalveolar lavage fluid do not distinguish idiopathic pulmonary fibrosis from other interstitial lung diseases. APMIS. 2007;115(8):969–75.
156. Neuringer IP, Mannon RB, Coffman TM, Parsons M, Burns K, Yankaskas JR, et al. Immune cells in a mouse airway model of obliterative bronchiolitis. Am J Respir Cell Mol Biol. 1998;19(3):379–86.
157. Stewart S, Fishbein MC, Snell GI, Berry GJ, Boehler A, Burke MM, et al. Revision of the 1996 working formulation for the standardization of nomenclature in the diagnosis of lung rejection. J Heart Lung Transplant. 2007;26(12):1229–42.
158. Fang X, Luo B, Yi X, Zeng Y, Liu F, Li H, et al. Unusual interstitial pneumonia coexisted with nonspecific interstitial pneumonia, whats the diagnosis? Diagn Pathol. 2012;7(1):167.

159. Flaherty KR, Travis WD, Colby TV, Toews GB, Kazerooni EA, Gross BH, et al. Histopathologic variability in usual and nonspecific interstitial pneumonias. Am J Respir Crit Care Med. 2001;164(9):1722–7.
160. Faé KC, da Silva DD, Oshiro SE, Tanaka AC, Pomerantzeff PM, Douay C, et al. Mimicry in recognition of cardiac myosin peptides by heart-intralesional T cell clones from rheumatic heart disease. J Immunol. 2006;176(9):5662–70.
161. Lu J, Basu A, Melenhorst J, Young NS, Brown KE. Analysis of T cell repertoire in hepatitis-associated aplastic anemia. Blood. 2004;103(12):4588–93.
162. Chen G, Zeng W, Green S, Young NS. Frequent HRPT mutations in paroxysmal nocturnal haemoglobinuria reflect T cell clonal expansion, not genomic instability. Br J Haematol. 2004;125(3):383–91.
163. Kottmann RM, Hogan CM, Phipps RP, Sime PJ. Determinants of initiation and progression of idiopathic pulmonary fibrosis. Respirology. 2009;14(7):917–33.
164. Taskar VS, Coutas DB. Is idiopathic pulmonary fibrosis an environmental disease? Proc Am Thorac Soc. 2006;3(4):293–8.
165. Moghaddam AE, Gartlan KH, Kong L, Sattentau QJ. Reactive carbonyls are a major Th2-inducing damage-associated molecular pattern generated by oxidative stress. J Immunol. 2011;187(4):1626–33.
166. Taillé C, Grootenboer-Mignot S, Boursier C, Michel L, Debray MP, Fagart J, et al. Identification of periplakin as a new target for autoreactivity in idiopathic pulmonary fibrosis. Am J Respir Crit Care Med. 2011;183(6):759–66.
167. Kurosu K, Takiguchi Y, Okada O, Yumoto N, Sakao S, Tada Y, et al. Identification of annexin 1 as a novel autoantigen in acute exacerbation of idiopathic pulmonary fibrosis. J Immunol. 2008;181(1):756–67.
168. Boon K, Bailey NW, Yang J, Steel MP, Groshong S, Kervitsky D, et al. Molecular phenotypes distinguish patients with relatively stable from progressive idiopathic pulmonary fibrosis (IPF). PLoS One. 2009;4(4):e5134.
169. Vallejo AN, Weyand CM, Goronzy JJ. T cell senescence: a culprit of immune abnormalities in chronic inflammation and persistent infection. Trends Mol Med. 2004;10(3):119–24.
170. Studer SM, George MP, Zhu X, Song Y, Valentine VG, Stoner MW, et al. CD28 down-regulation on CD4 T cells is a marker for graft dysfunction in lung transplant recipients. Am J Respir Crit Care Med. 2008;178(7):765–73.
171. Wang Y, Bai J, Li F, Wang H, Fu X, Zhao T, et al. Characteristics of expanded CD4+CD28null T cells in patients with chronic hepatitis B. Immunol Invest. 2009;38:434–46.
172. Fasth AE, Dastmalchi M, Rahbar A, Salomonsson S, Pandya JM, Lindroos E, et al. T cell infiltrates in the muscles of patients with dermatomyositis and polymyositis are dominated by CD28null T cells. J Immunol. 2009;183(7):4792–9.
173. Martens PB, Goronzy JJ, Schaid D, Weyand CM. Expansion of unusual CD4+ T cells in severe rheumatoid arthritis. Arthritis Rheum. 1997;40(6):1106–14.
174. Goronzy JJ, Weyand CM. Rheumatoid arthritis. Immunol Rev. 2005;204:55–73.
175. Thewissen M, Somers V, Hellings N, Fraussen J, Damoiseaux J, Stinissen P. CD4+CD28null T cells in autoimmune disease: pathogenic features and decreased susceptibility to immuno-regulation. J Immunol. 2007;179(10):6514–23.
176. Vallejo AN, Schirmer M, Weyand CM, Goronzy JJ. Clonality and longevity of CD4$^+$CD28$^{null}$ T cells are associated with defects in apoptotic pathways. J Immunol. 2000;165(11): 6301–7.
177. Schirmer M, Vallejo AN, Weyand CM, Goronzy JJ. Resistance to apoptosis and elevated expression of Bcl-$_2$ in clonally expanded CD4$^+$CD28$^-$ T cells from rheumatoid arthritis patients. J Immunol. 1998;161(2):1018–25.
178. Fasth AE, Cao D, van Vollenhoven R, Trollmo C, Malmström V. CD28nullCD4+ T cells–characterization of an effector memory T cell population in patients with rheumatoid arthritis. Scand J Immunol. 2004;60(1–2):199–208.
179. Nakajima T, Schulte S, Warrington KJ, Kopecky SL, Frye RL, Goronzy JJ, et al. T cell-mediated lysis of endothelial cells in acute coronary syndromes. Circulation. 2002;105(5):570–5.

180. Pinto-Medel MJ, García-León JA, Oliver-Martos B, López-Gómez C, Luque G, Arnáiz-Urrutia C, et al. The CD4+ T cell subset lacking expression of the CD28 costimulatory molecule is expanded and shows a higher activation state in multiple sclerosis. J Neuroimmunol. 2012;243(1–2):1–11.

181. Xue J, Duncan SR. Are telomere lengths of leukocytes from patients with pulmonary fibrosis really genetically determined? Am J Respir Crit Care Med. 2009;179(9):852.

182. Postlethwaite AE, Keski-Oja J, Moses HL, Kang AH. Stimulation of the chemotactic migration of human fibroblasts by transforming growth factor beta. J Exp Med. 1987;165(1):251–6.

183. Neilson EG, Jimenez SA, Phillips SM. Cell-mediated immunity in interstitial nephritis. III. T lymphocyte-mediated fibroblast proliferation and collagen synthesis: an immune mechanism for renal fibrogenesis. J Immunol. 1980;125(4):1708–14.

184. Casini A, Ricci OE, Paoletti F, Surrenti C. Immune mechanisms for hepatic fibrogenesis.T-lymphocyte-mediated stimulation of fibroblast collagen production in chronic active hepatitis. Liver. 1985;5(3):134–41.

185. Atamas SP, Luzina IG, Dai H, Wilt SG, White B. Synergy between CD40 ligation and IL-4 on fibroblast proliferation involves IL-4 receptor signaling. J Immunol. 2002;168:1139–45.

186. Sempowski GD, Chess PR, Phipps RP. CD40 is a functional activation antigen and B7-independent T cell costimulatory molecule on normal human lung fibroblasts. J Immunol. 1997;158(3):4670–7.

187. Yamamura Y, Gupta R, Morita Y, He X, Pai R, Endres J, et al. Effector function of resting T cells: activation of synovial fibroblasts. J Immunol. 2001;166(4):2270–5.

188. Miranda-Carus ME, Balsa A, Benito-Miguel M, de Ayala C, Martin-Mola E. IL-15 and the initiation of cell contact-depedent synovial fibroblast-T lymphocyte cross-talk in rheumatoid arthritis: effect of methotrexate. J Immunol. 2004;173(2):1463–76.

189. Quezada SA, Jarvinen LZ, Lind EF, Noelle RJ. CD40/CD154 interactions at the interface of tolerance and immunity. Annu Rev Immunol. 2004;22:307–28.

190. Distler JH, Jungel A, Caretto D, Schulze-Horsel U, Kowal-Bielecka O, Gay RE, et al. Monocyte chemoattractant protein 1 released from glycosaminoglycans mediates its profibrotic effects in systemic sclerosis via the release of interleukin-4 from T cells. Arthritis Rheum. 2006;54(1):214–5.

191. Alaibac M, Berti E, Chizzolini C, Fineschi S, Marzano AV, Pigozzi B, et al. Role of cellular immunity in the pathogenesis of autoimmune skin diseases. Clin Exp Rheumatol. 2006;24(1 Suppl 40):S14–9.

192. Kalogerou A, Gelou E, Mountantonakis S, Settas L, Zafiriou E, Sakkas L. Early T cell activation in the skin from patients with systemic sclerosis. Ann Rheum Dis. 2005;64(8):1233–5.

193. Marshall BG, Shaw RJ. T cells and fibrosis. Chem Immunol. 2000;78:148–58.

194. Wei L. Immunological aspect of cardiac remodeling: T lymphocyte subsets in inflammation-mediated cardiac fibrosis. Mol Pathol. 2011;90(1):74–8.

195. Marra F, Aleffi S, Galastri S, Provenzano A. Mononuclear cells in liver fibrosis. Semin Immunopathol. 2009;31(3):345–58.

196. O'Reilly S, Hügle T, van Laar JM. T cells in systemic sclerosis: a reappraisal. Rheumatology (Oxford). 2012;51(9):1540–9.

197. Sawai H, Park YW, He X, Goronzy JJ, Weyand CM. Fractalkine mediates T cell-dependent proliferation of synovial fibroblasts in rheumatoid arthritis. Arthritis Rheum. 2007;56(10):3215–25.

198. Bruijn JA, Roos A, de Geus B, de Heer E. Transforming growth factor-beta and the glomerular extracellular matrix in renal pathology. J Lab Clin Med. 1994;123(1):34–47.

199. Novobrantsevfa TI, Majeau GR, Amatucci A, Kogan S, Brenner I, Casola S, et al. Attenuated liver fibrosis in the absence of B cells. J Clin Invest. 2005;115(11):3072–82.

200. Selman M, Gonzalez G, Bravo M, Sullivan-Lopez J, Ramos C, Montano M, et al. Effect of lung T lymphocytes on fibroblasts in idiopathic pulmonary fibrosis and extrinsic allergic alveolitis. Thorax. 1990;45(6):451–5.

201. Hogaboam CM, Steinhauser ML, Chensue SW, Kunkel SL. Novel roles for chemokines and fibroblasts in interstitial fibrosis. Kidney Int. 1998;54(6):2152–9.
202. Humby F, Bombardieri M, Manzo A, Kelly S, Blades MC, Kirkham B, et al. Ectopic lymphoid structures support ongoing production of class-switched autoantibodies in rheumatoid synovium. PLoS Med. 2009;6(1):e1.
203. Hitchon CA, El-Gabalawy HS. The synovium in rheumatoid arthritis. Open Rheumatol J. 2011;5:107–14.
204. Perros F, Dorfmüller P, Montani D, Hammad H, Waelput W, Girerd B, et al. Pulmonary lymphoid neogenesis in idiopathic pulmonary arterial hypertension. Am J Respir Crit Care Med. 2012;185(3):311–21.
205. Pitsiou G, Papakosta D, Bouros D. Pulmonary hypertension in idiopathic pulmonary fibrosis: a review. Respiration. 2011;82(3):294–304.
206. Richards TJ, Kaminski N, Baribaud F, Flavin S, Brodmerkel C, Horowitz D, et al. Peripheral blood proteins predict mortality in idiopathic pulmonary fibrosis. Am J Respir Crit Care Med. 2012;185(1):67–76.
207. Cancro MP, D'Cruz DP, Khamashta MA. The role of B lymphocyte stimulator (BLyS) in systemic lupus erythematosus. J Clin Invest. 2009;119(5):1066–73.
208. Bossen C, Schneider P. BAFF, APRIL and their receptors: structure, function and signaling. Semin Immunol. 2006;18(5):263–75.
209. Dillon SR, Harder B, Lewis KB, Moore MD, Liu H, Bukowski TR, et al. B-lymphocyte stimulator/a proliferation-inducing ligand heterotrimers are elevated in the sera of patients with autoimmune disease and are neutralized by atacicept and B cell maturation antigen-immunoglobulin. Arthritis Res Ther. 2010;12(2):R48.
210. Jacobi AM, Reiter K, Mackay M, Aranow C, Hiepe F, Radbruch A, et al. Activated memory B cell subsets correlate with disease activity in systemic lupus erythematosus: delineation by expression of CD27, IgD, and CD95. Arthritis Rheum. 2008;58(6):1762–73.
211. Souto-Carneiro MM, Mahadevan V, Takada K, Fritsch-Stork R, Nanki T, Brown M, et al. Alterations in peripheral blood memory B cells in patients with active rheumatoid arthritis are dependent on the action of tumour necrosis factor. Arthritis Res Ther. 2009;11(3):R84.
212. Anolik JH, Barnard J, Cappione A, Pugh-Bernard AE, Felgar RE, Looney RJ, et al. Rituximab improves peripheral B cell abnormalities in human systemic lupus erythematosus. Arthritis Rheum. 2004;50(11):3580–90.
213. Hachem RR, Yusen RD, Meyers BF, Aloush AA, Mohanakumar T, Patterson A, et al. Anti-HLA antibodies and preemptive antibody directed therapy after lung transplantation. J Heart Lung Transplant. 2010;29(9):973–8.
214. Reverberi R, Reverberi L. Removal kinetics of therapeutic apheresis. Blood Transfus. 2007;5(3):164–74.
215. Nydegger UE, Sturzenegger M. Treatment of autoimmune disease: synergy between plasma exchange and intravenous immunoglobulin. Ther Apher. 2001;5(3):186–92.
216. Kim DS. Acute exacerbations of idiopathic pulmonary fibrosis. Clin Chest Med. 2012;33(1):59–68.
217. Donahoe M, Chien N, Gibson KF, Raval JS, Zhang Y, Duncan SR. Autoantibody-targeted treatments for acute exacerbations of idiopathic pulmonary fibrosis (abstract) (to be presented at American Thoracic Society International Conference May 2013).

# Chapter 8
# Mechanisms of Fibrosis in IPF

Nathan Sandbo

**Abstract** Idiopathic pulmonary fibrosis (IPF) is a disorder characterized by progressive destruction of normal lung architecture and replacement with abundant matrix that stiffens the lung and leads to respiratory failure. The pathobiology of IPF is characterized by the presence of alveolar epithelial cell (AEC) injury and apoptosis, which is accompanied by progressive fibrosis. Thus, while inflammatory signaling may still play a role in IPF, the previous paradigm of an *inflammation-driven* disorder (alveolitis) has been supplanted by the concept of IPF as a disorder of AEC injury accompanied by a non-resolving wound-healing response. AEC injury and apoptosis result in disordered cross talk between the epithelial and mesenchymal compartments via aberrant cell behavior, profibrotic signaling, and loss of inhibitory homeostatic signals. These aberrant signals lead to disruption of the alveolar basement membrane, formation of a provisional matrix, and recruitment of mesenchymal cells to form the fibroblastic focus, which serves as the site of new matrix accumulation in IPF. Myofibroblast differentiation, matrix synthesis and deposition, and tissue remodeling occur in response to transforming growth factor-β(beta) (TGF-β) and other growth factors. This remodeling process yields a stiffened, fibrotic matrix that independently perpetuates the fibrotic process via activation of TGF-β signaling and myofibroblast differentiation.

Despite this mechanistic understanding of the reparative process, the etiology for the lack of resolution in IPF compared to other responses to lung injury remains unknown. While an effective therapy for IPF remains elusive, approaches to therapy have begun to evolve toward targeted therapies directed at putative growth factors, receptors, and enzymes for which robust evidence now exists regarding their mechanistic involvement in matrix remodeling.

N. Sandbo, M.D. (✉)
Division of Allergy, Pulmonary, and Critical Care, University of Wisconsin,
5229 MFCB, 1685 Highland Ave, Madison, WI 53705, USA
e-mail: nsandbo@medicine.wisc.edu

K.C. Meyer and S.D. Nathan (eds.), *Idiopathic Pulmonary Fibrosis: A Comprehensive Clinical Guide*, Respiratory Medicine 9, DOI 10.1007/978-1-62703-682-5_8,
© Springer Science+Business Media New York 2014

**Keywords** Idiopathic pulmonary fibrosis • Fibrosis • Alveolar epithelial cell
• Apoptosis • Transforming growth factor-beta • Intracellular signaling • Fibroblast
• Extracellular matrix • Inflammation • Angiogenesis • Coagulation cascade

## Introduction

The normal reparative response to tissue injury is characterized by the orchestrated involvement of multiple cell types under the influence of myriad autocrine, paracrine, and inflammatory mediators with the goal of reestablishing tissue integrity and barrier function. Wound healing in the adult does not fully recapitulate embryologic developmental patterning, resulting in the formation of a scar at the site of injury [1, 2]. Resolution of the reparative response is important to preserve existing normal tissue architecture and involves the tight spatiotemporal regulation of the involved signals [3]. Fibrosis, characterized by excessive extracellular matrix accumulation and disruption of normal tissue architecture, can occur as a result of chronic injury, chronic inflammation, or dysregulation of the normal reparative process within a tissue bed.

The wall of the alveolus of the lung is formed by delicately apposed monolayers of alveolar epithelial cells (AECs) and endothelial cells, separated only by their respective basement membranes [4]. This delicate architecture forms the primary gas-exchanging interface of the lung, allowing rapid diffusion of oxygen and carbon dioxide between the alveolar airspace and the alveolar–capillary blood. The surrounding supporting interstitial spaces of the lung are comprised of a fine network of fibrillar proteins (collagens, fibronectin, elastin) in composite with hydrated glycosaminoglycans [5]. In pulmonary fibrosis, there is a dramatic disruption of this intricate structure, with expansion of the connective tissue compartment of the lung due to the accumulation of matrix components, associated alveolar obliteration and collapse, and progressive distortion of normal lung architecture [6]. These changes result in disturbances in gas exchange and, when progressive, respiratory failure and death.

Idiopathic pulmonary fibrosis (IPF) is one of several lung disorders that are characterized by pulmonary fibrosis. In contrast to several other forms of pulmonary fibrosis, such as the fibroproliferative phase of acute respiratory distress syndrome (diffuse AEC injury) or fibrotic sarcoidosis (exuberant granulomatous inflammation), the underlying etiology of the fibrotic response is not immediately apparent in IPF. The histopathology of IPF is defined by the usual interstitial pneumonia (UIP) pattern [7], which is characterized by spatial variegation of the fibrotic process [6, 8, 9] with normal-appearing areas of lung adjacent to areas characterized by severe scarring, architectural distortion, and the presence of microscopic honeycombing [6, 7].

Staining for early collagen forms, indicative of collagen synthesis, reveals that active, synthetic fibroblasts are present in clusters, termed fibroblastic foci, near the air–tissue interface [6]. The presence of these spatially discreet foci of "activated" fibroblasts in juxtaposition to areas of "old" scar containing fewer fibroblasts and more mature collagen along with normal-appearing alveoli suggests an indolent, but progressive, process. The presence of these various stages of fibrosis with the same pathologic specimen is termed "temporal heterogeneity" and is a required diagnostic element of the UIP pattern [7]. While areas of scarring may contain a mild, mixed inflammatory infiltrate as part of the UIP pattern, it does not predominate when compared to the fibrotic reaction.

The distinctive lesions of IPF, the fibroblastic foci, lend some insight into the underlying biology mediating this disorder. The fibroblastic foci are the site of "new fibrosis," with fibroblasts most proximal to the airspace demonstrating the greatest amount of collagen synthesis. Basal lamina remnants appear on the interstitial side of the fibroblastic focus, suggesting that this structure has developed within the previously normal airspace [6]. Supporting this concept, foci are often associated with a poorly adherent, hyperplastic epithelial cell layer on their luminal (airspace) side, with areas of epithelial sloughing. These structures form a reticulated network of fibrosis throughout the lung and are thought to represent the "leading edge" of new fibrosis [10]. The number of these structures present on surgical lung biopsy specimens correlates with survival [11, 12], consistent with their role in disease progression.

## An Overview of the Current and Evolving Model of IPF Pathogenesis

Given that several forms of pulmonary fibrosis are the result of a robust inflammatory response [13], it is not surprising that historically, IPF was originally viewed as a disorder primarily characterized by an early, macrophage-mediated alveolitis, with resultant progressive tissue fibrosis [14, 15]. The development of more precise classification schemes for the idiopathic interstitial pneumonias resulted in an improved appreciation of the lack of extensive inflammation in the histopathology of IPF [7] and called into question the role of inflammation in the disease process. It is now clear that broad inhibition of immune function using corticosteroids and azathioprine does not positively affect disease progression and patient outcomes [16–18]. Thus, the concept of IPF as a product of a robust, disordered inflammatory state has been supplanted by the current concept of IPF as a disorder resulting from repetitive AEC injury and an aberrant, non-resolving wound-healing response [19, 20].

The temporal relationships of the key pathogenic events of IPF are largely inferred from the knowledge gained from several decades of investigations into the mechanisms of epithelial cell injury and the reparative response of cells and tissues to such injury [2, 21, 22]. These processes have been most robustly studied in models of dermal wounding, and coupled with data from animal models of pulmonary fibrosis and correlative studies in IPF lungs specimens, these investigations have led to the current model of disease pathogenesis in IPF.

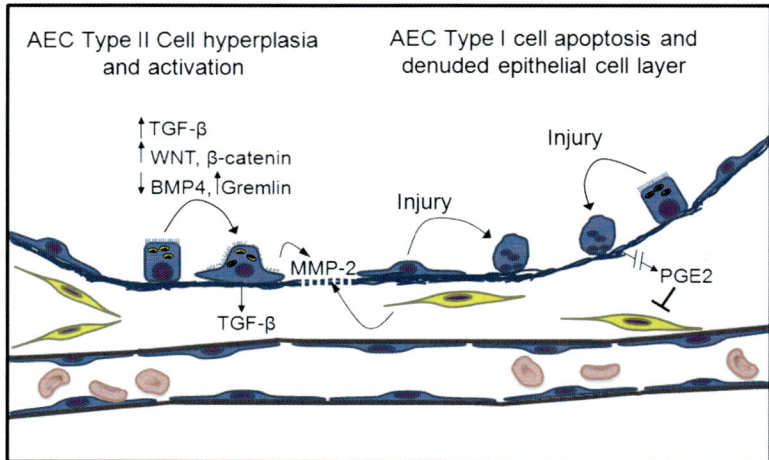

**Fig. 8.1** Epithelial injury and apoptosis initiate the fibrotic response in IPF. Epithelial cell injury leads to apoptosis and AEC dropout, resulting in a denuded basement membrane and loss of inhibitory signaling to fibroblasts via prostaglandin E2 (PGE2). Under the influence of TGF-β/BMP signaling and WNT/β-catenin signaling, residual AECs become activated and undergo EMT, resulting in the elaboration of multiple profibrotic cytokines, including TGF-β. Activation of MMPs adjacent to the basement membrane (from AECs or subbasement membrane fibroblasts) leads to disruption in the basement membrane (*broken lines*)

The initiation of IPF pathogenesis is thought to be the result of injury to the type I alveolar cells, which leads to AEC apoptosis and disruption of the AEC layer. Residual AECs are aberrantly activated and secrete profibrotic cytokines [especially transforming growth factor-β(beta) (TGF-β)], chemokines, and proteases that trigger the recruitment and activation of inflammatory cells and fibroblasts. The local elaboration of matrix metalloproteinases (MMPs) results in disruption of the basal lamina of the alveolus. These changes are summarized in Fig. 8.1. AEC injury is accompanied by the formation of a serum-derived fibrinous exudate that serves as a provisional matrix analogous to that of dermal wounds [23]. Chemokines and serum-derived factors present in the provisional matrix lead to the influx of fibroblasts from the local interstitial cell population, along with potential contributions from circulating cell populations and epithelial to mesenchymal transition (EMT) of local AECs (Fig. 8.2). Subsequent activation of these fibroblasts by TGF-β(beta) results in a highly contractile and synthetic fibroblast phenotype, termed the myofibroblast, which serves as the primary effector cell for matrix production and tissue remodeling. Myofibroblast activation and tissue remodeling persist in IPF, possibly due to failure to reestablish normal epithelialization or aberrant behavior of the myofibroblasts. Progressive matrix deposition and remodeling ensues, resulting in a severely disordered tissue architecture (honeycombing) and organ dysfunction (Fig. 8.3).

Several novel concepts that build upon this conceptual framework have emerged in recent years and are discussed in greater detail later. Repetitive epithelial cell

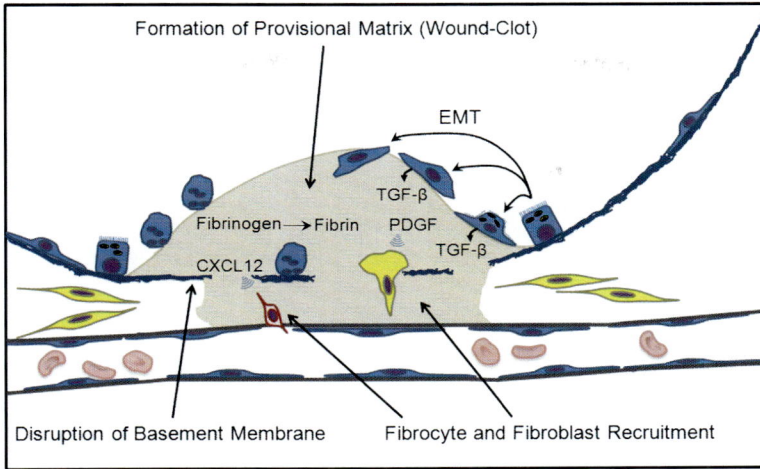

**Fig. 8.2** Formation of the provisional matrix and recruitment of mesenchymal cells in IPF. A serum-derived exudate forms within the alveolar airspace, presumably due to epithelial cell injury, basement membrane disruption, and changes in alveolar–capillary permeability. Activation of the coagulation cascade results in the conversion of fibrinogen to fibrin to form a provisional matrix. Serum-derived mediators present within the wound clot, such as platelet-derived growth factor (PDGF), recruit fibroblasts, while the CXCL12 and other chemokines may recruit circulating fibrocytes. AECs that have undergone EMT may account for some of the mesenchymal-type cells which populate the provisional matrix as well. Each of these cell types is activated by AEC-derived TGF-β, promoting the remodeling response

injury may be triggered by a combination of genetic/age-related factors that lead to increased susceptibility to AEC stress coupled with a "second hit" of exposure to environmental "triggers" such as tobacco smoke, gastroesophageal reflux, or viruses that trigger epithelial injury [24–26]. Global analysis of gene expression and non-coding microRNA in human subjects with IPF have demonstrated that signals associated with embryologic development and TGF-β(beta)-associated signals comprise a significant portion of the reparative gene expression response in IPF [27]. These pathways are linked to the epithelial cell responses to injury, repair of the disrupted alveolar cell layer, and myofibroblast activation in IPF. How differences between the developmental and reparative response in these signaling pathways lead to the propagation of fibrosis remains an area of investigation [28]. Finally, remodeled, fibrotic matrix is not merely the end result of the fibrotic response. Biomechanical features of the matrix environment, such as its stiffness, are an independent determinant of fibroblast response and fibrotic progression, suggesting a new mechanism of aberrant cell behavior/function in IPF. In total, these mechanisms result in a mutually reinforcing cycle of fibrotic signaling that leads to non-resolving tissue fibrosis (Fig. 8.4). The subsequent sections explore these concepts in detail.

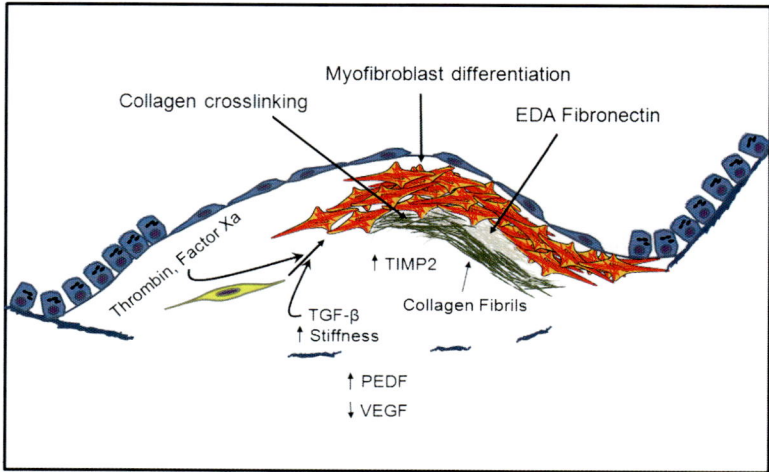

**Fig. 8.3** Formation of the fibroblastic focus and mechanisms of tissue remodeling in IPF. Fibroblasts undergo activation by TGF-β, thrombin, and other growth factors, increasing the production of EDA fibronectin, collagen isoforms, and other matrix components. Deposition of EDA fibronectin by myofibroblasts serves as a template for collagen fibril incorporation. Collagen fibrils are then cross-linked via the action of lysyl oxidases (LOXL2), contributing to increases in matrix stiffness (elasticity). Persistence of newly synthesized matrix is promoted by local increases in TIMP2, inhibiting degradation. Increases in tissue stiffness independently promote myofibroblast activation and differentiation, perpetuating the fibrotic response. Vascular obliteration and inhibition of neovascularization in the area of the fibroblastic focus is potentiated by an anti-angiogenic environment, with elevated PEDF and low VEGF levels. Progressive remodeling of this lesion results in architectural distortion and honeycombing

# Alveolar Epithelial Cell Injury

## *Alveolar Epithelial Cell Injury and Apoptosis*

The normal alveolar epithelial lining of the lung is comprised of two types of epithelial cells, type I and type II, which form a layer of single cell thickness. Type I cells are flat, highly specialized cells whose membrane comprises the bulk of the alveolar–capillary interface in normal lung tissue [29]. Type II cells have a cuboidal morphology, with intracellular lamellar bodies. Type II cells secrete surfactant proteins, retain proliferative capacity, and are responsible for the regeneration of epithelium after injury [30], including trans-differentiation to type I cells [31]. In IPF, AEC morphology is severely deranged, with overt epithelial cell necrosis and denudation of the capillary basement membrane [32] as well as extensive type II pneumocyte apoptosis [33]. Alveolar spaces that have been disrupted by extensive fibrotic changes in IPF lungs are lined with numerous, hyperplastic type II pneumocytes that may be derived from the adjacent bronchiolar lining cells [34] and elongated epithelial cells that are abnormal in appearance [35]. The presence of

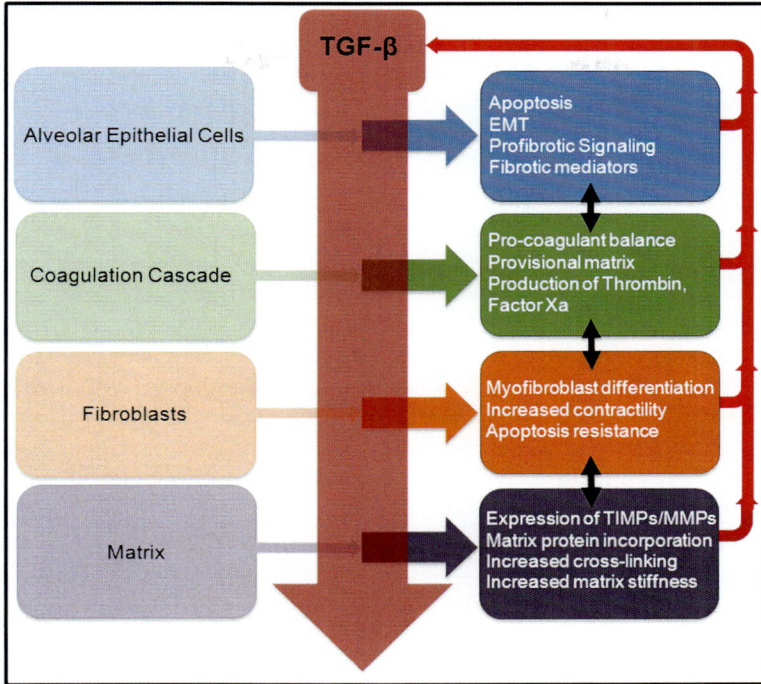

**Fig. 8.4** Mutually reinforcing reciprocal signaling in pulmonary fibrosis. The pathobiology of IPF is characterized by AEC injury, activation of the coagulation cascade, fibroblast activation, and reorganization of the matrix. During pulmonary fibrosis, mutually reinforcing signals across compartments contribute to the propagation of the reparative response. Transforming growth factor-β is a central coordinator, integrator, and amplifier of the fibrotic response via its cell- and compartment-specific effects

these abnormal epithelial phenotypes in areas that normally contain predominately type I epithelial cells is suggestive of a failure of normal re-epithelialization after injury [36].

While AEC injury could be consequent to the development of a fibrotic response, several lines of evidence suggest that AEC injury may be an inciting event. In IPF, AEC apoptosis is present in areas without significant interstitial fibrosis, suggesting that this process may be a primary inciting factor [33]. Several exogenous agents that could trigger alveolar epithelial injury are associated with the development of IPF. Gastroesophageal reflux disease is present in up to 90 % of patients with IPF [37, 38], and coexisting treatment with proton pump inhibitors or Nissen fundoplication has been associated with longer patient survival [39, 40]. Approximately 70 % of IPF patients are current or former cigarette smokers [41], and current or former cigarette smoking is a powerful risk factor for the development of both IPF and familial pulmonary fibrosis [42, 43]. Workplace exposures are less robustly linked [44] but may contribute to risk in a cohort of IPF patients. Several viruses that are trophic for the lung epithelium have been identified in IPF lungs [45], with the family of herpes viruses having the strongest association. A high prevalence of herpes virus DNA has been identified in the AECs and immune cells of the IPF lung [46–48]. The presence of herpes viral antigens has also been associated with signs of endoplasmic reticulum (ER) stress in the AECs [49], suggesting another possible mechanism of injury.

AECs from patients with IPF may have an intrinsic defect conferring susceptibility to injury and apoptosis. Several rare mutations in surfactant protein C (SP-C), a protein produced by the AEC type II cells, have been identified in patients with the familial form of pulmonary fibrosis [50, 51], which can have an identical histopathology to sporadic IPF. These mutations alter the processing of SP-C by AEC type II cells, leading to deficient expression and secretion, endoplasmic reticulum stress, and apoptosis [51–53]. Mice with germ-line deletion of SP-C develop interstitial lung disease as adults [54], suggesting a causal relationship for disordered SP-C biology. Rare mutations in surfactant protein A2 have also been identified in patients from two kindreds with familial pulmonary fibrosis, and these mutations result in a similar defect in protein stability, defective secretion, and a subsequent increase in ER stress-associated signaling [55].

Several mutations in the two components of telomerase, telomerase reverse transcriptase (hTERT) and the RNA component of telomerase (hTR) [56, 57], have been identified in patients with familial pulmonary fibrosis. Chromosomal telomere shortening, which occurs with cell division and aging, is associated with the development of cell senescence and susceptibility to apoptosis [58]. Telomerase is present in progenitor cells, where it counteracts telomere shortening, preserving proliferative potential [59]. When compared to age-matched family members without the mutation, family members with hTERT and hTR loss of function mutations had shorter telomeres and an increased risk for the development of pulmonary fibrosis [56]. The presence of these mutations has been associated with a penetrance of pulmonary fibrosis of 40 % in affected individuals [60]. However, the mutations identified are rare and have only been identified in a small percentage of patients with sporadic IPF [61]. The concept of telomere length-dependent susceptibility to alveolar epithelial injury and the development of pulmonary fibrosis is supported by the identification of short telomeres as an independent risk factor for the development of sporadic IPF [62]. Additionally, a genome-wide association study (GWAS) has identified a common single nucleotide polymorphism (SNP) in the hTERT gene that confers risk for the development of IPF [63].

Linkage analysis of a cohort of Finnish families with familial pulmonary fibrosis identified the gene ELMO domain containing 2 (ELMOD2) [64, 65] as a candidate gene associated with the development of pulmonary fibrosis. ELMOD2 is normally expressed in epithelial cells and macrophages of the lung, but ELMOD2 expression was significantly decreased in lungs of patients with pulmonary fibrosis. ELMOD2 may play a role in the response of epithelial cells and macrophages to viral infection [64], potentially linking an environmental and genetic trigger in this disorder.

Two large genome-wide association studies (GWAS) have identified a SNP in the promoter region of the mucin 5B gene (MUC5B) that is strongly associated with the development of familial and sporadic forms of pulmonary fibrosis [66, 67].

The minor (risk-conferring) allele was present in 34–38.5 % of IPF cases and 9–11 % of controls. The presence of homozygosity for the minor allele confers a ten- to twenty-fold increase in the risk for developing IPF. MUC5B is present at increased levels in fibrotic areas of IPF lungs, and the mutant allele for this gene is associated with significantly increased expression of MUC5B in lungs of subjects without pulmonary fibrosis when compared to counterparts homozygous for the wild-type allele. This suggests that the MUC5B SNP results in alterations in gene expression that may contribute to the development of IPF.

Finally, ER stress is present in the epithelial cells of lungs from patients with sporadic IPF, independent of known genetic defects. The ER stress markers ATF4, ATF6, and CHOP are preferentially localized to the epithelial cells of patients with sporadic IPF, in contrast to normal lungs or lungs from patients with chronic obstructive pulmonary disease [68]. These changes were often localized to areas with significant fibrosis and co-localized with markers of apoptosis, suggesting a role for ER stress and cellular apoptosis in the fibrotic process [68].

These observations provide conceptual evidence that intrinsic epithelial defects may render the epithelial cell susceptible to repetitive injury, possibly from the environmental factors listed above, which could lead to perpetuation of the wound-healing response. Several of these observations shed light on potential mechanisms mediating the age-related incidence of IPF, as aging is associated with shortened telomeres [58] and increased markers of ER stress [69], potentially increasing the susceptibility to repetitive epithelial cell injury with advancing age.

## *Aberrant Epithelial Cell Signaling*

AEC injury is a key inciting factor in the initiation of the reparative response in the lung. This concept has been experimentally demonstrated by targeted injury to type II AECs in mice via transgenic expression of SP-C-driven diphtheria toxin receptor expression, followed by intraperitoneal diphtheria toxin administration. Changes in AEC gene expression and function were present in the transgenic animals, and repeated exposure to diphtheria toxin resulted in the development of alveolar interstitial fibrosis without induction of inflammation [70].

Several potential mechanisms likely account for the development of fibrosis in response to AEC injury, including the loss of homeostatic signaling, aberrant function of residual, activated epithelial cells, and the elaboration of local profibrotic cytokines (see Fig. 8.1). Type II AECs maintain normal alveolar homeostasis via the production of surfactant, the regulation of fluid balance, and the interaction with other structural cells of the alveolus [71]. AECs also maintain cell–cell contact with the fibroblasts of the alveolar wall under normal conditions [72], but the function of these connections remains obscure. Under normal conditions, AECs have an inhibitory effect on fibroblasts [73]. In IPF, loss of inhibitory signaling from the AEC to the mesenchyme may result from AEC dropout. One potential mediator of mesenchymal inhibition is prostaglandin E2 (PGE2). PGE2 is a product of cyclooxygenase and prostaglandin E synthases that is produced by local AECs, monocytes, and other structural cells of the lung [74, 75]. PGE2 has shown to have an inhibitory effect on fibroblast proliferation [76, 77], migration [78], and collagen synthesis [79, 80]. In IPF, levels of PGE2 are decreased in bronchoalveolar lavage (BAL) [81], and EP2 prostaglandin receptor expression and signaling in fibroblasts is diminished [82]. Thus, AEC injury may result in the loss of the PGE2 production by AECs, leading to fibroblast activation during pulmonary fibrosis.

In response to an acute injury, the alveolar epithelium rapidly regenerates with reestablishment of the normal AEC layer via proliferation of type II AEC and subsequent trans-differentiation to type I AECs [83]. This process may serve to reestablish the homeostatic function of the epithelium and participate in resolution of the reparative response during normal wound healing. Experiments performed in an ex vivo model of hyperoxia-mediated AEC injury support the importance of this process in regulating the fibrotic process, as lungs that exhibit decreased rates of epithelial cell proliferation develop fibrosis, while lungs that rapidly re-epithelialize revert to normal [83]. Similarly, utilizing diphtheria toxin-mediated depletion of airway progenitor (Clara) cells, Perl and colleagues [84] demonstrated that chronic depletion of Clara cells results in incomplete and aberrant re-epithelialization of the bronchiolar airway and the development of peribronchiolar fibrosis, while acute depletion, which presumably leaves a reserve of Clara cell progenitors, results in normal re-epithelialization and does not lead to fibrosis.

IPF is characterized by a failure of re-epithelialization and a disordered epithelial layer. This is characterized by the proliferation of bronchiolar basilar epithelial cells, which exhibit signs of epithelial stress and atypia [85] as well as the presence of AECs that exhibit an intermediate phenotype with traits of both type I and type II cells [36]. The receptor for advanced glycation end products (RAGE) is a transmembrane receptor that is a specific marker for differentiated type I epithelial cells [86]. The expression of RAGE in type I cells likely plays a role in their differentiation and homeostasis by promoting cell spreading and attachment to the basement membrane [87, 88]. IPF lungs demonstrate abnormally low expression of RAGE [88, 89] consistent with the presence of disrupted re-epithelialization. Dysfunctional RAGE expression may also play a role in mediating the fibrotic process. In this regard, RAGE-null mice develop more severe experimental pulmonary fibrosis and spontaneously develop fibro-like lesions as they age [89].

## Epithelial–Mesenchymal Transition

In IPF, the AECs tend to have a flattened morphology, which may represent promigratory phenotypes that facilitate re-epithelialization of the alveolar space after injury [35]. This morphology is similar to epithelial cells that are undergoing epithelial–mesenchymal transition (EMT). EMT is the process by which epithelial cells lose attributes of full epithelial differentiation (cuboidal shape, apical-basal polarization, cell–cell contacts, epithelial gene repertoire) and take on attributes of mesenchymal cell lineages (spindle morphology, loss of cell contacts, mesenchymal gene expression). EMT is accompanied by the loss of several epithelial markers such as E-cadherin, the acquisition of mesenchymal markers such as N-cadherin and vimentin, and the upregulation of transcription factors implicated in EMT such as Twist, SNAI1 (snail), and SNAI2 (Slug) [90]. EMT is critical for gastrulation during embryogenesis [91], and epithelial cells that have undergone EMT have an augmented ability to metastasize [92]. Several forms of tissue injury and repair demonstrate the presence of EMT as part of their pathogenesis [93]—for example, the deletion of snail protects from the development of hepatic fibrosis [94], suggesting a mechanistic role in the propagation of tissue fibrosis. Tissue sections from established models of experimental pulmonary fibrosis, such as the bleomycin mouse model [95], also demonstrate evidence of EMT [96–98], while lung tissue from patients with IPF demonstrates increased expression of Twist and Snail, suggesting the presence of EMT-associated signaling in human IPF [99, 100]. These data suggest that EMT and associated signaling is present in IPF and that this may be the source of significant profibrotic signals.

Regulation of EMT during development is regulated, in part, by family members of the transforming growth factor-β(beta) superfamily of cytokines [91], which includes TGF-β1, -β2, -β3, and bone morphogenic proteins (BMPs). TGF-β/BMP balance is important in the development of the mesodermal/epithelial compartment during development and regulates EMT [101, 102]. TGF-β induces EMT in both developmental and fibrotic contexts [103], and it is a potent inducer of EMT in ex vivo epithelial cell cultures [104, 105], although cell contact and integrin-mediated signaling can modify this response [106, 107]. Several BMPs are implicated in the reverse process, mesenchymal to epithelial transition, and can antagonize TGF-β-dependent signaling. Interestingly, the expression of two of these BMPs, BMP-2 and BMP-4, is altered in IPF [28], and the inhibitor of BMP signaling, gremlin, is increased in IPF lungs [108], implicating dysregulated TGF-β/BMP signaling balance in the pathogenesis of the disorder.

The WNT/β(beta)-catenin signaling pathway has also been implicated in mediating altered epithelial cell function during lung injury and fibrosis. WNT/β-catenin signaling mediates branching morphogenesis during lung development and the maintenance of progenitor cells [109]. WNT proteins are secreted glycoproteins that can signal in a paracrine or autocrine factor through their receptors (Frizzled proteins) and co-receptors (LRPs) to stabilize β(beta)-catenin, leading to its nuclear translocation. In the adult lung, WNT/β-catenin signaling is involved in epithelial cell proliferation, differentiation, and cell–cell adhesion in the lung [109, 110]. A common finding from recent, unbiased gene expression screens of lung tissue from patients with IPF is upregulation of many developmental pathways, including markers of the WNT/β-catenin pathway [28, 111–113]. WNT genes WNT2 and WNT5a and the WNT receptors Frizzled 7 and Frizzled 10 are increased in the lungs of patients with IPF [28, 111, 114]. Patients with IPF have increases in nuclear localization of β-catenin in the hyperplastic epithelium adjacent to fibrotic lesions [115] as well as increased phosphorylation of the Wnt/LRP receptors, suggesting activation of this pathway [116]. Consistent with the role of this pathway in pulmonary fibrosis, several WNT/β-catenin-dependent genes are upregulated in IPF [112, 113, 117], and disruption of signaling via the WNT target gene, WNT-induced signaling protein (WISP), inhibits both markers of EMT and the development of fibrosis in response to bleomycin [117].

Finally, AECs are an important source of profibrotic mediators that can signal to the surrounding mesenchyme, to promote fibroblast recruitment and induction of matrix production [36]. Several profibrotic growth factors are localized to the epithelial cells in IPF, including TGF-β1 [118, 119], platelet-derived growth factor (PDGF) [120], monocyte chemoattractant protein-1 (MCP-1) [121], connective tissue growth factor (CTGF) [122], endothelin-1 [123], and tumor necrosis factor-α(alpha) (TNF-α) [118, 124, 125]. AECs are also the source of several MMPs and tissue inhibitors of matrix metalloproteinases (TIMPs) implicated in IPF [126].

## The Provisional Matrix and Coagulant Balance

The fibroblastic foci of UIP are found on the luminal side of the alveolar basement membrane in association with disruptions in the basement membrane [6]. These structures are morphologically analogous to the fibroblast collections that organize fibrinous alveolar exudates during the fibroproliferative phase of acute lung injury and the Masson bodies of organizing pneumonia. IPF lungs demonstrate evidence of endothelial injury, with swelling of endothelial cells, reduplication of the endothelial cell capillary basement membrane [127], and increased trans-endothelial permeability [128]. Interestingly, the degree of capillary permeability in IPF also correlates with prognosis [128, 129]. These observations suggest that the initial injury to the AEC layer in IPF is accompanied by the exudation of serum-derived factors into the alveolar airspace to form the provisional matrix [6, 130]. AECs and macrophages express tissue factor [131, 132], which interacts with coagulation factors present in the alveolar exudate and activates the extrinsic coagulation pathway. Activation of the coagulation cascade results in the generation of thrombin, and subsequent thrombin-mediated conversion of serum-derived fibrinogen to fibrin forms the provisional matrix [133]. The provisional matrix also contains serum-derived fibronectin [6, 127] and growth factors, such as PDGF, which facilitate subsequent fibroblast recruitment, migration, and matrix organization [134] (see Fig. 8.2).

Stabilization of the nascent fibrin-containing provisional matrix in healing wounds would be predicted to require the presence of an increased procoagulant balance, as normal lung tissue expresses proteases such as the plasminogen activator, urokinase, that promote local fibrinolysis [135]. Immunohistochemical staining of IPF lungs demonstrates the deposition of fibrin localized in the alveolar space in areas that are adjacent to the epithelial cell layer [136]. Additionally, BAL samples from patients with IPF demonstrate increased levels of plasminogen activator inhibitor-1 and plasminogen activator inhibitor-2 (PAI-1, PAI-2) and a reduction in urokinase activity [132, 137, 138], suggesting the presence of increased procoagulant balance.

Increased procoagulant activity also contributes to profibrotic signaling via the entrapment of serum-derived mediators present within the provisional matrix, forming a reservoir of growth factors that can be activated as the provisional matrix is remodeled [139]. The importance of procoagulant signaling is supported by studies in experimental models of pulmonary fibrosis that have shown protection from the development of fibrosis in PAI-1-deficient mice and potentiation of the fibrotic response by transgenic overexpression of PAI-1 [140].

Products of activation of the coagulation cascade, such as thrombin, also act as growth factors for fibroblasts. Thrombin is produced from the conversion of prothrombin to thrombin by Factor Va and Factor Xa and can signal through proteinase-activated receptors (PAR) found on epithelial cells and fibroblasts in the lung. Thrombin signaling occurs via proteolytic activation of its high-affinity receptor, PAR-1, leading to the expression of profibrotic cytokines, activation of TGF-β, and myofibroblast differentiation [133]. Germ-line deletion of the PAR1 receptor is protective against the development of bleomycin-induced pulmonary fibrosis [141]. Other coagulation proteinases may play a role in coagulation-dependent signaling as well. Factor X co-localizes to the alveolar epithelia of IPF lungs and can signal via PAR-1 [142]. Factor VIIa is also found in abundance on tissue biopsies from IPF lung and, in combination with tissue factor, can mediate PAR-2-dependent proliferation of fibroblasts [143].

Despite the robust evidence supporting a key role for coagulation imbalance in the pathogenesis of fibrosis, a recent large, randomized clinical trial of systemic anticoagulation with warfarin for patients with IPF did not show clinical benefit, and the trial was terminated early due to increased risk of death in the treatment arm [144]. Nonetheless, pharmacotherapy directed at specific targets and coagulation-associated signaling still remain potential strategies for therapy.

## Myofibroblasts: Effector Cells of Fibrosis

### *Concept of the Myofibroblast*

The primary effector cell for connective tissue remodeling is the myofibroblast, a mechanically active, matrix-producing mesenchymal cell with distinct morphologic features that differ from normal resident fibroblasts. Myofibroblasts are characterized by the presence of large, bundled microfilaments and enlarged focal adhesions [145]. Myofibroblast differentiation has been historically defined by the expression of both contractile proteins, such as the α(alpha)-isoform of smooth muscle actin (α-SMA), and matrix proteins, such as collagens and the extra type III domain A (EDA) splice isoform of fibronectin [146]. A(alpha)-SMA(+) myofibroblasts are not thought to be present in the normal tissue of the lung, although niche populations of microfilament containing α-SMA(−) myofibroblasts have been identified [147]. In contrast, α-SMA(+) myofibroblasts are invariably found in granulation tissue of wounds [148] and in scarring diseases in other organs [149, 150]. They act as central mediators of connective tissue remodeling via their production of matrix proteins, pro- and anti-proteinase proteins, and modulation of matrix organization and tension [145, 151, 152] (see Fig. 8.3). Their presence in the lung is associated with the formation of a dense collagen matrix and progression of pulmonary fibrosis [153].

## Origins of Myofibroblasts

The potential origins of myofibroblasts are diverse, with several cellular precursors implicated in the expansion of the myofibroblast population during tissue remodeling and fibrosis [145]. Potential myofibroblast precursors include the resident fibroblasts of the alveolar interstitium, AECs that have undergone EMT, and circulating, bone marrow-derived progenitors that are termed "fibrocytes" [154].

Fibrocytes are circulating progenitor cells that express hematopoietic surface antigens CD34 and CD45, along with fibroblast-associated proteins such as collagen I (Col I), collagen III, and collagen IV [155]. Fibrocytes were originally identified in a model of dermal wound healing [156] and are derived from bone marrow precursors [157]. Subsequently, studies using chimeric mice with green-fluorescing protein (GFP)-labeled bone marrow precursors demonstrated the accumulation of GFP+, Col I+ cells in the lungs after the induction of bleomycin-induced pulmonary fibrosis [155, 158]. Fibrocytes express the chemokine receptor, CXCR4, and fibrocyte recruitment to the lung is dependent on the CXCR4 receptor ligand, CXCL12 [159]. Several other studies in murine models of pulmonary fibrosis have demonstrated that circulating fibrocytes can express additional fibroblast-associated markers (e.g., S100A, vimentin, $\alpha$-SMA) in the context of their recruitment to the lung [97, 155, 159, 160]. However, conflicting data exist as to the potential of these cells to contribute to the myofibroblast ($\alpha$-SMA expressing) population in vivo, with several studies demonstrating no evidence of an $\alpha$-SMA+ fibrocyte population during experimental fibrosis [158, 161] and an inability of fibrocytes to express $\alpha$-SMA [162]. Regardless of the ability of fibrocytes to become "fully differentiated" myofibroblasts, they may promote fibrosis via other paracrine effects, such as the production of profibrotic cytokines [163]. Fibrocytes and elevations in CXCL12 are present in the blood of patients with IPF [164] as well as in ex vivo preparations of lung specimens from patients with IPF [165]. Elevations in the number of circulating fibrocytes are a marker of disease progression in human IPF [63], and neutralizing antibodies against CXCL12 ameliorate bleomycin-induced pulmonary fibrosis [159].

The process of EMT can provide an additional potential source of myofibroblasts. As previously discussed, a substantial amount of evidence supports the presence of aberrant epithelial signaling, including EMT-associated signaling, in IPF and experimental pulmonary fibrosis [166, 167]. Additionally, lineage-marking techniques that broadly label distal airway and AECs during gestation provide evidence that epithelial cells can express mesenchymal cell markers during experimental lung fibrosis [96, 97]. In contrast, a more restricted lineage-marking strategy of adult AEC type II cells and terminal bronchial epithelial cells found that no α-SMA+ cell population was derived from these epithelial lineages in the bleomycin model of pulmonary fibrosis [167]. Discrepancies between these studies could be explained by technical differences in marking techniques, or through the presence of a discrete epithelial progenitor population, that evaded lineage-marking in the adult murine lung, but could differentiate into type II cells or undergo EMT directly in response to injury [168]. Recent evidence supports the existence of such a population [169]. Thus, while EMT-associated signaling programs are present in pulmonary fibrosis and appear to mediate important profibrotic cross talk between the epithelial and mesenchymal compartments, it remains unclear to what extent epithelial-derived cells are a significant contributor to the contractile and matrix-producing cells of the parenchyma in pulmonary fibrosis.

These data suggest that the resident fibroblast population within the lung remains a predominant source of myofibroblasts during tissue fibrosis. The resident mesenchymal precursor population is a mixed population of several different mesenchymal cell subtypes that are important for the normal homeostatic maintenance and turnover of the lung connective tissue scaffold. These cells can proliferate and expand in response to injury and upon exposure to profibrotic signals, such as cell, serum, or matrix-derived TGF-β, can differentiate into myofibroblasts [72, 147, 167, 170, 171].

Upon expansion in response to pulmonary injury and fibrosis, the fibroblast population exhibits significant heterogeneity, and several different sub-phenotypes appear to be present [172, 173]. Myofibroblasts are defined by the expression of α-SMA and collagen production, but a significant subset lacks the cell surface marker Thy-1 [174], which conveys a more fibrotic phenotype [175]. It is unclear whether there is linkage between subpopulations of precursor cells and the development of these fibroblast subsets as the fibrotic process evolves.

## *Aberrant Fibroblast Behavior*

Deranged fibroblast biology likely plays an important role in the propagation of pulmonary fibrosis by enabling a disproportionate and non-resolving fibrotic response to epithelial injury. Populations of lung fibroblasts isolated from patients with IPF demonstrate differences in global gene expression [176], proliferative capacity [59, 177], resistance to apoptosis [178], anchorage-independent growth [179], and deficits in translational control [180] when compared to normal lung fibroblasts.

The putative mechanisms mediating some of these disordered functions have begun to be elucidated. Phosphatase and tensin homolog deleted on chromosome ten (PTEN) is a lipid/protein phosphatase that can act as a tumor suppressor via inhibition of the phosphoinositide 3-kinase (PI3K)/Akt signaling pathway. Levels of PTEN are nearly absent in the fibroblastic foci of IPF lungs and in ex vivo IPF fibroblast cultures, in contrast with normal lung tissue and fibroblasts [177, 181]. Disordered PTEN activity in IPF fibroblasts conveys an abnormal proliferative response to polymerized collagen matrices via increases in PI3K/ Akt signaling. Additionally, PTEN-deficient mice develop an accentuated fibro-proliferative wound-healing response and more severe bleomycin-induced pulmonary fibrosis [177].

Caveolin-1 (cav-1) serves as a scaffolding protein and can inhibit the responses to growth factor signaling [182, 183]. The fibroblastic foci of IPF lungs lack cav-1 staining, and cav-1 expression by fibroblasts decreases in response to TGF-β. In contrast, overexpression of cav-1 disrupts TGF-β signaling and matrix protein induction, and cav-1 overexpression attenuates bleomycin-induced pulmonary fibrosis [184]. The loss of cav-1 in IPF myofibroblasts also results in decreases in PTEN expression [169].

Finally, myofibroblasts from IPF lungs manifest deficits in responses to the anti-fibrotic cytokine PGE2 [82]. The mechanism mediating PGE2 "resistance" has been linked to decreased expression of the PGE2 receptor, EP2, by IPF myofibroblasts [185]. This is partially via hypermethylation of the promoter region for the EP2 receptor, which leads to decreased EP2 expression [186].

# Paracrine Mediators of Tissue Fibrosis

## Growth Factors

Transforming growth factor-β(beta) (TGF-β) was one of the first cytokines implicated in the normal wound-healing response [187], and TGF-β plays a central role in the pathobiology of tissue fibrosis [188–190]. Patients with IPF have increased immunolocalization of TGF-β in epithelial cells, macrophages, and myofibroblasts in areas of active fibrosis (fibroblastic foci) [191, 192], while inhibition of TGF-β signaling protects against progression of fibrosis in experimental models of pulmonary fibrosis [188, 193, 194].

TGF-β is secreted as a latent protein, which is then dimerized, and subsequently forms a complex with latent binding protein-1 (LTBP-1) via its latency-associated peptide (LAP) [195]. As part of this complex, it is tethered to matrix elements such as fibrillin and fibronectin [196] and is thus unable to activate the TGF-β receptor on neighboring cells [197]. Activation of latent TGF-βs may occur via direct proteolytic cleavage by several proteinases (including MMP-2 and MMP-9) or via interactions with α(alpha)$_v$-containing integrins [198]. In the lung, $\alpha_v\beta_6$ integrins expressed on the surface of epithelial cells bind the LAP of the latent TGF-β complex and facilitate its activation by G protein-coupled receptor agonists via the generation of cell-mediated mechanical tension. Examples of such agonists include thrombin and lysophosphatidic acid [1, 199]. The application of tension to the $\alpha_v\beta_6$ integrin releases TGF-β from the latent complex, allowing it to interact with its cognate receptor complex on the surface of adjacent cells, such as fibroblasts [200].

The TGF-β receptor complex is a heterodimer comprised of a TGF-β type I receptor (TGF-βR1) and a type II receptor (TGF-βR2), with TGF-βR1 having serine–threonine kinase activity. Upon activation, TGF-βR1 phosphorylates receptor-activated SMAD effector proteins (SMAD2 and SMAD3) associate with the common mediator smad, SMAD4, and translocate to the nucleus with activation of SMAD target genes. Signaling via this pathway appears to be critical during fibrogenesis, as SMAD 3 null mice are protected from experimental pulmonary fibrosis [188], and depletion of the high-affinity type II TGF-beta receptor in resident fibroblasts inhibits experimental pulmonary fibrosis [201].

TGF-β receptor activation also results in the activation of several noncanonical signaling pathways that promote myofibroblast differentiation and resistance to apoptosis. Downstream targets of TGF-β include activation of mitogen-associated kinase pathways [202], TGF-activated kinase [203], PTEN/PI3kinase/Akt [203], focal adhesion kinase [205, 206], the tyrosine kinase, c-Abelson [207], the small GTPase rho/cytoskeletal-dependent signals [208, 209], oxidant-mediated signaling [210], as well as other moieties and pathways. Activation of these pathways results in cell shape change and the regulation of gene programs that mediate fibroblast phenotypic differentiation and survival [211, 212].

Functionally, TGF-β results in pleiotropic effects that promote a coordinated fibrotic response (see Fig. 8.4). Treatment of AECs with TGF-β can result in the induction of apoptosis or the induction of EMT, depending upon the matrix substrate that is present [96, 105]. In fibroblasts, TGF-β results in myofibroblast differentiation [171], apoptosis resistance [212], and the marked upregulation of expression of matrix components [146, 213, 214]. Finally, TGF-β mediates the epigenetic regulation of gene expression via the induction of several microRNAs that mediate the fibrotic response, which are also differentially regulated in IPF and include mir-21 and let-7d [215, 216].

Lysophosphatidic acid (LPA) is a lipid-derived mediator that can be produced by platelets, membrane phospholipids, and lung surfactant [217]. LPA signals through several G-protein-coupled receptors to exert its biologic effects. In the context of pulmonary fibrosis, LPA appears to promote the fibrotic response via induction of epithelial cell apoptosis [218], increased endothelial cell permeability [219], as well as increased fibroblast migration [219, 220] and survival [218]. Elevated levels of LPA have been found in the BAL from patients with IPF, and $LPA_1$ receptor knockout mice are protected from the development of pulmonary fibrosis [219].

Multiple other growth factors, including endothelin-1 [221], angiotensin II [222], PDGF [223], and TGF-α [224], have been identified as playing a role in the fibrotic response. Since they are implicated in the pathogenesis of IPF, these growth factors may serve as targets for therapy.

## *Inflammatory Mediators*

Early studies in IPF lungs identified significant alteration in levels of several cytokines and chemokines typically involved in mediating an inflammatory response. Despite the lack of therapeutic benefit of broad immunosuppression in patients with IPF, inflammatory cells and their associated signaling may still play a role in the pathobiology of IPF, potentially via the modulation of the fibrotic response. The inflammatory cytokines, TNF-α and interleukin-1β (IL-1β), both localize to epithelial cells at sites of fibrosis in IPF [125, 225] and are both released by macrophages from patients with IPF [226]. Similarly, a downstream target of IL-1β, interleukin-17A (IL-17A), is increased in the BAL fluid of patients with IPF and mediates the fibrotic response in the bleomycin murine model [227]. Markers of the Th2 immune response—interleukin-4 (IL-4), interleukin-5 (IL-5), and interleukin-13 (IL-13)—have also been found in increased levels in the disorder [228]. IL-13 plays a key role in inducing Th2 responses in the lung in chronic inflammation [229], while IL-13 levels and IL-13 receptor expression correlate with disease severity [230].

Chemokines play a role in IPF via the recruitment of monocytes, leukocytes, and fibrocytes to the injured lung, as well as in the angiogenic remodeling that occurs in fibrotic lung disease. CCL-12 and its receptor CXCR4 are strongly implicated in fibrocyte recruitment to the lung [155] along with monocyte chemotactic protein-1 (MCP-1/CCL-2) and its receptor CCR2 [231]. Macrophage inflammatory protein-1α (MIP-1α/CCL-3) and MCP-1/CCL-2 are increased in tissue and BAL [232–237] in human IPF and likely participate in macrophage recruitment. This can amplify the fibrotic response through the production of profibrotic cytokines and the recruitment of additional inflammatory cells via secreted chemokines [238]. Production of CCL-18 by macrophages has also been implicated in the progression of pulmonary fibrosis, and indeed, circulating levels of CCL-18 correlate with survival in IPF [239]. Conversely, macrophages may facilitate resolution of the fibrotic response via phagocytosis of apoptotic cells and the production of MMPs [229]. Alternatively, activated macrophages, which represent the majority of macrophages in IPF lungs, may play a role in this process, as depletion of this cell cohort attenuates the fibrotic response in bleomycin-induced pulmonary fibrosis [240].

Despite the abundance of inflammatory mediators implicated in IPF, it remains unclear how these varied pathways intersect with the other components of the fibrotic process. An improved understanding of these interactions may allow for a more rational approach to targeting these pathways for therapeutic benefit in the future.

## Tissue Remodeling and Failure to Resolve the Wound

Angiogenesis, the formation of new blood vessels, is an important component of the wound-healing response in several tissue beds. In dermal wounds, the angiogenic response potentiates the influx of inflammatory mediators that participate in the tissue remodeling process. Insofar as the pathobiology of IPF is an extrapolation of many of the mechanisms that mediate other forms of wound healing, it would not be surprising to detect an angiogenic response. Indeed, the pathology of IPF does demonstrate areas of neovascularization along with the presence of pulmonary-systemic anastomoses, which are often in a sub-pleural location [241]. Additionally, circulating levels of the angiogenic cytokines, interleukin-8 (IL-8/CXCL8) and endothelin-1, are elevated in patients with IPF compared to normal controls, and these tend to correlate with disease progression [242].

However, there is significant spatial heterogeneity of neovascularization and vascular density in IPF tissue biopsies when compared to normal lung tissue. When carefully quantified using endothelial cell markers, the level of neovascularization present within an area of IPF lung is inversely correlated with the degree of parenchymal fibrosis in that area [243–245]. Furthermore, complete vascular obliteration is often seen in areas of dense parenchymal fibrosis. Most often, areas of neovascularization are present adjacent to intact AECs, which might indicate an angiogenic response to reestablish the normal alveolar/capillary interface [244]. This suggests the presence of significant spatial heterogeneity to the angiogenic response in IPF, with areas of angiogenic signaling alternating with areas defined by a predominance of angiostatic signaling.

Corroborating these observations, the angiostatic cytokine, endostatin, has been found to be elevated in the serum of IPF patients [246], while serum levels of vascular endothelial growth factor (VEGF) have been observed to be decreased. Clarifying the issue significantly, it has been shown that local VEGF expression is absent in areas of dense fibrosis, while the angiostatic protein, pigment epithelium-derived factor (PEDF), a VEGF antagonist, has increased expression in the fibroblastic foci of IPF lungs [247]. PEDF is a TGF-β target gene, suggesting that the local environment of the fibroblastic focus is characterized by an angiostatic environment. Whether the angiostatic environment of areas of fibrosis is a cause or consequence of the fibrotic response is unclear. Similarly, the role of the scattered areas of neovascularization in adjacent lung tissue remains undetermined.

## Role of Matrix Remodeling on Fibrotic Progression

The normal lung architecture and matrix environment are maintained by the constant and tightly regulated control of cell activation, matrix production, and extracellular matrix (ECM) proteolysis [5]. During fibrosis, matrix organization is severely altered with increased accumulation of multiple matrix components, including EDA fibronectin, hyaluronic acid, and collagen isoforms. In response to TGF-β, other growth factors and environmental cues, there is an induction of collagen synthesis and secretion by fibroblasts and myofibroblasts. Collagens are secreted as a soluble pro-molecule, which then self-assembles to form insoluble collagen fibrils that are relatively resistant to degradation by proteases [126]. Studies of the collagen content of IPF lungs have demonstrated that collagen III is the primary component in areas of alveolar septal fibrosis, and collagen I predominates in areas of mature fibrosis [248, 249].

Extracellular matrix turnover is tightly regulated by several families of proteinases and their respective inhibitors [22]. MMPs comprise a family of proteinases that can target collagen and other matrix components for degradation. Given the role of these molecules in maintaining the balance of matrix molecules during normal tissue homeostasis, a defect in the balance of these factors might be expected in disorders characterized by matrix accumulation, such as IPF. In line with this expectation, several TIMPs are locally expressed in pulmonary fibrosis [250], and overall collagenase inhibitory activity is elevated in IPF patients when compared to controls [251]. However, total collagenase activity is also increased in IPF [252], and several MMPs, including MMP-1, MMP-2, and MMP-7, have been identified as highly enriched genes in IPF lung tissue [111, 253]. Interestingly, an assessment of global gene expression in IPF lungs found a strong bias toward increased protease expression, supporting a net degradative environment [254]. Given this observation, the spectrum of spatial localization of protease/antiprotease expression is likely not reflected by global assessments of protease/antiprotease "balance."

Analysis of MMP expression demonstrates the importance of spatial localization in IPF. MMP-1 is increased in IPF [111] and localizes to the alveolar epithelium [250], where it participates in the processing of cytokines, in contrast to its role in collagen fibril degradation [126]. MMP-7 (matrilysin) is a highly upregulated gene in IPF lungs, and MMP-7 levels in BAL fluid correlate with survival in IPF patients [129]. MMP-7 also localizes to the AECs [112], but it has diverse roles relevant to tissue remodeling that are distinct from its degrading effect on matrix proteins. In particular, MMP-7 can activate other MMPs, regulate TGF-β activation, and activate osteopontin [113, 255]. MMP-2 is a gelatinase that targets collagen IV as a substrate [256]. MMP-2 is increased in the BAL fluid of IPF patients [250] and is localized to AECs [257, 258], where it may contribute to alveolar basement membrane degradation. MMP-9 is also expressed by epithelial cells and inflammatory cells [259], has increased expression in patients with IPF [260], and has been associated with increases in endothelial permeability, neutrophil activation, and rapidly progressive disease [129, 261]. TIMPs also have differential localization, with TIMP-2 predominating in the fibroblastic foci, where it may facilitate matrix stabilization and accumulation [250].

MMPs can also modify the matrix remodeling response via the cleavage of matrix proteins, yielding fragments that can act as cell signaling ligands [22]. Additionally, MMPs and TIMPs can themselves mediate profibrotic signaling via proteolytic activation of growth factors, chemokines, and shedding of membrane-associated ligands [256]. These profibrotic effects of MMPs may predominate in IPF, making inferences concerning the net effect of increased MMP expression on matrix accumulation difficult.

Matrix composition and organization play key roles modifying cell behavior, and indeed, dysregulation of matrix cues has been implicated in various disease states including tumor progression [262]. In the context of IPF, individual ECM components can significantly modify the response to soluble and matrix-derived mediators.

For example, primary AECs cultured on fibrinogen or fibrin and treated with TGF-β will undergo EMT, while the same cells cultured on matrigel (collagen and laminin) and similarly treated with TGF-β will undergo apoptosis [96]. Myofibroblast differentiation is also dependent on the presence of several matrix cues. The extra type III domain A isoform of fibronectin (EDA FN) is preferentially expressed in healing wounds, and its presence is required for TGF-β-induced myofibroblast differentiation [146]. Mice deficient in this isoform are protected from bleomycin-induced pulmonary fibrosis [263]. De novo expression of the matrix protein, periostin, has been implicated in the fibrotic remodeling that occurs with asthma [264]. Periostin is also highly expressed in the fibroblastic foci and serum of patients with IPF [265], and periostin-deficient mice are protected from bleomycin-induced pulmonary fibrosis [266]. Matrix-associated proteoglycans, such as hyaluronic acid, have increased expression in the fibrotic lung and participate in the fibrotic process, likely via recruitment of inflammatory cells and by facilitating fibroblast migration through cognate receptors such as CD44 [267]. Thus, while the in vivo details of matrix-dependent signaling are currently lacking, it is likely that altered expression of these and other matrix components facilitate and perpetuate the fibrotic response in IPF.

Incorporation of new matrix elements is not merely a result of haphazard matrix protein accumulation and proceeds in an orderly fashion [21]. Newly synthesized fibronectin is desolubilized by integrin-mediated incorporation [99], subsequently serving as a scaffold for collagen and other matrix protein deposition [268]. Newly deposited collagen and elastin are cross-linked via the action of tissue transglutaminases and lysyl oxidases [269], which increases tissue stiffness. Lysyl oxidase 2 (LOXL2) may play an important role in the aberrant tissue remodeling. This mediator displays differentially increased expression in tumor-associated desmoplastic tissue when compared to other lysyl oxidase family members [270]. In liver fibrosis, cross-linking by lysyl oxidase 2 (LOXL2) leads to the development increased tissue stiffness, which precedes the accumulation of matrix components [271]. In IPF, LOXL2 is increased in the fibroblastic foci, and inhibition of its activity using a monoclonal antibody (AB0023) attenuates experimental pulmonary fibrosis [270]. Similarly, tissue transglutaminase-2 expression and activity is upregulated in IPF, and germ-line knockout of this protein prevents the development of experimental pulmonary fibrosis [272].

Alterations in the biomechanical characteristics of the ECM during fibrosis, such as increased tissue elasticity (stiffness), can independently modify cell behaviors and phenotype determination. Tissue stiffness is quantified by its shear modulus, which is typically determined via atomic force microscopy [273]. Careful determinations demonstrate that normal lung tissue has a shear modulus of 0.5 kPa, whereas in fibrotic lung, the median shear modulus increases to 6 kPa [274]. However, significant spatial heterogeneity of tissue stiffness exists within fibrotic lung, with uninvolved areas retaining near-normal shear modulus and areas of dense fibrosis having a shear modulus that surpasses 15 kPa.

All cell types likely sense and respond to alterations in the biomechanical features of the matrix [275]. The development of tension across a healing wound modifies myofibroblast differentiation [276, 277], and release of this tension leads to the induction of myofibroblast apoptosis [278]. Similarly, stiff matrices induce fibroblast to myofibroblast transition [279, 280], which is accompanied by the augmentation of matrix protein expression [274]. The development of matrix tension and stiffness also modifies cellular responses to TGF-β. TGF-β bioavailability is directly modified by the transmission of tension to its associated LTBP, via $\alpha_v$-containing integrins [281, 282]. As a result, myofibroblast differentiation by soluble TGF-β requires the development of matrix-derived tension across the cell [283, 284].

Functionally, increases in matrix stiffness that mimic fibrotic lung result in augmentation of traction forces by lung fibroblasts in response to TGF-β, whereas normal matrix stiffness does not [285]. Epithelial cells toggle their response to TGF-β stimulation dependent on the matrix stiffness of their environment, undergoing apoptosis on low-stiffness substrates and EMT on high stiffness substrates [286]. Some matrix stiffness-dependent effects on cells may be durable, as fibroblasts retain the "programmed" behavior imparted by culture on a stiff matrix, even after subsequent prolonged culture on matrix with "normal" stiffness [287]. Similarly, adoptive transfer of lung fibroblasts from patients with pulmonary fibrosis induces the development of fibrotic lung lesions in mice, while those from normal lungs do not [288, 289]. The acquisition of these durable aberrant behaviors from the matrix environment may be due to epigenetic "programming," although this has not been formally demonstrated as of yet.

These observations strongly suggest that ECM and its cellular constituents participate in reciprocal signaling during fibrosis that provides a "feed-forward" mechanism for fibrotic progression (Fig. 8.5). How matrix-derived signaling varies between fibrosis and normal wound healing is an area of ongoing investigation.

## Targets for Therapeutic Agents

As our understanding of the pathogenesis of IPF has shifted over time, pharmacologic strategies aimed at halting the progression of the disease have also evolved (Table 8.1). Previous clinical trials have targeted inflammatory activation with the use of agents such as prednisone and azathioprine. The inadequacy of this approach was highlighted by the recent publication of the NIH-sponsored PANTHER study, which halted enrollment in the prednisone/azathioprine/N-acetyl-cysteine (NAC) treatment arm due to the significantly increased risk of death and hospitalization amongst the patients randomized to this triple therapy [16]. A refinement in approach via selective targeting of potential inflammatory mediators in IPF (e.g., TNF-α, IFNγ-1b) has also yielded disappointing results [292, 293]. Additionally, therapies directed at putative signaling mechanisms in IPF pathogenesis, such as endothelin-1 receptors [290, 291], the coagulation cascade [144], and receptor tyrosine kinases [294], have also thus far not led to improved patient outcomes. Several other potential antifibrotic agents have demonstrated mixed evidence of efficacy and remain under investigation, such as pirfenidone, an antifibrotic agent with pleiotropic

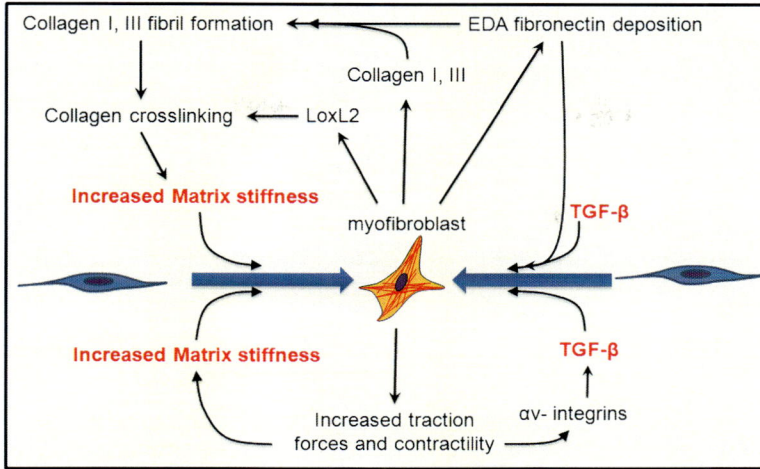

**Fig. 8.5** A model of matrix-dependent feed-forward signaling in fibrotic progression. The myofibroblast is a central effector of tissue remodeling in pulmonary fibrosis. Both matrix stiffness and TGF-β induce myofibroblast activation and differentiation, resulting in increases in matrix protein production (collagen I, III, EDA fibronectin, and others), LOXL2 expression, and the generation of increased traction forces by myofibroblasts. After deposition of collagen fibrils onto a scaffold of EDA fibronectin fibrils, LOXL2 cross-links collagen fibrils, resulting in increased tissue stiffness. Additionally, increased contractility due to myofibroblast differentiation results in the generation of increased tension within the ECM (*lower left quadrant*) and activation of TGF-β via integrin-mediated force transmission (*lower right quadrant*). These processes (EDA FN generation, increased matrix stiffness, TGF-β activation) are thus reinforcing and facilitating and promoting additional myofibroblast differentiation

effects [295–298]; NAC, an antioxidant [303]; sildenafil [304]; and the tyrosine kinase receptor inhibitor, BIBF 1120 (Boehringer-Ingelheim, UK) [299] (see Table 8.1).

Drugs in development continue to target the growing list of mediators/mechanisms involved in tissue fibrosis. TGF-β is a natural target for antifibrotic therapy given its central role in tissue fibrosis. To this end, antibodies against TGF-β isoforms are under development and have undergone phase I testing (CAT-192, Genzyme, USA). However, given the multiple homeostatic roles of TGF-β, broad inhibition of its function may have undesirable side effects. Targeting $\alpha_v\beta_6$ integrin-dependent activation of TGF-β, which is a preferential mechanism of activation during tissue fibrosis, is one potential approach that can be taken to address this issue, In this regard, a humanized monoclonal antibody against $\alpha_v\beta_6$, STX-100 (Stromedix, USA), is currently under investigation as a potential therapeutic agent for IPF. Other antifibrotic targets include CTGF, which is a downstream target of TGF-β activation. CTGF mediates its own profibrotic effects, and a small-molecule inhibitor of CTGF has been developed that is currently under investigation (FG-3019, Fibrogen, USA). Likewise, drug development efforts have also focused on other soluble mediators of the fibrotic response such as lysophosphatidic acid (LPA1 Receptor antagonist, IM152) and CCL2 (CNTO-888, Centocor Inc, USA).

**Table 8.1** Mechanistic targets of therapy for IPF

| Previously evaluated targets of therapy with no clinical benefit | Agent (references) |
|---|---|
| Immune response | Prednisone [16] |
| | Azathioprine [16] |
| Endothelin-1 receptor | Bosentan [290, 291] |
| | Ambrisentan [290, 291] |
| TNF-α | Etanercept [292] |
| Th1/Th2 balance | Interferon γ-1b [293] |
| Coagulation cascade | Warfarin [144] |
| Receptor tyrosine kinases | Imatinib [294] |
| *Targets under evaluation* | *Agent* |
| Oxidative stress | *N*-acetyl cysteine [16] |
| Pirfenidone | Pirfenidone [295–298] |
| Receptor tyrosine kinases | BIBF 1120 [299] |
| PDE5 | Sildenafil [300] |
| CTGF | FG-3019 [301] |
| *Future targets* | *Agent* |
| TGF-β | GC1008 |
| $\alpha_v\beta_6$ | STX-100 [302] |
| LPA1 receptor | AM152 |
| LoxL2 | AB0023 [270] |

Therapeutic approaches directed at reestablishing the normal, epithelial-derived inhibitory signaling to mesenchyme via the use of prostaglandin E2 analogs may represent a useful strategy in the future. Alternatively, interrupting the cellular and enzymatic processes involved in the formation of a stiff, fibrotic matrix may help interrupt the feed-forward loop of signaling that is driven by matrix remodeling. A monoclonal antibody against the collagen cross-linking enzyme, LOXL2 (AB0023, Gilead Sciences, USA), is currently under development as a therapeutic agent for treating IPF. Finally, given the downside of targeting TGF-β receptor ligation and proximal signaling, alternative methods to interrupt TGF-β-dependent fibrotic signals need to be developed. One particularly appealing approach is the inhibition of the discrete sets of TGF-β-dependent genes through the use of oligomers (antagomirs) that can bind to and inactivate microRNAs [305, 306]. This technology is currently under development and would allow for the selective inhibition of critical microRNAs differentially regulated in IPF [215, 216]. However, significant technical hurdles remain to overcome the inherent difficulty of delivering oligonucleotides to the interior of target cells in vivo, hampering the current feasibility of this approach.

## New Directions

The use of genome-wide assessments of gene expression patterns and genetic linkage analysis has provided investigators with powerful new tools to facilitate pathway discovery for complex disorders such as IPF. In the past several years, publication of many of these studies has led to new insights into disease pathogenesis.

## *mRNA Expression Profiling*

Several unbiased, high-throughput analyses of RNA expression profiles using oligonucleotide microarray technology have been performed in IPF patient cohorts. These have demonstrated increased gene expression of developmental signals, adhesion proteins, extracellular matrix proteins, and smooth contractile proteins in IPF lungs as compared to normal lungs or other interstitial lung diseases [99, 111, 112, 307]. Subsequent global analysis of cumulative datasets demonstrates that WNT and TGF-β signaling pathways are highly enriched in IPF lungs [28]. Finally, mRNA expression profiling has yielded insight into potential mechanistic differences in sub-phenotypes of IPF, demonstrating distict patterns of gene expression in IPF patients with secondary pulmonary hypertension [305], progressive disease [308, 309], and acute exacerbations [310]. In addition to providing insight into disease pathogenesis, a major potential use of gene expression profiling is the development of diagnostic, prognostic, and disease activity biomarkers. Several candidates have been identified [306], but validation of these approaches and translation to clinical practice remain future goals.

## *Genome-Wide Association Studies*

Several large GWAS have been performed in patients with sporadic IPF with the identification of SNPs that confer an increased risk for the development of IPF [57, 63]. The SNPs identified reside within the TERT, ELMOD2, and MUC5B genes (see previous discussion). Each of these proteins has putative effects on AEC susceptibility to injury. However, the mechanistic basis for each of these genes in the pathogenesis of IPF remains to be determined and is the focus of ongoing investigation.

## *Epigenetic Regulation*

From a mechanistic perspective, the evolving understanding of epigenetic regulation of gene expression has opened a new area of investigation into the pathogenesis of pulmonary fibrosis. Epigenetic gene regulation refers to regulation of gene expression, which occurs outside of changes in DNA germ-line coding. Epigenetic regulation occurs via three main mechanisms: histone modifications, DNA methylation, and noncoding RNAs (microRNAs).

Unbiased oligonucleotide microarray screens to determine microRNA expression profiling have demonstrated that approximately 10 % of microRNAs are differentially regulated in IPF [27]. The first reports of differentially regulated microRNAs in IPF focused on let-7d [215] and mir-21 [216]. Let7d is a microRNA that is downregulated by TGF-β, and it is decreased in the lungs of patients with IPF

[215]. Let-7d is localized to the alveolar epithelium in normal lungs and is involved in the regulation of EMT [215]. Mir-21 expression is induced by TGF-β, and elevated levels of mir-21 are found in the lungs of IPF patients compared to controls [216]. In contrast to let-7d, mir-21 localizes to myofibroblasts, and it is known to mediate many of the effects of TGF-β, including regulating expression levels of PTEN [311].

DNA modifications are a mechanism by which somatic cells can "program" gene expression and pass this information on to daughter cells. One of the most common modifications that can alter gene expression is gene silencing by methylation at CpG islands [312]. Hypo- and hypermethylation of critical genes have been implicated in the development of cancers [313], but until recently, there have been limited reports of gene methylation in tissue fibrosis. In the context of pulmonary fibrosis, widespread alterations in epigenetic patterning are present in IPF [291, 314], and upregulation of DNA methyltransferase 3a in the hyperplastic epithelium of IPF lung has been reported [291]. Several fibroblast-related genes exhibit hypermethylation and silencing in fibrosis, including the prostaglandin E2 receptor (PTGER2) [186], IP-10 [315], and Thy-1 [316]. Interestingly, the α-SMA promoter is hypermethylated at several CpG islands in epithelial cells, whereas decreased methylation occurs in fibroblasts [317].

These results suggest that IPF is characterized by severe derangements in the regulatory control of gene expression. Further investigation is needed to understand the origins and implications of many of these observations on the mechanisms of disease pathogenesis. However, several of these technologies have exciting therapeutic and diagnostic potential. The identification of key gene expression profiles may lead to the development of individual biomarkers or gene sets that may obviate the need for a surgical lung biopsy, allow for more precise classification of IPF phenotypes, and identify patients at high risk for disease progression. The discovery of key microRNAs involved in IPF may allow for a novel mode of targeting deranged signaling in IPF, as a single microRNA can target many different genes from divergent signaling pathways. Implementation of this strategy will require a more detailed understanding of the relationships between downstream signaling pathways, along with the development of drug-delivery technology to enable this novel mode of targeting.

# Summary

IPF is a disorder characterized by the presence of extensive AEC injury accompanied by a robust, non-resolving wound-healing response. While the mechanistic triggers for the development of IPF still need to be fully elucidated, the results of numerous investigations in both familial pulmonary fibrosis and sporadic IPF strongly suggest that AEC susceptibility to injury and apoptosis coupled with an environmental trigger may be an initiating event. AEC injury is a key driver of the fibrotic response, and several important mechanisms mediating aberrant epithelial cell signaling have been identified, including TGF-β and WNT signaling. The reparative response in IPF is characterized by activation of the coagulation cascade and formation of a provisional matrix. There is recruitment and activation of epithelial cells, fibroblasts, and fibrocytes within the provisional matrix and differentiation of myofibroblasts that form the fibroblastic foci. TGF-β is a central regulator of the reparative response via its pleiotropic effects on epithelial cells, fibroblasts, and matrix remodeling. Matrix remodeling and myofibroblast-mediated increases in tension yield a stiffened, fibrotic matrix that promotes ongoing myofibroblast differentiation and TGF-β activation, respectively.

While an effective therapy for IPF remains elusive, approaches to treatment have begun to evolve toward targeted therapies directed at putative growth factors, receptors, and enzymes that have evidence for mechanistic involvement in matrix remodeling. Significant gaps in our understanding of IPF pathogenesis remain, including identification of the mechanisms that are responsible for either the success or failure of the reparative response to resolve and other key elements that might foster the development of lung fibrosis.

# References

1. Martin P. Wound healing–aiming for perfect skin regeneration. Science. 1997;276(5309):75–81 [Research Support, Non-U.S. Gov't Review].
2. Beers MF, Morrisey EE. The three R's of lung health and disease: repair, remodeling, and regeneration. J Clin Invest. 2011;121(6):2065–73 [Research Support, N.I.H., Extramural Review].
3. Shaw TJ, Martin P. Wound repair at a glance. J Cell Sci. 2009;122(Pt 18):3209–13 [Research Support, Non-U.S. Gov't Review].
4. West JB, Mathieu-Costello O. Structure, strength, failure, and remodeling of the pulmonary blood-gas barrier. Annu Rev Physiol. 1999;61:543–72.
5. Frantz C, Stewart KM, Weaver VM. The extracellular matrix at a glance. J Cell Sci. 2010;123(Pt 24):4195–200 [Research Support, N.I.H., Extramural Research Support, U.S. Gov't, Non-P.H.S. Review].
6. Kuhn 3rd C, Boldt J, King Jr TE, Crouch E, Vartio T, McDonald JA. An immunohistochemical study of architectural remodeling and connective tissue synthesis in pulmonary fibrosis. Am Rev Respir Dis. 1989;140(6):1693–703 [Research Support, U.S. Gov't, P.H.S.].
7. Katzenstein AL, Myers JL. Idiopathic pulmonary fibrosis: clinical relevance of pathologic classification. Am J Respir Crit Care Med. 1998;157(4 Pt 1):1301–15.
8. American Thoracic Society. Idiopathic pulmonary fibrosis: diagnosis and treatment. International consensus statement. American Thoracic Society (ATS), and the European Respiratory Society (ERS). Am J Respir Crit Care Med. 2000;161(2 Pt 1):646–64.
9. American Thoracic Society, European Respiratory Society. American Thoracic Society/European Respiratory Society International Multidisciplinary Consensus Classification of the Idiopathic Interstitial Pneumonias. This joint statement of the American Thoracic Society (ATS), and the European Respiratory Society (ERS) was adopted by the ATS board of directors, June 2001 and by the ERS Executive Committee, June 2001. Am J Respir Crit Care Med. 2002;165(2):277–304.
10. Cool CD, Groshong SD, Rai PR, Henson PM, Stewart JS, Brown KK. Fibroblast foci are not discrete sites of lung injury or repair: the fibroblast reticulum. Am J Respir Crit Care Med. 2006;174(6):654–8 [Comparative Study In Vitro Research Support, N.I.H., Extramural].

11. King Jr TE, Schwarz MI, Brown K, Tooze JA, Colby TV, Waldron Jr JA, et al. Idiopathic pulmonary fibrosis: relationship between histopathologic features and mortality. Am J Respir Crit Care Med. 2001;164(6):1025–32 [Comparative Study Research Support, U.S. Gov't, P.H.S.].

12. Nicholson AG, Fulford LG, Colby TV, du Bois RM, Hansell DM, Wells AU. The relationship between individual histologic features and disease progression in idiopathic pulmonary fibrosis. Am J Respir Crit Care Med. 2002;166(2):173–7.

13. Wynn TA. Common and unique mechanisms regulate fibrosis in various fibroproliferative diseases. J Clin Invest. 2007;117(3):524–9.

14. Keogh BA, Crystal RG. Alveolitis: the key to the interstitial lung disorders. Thorax. 1982;37(1):1–10.

15. Crystal RG, Bitterman PB, Rennard SI, Hance AJ, Keogh BA. Interstitial lung diseases of unknown cause. Disorders characterized by chronic inflammation of the lower respiratory tract (first of two parts). N Engl J Med. 1984;310(3):154–66.

16. Raghu G, Anstrom KJ, King Jr TE, Lasky JA, Martinez FJ. Prednisone, azathioprine, and N-acetylcysteine for pulmonary fibrosis. N Engl J Med. 2012;366(21):1968–77 [Comparative Study Multicenter Study Randomized Controlled Trial Research Support, N.I.H., Extramural Research Support, Non-U.S. Gov't].

17. Davies HR, Richeldi L, Walters EH. Immunomodulatory agents for idiopathic pulmonary fibrosis. Cochrane Database Syst Rev. 2003;(3):CD003134.

18. Richeldi L, Davies HR, Ferrara G, Franco F. Corticosteroids for idiopathic pulmonary fibrosis. Cochrane Database Syst Rev. 2003;(3):CD002880.

19. Thannickal VJ, Toews GB, White ES, Lynch 3rd JP, Martinez FJ. Mechanisms of pulmonary fibrosis. Annu Rev Med. 2004;55:395–417.

20. Selman M, King TE, Pardo A. Idiopathic pulmonary fibrosis: prevailing and evolving hypotheses about its pathogenesis and implications for therapy. Ann Intern Med. 2001;134(2):136–51 [Consensus Development Conference Review].

21. Daley WP, Peters SB, Larsen M. Extracellular matrix dynamics in development and regenerative medicine. J Cell Sci. 2008;121(Pt 3):255–64.

22. Lu P, Takai K, Weaver VM, Werb Z. Extracellular matrix degradation and remodeling in development and disease. Cold Spring Harb Perspect Biol. 2011;3(12):Pii: a005058 [Research Support, N.I.H., Extramural Research Support, Non-U.S. Gov't Review].

23. Clark RA. Fibrin and wound healing. Ann N Y Acad Sci. 2001;936:355–67 [Research Support, U.S. Gov't, P.H.S. Review].

24. Zoz DF, Lawson WE, Blackwell TS. Idiopathic pulmonary fibrosis: a disorder of epithelial cell dysfunction. Am J Med Sci. 2011;341(6):435–8 [Research Support, N.I.H., Extramural Research Support, Non-U.S. Gov't Research Support, U.S. Gov't, Non-P.H.S.].

25. Selman M, Pardo A. Role of epithelial cells in idiopathic pulmonary fibrosis: from innocent targets to serial killers. Proc Am Thorac Soc. 2006;3(4):364–72.

26. Macneal K, Schwartz DA. The genetic and environmental causes of pulmonary fibrosis. Proc Am Thorac Soc. 2012;9(3):120–5.

27. Pandit KV, Milosevic J, Kaminski N. MicroRNAs in idiopathic pulmonary fibrosis. Transl Res. 2011;157(4):191–9 [Research Support, N.I.H., Extramural Research Support, Non-U.S. Gov't Review].

28. Selman M, Pardo A, Kaminski N. Idiopathic pulmonary fibrosis: aberrant recapitulation of developmental programs? PLoS Med. 2008;5(3):e62 [Research Support, N.I.H., Extramural Research Support, Non-U.S. Gov't].

29. Mason RJ. Biology of alveolar type II cells. Respirology. 2006;11(Suppl):S12–5 [Research Support, N.I.H., Extramural Research Support, U.S. Gov't, Non-P.H.S. Review].

30. Adamson IY, Bowden DH. The pathogenesis of bleomycin-induced pulmonary fibrosis in mice. Am J Pathol. 1974;77(2):185–97.

31. Bhaskaran M, Kolliputi N, Wang Y, Gou D, Chintagari NR, Liu L. Trans-differentiation of alveolar epithelial type II cells to type I cells involves autocrine signaling by transforming

growth factor beta 1 through the Smad pathway. J Biol Chem. 2007;282(6):3968–76 [Research Support, N.I.H., Extramural].
32. Myers JL, Katzenstein AL. Epithelial necrosis and alveolar collapse in the pathogenesis of usual interstitial pneumonia. Chest. 1988;94(6):1309–11.
33. Barbas-Filho JV, Ferreira MA, Sesso A, Kairalla RA, Carvalho CR, Capelozzi VL. Evidence of type II pneumocyte apoptosis in the pathogenesis of idiopathic pulmonary fibrosis (IFP)/ usual interstitial pneumonia (UIP). J Clin Pathol. 2001;54(2):132–8 [Research Support, Non-U.S. Gov't].
34. Kawanami O, Ferrans VJ, Crystal RG. Structure of alveolar epithelial cells in patients with fibrotic lung disorders. Lab Invest. 1982;46(1):39–53.
35. Brody AR, Soler P, Basset F, Haschek WM, Witschi H. Epithelial-mesenchymal associations of cells in human pulmonary fibrosis and in BHT-oxygen-induced fibrosis in mice. Exp Lung Res. 1981;2(3):207–20 [Research Support, Non-U.S. Gov't Research Support, U.S. Gov't, P.H.S.].
36. Kasper M, Haroske G. Alterations in the alveolar epithelium after injury leading to pulmonary fibrosis. Histol Histopathol. 1996;11(2):463–83 [Research Support, Non-U.S. Gov't Review].
37. Raghu G, Freudenberger TD, Yang S, Curtis JR, Spada C, Hayes J, et al. High prevalence of abnormal acid gastro-oesophageal reflux in idiopathic pulmonary fibrosis. Eur Respir J. 2006;27(1):136–42.
38. Tobin RW, Pope 2nd CE, Pellegrini CA, Emond MJ, Sillery J, Raghu G. Increased prevalence of gastroesophageal reflux in patients with idiopathic pulmonary fibrosis. Am J Respir Crit Care Med. 1998;158(6):1804–8.
39. Raghu G, Meyer KC. Silent gastro-oesophageal reflux and microaspiration in IPF: mounting evidence for anti-reflux therapy? Eur Respir J. 2012;39(2):242–5.
40. Lee JS, Ryu JH, Elicker BM, Lydell CP, Jones KD, Wolters PJ, et al. Gastroesophageal reflux therapy is associated with longer survival in patients with idiopathic pulmonary fibrosis. Am J Respir Crit Care Med. 2011;184(12):1390–4 [Research Support, N.I.H., Extramural].
41. Oh CK, Murray LA, Molfino NA. Smoking and idiopathic pulmonary fibrosis. Pulm Med. 2012;2012:808260.
42. Baumgartner KB, Samet JM, Stidley CA, Colby TV, Waldron JA. Cigarette smoking: a risk factor for idiopathic pulmonary fibrosis. Am J Respir Crit Care Med. 1997;155(1):242–8 [Multicenter Study Research Support, U.S. Gov't, P.H.S.].
43. Steele MP, Speer MC, Loyd JE, Brown KK, Herron A, Slifer SH, et al. Clinical and pathologic features of familial interstitial pneumonia. Am J Respir Crit Care Med. 2005;172(9):1146–52 [Research Support, N.I.H., Extramural Research Support, U.S. Gov't, Non-P.H.S.].
44. Taskar VS, Coultas DB. Is idiopathic pulmonary fibrosis an environmental disease? Proc Am Thorac Soc. 2006;3(4):293–8.
45. Naik PK, Moore BB. Viral infection and aging as cofactors for the development of pulmonary fibrosis. Expert Rev Respir Med. 2010;4(6):759–71 [Research Support, N.I.H., Extramural Review].
46. Lasithiotaki I, Antoniou KM, Vlahava VM, Karagiannis K, Spandidos DA, Siafakas NM, et al. Detection of herpes simplex virus type-1 in patients with fibrotic lung diseases. PLoS One. 2011;6(12):e27800 [Research Support, Non-U.S. Gov't].
47. Pulkkinen V, Salmenkivi K, Kinnula VL, Sutinen E, Halme M, Hodgson U, et al. A novel screening method detects herpesviral DNA in the idiopathic pulmonary fibrosis lung. Ann Med. 2012;44(2):178–86 [Research Support, Non-U.S. Gov't].
48. Tang YW, Johnson JE, Browning PJ, Cruz-Gervis RA, Davis A, Graham BS, et al. Herpesvirus DNA is consistently detected in lungs of patients with idiopathic pulmonary fibrosis. J Clin Microbiol. 2003;41(6):2633–40.
49. Lawson WE, Crossno PF, Polosukhin VV, Roldan J, Cheng DS, Lane KB, et al. Endoplasmic reticulum stress in alveolar epithelial cells is prominent in IPF: association with altered surfactant protein processing and herpesvirus infection. Am J Physiol Lung Cell Mol Physiol.

2008;294(6):L1119–26 [Research Support, N.I.H., Extramural Research Support, Non-U.S. Gov't].

50. Nogee LM, Dunbar 3rd AE, Wert SE, Askin F, Hamvas A, Whitsett JA. A mutation in the surfactant protein C gene associated with familial interstitial lung disease. N Engl J Med. 2001;344(8):573–9 [Case Reports Research Support, Non-U.S. Gov't Research Support, U.S. Gov't, P.H.S.].

51. Thomas AQ, Lane K, Phillips 3rd J, Prince M, Markin C, Speer M, et al. Heterozygosity for a surfactant protein C gene mutation associated with usual interstitial pneumonitis and cellular nonspecific interstitial pneumonitis in one kindred. Am J Respir Crit Care Med. 2002;165(9):1322–8 [Research Support, Non-U.S. Gov't Research Support, U.S. Gov't, P.H.S.].

52. Mulugeta S, Maguire JA, Newitt JL, Russo SJ, Kotorashvili A, Beers MF. Misfolded BRICHOS SP-C mutant proteins induce apoptosis via caspase-4- and cytochrome c-related mechanisms. Am J Physiol Lung Cell Mol Physiol. 2007;293(3):L720–9 [Research Support, N.I.H., Extramural Research Support, Non-U.S. Gov't].

53. Mulugeta S, Nguyen V, Russo SJ, Muniswamy M, Beers MF. A surfactant protein C precursor protein BRICHOS domain mutation causes endoplasmic reticulum stress, proteasome dysfunction, and caspase 3 activation. Am J Respir Cell Mol Biol. 2005;32(6):521–30 [Research Support, N.I.H., Extramural Research Support, Non-U.S. Gov't Research Support, U.S. Gov't, P.H.S.].

54. Glasser SW, Detmer EA, Ikegami M, Na CL, Stahlman MT, Whitsett JA. Pneumonitis and emphysema in sp-C gene targeted mice. J Biol Chem. 2003;278(16):14291–8 [Research Support, U.S. Gov't, P.H.S.].

55. Wang Y, Kuan PJ, Xing C, Cronkhite JT, Torres F, Rosenblatt RL, et al. Genetic defects in surfactant protein A2 are associated with pulmonary fibrosis and lung cancer. Am J Hum Genet. 2009;84(1):52–9 [Research Support, N.I.H., Extramural Research Support, Non-U.S. Gov't].

56. Tsakiri KD, Cronkhite JT, Kuan PJ, Xing C, Raghu G, Weissler JC, et al. Adult-onset pulmonary fibrosis caused by mutations in telomerase. Proc Natl Acad Sci USA. 2007;104(18):7552–7 [Research Support, N.I.H., Extramural Research Support, Non-U.S. Gov't Research Support, U.S. Gov't, Non-P.H.S.].

57. Armanios MY, Chen JJ, Cogan JD, Alder JK, Ingersoll RG, Markin C, et al. Telomerase mutations in families with idiopathic pulmonary fibrosis. N Engl J Med. 2007;356(13):1317–26 [Research Support, N.I.H., Extramural Research Support, Non-U.S. Gov't].

58. Hornsby PJ. Telomerase and the aging process. Exp Gerontol. 2007;42(7):575–81 [Research Support, N.I.H., Extramural Research Support, Non-U.S. Gov't Review].

59. Moodley YP, Scaffidi AK, Misso NL, Keerthisingam C, McAnulty RJ, Laurent GJ, et al. Fibroblasts isolated from normal lungs and those with idiopathic pulmonary fibrosis differ in interleukin-6/gp130-mediated cell signaling and proliferation. Am J Pathol. 2003;163(1):345–54 [Research Support, Non-U.S. Gov't].

60. Diaz de Leon A, Cronkhite JT, Katzenstein AL, Godwin JD, Raghu G, Glazer CS, et al. Telomere lengths, pulmonary fibrosis and telomerase (TERT) mutations. PLoS One. 2010;5(5):e10680 [Research Support, N.I.H., Extramural Research Support, Non-U.S. Gov't].

61. Cronkhite JT, Xing C, Raghu G, Chin KM, Torres F, Rosenblatt RL, et al. Telomere shortening in familial and sporadic pulmonary fibrosis. Am J Respir Crit Care Med. 2008;178(7):729–37 [Research Support, N.I.H., Extramural].

62. Alder JK, Chen JJ, Lancaster L, Danoff S, Su SC, Cogan JD, et al. Short telomeres are a risk factor for idiopathic pulmonary fibrosis. Proc Natl Acad Sci USA. 2008;105(35):13051–6 [Research Support, N.I.H., Extramural Research Support, Non-U.S. Gov't].

63. Moeller A, Gilpin SE, Ask K, Cox G, Cook D, Gauldie J, et al. Circulating fibrocytes are an indicator of poor prognosis in idiopathic pulmonary fibrosis. Am J Respir Crit Care Med. 2009;179(7):588–94 [Research Support, Non-U.S. Gov't].

64. Pulkkinen V, Bruce S, Rintahaka J, Hodgson U, Laitinen T, Alenius H, et al. ELMOD2, a candidate gene for idiopathic pulmonary fibrosis, regulates antiviral responses. FASEB J. 2010;24(4):1167–77 [Research Support, Non-U.S. Gov't].
65. Hodgson U, Pulkkinen V, Dixon M, Peyrard-Janvid M, Rehn M, Lahermo P, et al. ELMOD2 is a candidate gene for familial idiopathic pulmonary fibrosis. Am J Hum Genet. 2006;79(1):149–54 [Research Support, Non-U.S. Gov't].
66. Seibold MA, Wise AL, Speer MC, Steele MP, Brown KK, Loyd JE, et al. A common MUC5B promoter polymorphism and pulmonary fibrosis. N Engl J Med. 2011;364(16):1503–12 [Research Support, N.I.H., Extramural Research Support, N.I.H., Intramural Research Support, Non-U.S. Gov't].
67. Zhang Y, Noth I, Garcia JG, Kaminski N. A variant in the promoter of MUC5B and idiopathic pulmonary fibrosis. N Engl J Med. 2011;364(16):1576–7 [Letter Research Support, N.I.H., Extramural].
68. Korfei M, Ruppert C, Mahavadi P, Henneke I, Markart P, Koch M, et al. Epithelial endoplasmic reticulum stress and apoptosis in sporadic idiopathic pulmonary fibrosis. Am J Respir Crit Care Med. 2008;178(8):838–46 [Comparative Study Research Support, N.I.H., Extramural Research Support, Non-U.S. Gov't].
69. Naidoo N. The endoplasmic reticulum stress response and aging. Rev Neurosci. 2009;20(1):23–37.
70. Sisson TH, Mendez M, Choi K, Subbotina N, Courey A, Cunningham A, et al. Targeted injury of type II alveolar epithelial cells induces pulmonary fibrosis. Am J Respir Crit Care Med. 2010;181(3):254–63 [Comparative Study Research Support, N.I.H., Extramural Research Support, Non-U.S. Gov't Research Support, U.S. Gov't, Non-P.H.S.].
71. Fehrenbach H. Alveolar epithelial type II cell: defender of the alveolus revisited. Respir Res. 2001;2(1):33–46 [Research Support, Non-U.S. Gov't Review].
72. Sirianni FE, Chu FS, Walker DC. Human alveolar wall fibroblasts directly link epithelial type 2 cells to capillary endothelium. Am J Respir Crit Care Med. 2003;168(12):1532–7 [Research Support, U.S. Gov't, P.H.S.].
73. Portnoy J, Pan T, Dinarello CA, Shannon JM, Westcott JY, Zhang L, et al. Alveolar type II cells inhibit fibroblast proliferation: role of IL-1alpha. Am J Physiol Lung Cell Mol Physiol. 2006;290(2):L307–16 [Research Support, N.I.H., Extramural].
74. Chauncey JB, Peters-Golden M, Simon RH. Arachidonic acid metabolism by rat alveolar epithelial cells. Lab Invest. 1988;58(2):133–40 [Research Support, Non-U.S. Gov't Research Support, U.S. Gov't, Non-P.H.S. Research Support, U.S. Gov't, P.H.S.].
75. Lipchik RJ, Chauncey JB, Paine R, Simon RH, Peters-Golden M. Arachidonate metabolism increases as rat alveolar type II cells differentiate in vitro. Am J Physiol. 1990;259(2 Pt 1):L73–80.
76. Lama V, Moore BB, Christensen P, Toews GB, Peters-Golden M. Prostaglandin E2 synthesis and suppression of fibroblast proliferation by alveolar epithelial cells is cyclooxygenase-2-dependent. Am J Respir Cell Mol Biol. 2002;27(6):752–8 [Research Support, U.S. Gov't, P.H.S.].
77. Bitterman PB, Wewers MD, Rennard SI, Adelberg S, Crystal RG. Modulation of alveolar macrophage-driven fibroblast proliferation by alternative macrophage mediators. J Clin Invest. 1986;77(3):700–8.
78. Kohyama T, Ertl RF, Valenti V, Spurzem J, Kawamoto M, Nakamura Y, et al. Prostaglandin E(2) inhibits fibroblast chemotaxis. Am J Physiol Lung Cell Mol Physiol. 2001;281(5):L1257–63 [Research Support, Non-U.S. Gov't].
79. Korn JH, Halushka PV, LeRoy EC. Mononuclear cell modulation of connective tissue function: suppression of fibroblast growth by stimulation of endogenous prostaglandin production. J Clin Invest. 1980;65(2):543–54 [Research Support, U.S. Gov't, P.H.S.].
80. Goldstein RH, Polgar P. The effect and interaction of bradykinin and prostaglandins on protein and collagen production by lung fibroblasts. J Biol Chem. 1982;257(15):8630–3 [Research Support, U.S. Gov't, P.H.S.].

81. Borok Z, Gillissen A, Buhl R, Hoyt RF, Hubbard RC, Ozaki T, et al. Augmentation of functional prostaglandin E levels on the respiratory epithelial surface by aerosol administration of prostaglandin E. Am Rev Respir Dis. 1991;144(5):1080–4 [Comparative Study Research Support, Non-U.S. Gov't].

82. Huang SK, Wettlaufer SH, Hogaboam CM, Flaherty KR, Martinez FJ, Myers JL, et al. Variable prostaglandin E2 resistance in fibroblasts from patients with usual interstitial pneumonia. Am J Respir Crit Care Med. 2008;177(1):66–74 [Research Support, N.I.H., Extramural].

83. Adamson IY, Young L, Bowden DH. Relationship of alveolar epithelial injury and repair to the induction of pulmonary fibrosis. Am J Pathol. 1988;130(2):377–83 [Research Support, Non-U.S. Gov't].

84. Perl AK, Riethmacher D, Whitsett JA. Conditional depletion of airway progenitor cells induces peribronchiolar fibrosis. Am J Respir Crit Care Med. 2011;183(4):511–21 [Research Support, N.I.H., Extramural Research Support, Non-U.S. Gov't].

85. Chilosi M, Poletti V, Murer B, Lestani M, Cancellieri A, Montagna L, et al. Abnormal re-epithelialization and lung remodeling in idiopathic pulmonary fibrosis: the role of deltaN-p63. Lab Invest. 2002;82(10):1335–45 [Research Support, Non-U.S. Gov't].

86. Fehrenbach H, Kasper M, Tschernig T, Shearman MS, Schuh D, Muller M. Receptor for advanced glycation endproducts (RAGE) exhibits highly differential cellular and subcellular localisation in rat and human lung. Cell Mol Biol (Noisy-le-Grand). 1998;44(7):1147–57 [Research Support, Non-U.S. Gov't].

87. Demling N, Ehrhardt C, Kasper M, Laue M, Knels L, Rieber EP. Promotion of cell adherence and spreading: a novel function of RAGE, the highly selective differentiation marker of human alveolar epithelial type I cells. Cell Tissue Res. 2006;323(3):475–88.

88. Queisser MA, Kouri FM, Konigshoff M, Wygrecka M, Schubert U, Eickelberg O, et al. Loss of RAGE in pulmonary fibrosis: molecular relations to functional changes in pulmonary cell types. Am J Respir Cell Mol Biol. 2008;39(3):337–45 [Research Support, Non-U.S. Gov't].

89. Englert JM, Hanford LE, Kaminski N, Tobolewski JM, Tan RJ, Fattman CL, et al. A role for the receptor for advanced glycation end products in idiopathic pulmonary fibrosis. Am J Pathol. 2008;172(3):583–91 [Research Support, N.I.H., Extramural Research Support, Non--U.S. Gov't].

90. Zavadil J, Bottinger EP. TGF-beta and epithelial-to-mesenchymal transitions. Oncogene. 2005;24(37):5764–74 [Research Support, N.I.H., Extramural Research Support, U.S. Gov't, P.H.S. Review].

91. Thiery JP, Sleeman JP. Complex networks orchestrate epithelial-mesenchymal transitions. Nat Rev Mol Cell Biol. 2006;7(2):131–42 [Research Support, Non-U.S. Gov't Review].

92. Thiery JP. Epithelial-mesenchymal transitions in tumour progression. Nat Rev Cancer. 2002;2(6):442–54.

93. Iwano M, Plieth D, Danoff TM, Xue C, Okada H, Neilson EG. Evidence that fibroblasts derive from epithelium during tissue fibrosis. J Clin Invest. 2002;110(3):341–50 [Research Support, U.S. Gov't, P.H.S.].

94. Rowe RG, Lin Y, Shimizu-Hirota R, Hanada S, Neilson EG, Greenson JK, et al. Hepatocyte-derived Snail1 propagates liver fibrosis progression. Mol Cell Biol. 2011;31(12):2392–403 [Research Support, N.I.H., Extramural].

95. Moore BB, Hogaboam CM. Murine models of pulmonary fibrosis. Am J Physiol Lung Cell Mol Physiol. 2008;294(2):L152–60.

96. Kim KK, Kugler MC, Wolters PJ, Robillard L, Galvez MG, Brumwell AN, et al. Alveolar epithelial cell mesenchymal transition develops in vivo during pulmonary fibrosis and is regulated by the extracellular matrix. Proc Natl Acad Sci USA. 2006;103(35):13180–5 [Research Support, N.I.H., Extramural].

97. Tanjore H, Xu XC, Polosukhin VV, Degryse AL, Li B, Han W, et al. Contribution of epithelial-derived fibroblasts to bleomycin-induced lung fibrosis. Am J Respir Crit Care Med. 2009;180(7):657–65 [Research Support, N.I.H., Extramural Research Support, Non-U.S. Gov't].

98. Marmai C, Sutherland RE, Kim KK, Dolganov GM, Fang X, Kim SS, et al. Alveolar epithelial cells express mesenchymal proteins in patients with idiopathic pulmonary fibrosis. Am J Physiol Lung Cell Mol Physiol. 2011;301(1):L71–8 [Research Support, N.I.H., Extramural Research Support, Non-U.S. Gov't].

99. Bridges RS, Kass D, Loh K, Glackin C, Borczuk AC, Greenberg S. Gene expression profiling of pulmonary fibrosis identifies Twist1 as an antiapoptotic molecular "rectifier" of growth factor signaling. Am J Pathol. 2009;175(6):2351–61 [Research Support, N.I.H., Extramural Research Support, Non-U.S. Gov't].

100. Jayachandran A, Konigshoff M, Yu H, Rupniewska E, Hecker M, Klepetko W, et al. SNAI transcription factors mediate epithelial-mesenchymal transition in lung fibrosis. Thorax. 2009;64(12):1053–61 [Research Support, Non-U.S. Gov't].

101. Shannon JM, Hyatt BA. Epithelial-mesenchymal interactions in the developing lung. Annu Rev Physiol. 2004;66:625–45 [Research Support, Non-U.S. Gov't Research Support, U.S. Gov't, P.H.S.Review].

102. Cardoso WV. Molecular regulation of lung development. Annu Rev Physiol. 2001;63:471–94 [Research Support, U.S. Gov't, P.H.S. Review].

103. Thiery JP, Acloque H, Huang RY, Nieto MA. Epithelial-mesenchymal transitions in development and disease. Cell. 2009;139(5):871–90 [Research Support, Non-U.S. Gov't Review].

104. Xu J, Lamouille S, Derynck R. TGF-beta-induced epithelial to mesenchymal transition. Cell Res. 2009;19(2):156–72.

105. Willis BC, Borok Z. TGF-beta-induced EMT: mechanisms and implications for fibrotic lung disease. Am J Physiol Lung Cell Mol Physiol. 2007;293(3):L525–34 [Research Support, N.I.H., Extramural Research Support, Non-U.S. Gov't Review].

106. Kim KK, Wei Y, Szekeres C, Kugler MC, Wolters PJ, Hill ML, et al. Epithelial cell alpha-3beta1 integrin links beta-catenin and Smad signaling to promote myofibroblast formation and pulmonary fibrosis. J Clin Invest. 2009;119(1):213–24 [Research Support, N.I.H., Extramural].

107. Masszi A, Fan L, Rosivall L, McCulloch CA, Rotstein OD, Mucsi I, et al. Integrity of cell-cell contacts is a critical regulator of TGF-beta 1-induced epithelial-to-myofibroblast transition: role for beta-catenin. Am J Pathol. 2004;165(6):1955–67 [Research Support, Non-U.S. Gov't].

108. Koli K, Myllarniemi M, Vuorinen K, Salmenkivi K, Ryynanen MJ, Kinnula VL, et al. Bone morphogenetic protein-4 inhibitor gremlin is overexpressed in idiopathic pulmonary fibrosis. Am J Pathol. 2006;169(1):61–71 [Research Support, Non-U.S. Gov't].

109. Konigshoff M, Eickelberg O. WNT signaling in lung disease: a failure or a regeneration signal? Am J Respir Cell Mol Biol. 2010;42(1):21–31 [Research Support, Non-U.S. Gov't Review].

110. Mucenski ML, Nation JM, Thitoff AR, Besnard V, Xu Y, Wert SE, et al. Beta-catenin regulates differentiation of respiratory epithelial cells in vivo. Am J Physiol Lung Cell Mol Physiol. 2005;289(6):L971–9 [Research Support, N.I.H., Extramural Research Support, Non-U.S. Gov't].

111. Selman M, Pardo A, Barrera L, Estrada A, Watson SR, Wilson K, et al. Gene expression profiles distinguish idiopathic pulmonary fibrosis from hypersensitivity pneumonitis. Am J Respir Crit Care Med. 2006;173(2):188–98 [Clinical Trial Research Support, N.I.H., Extramural Research Support, Non-U.S. Gov't].

112. Zuo F, Kaminski N, Eugui E, Allard J, Yakhini Z, Ben-Dor A, et al. Gene expression analysis reveals matrilysin as a key regulator of pulmonary fibrosis in mice and humans. Proc Natl Acad Sci USA. 2002;99(9):6292–7 [Research Support, Non-U.S. Gov't].

113. Pardo A, Gibson K, Cisneros J, Richards TJ, Yang Y, Becerril C, et al. Up-regulation and profibrotic role of osteopontin in human idiopathic pulmonary fibrosis. PLoS Med. 2005;2(9):e251.

114. Yang IV, Burch LH, Steele MP, Savov JD, Hollingsworth JW, McElvania-Tekippe E, et al. Gene expression profiling of familial and sporadic interstitial pneumonia. Am J Respir Crit Care Med. 2007;175(1):45–54 [Comparative Study Research Support, N.I.H., Extramural Research Support, N.I.H., Intramural].

115. Chilosi M, Poletti V, Zamo A, Lestani M, Montagna L, Piccoli P, et al. Aberrant Wnt/beta-catenin pathway activation in idiopathic pulmonary fibrosis. Am J Pathol. 2003;162(5):1495–502 [Research Support, Non-U.S. Gov't].
116. Konigshoff M, Balsara N, Pfaff EM, Kramer M, Chrobak I, Seeger W, et al. Functional Wnt signaling is increased in idiopathic pulmonary fibrosis. PLoS One. 2008;3(5):e2142 [Research Support, Non-U.S. Gov't].
117. Konigshoff M, Kramer M, Balsara N, Wilhelm J, Amarie OV, Jahn A, et al. WNT1-inducible signaling protein-1 mediates pulmonary fibrosis in mice and is upregulated in humans with idiopathic pulmonary fibrosis. J Clin Invest. 2009;119(4):772–87 [Research Support, Non-U.S. Gov't].
118. Kapanci Y, Desmouliere A, Pache JC, Redard M, Gabbiani G. Cytoskeletal protein modulation in pulmonary alveolar myofibroblasts during idiopathic pulmonary fibrosis. Possible role of transforming growth factor beta and tumor necrosis factor alpha. Am J Respir Crit Care Med. 1995;152(6 Pt 1):2163–9 [Research Support, Non-U.S. Gov't].
119. Khalil N, O'Connor RN, Flanders KC, Unruh H. TGF-beta 1, but not TGF-beta 2 or TGF-beta 3, is differentially present in epithelial cells of advanced pulmonary fibrosis: an immunohistochemical study. Am J Respir Cell Mol Biol. 1996;14(2):131–8 [Research Support, Non-U.S. Gov't].
120. Antoniades HN, Bravo MA, Avila RE, Galanopoulos T, Neville-Golden J, Maxwell M, et al. Platelet-derived growth factor in idiopathic pulmonary fibrosis. J Clin Invest. 1990;86(4):1055–64 [Research Support, Non-U.S. Gov't Research Support, U.S. Gov't, P.H.S.].
121. Antoniades HN, Neville-Golden J, Galanopoulos T, Kradin RL, Valente AJ, Graves DT. Expression of monocyte chemoattractant protein 1 mRNA in human idiopathic pulmonary fibrosis. Proc Natl Acad Sci USA. 1992;89(12):5371–5 [Research Support, Non-U.S. Gov't Research Support, U.S. Gov't, P.H.S.].
122. Pan LH, Yamauchi K, Uzuki M, Nakanishi T, Takigawa M, Inoue H, et al. Type II alveolar epithelial cells and interstitial fibroblasts express connective tissue growth factor in IPF. Eur Respir J. 2001;17(6):1220–7 [Research Support, Non-U.S. Gov't].
123. Giaid A, Michel RP, Stewart DJ, Sheppard M, Corrin B, Hamid Q. Expression of endothelin-1 in lungs of patients with cryptogenic fibrosing alveolitis. Lancet. 1993;341(8860):1550–4 [Research Support, Non-U.S. Gov't].
124. Nash JR, McLaughlin PJ, Butcher D, Corrin B. Expression of tumour necrosis factor-alpha in cryptogenic fibrosing alveolitis. Histopathology. 1993;22(4):343–7.
125. Piguet PF, Ribaux C, Karpuz V, Grau GE, Kapanci Y. Expression and localization of tumor necrosis factor-alpha and its mRNA in idiopathic pulmonary fibrosis. Am J Pathol. 1993;143(3):651–5 [Research Support, Non-U.S. Gov't].
126. Dancer RC, Wood AM, Thickett DR. Metalloproteinases in idiopathic pulmonary fibrosis. Eur Respir J. 2011;38(6):1461–7.
127. Corrin B, Dewar A, Rodriguez-Roisin R, Turner-Warwick M. Fine structural changes in cryptogenic fibrosing alveolitis and asbestosis. J Pathol. 1985;147(2):107–19.
128. Mogulkoc N, Brutsche MH, Bishop PW, Murby B, Greaves MS, Horrocks AW, et al. Pulmonary (99m)Tc-DTPA aerosol clearance and survival in usual interstitial pneumonia (UIP). Thorax. 2001;56(12):916–23.
129. McKeown S, Richter AG, O'Kane C, McAuley DF, Thickett DR. MMP expression and abnormal lung permeability are important determinants of outcome in IPF. Eur Respir J. 2009;33(1):77–84 [Research Support, Non-U.S. Gov't].
130. Basset F, Ferrans VJ, Soler P, Takemura T, Fukuda Y, Crystal RG. Intraluminal fibrosis in interstitial lung disorders. Am J Pathol. 1986;122(3):443–61.
131. Gross TJ, Simon RH, Sitrin RG. Tissue factor procoagulant expression by rat alveolar epithelial cells. Am J Respir Cell Mol Biol. 1992;6(4):397–403 [Research Support, Non-U.S. Gov't Research Support, U.S. Gov't, P.H.S.].
132. Kotani I, Sato A, Hayakawa H, Urano T, Takada Y, Takada A. Increased procoagulant and antifibrinolytic activities in the lungs with idiopathic pulmonary fibrosis. Thromb Res. 1995;77(6):493–504.

133. Chambers RC, Scotton CJ. Coagulation cascade proteinases in lung injury and fibrosis. Proc Am Thorac Soc. 2012;9(3):96–101.
134. Chapman HA. Disorders of lung matrix remodeling. J Clin Invest. 2004;113(2):148–57 [Research Support, U.S. Gov't, P.H.S. Review].
135. Marshall BC, Brown BR, Rothstein MA, Rao NV, Hoidal JR, Rodgers GM. Alveolar epithelial cells express both plasminogen activator and tissue factor. Potential role in repair of lung injury. Chest. 1991;99(3 Suppl):25S–7 [Research Support, U.S. Gov't, Non-P.H.S. Research Support, U.S. Gov't, P.H.S.].
136. Imokawa S, Sato A, Hayakawa H, Kotani M, Urano T, Takada A. Tissue factor expression and fibrin deposition in the lungs of patients with idiopathic pulmonary fibrosis and systemic sclerosis. Am J Respir Crit Care Med. 1997;156(2 Pt 1):631–6.
137. Gunther A, Mosavi P, Ruppert C, Heinemann S, Temmesfeld B, Velcovsky HG, et al. Enhanced tissue factor pathway activity and fibrin turnover in the alveolar compartment of patients with interstitial lung disease. Thromb Haemost. 2000;83(6):853–60 [Comparative Study Research Support, Non-U.S. Gov't].
138. Fujii M, Hayakawa H, Urano T, Sato A, Chida K, Nakamura H, et al. Relevance of tissue factor and tissue factor pathway inhibitor for hypercoagulable state in the lungs of patients with idiopathic pulmonary fibrosis. Thromb Res. 2000;99(2):111–7.
139. Grainger DJ, Wakefield L, Bethell HW, Farndale RW, Metcalfe JC. Release and activation of platelet latent TGF-beta in blood clots during dissolution with plasmin. Nat Med. 1995;1(9):932–7 [Research Support, Non-U.S. Gov't].
140. Eitzman DT, McCoy RD, Zheng X, Fay WP, Shen T, Ginsburg D, et al. Bleomycin-induced pulmonary fibrosis in transgenic mice that either lack or overexpress the murine plasminogen activator inhibitor-1 gene. J Clin Invest. 1996;97(1):232–7 [Research Support, Non-U.S. Gov't Research Support, U.S. Gov't, P.H.S.].
141. Howell DC, Johns RH, Lasky JA, Shan B, Scotton CJ, Laurent GJ, et al. Absence of proteinase-activated receptor-1 signaling affords protection from bleomycin-induced lung inflammation and fibrosis. Am J Pathol. 2005;166(5):1353–65 [Research Support, Non-U.S. Gov't].
142. Scotton CJ, Krupiczojc MA, Konigshoff M, Mercer PF, Lee YC, Kaminski N, et al. Increased local expression of coagulation factor X contributes to the fibrotic response in human and murine lung injury. J Clin Invest. 2009;119(9):2550–63 [Research Support, Non-U.S. Gov't].
143. Wygrecka M, Kwapiszewska G, Jablonska E, von Gerlach S, Henneke I, Zakrzewicz D, et al. Role of protease-activated receptor-2 in idiopathic pulmonary fibrosis. Am J Respir Crit Care Med. 2011;183(12):1703–14 [In Vitro Research Support, Non-U.S. Gov't].
144. Noth I, Anstrom KJ, Calvert SB, de Andrade J, Flaherty KR, Glazer C, et al. A Placebo-controlled randomized trial of warfarin in idiopathic pulmonary fibrosis. Am J Respir Crit Care Med. 2012;186(1):88–95.
145. Hinz B, Phan SH, Thannickal VJ, Galli A, Bochaton-Piallat ML, Gabbiani G. The myofibroblast. one function, multiple origins. Am J Pathol. 2007;170(6):1807–16.
146. Serini G, Bochaton-Piallat ML, Ropraz P, Geinoz A, Borsi L, Zardi L, et al. The fibronectin domain ED-A is crucial for myofibroblastic phenotype induction by transforming growth factor-beta1. J Cell Biol. 1998;142(3):873–81.
147. Kapanci Y, Ribaux C, Chaponnier C, Gabbiani G. Cytoskeletal features of alveolar myofibroblasts and pericytes in normal human and rat lung. J Histochem Cytochem. 1992;40(12):1955–63 [Research Support, Non-U.S. Gov't].
148. Darby I, Skalli O, Gabbiani G. Alpha-smooth muscle actin is transiently expressed by myofibroblasts during experimental wound healing. Lab Invest. 1990;63(1):21–9.
149. Ehrlich HP, Desmouliere A, Diegelmann RF, Cohen IK, Compton CC, Garner WL, et al. Morphological and immunochemical differences between keloid and hypertrophic scar. Am J Pathol. 1994;145(1):105–13.
150. Gabbiani G. The myofibroblast in wound healing and fibrocontractive diseases. J Pathol. 2003;200(4):500–3.

151. Powell DW, Mifflin RC, Valentich JD, Crowe SE, Saada JI, West AB. Myofibroblasts I. Paracrine cells important in health and disease. Am J Physiol. 1999;277(1 Pt 1):C1–9.
152. Hinz B, Phan SH, Thannickal VJ, Prunotto M, Desmouliere A, Varga J, et al. Recent developments in myofibroblast biology: paradigms for connective tissue remodeling. Am J Pathol. 2012;180(4):1340–55 [Research Support, N.I.H., Extramural Research Support, Non-U.S. Gov't Review].
153. Kuhn C, McDonald JA. The roles of the myofibroblast in idiopathic pulmonary fibrosis. Ultrastructural and immunohistochemical features of sites of active extracellular matrix synthesis. Am J Pathol. 1991;138(5):1257–65.
154. Phan SH. Genesis of the myofibroblast in lung injury and fibrosis. Proc Am Thorac Soc. 2012;9(3):148–52.
155. Strieter RM, Keeley EC, Hughes MA, Burdick MD, Mehrad B. The role of circulating mesenchymal progenitor cells (fibrocytes) in the pathogenesis of pulmonary fibrosis. J Leukoc Biol. 2009;86(5):1111–8 [Research Support, N.I.H., Extramural Review].
156. Bucala R, Spiegel LA, Chesney J, Hogan M, Cerami A. Circulating fibrocytes define a new leukocyte subpopulation that mediates tissue repair. Mol Med. 1994;1(1):71–81 [Research Support, Non-U.S. Gov't Research Support, U.S. Gov't, P.H.S.].
157. Ebihara Y, Masuya M, Larue AC, Fleming PA, Visconti RP, Minamiguchi H, et al. Hematopoietic origins of fibroblasts: II. In vitro studies of fibroblasts, CFU-F, and fibrocytes. Exp Hematol. 2006;34(2):219–29 [In Vitro Research Support, N.I.H., Extramural Research Support, U.S. Gov't, Non-P.H.S.].
158. Hashimoto N, Jin H, Liu T, Chensue SW, Phan SH. Bone marrow-derived progenitor cells in pulmonary fibrosis. J Clin Invest. 2004;113(2):243–52 [Research Support, U.S. Gov't, P.H.S.].
159. Phillips RJ, Burdick MD, Hong K, Lutz MA, Murray LA, Xue YY, et al. Circulating fibrocytes traffic to the lungs in response to CXCL12 and mediate fibrosis. J Clin Invest. 2004;114(3):438–46 [Research Support, U.S. Gov't, P.H.S.].
160. Epperly MW, Guo H, Gretton JE, Greenberger JS. Bone marrow origin of myofibroblasts in irradiation pulmonary fibrosis. Am J Respir Cell Mol Biol. 2003;29(2):213–24 [Research Support, U.S. Gov't, P.H.S.].
161. Humphreys BD, Lin SL, Kobayashi A, Hudson TE, Nowlin BT, Bonventre JV, et al. Fate tracing reveals the pericyte and not epithelial origin of myofibroblasts in kidney fibrosis. Am J Pathol. 2010;176(1):85–97 [Research Support, N.I.H., Extramural Research Support, U.S. Gov't, Non-P.H.S.].
162. Yokota T, Kawakami Y, Nagai Y, Ma JX, Tsai JY, Kincade PW, et al. Bone marrow lacks a transplantable progenitor for smooth muscle type alpha-actin-expressing cells. Stem Cells. 2006;24(1):13–22 [Research Support, N.I.H., Extramural].
163. Strieter RM. Pathogenesis and natural history of usual interstitial pneumonia: the whole story or the last chapter of a long novel. Chest. 2005;128(5 Suppl 1):526S–32.
164. Mehrad B, Burdick MD, Zisman DA, Keane MP, Belperio JA, Strieter RM. Circulating peripheral blood fibrocytes in human fibrotic interstitial lung disease. Biochem Biophys Res Commun. 2007;353(1):104–8 [Research Support, N.I.H., Extramural Research Support, Non-U.S. Gov't].
165. Andersson-Sjoland A, de Alba CG, Nihlberg K, Becerril C, Ramirez R, Pardo A, et al. Fibrocytes are a potential source of lung fibroblasts in idiopathic pulmonary fibrosis. Int J Biochem Cell Biol. 2008;40(10):2129–40 [Research Support, Non-U.S. Gov't].
166. Willis BC, Liebler JM, Luby-Phelps K, Nicholson AG, Crandall ED, du Bois RM, et al. Induction of epithelial-mesenchymal transition in alveolar epithelial cells by transforming growth factor-beta1: potential role in idiopathic pulmonary fibrosis. Am J Pathol. 2005;166(5):1321–32 [Research Support, N.I.H., Extramural Research Support, Non-U.S. Gov't Research Support, U.S. Gov't, P.H.S.].
167. Rock JR, Barkauskas CE, Cronce MJ, Xue Y, Harris JR, Liang J, et al. Multiple stromal populations contribute to pulmonary fibrosis without evidence for epithelial to mesenchymal

transition. Proc Natl Acad Sci USA. 2011;108(52):E1475–83 [Comparative Study Research Support, N.I.H., Extramural].

168. Chapman HA. Epithelial responses to lung injury: role of the extracellular matrix. Proc Am Thorac Soc. 2012;9(3):89–95.

169. Chapman HA, Li X, Alexander JP, Brumwell A, Lorizio W, Tan K, et al. Integrin alpha6beta4 identifies an adult distal lung epithelial population with regenerative potential in mice. J Clin Invest. 2011;121(7):2855–62 [Research Support, N.I.H., Extramural Research Support, Non-U.S. Gov't].

170. Zhang K, Rekhter MD, Gordon D, Phan SH. Myofibroblasts and their role in lung collagen gene expression during pulmonary fibrosis. A combined immunohistochemical and in situ hybridization study. Am J Pathol. 1994;145(1):114–25 [Research Support, U.S. Gov't, P.H.S.].

171. Desmouliere A, Geinoz A, Gabbiani F, Gabbiani G. Transforming growth factor-beta 1 induces alpha-smooth muscle actin expression in granulation tissue myofibroblasts and in quiescent and growing cultured fibroblasts. J Cell Biol. 1993;122(1):103–11.

172. Phan SH. Fibroblast phenotypes in pulmonary fibrosis. Am J Respir Cell Mol Biol. 2003;29(3 Suppl):S87–92.

173. Hagood JS, Lasky JA, Nesbitt JE, Segarini P. Differential expression, surface binding, and response to connective tissue growth factor in lung fibroblast subpopulations. Chest. 2001;120(1 Suppl):64S–6 [Research Support, U.S. Gov't, P.H.S.].

174. Hagood JS, Prabhakaran P, Kumbla P, Salazar L, MacEwen MW, Barker TH, et al. Loss of fibroblast Thy-1 expression correlates with lung fibrogenesis. Am J Pathol. 2005;167(2):365–79 [Research Support, N.I.H., Extramural Research Support, Non-U.S. Gov't Research Support, U.S. Gov't, P.H.S.].

175. Sanders YY, Kumbla P, Hagood JS. Enhanced myofibroblastic differentiation and survival in Thy-1(−) lung fibroblasts. Am J Respir Cell Mol Biol. 2007;36(2):226–35 [Research Support, N.I.H., Extramural Research Support, Non-U.S. Gov't].

176. Emblom-Callahan MC, Chhina MK, Shlobin OA, Ahmad S, Reese ES, Iyer EP, et al. Genomic phenotype of non-cultured pulmonary fibroblasts in idiopathic pulmonary fibrosis. Genomics. 2010;96(3):134–45.

177. Xia H, Diebold D, Nho R, Perlman D, Kleidon J, Kahm J, et al. Pathological integrin signaling enhances proliferation of primary lung fibroblasts from patients with idiopathic pulmonary fibrosis. J Exp Med. 2008;205(7):1659–72 [Research Support, N.I.H., Extramural].

178. Ramos C, Montano M, Garcia-Alvarez J, Ruiz V, Uhal BD, Selman M, et al. Fibroblasts from idiopathic pulmonary fibrosis and normal lungs differ in growth rate, apoptosis, and tissue inhibitor of metalloproteinases expression. Am J Respir Cell Mol Biol. 2001;24(5):591–8.

179. Torry DJ, Richards CD, Podor TJ, Gauldie J. Anchorage-independent colony growth of pulmonary fibroblasts derived from fibrotic human lung tissue. J Clin Invest. 1994;93(4):1525–32 [Research Support, Non-U.S. Gov't].

180. Larsson O, Diebold D, Fan D, Peterson M, Nho RS, Bitterman PB, et al. Fibrotic myofibroblasts manifest genome-wide derangements of translational control. PLoS One. 2008;3(9):e3220 [Research Support, N.I.H., Extramural Research Support, Non-U.S. Gov't].

181. White ES, Atrasz RG, Hu B, Phan SH, Stambolic V, Mak TW, et al. Negative regulation of myofibroblast differentiation by PTEN (Phosphatase and Tensin Homolog Deleted on chromosome 10). Am J Respir Crit Care Med. 2006;173(1):112–21 [Research Support, N.I.H., Extramural].

182. Okamoto T, Schlegel A, Scherer PE, Lisanti MP. Caveolins, a family of scaffolding proteins for organizing "preassembled signaling complexes" at the plasma membrane. J Biol Chem. 1998;273(10):5419–22 [Research Support, Non-U.S. Gov't Research Support, U.S. Gov't, P.H.S. Review].

183. Liu P, Ying Y, Ko YG, Anderson RG. Localization of platelet-derived growth factor-stimulated phosphorylation cascade to caveolae. J Biol Chem. 1996;271(17):10299–303 [Research Support, Non-U.S. Gov't Research Support, U.S. Gov't, P.H.S.].

184. Wang XM, Zhang Y, Kim HP, Zhou Z, Feghali-Bostwick CA, Liu F, et al. Caveolin-1: a critical regulator of lung fibrosis in idiopathic pulmonary fibrosis. J Exp Med. 2006;203(13):2895–906 [Research Support, N.I.H., Extramural Research Support, Non-U.S. Gov't].
185. Sagana RL, Yan M, Cornett AM, Tsui JL, Stephenson DA, Huang SK, et al. Phosphatase and tensin homologue on chromosome 10 (PTEN) directs prostaglandin E2-mediated fibroblast responses via regulation of E prostanoid 2 receptor expression. J Biol Chem. 2009;284(47): 32264–71 [Research Support, N.I.H., Extramural].
186. Huang SK, Fisher AS, Scruggs AM, White ES, Hogaboam CM, Richardson BC, et al. Hypermethylation of PTGER2 confers prostaglandin E2 resistance in fibrotic fibroblasts from humans and mice. Am J Pathol. 2010;177(5):2245–55 [Research Support, N.I.H., Extramural Research Support, Non-U.S. Gov't].
187. Kane CJ, Hebda PA, Mansbridge JN, Hanawalt PC. Direct evidence for spatial and temporal regulation of transforming growth factor beta 1 expression during cutaneous wound healing. J Cell Physiol. 1991;148(1):157–73 [Research Support, Non-U.S. Gov't Research Support, U.S. Gov't, P.H.S.].
188. Gauldie J, Bonniaud P, Sime P, Ask K, Kolb M. TGF-beta, Smad3 and the process of progressive fibrosis. Biochem Soc Trans. 2007;35(Pt 4):661–4.
189. Leask A, Abraham DJ. TGF-beta signaling and the fibrotic response. FASEB J. 2004;18(7):816–27.
190. Sheppard D. Transforming growth factor beta: a central modulator of pulmonary and airway inflammation and fibrosis. Proc Am Thorac Soc. 2006;3(5):413–7 [Research Support, N.I.H., Extramural Research Support, Non-U.S. Gov't Review].
191. Broekelmann TJ, Limper AH, Colby TV, McDonald JA. Transforming growth factor beta 1 is present at sites of extracellular matrix gene expression in human pulmonary fibrosis. Proc Natl Acad Sci USA. 1991;88(15):6642–6.
192. Khalil N, O'Connor RN, Unruh HW, Warren PW, Flanders KC, Kemp A, et al. Increased production and immunohistochemical localization of transforming growth factor-beta in idiopathic pulmonary fibrosis. Am J Respir Cell Mol Biol. 1991;5(2):155–62 [Research Support, Non-U.S. Gov't].
193. Giri SN, Hyde DM, Hollinger MA. Effect of antibody to transforming growth factor beta on bleomycin induced accumulation of lung collagen in mice. Thorax. 1993;48(10):959–66.
194. Wang Q, Wang Y, Hyde DM, Gotwals PJ, Koteliansky VE, Ryan ST, et al. Reduction of bleomycin induced lung fibrosis by transforming growth factor beta soluble receptor in hamsters. Thorax. 1999;54(9):805–12.
195. Annes JP, Munger JS, Rifkin DB. Making sense of latent TGFbeta activation. J Cell Sci. 2003;116(Pt 2):217–24 [Research Support, Non-U.S. Gov't Research Support, U.S. Gov't, P.H.S. Review].
196. Hynes RO. The extracellular matrix: not just pretty fibrils. Science. 2009;326(5957):1216–9 [Research Support, N.I.H., Extramural Research Support, Non-U.S. Gov't Review].
197. Rifkin DB. Latent transforming growth factor-beta (TGF-beta) binding proteins: orchestrators of TGF-beta availability. J Biol Chem. 2005;280(9):7409–12.
198. Jenkins G. The role of proteases in transforming growth factor-beta activation. Int J Biochem Cell Biol. 2008;40(6–7):1068–78.
199. Xu MY, Porte J, Knox AJ, Weinreb PH, Maher TM, Violette SM, et al. Lysophosphatidic acid induces alphavbeta6 integrin-mediated TGF-beta activation via the LPA2 receptor and the small G protein G alpha(q). Am J Pathol. 2009;174(4):1264–79 [Research Support, N.I.H., Extramural Research Support, Non-U.S. Gov't].
200. Hinz B. Mechanical aspects of lung fibrosis: a spotlight on the myofibroblast. Proc Am Thorac Soc. 2012;9(3):137–47.
201. Hoyles RK, Derrett-Smith EC, Khan K, Shiwen X, Howat SL, Wells AU, et al. An essential role for resident fibroblasts in experimental lung fibrosis is defined by lineage-specific deletion of high-affinity type II transforming growth factor beta receptor. Am J Respir Crit Care Med. 2011;183(2):249–61 [Research Support, Non-U.S. Gov't].
202. Hashimoto S, Gon Y, Takeshita I, Matsumoto K, Maruoka S, Horie T. Transforming growth Factor-beta1 induces phenotypic modulation of human lung fibroblasts to myofibroblast

through a c-Jun-NH2-terminal kinase-dependent pathway. Am J Respir Crit Care Med. 2001;163(1):152–7.

203. Shi-wen X, Parapuram SK, Pala D, Chen Y, Carter DE, Eastwood M, et al. Requirement of transforming growth factor beta-activated kinase 1 for transforming growth factor beta-induced alpha-smooth muscle actin expression and extracellular matrix contraction in fibroblasts. Arthritis Rheum. 2009;60(1):234–41.

204. Wilkes MC, Mitchell H, Penheiter SG, Dore JJ, Suzuki K, Edens M, et al. Transforming growth factor-beta activation of phosphatidylinosital 3-kinase is independent of Smad2 and Smad3 and regulates fibroblast responses via p21-activated kinase-2. Cancer Res. 2005;65(22):10431–40 [Research Support, N.I.H., Extramural Research Support, Non-U.S. Gov't].

205. Horowitz JC, Rogers DS, Sharma V, Vittal R, White ES, Cui Z, et al. Combinatorial activation of FAK and AKT by transforming growth factor-beta1 confers an anoikis-resistant phenotype to myofibroblasts. Cell Signal. 2007;19(4):761–71 [Research Support, N.I.H., Extramural Research Support, Non-U.S. Gov't].

206. Thannickal VJ, Lee DY, White ES, Cui Z, Larios JM, Chacon R, et al. Myofibroblast differentiation by transforming growth factor-beta1 is dependent on cell adhesion and integrin signaling via focal adhesion kinase. J Biol Chem. 2003;278(14):12384–9.

207. Daniels CE, Wilkes MC, Edens M, Kottom TJ, Murphy SJ, Limper AH, et al. Imatinib mesylate inhibits the profibrogenic activity of TGF-beta and prevents bleomycin-mediated lung fibrosis. J Clin Invest. 2004;114(9):1308–16 [Research Support, Non-U.S. Gov't Research Support, U.S. Gov't, P.H.S.].

208. Derynck R, Zhang YE. Smad-dependent and Smad-independent pathways in TGF-beta family signalling. Nature. 2003;425(6958):577–84.

209. Sandbo N, Lau A, Kach J, Ngam C, Yau D, Dulin NO. Delayed stress fiber formation mediates pulmonary myofibroblast differentiation in response to TGF-beta. Am J Physiol Lung Cell Mol Physiol. 2011;301(5):L656–66 [Research Support, N.I.H., Extramural Research Support, Non-U.S. Gov't].

210. Hecker L, Vittal R, Jones T, Jagirdar R, Luckhardt TR, Horowitz JC, et al. NADPH oxidase-4 mediates myofibroblast activation and fibrogenic responses to lung injury. Nat Med. 2009;15(9):1077–81 [Research Support, N.I.H., Extramural].

211. Sandbo N, Dulin N. Actin cytoskeleton in myofibroblast differentiation: ultrastructure defining form and driving function. Transl Res. 2011;158(4):181–96 [Research Support, N.I.H., Extramural Research Support, Non-U.S. Gov't Review].

212. Horowitz JC, Lee DY, Waghray M, Keshamouni VG, Thomas PE, Zhang H, et al. Activation of the pro-survival phosphatidylinosital 3-kinase/AKT pathway by transforming growth factor-beta1 in mesenchymal cells is mediated by p38 MAPK-dependent induction of an autocrine growth factor. J Biol Chem. 2004;279(2):1359–67.

213. Varga J, Jimenez SA. Stimulation of normal human fibroblast collagen production and processing by transforming growth factor-beta. Biochem Biophys Res Commun. 1986;138(2):974–80 [Research Support, Non-U.S. Gov't Research Support, U.S. Gov't, P.H.S.].

214. Ignotz RA, Massague J. Transforming growth factor-beta stimulates the expression of fibronectin and collagen and their incorporation into the extracellular matrix. J Biol Chem. 1986;261(9):4337–45.

215. Pandit KV, Corcoran D, Yousef H, Yarlagadda M, Tzouvelekis A, Gibson KF, et al. Inhibition and role of let-7d in idiopathic pulmonary fibrosis. Am J Respir Crit Care Med. 2010;182(2):220–9 [Clinical Trial Research Support, N.I.H., Extramural].

216. Liu G, Friggeri A, Yang Y, Milosevic J, Ding Q, Thannickal VJ, et al. Mir-21 mediates fibrogenic activation of pulmonary fibroblasts and lung fibrosis. J Exp Med. 2010;207(8):1589–97 [Research Support, N.I.H., Extramural].

217. Aoki J. Mechanisms of lysophosphatidic acid production. Semin Cell Dev Biol. 2004;15(5):477–89.

218. Funke M, Zhao Z, Xu Y, Chun J, Tager AM. The lysophosphatidic acid receptor LPA1 promotes epithelial cell apoptosis after lung injury. Am J Respir Cell Mol Biol. 2012;46(3):355–64 [Research Support, N.I.H., Extramural].

219. Tager AM, LaCamera P, Shea BS, Campanella GS, Selman M, Zhao Z, et al. The lysophosphatidic acid receptor LPA1 links pulmonary fibrosis to lung injury by mediating fibroblast recruitment and vascular leak. Nat Med. 2008;14(1):45–54 [Research Support, N.I.H., Extramural Research Support, Non-U.S. Gov't].

220. Sakai T, Peyruchaud O, Fassler R, Mosher DF. Restoration of beta1A integrins is required for lysophosphatidic acid-induced migration of beta1-null mouse fibroblastic cells. J Biol Chem. 1998;273(31):19378–82 [Research Support, Non-U.S. Gov't Research Support, U.S. Gov't, P.H.S.].

221. Fonseca C, Abraham D, Renzoni EA. Endothelin in pulmonary fibrosis. Am J Respir Cell Mol Biol. 2011;44(1):1–10.

222. Uhal BD, Li X, Piasecki CC, Molina-Molina M. Angiotensin signalling in pulmonary fibrosis. Int J Biochem Cell Biol. 2012;44(3):465–8.

223. Trojanowska M. Role of PDGF in fibrotic diseases and systemic sclerosis. Rheumatology (Oxford). 2008;47 Suppl 5:v2–4.

224. Hardie WD, Hagood JS, Dave V, Perl AK, Whitsett JA, Korfhagen TR, et al. Signaling pathways in the epithelial origins of pulmonary fibrosis. Cell Cycle. 2010;9(14):2769–76 [Research Support, N.I.H., Extramural Review].

225. Pan LH, Ohtani H, Yamauchi K, Nagura H. Co-expression of TNF alpha and IL-1 beta in human acute pulmonary fibrotic diseases: an immunohistochemical analysis. Pathol Int. 1996;46(2):91–9.

226. Zhang Y, Lee TC, Guillemin B, Yu MC, Rom WN. Enhanced IL-1 beta and tumor necrosis factor-alpha release and messenger RNA expression in macrophages from idiopathic pulmonary fibrosis or after asbestos exposure. J Immunol. 1993;150(9):4188–96 [Research Support, Non-U.S. Gov't Research Support, U.S. Gov't, P.H.S.].

227. Wilson MS, Madala SK, Ramalingam TR, Gochuico BR, Rosas IO, Cheever AW, et al. Bleomycin and IL-1beta-mediated pulmonary fibrosis is IL-17A dependent. J Exp Med. 2010;207(3):535–52 [Research Support, N.I.H., Intramural].

228. Wallace WA, Ramage EA, Lamb D, Howie SE. A type 2 (Th2-like) pattern of immune response predominates in the pulmonary interstitium of patients with cryptogenic fibrosing alveolitis (CFA). Clin Exp Immunol. 1995;101(3):436–41 [Research Support, Non-U.S. Gov't].

229. Wynn TA. Integrating mechanisms of pulmonary fibrosis. J Exp Med. 2011;208(7):1339–50 [Research Support, N.I.H., Intramural Review].

230. Park SW, Ahn MH, Jang HK, Jang AS, Kim DJ, Koh ES, et al. Interleukin-13 and its receptors in idiopathic interstitial pneumonia: clinical implications for lung function. J Korean Med Sci. 2009;24(4):614–20 [Research Support, Non-U.S. Gov't].

231. Moore BB, Kolodsick JE, Thannickal VJ, Cooke K, Moore TA, Hogaboam C, et al. CCR2-mediated recruitment of fibrocytes to the alveolar space after fibrotic injury. Am J Pathol. 2005;166(3):675–84 [Research Support, U.S. Gov't, P.H.S.].

232. Agostini C, Gurrieri C. Chemokine/cytokine cocktail in idiopathic pulmonary fibrosis. Proc Am Thorac Soc. 2006;3(4):357–63 [Research Support, Non-U.S. Gov't Review].

233. Baran CP, Opalek JM, McMaken S, Newland CA, O'Brien Jr JM, Hunter MG, et al. Important roles for macrophage colony-stimulating factor, CC chemokine ligand 2, and mononuclear phagocytes in the pathogenesis of pulmonary fibrosis. Am J Respir Crit Care Med. 2007;176(1):78–89 [Research Support, N.I.H., Extramural].

234. Car BD, Meloni F, Luisetti M, Semenzato G, Gialdroni-Grassi G, Walz A. Elevated IL-8 and MCP-1 in the bronchoalveolar lavage fluid of patients with idiopathic pulmonary fibrosis and pulmonary sarcoidosis. Am J Respir Crit Care Med. 1994;149(3 Pt 1):655–9 [Comparative Study Research Support, Non-U.S. Gov't].

235. Standiford TJ, Kunkel SL, Liebler JM, Burdick MD, Gilbert AR, Strieter RM. Gene expression of macrophage inflammatory protein-1 alpha from human blood monocytes and alveolar macrophages is inhibited by interleukin-4. Am J Respir Cell Mol Biol. 1993;9(2):192–8 [Research Support, Non-U.S. Gov't Research Support, U.S. Gov't, P.H.S.].

236. Standiford TJ, Rolfe MR, Kunkel SL, Lynch 3rd JP, Becker FS, Orringer MB, et al. Altered production and regulation of monocyte chemoattractant protein-1 from pulmonary fibroblasts isolated from patients with idiopathic pulmonary fibrosis. Chest. 1993;103(2 Suppl):121S.

237. Standiford TJ, Rolfe MW, Kunkel SL, Lynch 3rd JP, Burdick MD, Gilbert AR, et al. Macrophage inflammatory protein-1 alpha expression in interstitial lung disease. J Immunol. 1993;151(5):2852–63 [Research Support, Non-U.S. Gov't Research Support, U.S. Gov't, P.H.S.].

238. Wynn TA, Barron L. Macrophages: master regulators of inflammation and fibrosis. Semin Liver Dis. 2010;30(3):245–57.

239. Prasse A, Probst C, Bargagli E, Zissel G, Toews GB, Flaherty KR, et al. Serum CC-chemokine ligand 18 concentration predicts outcome in idiopathic pulmonary fibrosis. Am J Respir Crit Care Med. 2009;179(8):717–23.

240. Gibbons MA, MacKinnon AC, Ramachandran P, Dhaliwal K, Duffin R, Phythian-Adams AT, et al. Ly6Chi monocytes direct alternatively activated profibrotic macrophage regulation of lung fibrosis. Am J Respir Crit Care Med. 2011;184(5):569–81 [Comparative Study Research Support, Non-U.S. Gov't].

241. Turner-Warwick M. Precapillary systemic-pulmonary anastomoses. Thorax. 1963;18: 225–37.

242. Simler NR, Brenchley PE, Horrocks AW, Greaves SM, Hasleton PS, Egan JJ. Angiogenic cytokines in patients with idiopathic interstitial pneumonia. Thorax. 2004;59(7):581–5 [Clinical Trial Comparative Study Controlled Clinical Trial].

243. Parra ER, David YR, da Costa LR, Ab'Saber A, Sousa R, Kairalla RA, et al. Heterogeneous remodeling of lung vessels in idiopathic pulmonary fibrosis. Lung. 2005;183(4):291–300 [Research Support, Non-U.S. Gov't].

244. Ebina M, Shimizukawa M, Shibata N, Kimura Y, Suzuki T, Endo M, et al. Heterogeneous increase in CD34-positive alveolar capillaries in idiopathic pulmonary fibrosis. Am J Respir Crit Care Med. 2004;169(11):1203–8 [Comparative Study Evaluation Studies Research Support, Non-U.S. Gov't].

245. Renzoni EA, Walsh DA, Salmon M, Wells AU, Sestini P, Nicholson AG, et al. Interstitial vascularity in fibrosing alveolitis. Am J Respir Crit Care Med. 2003;167(3):438–43.

246. Sumi M, Satoh H, Kagohashi K, Ishikawa H, Sekizawa K. Increased serum levels of endostatin in patients with idiopathic pulmonary fibrosis. J Clin Lab Anal. 2005;19(4):146–9.

247. Cosgrove GP, Brown KK, Schiemann WP, Serls AE, Parr JE, Geraci MW, et al. Pigment epithelium-derived factor in idiopathic pulmonary fibrosis: a role in aberrant angiogenesis. Am J Respir Crit Care Med. 2004;170(3):242–51 [Research Support, Non-U.S. Gov't Research Support, U.S. Gov't, P.H.S.].

248. Raghu G, Striker LJ, Hudson LD, Striker GE. Extracellular matrix in normal and fibrotic human lungs. Am Rev Respir Dis. 1985;131(2):281–9 [Research Support, U.S. Gov't, P.H.S.].

249. Kaarteenaho-Wiik R, Lammi L, Lakari E, Kinnula VL, Risteli J, Ryhanen L, et al. Localization of precursor proteins and mRNA of type I and III collagens in usual interstitial pneumonia and sarcoidosis. J Mol Histol. 2005;36(6–7):437–46 [Research Support, Non-U.S. Gov't].

250. Selman M, Ruiz V, Cabrera S, Segura L, Ramirez R, Barrios R, et al. TIMP-1, -2, -3, and −4 in idiopathic pulmonary fibrosis. A prevailing nondegradative lung microenvironment? Am J Physiol Lung Cell Mol Physiol. 2000;279(3):L562–74 [Research Support, Non-U.S. Gov't].

251. Montano M, Ramos C, Gonzalez G, Vadillo F, Pardo A, Selman M. Lung collagenase inhibitors and spontaneous and latent collagenase activity in idiopathic pulmonary fibrosis and hypersensitivity pneumonitis. Chest. 1989;96(5):1115–9.

252. Gadek JE, Kelman JA, Fells G, Weinberger SE, Horwitz AL, Reynolds HY, et al. Collagenase in the lower respiratory tract of patients with idiopathic pulmonary fibrosis. N Engl J Med. 1979;301(14):737–42.

253. Garcia-Alvarez J, Ramirez R, Sampieri CL, Nuttall RK, Edwards DR, Selman M, et al. Membrane type-matrix metalloproteinases in idiopathic pulmonary fibrosis. Sarcoidosis

Vasc Diffuse Lung Dis. 2006;23(1):13–21 [Comparative Study Research Support, Non-U.S. Gov't].

254. Pardo A, Selman M, Kaminski N. Approaching the degradome in idiopathic pulmonary fibrosis. Int J Biochem Cell Biol. 2008;40(6–7):1141–55.
255. Agnihotri R, Crawford HC, Haro H, Matrisian LM, Havrda MC, Liaw L. Osteopontin, a novel substrate for matrix metalloproteinase-3 (stromelysin-1) and matrix metalloproteinase-7 (matrilysin). J Biol Chem. 2001;276(30):28261–7 [Research Support, Non-U.S. Gov't Research Support, U.S. Gov't, P.H.S.].
256. Loffek S, Schilling O, Franzke CW. Series "matrix metalloproteinases in lung health and disease": Biological role of matrix metalloproteinases: a critical balance. Eur Respir J. 2011;38(1):191–208 [Research Support, Non-U.S. Gov't Review].
257. Fukuda Y, Ishizaki M, Kudoh S, Kitaichi M, Yamanaka N. Localization of matrix metalloproteinases-1, -2, and -9 and tissue inhibitor of metalloproteinase-2 in interstitial lung diseases. Lab Invest. 1998;78(6):687–98 [Research Support, Non-U.S. Gov't].
258. Hayashi T, Stetler-Stevenson WG, Fleming MV, Fishback N, Koss MN, Liotta LA, et al. Immunohistochemical study of metalloproteinases and their tissue inhibitors in the lungs of patients with diffuse alveolar damage and idiopathic pulmonary fibrosis. Am J Pathol. 1996;149(4):1241–56.
259. Atkinson JJ, Senior RM. Matrix metalloproteinase-9 in lung remodeling. Am J Respir Cell Mol Biol. 2003;28(1):12–24 [Research Support, Non-U.S. Gov't Research Support, U.S. Gov't, P.H.S. Review].
260. Lemjabbar H, Gosset P, Lechapt-Zalcman E, Franco-Montoya ML, Wallaert B, Harf A, et al. Overexpression of alveolar macrophage gelatinase B (MMP-9) in patients with idiopathic pulmonary fibrosis: effects of steroid and immunosuppressive treatment. Am J Respir Cell Mol Biol. 1999;20(5):903–13.
261. Suga M, Iyonaga K, Okamoto T, Gushima Y, Miyakawa H, Akaike T, et al. Characteristic elevation of matrix metalloproteinase activity in idiopathic interstitial pneumonias. Am J Respir Crit Care Med. 2000;162(5):1949–56 [Research Support, Non-U.S. Gov't].
262. Egeblad M, Nakasone ES, Werb Z. Tumors as organs: complex tissues that interface with the entire organism. Dev Cell. 2010;18(6):884–901 [Research Support, N.I.H., Extramural Research Support, Non-U.S. Gov't Review].
263. Muro AF, Moretti FA, Moore BB, Yan M, Atrasz RG, Wilke CA, et al. An essential role for fibronectin extra type III domain A in pulmonary fibrosis. Am J Respir Crit Care Med. 2008;177(6):638–45 [Research Support, N.I.H., Extramural Research Support, Non-U.S. Gov't].
264. Woodruff PG, Boushey HA, Dolganov GM, Barker CS, Yang YH, Donnelly S, et al. Genome-wide profiling identifies epithelial cell genes associated with asthma and with treatment response to corticosteroids. Proc Natl Acad Sci USA. 2007;104(40):15858–63 [Randomized Controlled Trial Research Support, N.I.H., Extramural Research Support, Non-U.S. Gov't].
265. Okamoto M, Hoshino T, Kitasato Y, Sakazaki Y, Kawayama T, Fujimoto K, et al. Periostin, a matrix protein, is a novel biomarker for idiopathic interstitial pneumonias. Eur Respir J. 2011;37(5):1119–27 [Research Support, Non-U.S. Gov't].
266. Uchida M, Shiraishi H, Ohta S, Arima K, Taniguchi K, Suzuki S, et al. Periostin, a matricellular protein, plays a role in the induction of chemokines in pulmonary fibrosis. Am J Respir Cell Mol Biol. 2012;46(5):677–86 [Research Support, N.I.H., Extramural Research Support, Non-U.S. Gov't].
267. Li Y, Jiang D, Liang J, Meltzer EB, Gray A, Miura R, et al. Severe lung fibrosis requires an invasive fibroblast phenotype regulated by hyaluronan and CD44. J Exp Med. 2011;208(7):1459–71 [Research Support, N.I.H., Extramural Research Support, Non-U.S. Gov't].
268. Sottile J, Hocking DC. Fibronectin polymerization regulates the composition and stability of extracellular matrix fibrils and cell-matrix adhesions. Mol Biol Cell. 2002;13(10):3546–59 [Research Support, U.S. Gov't, P.H.S.].

269. Lucero HA, Kagan HM. Lysyl oxidase: an oxidative enzyme and effector of cell function. Cell Mol Life Sci. 2006;63(19–20):2304–16 [Research Support, N.I.H., Extramural Review].

270. Barry-Hamilton V, Spangler R, Marshall D, McCauley S, Rodriguez HM, Oyasu M, et al. Allosteric inhibition of lysyl oxidase-like-2 impedes the development of a pathologic micro-environment. Nat Med. 2010;16(9):1009–17.

271. Georges PC, Hui JJ, Gombos Z, McCormick ME, Wang AY, Uemura M, et al. Increased stiffness of the rat liver precedes matrix deposition: implications for fibrosis. Am J Physiol Gastrointest Liver Physiol. 2007;293(6):G1147–54 [Research Support, N.I.H., Extramural].

272. Olsen KC, Sapinoro RE, Kottmann RM, Kulkarni AA, Iismaa SE, Johnson GV, et al. Transglutaminase 2 and its role in pulmonary fibrosis. Am J Respir Crit Care Med. 2011;184(6):699–707 [Research Support, N.I.H., Extramural].

273. Liu F, Tschumperlin DJ. Micro-mechanical characterization of lung tissue using atomic force microscopy. J Vis Exp. 2011;(54):pii: 2911 [Research Support, N.I.H., Extramural Research Support, U.S. Gov't, Non-P.H.S. Video-Audio Media].

274. Liu F, Mih JD, Shea BS, Kho AT, Sharif AS, Tager AM, et al. Feedback amplification of fibrosis through matrix stiffening and COX-2 suppression. J Cell Biol. 2010;190(4):693–706 [Research Support, N.I.H., Extramural Research Support, Non-U.S. Gov't Research Support, U.S. Gov't, Non-P.H.S.].

275. Discher DE, Janmey P, Wang YL. Tissue cells feel and respond to the stiffness of their substrate. Science. 2005;310(5751):1139–43.

276. Hinz B, Mastrangelo D, Iselin CE, Chaponnier C, Gabbiani G. Mechanical tension controls granulation tissue contractile activity and myofibroblast differentiation. Am J Pathol. 2001;159(3):1009–20.

277. Tomasek JJ, Gabbiani G, Hinz B, Chaponnier C, Brown RA. Myofibroblasts and mechano-regulation of connective tissue remodelling. Nat Rev Mol Cell Biol. 2002;3(5):349–63.

278. Grinnell F, Zhu M, Carlson MA, Abrams JM. Release of mechanical tension triggers apoptosis of human fibroblasts in a model of regressing granulation tissue. Exp Cell Res. 1999;248(2):608–19 [Research Support, U.S. Gov't, P.H.S.].

279. Huang X, Yang N, Fiore VF, Barker TH, Sun Y, Morris SW, et al. Matrix stiffness-induced myofibroblast differentiation is mediated by intrinsic mechanotransduction. Am J Respir Cell Mol Biol. 2012;47(3):340–8.

280. Goffin JM, Pittet P, Csucs G, Lussi JW, Meister JJ, Hinz B. Focal adhesion size controls tension-dependent recruitment of alpha-smooth muscle actin to stress fibers. J Cell Biol. 2006;172(2):259–68.

281. Maeda T, Sakabe T, Sunaga A, Sakai K, Rivera AL, Keene DR, et al. Conversion of mechanical force into TGF-beta-mediated biochemical signals. Curr Biol. 2011;21(11):933–41 [Research Support, N.I.H., Extramural Research Support, Non-U.S. Gov't].

282. Shi M, Zhu J, Wang R, Chen X, Mi L, Walz T, et al. Latent TGF-beta structure and activation. Nature. 2011;474(7351):343–9 [Research Support, Non-U.S. Gov't].

283. Arora PD, Narani N, McCulloch CA. The compliance of collagen gels regulates transforming growth factor-beta induction of alpha-smooth muscle actin in fibroblasts. Am J Pathol. 1999;154(3):871–82.

284. Li Z, Dranoff JA, Chan EP, Uemura M, Sevigny J, Wells RG. Transforming growth factor-beta and substrate stiffness regulate portal fibroblast activation in culture. Hepatology. 2007;46(4):1246–56 [Comparative Study Research Support, N.I.H., Extramural Research Support, Non-U.S. Gov't].

285. Marinkovic A, Mih JD, Park JA, Liu F, Tschumperlin DJ. Improved throughput traction microscopy reveals pivotal role for matrix stiffness in fibroblast contractility and TGF-beta responsiveness. Am J Physiol Lung Cell Mol Physiol. 2012;303(3):L169–80.

286. Leight JL, Wozniak MA, Chen S, Lynch ML, Chen CS. Matrix rigidity regulates a switch between TGF-beta1-induced apoptosis and epithelial-mesenchymal transition. Mol Biol Cell. 2012;23(5):781–91 [Research Support, N.I.H., Extramural Research Support, Non-U.S. Gov't Research Support, U.S. Gov't, Non-P.H.S.].

287. Balestrini JL, Chaudhry S, Sarrazy V, Koehler A, Hinz B. The mechanical memory of lung myofibroblasts. Integr Biol (Camb). 2012;4(4):410–21 [Research Support, Non-U.S. Gov't].
288. Trujillo G, Meneghin A, Flaherty KR, Sholl LM, Myers JL, Kazerooni EA, et al. TLR9 differentiates rapidly from slowly progressing forms of idiopathic pulmonary fibrosis. Sci Transl Med. 2010;2(57):57ra82 [Research Support, N.I.H., Extramural].
289. Pierce EM, Carpenter K, Jakubzick C, Kunkel SL, Flaherty KR, Martinez FJ, et al. Therapeutic targeting of CC ligand 21 or CC chemokine receptor 7 abrogates pulmonary fibrosis induced by the adoptive transfer of human pulmonary fibroblasts to immunodeficient mice. Am J Pathol. 2007;170(4):1152–64 [Research Support, N.I.H., Extramural].
290. King Jr TE, Brown KK, Raghu G, du Bois RM, Lynch DA, Martinez F, et al. BUILD-3: a randomized, controlled trial of bosentan in idiopathic pulmonary fibrosis. Am J Respir Crit Care Med. 2011;184(1):92–9 [Multicenter Study Randomized Controlled Trial Research Support, Non-U.S. Gov't].
291. Raghu G, Behr J, Brown K, Egan J, Kawut S, Flaherty, K, et al. A Placebo-Controlled Trial of Ambrisentan in Idiopathic Pulmonary Fibrosis. Am J Respir Crit Care Med. 2912;185:A:3632 [Abstract].
292. Raghu G, Brown KK, Costabel U, Cottin V, du Bois RM, Lasky JA, et al. Treatment of idiopathic pulmonary fibrosis with etanercept: an exploratory, placebo-controlled trial. Am J Respir Crit Care Med. 2008;178(9):948–55 [Clinical Trial, Phase II Multicenter Study Randomized Controlled Trial Research Support, Non-U.S. Gov't].
293. King Jr TE, Albera C, Bradford WZ, Costabel U, Hormel P, Lancaster L, et al. Effect of interferon gamma-1b on survival in patients with idiopathic pulmonary fibrosis (INSPIRE): a multicentre, randomised, placebo-controlled trial. Lancet. 2009;374(9685):222–8 [Multicenter Study Randomized Controlled Trial Research Support, Non-U.S. Gov't].
294. Daniels CE, Lasky JA, Limper AH, Mieras K, Gabor E, Schroeder DR. Imatinib treatment for idiopathic pulmonary fibrosis: randomized placebo-controlled trial results. Am J Respir Crit Care Med. 2010;181(6):604–10 [Clinical Trial, Phase II Multicenter Study Randomized Controlled Trial Research Support, Non-U.S. Gov't].
295. Maher TM. Pirfenidone in idiopathic pulmonary fibrosis. Drugs Today (Barc). 2010;46(7):473–82 [Research Support, Non-U.S. Gov't Review].
296. Azuma A, Nukiwa T, Tsuboi E, Suga M, Abe S, Nakata K, et al. Double-blind, placebo-controlled trial of pirfenidone in patients with idiopathic pulmonary fibrosis. Am J Respir Crit Care Med. 2005;171(9):1040–7 [Clinical Trial Multicenter Study Randomized Controlled Trial Research Support, Non-U.S. Gov't].
297. Noble PW, Albera C, Bradford WZ, Costabel U, Glassberg MK, Kardatzke D, et al. Pirfenidone in patients with idiopathic pulmonary fibrosis (CAPACITY): two randomised trials. Lancet. 2011;377(9779):1760–9 [Comparative Study Multicenter Study Randomized Controlled Trial Research Support, Non-U.S. Gov't].
298. Taniguchi H, Ebina M, Kondoh Y, Ogura T, Azuma A, Suga M, et al. Pirfenidone in idiopathic pulmonary fibrosis. Eur Respir J. 2010;35(4):821–9 [Clinical Trial, Phase III Multicenter Study Randomized Controlled Trial Research Support, Non-U.S. Gov't].
299. Richeldi L, Costabel U, Selman M, Kim DS, Hansell DM, Nicholson AG, et al. Efficacy of a tyrosine kinase inhibitor in idiopathic pulmonary fibrosis. N Engl J Med. 2011;365(12):1079–87 [Clinical Trial, Phase II Multicenter Study Randomized Controlled Trial Research Support, Non-U.S. Gov't].
300. Rossi GP, Seccia TM. Sildenafil in idiopathic pulmonary fibrosis. N Engl J Med. 2010;363(22):2169–70. author reply 70–1.
301. Wang Q, Usinger W, Nichols B, Gray J, Xu L, Seeley TW, et al. Cooperative interaction of CTGF and TGF-beta in animal models of fibrotic disease. Fibrogenesis Tissue Repair. 2011;4(1):4.
302. ClinicalTrials.gov. STX-100 in patients with idiopathic pulmonary fibrosis (IPF) Identifier: NCT01371305. [updated 5/9/128/28/12].
303. Demedts M, Behr J, Buhl R, Costabel U, Dekhuijzen R, Jansen HM, et al. High-dose acetylcysteine in idiopathic pulmonary fibrosis. N Engl J Med. 2005;353(21):2229–42 [Multicenter Study Randomized Controlled Trial Research Support, Non-U.S. Gov't].

304. Zisman DA, Schwarz M, Anstrom KJ, Collard HR, Flaherty KR, Hunninghake GW. A controlled trial of sildenafil in advanced idiopathic pulmonary fibrosis. N Engl J Med. 2010;363(7):620–8 [Multicenter Study Randomized Controlled Trial Research Support, N.I.H., Extramural Research Support, Non-U.S. Gov't].

305. Rajkumar R, Konishi K, Richards TJ, Ishizawar DC, Wiechert AC, Kaminski N, et al. Genomewide RNA expression profiling in lung identifies distinct signatures in idiopathic pulmonary arterial hypertension and secondary pulmonary hypertension. Am J Physiol Heart Circ Physiol. 2010;298(4):H1235–48 [Research Support, N.I.H., Extramural Research Support, Non-U.S. Gov't].

306. Rosas IO, Richards TJ, Konishi K, Zhang Y, Gibson K, Lokshin AE, et al. MMP1 and MMP7 as potential peripheral blood biomarkers in idiopathic pulmonary fibrosis. PLoS Med. 2008;5(4):e93 [Research Support, N.I.H., Extramural Research Support, N.I.H., Intramural Research Support, Non-U.S. Gov't].

307. Chadalavada RS, Korkola JE, Houldsworth J, Olshen AB, Bosl GJ, Studer L, et al. Constitutive gene expression predisposes morphogen-mediated cell fate responses of NT2/D1 and 27X-1 human embryonal carcinoma cells. Stem Cells. 2007;25(3):771–8 [Research Support, N.I.H., Extramural Research Support, Non-U.S. Gov't].

308. Selman M, Carrillo G, Estrada A, Mejia M, Becerril C, Cisneros J, et al. Accelerated variant of idiopathic pulmonary fibrosis: clinical behavior and gene expression pattern. PLoS One. 2007;2(5):e482 [Research Support, N.I.H., Extramural Research Support, Non-U.S. Gov't].

309. Boon K, Bailey NW, Yang J, Steel MP, Groshong S, Kervitsky D, et al. Molecular phenotypes distinguish patients with relatively stable from progressive idiopathic pulmonary fibrosis (IPF). PLoS One. 2009;4(4):e5134.

310. Konishi K, Gibson KF, Lindell KO, Richards TJ, Zhang Y, Dhir R, et al. Gene expression profiles of acute exacerbations of idiopathic pulmonary fibrosis. Am J Respir Crit Care Med. 2009;180(2):167–75 [Research Support, N.I.H., Extramural Research Support, Non-U.S. Gov't].

311. Dey N, Ghosh-Choudhury N, Kasinath BS, Choudhury GG. TGFbeta-stimulated MicroRNA-21 utilizes PTEN to orchestrate AKT/mTORC1 signaling for mesangial cell hypertrophy and matrix expansion. PLoS One. 2012;7(8):e42316.

312. Jones PA, Takai D. The role of DNA methylation in mammalian epigenetics. Science. 2001;293(5532):1068–70 [Research Support, U.S. Gov't, P.H.S.].

313. Rauch TA, Zhong X, Wu X, Wang M, Kernstine KH, Wang Z, et al. High-resolution mapping of DNA hypermethylation and hypomethylation in lung cancer. Proc Natl Acad Sci USA. 2008;105(1):252–7 [Research Support, N.I.H., Extramural].

314. Rabinovich EI, Kapetanaki MG, Steinfeld I, Gibson KF, Pandit KV, Yu G, et al. Global methylation patterns in idiopathic pulmonary fibrosis. PLoS One. 2012;7(4):e33770 [Research Support, N.I.H., Extramural Research Support, Non-U.S. Gov't].

315. Coward WR, Watts K, Feghali-Bostwick CA, Jenkins G, Pang L. Repression of IP-10 by interactions between histone deacetylation and hypermethylation in idiopathic pulmonary fibrosis. Mol Cell Biol. 2010;30(12):2874–86 [Research Support, Non-U.S. Gov't].

316. Ramirez G, Hagood JS, Sanders Y, Ramirez R, Becerril C, Segura L, et al. Absence of Thy-1 results in TGF-beta induced MMP-9 expression and confers a profibrotic phenotype to human lung fibroblasts. Lab Invest. 2011;91(8):1206–18 [Research Support, N.I.H., Extramural Research Support, Non-U.S. Gov't].

317. Hu B, Gharaee-Kermani M, Wu Z, Phan SH. Epigenetic regulation of myofibroblast differentiation by DNA methylation. Am J Pathol. 2010;177(1):21–8 [Research Support, N.I.H., Extramural].

# Chapter 9
# The Genetics of Pulmonary Fibrosis

Sonye K. Danoff and Cheilonda Johnson

**Abstract** The past two decades have been marked by a dramatic increase in the knowledge of the genetics of human disease. The field of interstitial lung disease (ILD) genetics has expanded as well. Much of the early understanding of ILD genetics came from rare Mendelian disorders that were associated with premature onset of disease. Other information came from single-gene multisystem disorders in which lung disease was variably present. More recently, the major advances in ILD genetics have come from focused analysis of familial pulmonary fibrosis. These rare families with multiple members affected by ILD have provided critical new insight into the possible mechanism of sporadic as well as inherited disease. Both linkage studies and large-scale, genome-wide association studies (GWAS) have identified genetic loci implicated in susceptibility to idiopathic pulmonary fibrosis (IPF). The next two decades will surely produce not only new risk alleles but also a more extensive understanding of genetics based on patient molecular phenotyping. In addition, epigenetics remains an area of potential discovery.

**Keywords** Genetics • Pulmonary fibrosis • Interstitial lung disease • Mutations • Inherited disorders

S.K. Danoff, M.D., Ph.D. (✉)
Department of Medicine, Division of Pulmonary and Critical Care Medicine,
Johns Hopkins University School of Medicine, 1830 E. Monument Street,
Suite 500, Baltimore, MD 21205, USA
e-mail: sdanoff@jhmi.edu

C. Johnson, M.D., M.H.S.
Department of Medicine, Johns Hopkins University, Baltimore, MD, USA

K.C. Meyer and S.D. Nathan (eds.), *Idiopathic Pulmonary Fibrosis: A Comprehensive Clinical Guide*, Respiratory Medicine 9, DOI 10.1007/978-1-62703-682-5_9,
© Springer Science+Business Media New York 2014

# Overview of Inherited Forms of Pulmonary Fibrosis

As is true for most complex disorders, genetic susceptibility contributes to the development of ILD. The association of ILD with rare Mendelian-inherited disorders provided some of the first evidence for a genetic basis of ILD. This evidence was bolstered by clustering of IPF cases in families and monozygotic twin studies. This section discusses inherited forms of pulmonary fibrosis associated with known genetic mutations. Heritable lung diseases fall into two categories: those with primarily lung involvement, such as familial pulmonary fibrosis, and those with systemic/multiorgan system involvement (Table 9.1) [1]. We will focus on the latter group in the following section.

**Table 9.1** Inherited pulmonary fibrosis[a]

| Disorder | Gene(s) | Inheritance pattern | Proposed pathogenesis | Presentation |
|---|---|---|---|---|
| Birt-Hogg-Dubé syndrome | *FLCN* | AD | Loss of folliculin | Multiple cysts |
| Dyskeratosis congenita | *DKC1* *TERC* *TERT* *TINF2* | XLR AD | Telomere shortening | ILD |
| Familial hypocalciuric hypercalcemia | *CaSR* | AD | Altered calcium homeostasis | ILD |
| Familial pulmonary fibrosis | *MUC5B* *TERC* *TERT* *SFTPA2* *SFTPC* | AD | MUC5B production Telomere shortening ER stress/SP-C deficiency | ILD |
| Gaucher disease | *GBA* | AR | β(beta)-glucosidase deficiency | ILD, PAH |
| Hermansky-Pudlak syndrome | *HPS1* *HPS4* | AR | Cytoplasmic organelle defects | ILD |
| Hyper-IgE syndrome | *STAT3* | AD | Lack of TH17 | Pneumatoceles, bronchiectasis |
| Lysinuric protein intolerance | *SLC7A7* | AR | Cationic amino acid transport defects | PAP, ILD |
| Niemann-Pick disease | *SMPD1* | AR | Sphingomyelinase deficiency | ILD |
| Neurofibromatosis type I | *NF1* | AD | Loss of tumor suppressor function | ILD, bullae |
| Tuberous sclerosis/ LAM | *TSC1* *TSC2* | AD | Proliferation of LAM cells | Multiple cysts |

*AD* autosomal dominant, *AR* autosomal recessive, *XLR* X-linked recessive, *ILD* interstitial lung disease, *PAP* protein alveolar proteinosis, *PAH* pulmonary arterial hypertension
[a]Adapted from [1]

# Pulmonary Fibrosis with Systemic/Multiorgan System Involvement

## *Birt-Hogg-Dubé Syndrome*

Birt-Hogg-Dubé syndrome (BHDS) is a rare autosomal dominant disorder characterized by multiple benign skin tumors (fibrofolliculomas and trichodiscomas), pulmonary cysts, and renal neoplasms [1, 2]. BHDS is the result of a loss-of-function mutation in the gene for the tumor suppressor protein folliculin (*FLCN*) [1, 2]. The hallmark of the pulmonary presentation is bilateral mid- and lower lung zone pulmonary cysts complicated by spontaneous pneumothorax [1]. A high index of suspicion is needed to establish the diagnosis [3]. Since skin and renal tumors typically appear later in life, spontaneous pneumothoraces are often the first overt manifestation of the disease [1, 3]. BHDS should be suspected in any individual with multiple facial or truncal papules, numerous renal tumors, or a family history of spontaneous pneumothorax [1].

## *Dyskeratosis Congenita*

Dyskeratosis congenita (DC) is a rare inherited disorder of defective telomere length maintenance with significant clinical and genetic heterogeneity [4, 5]. Classically, DC is described as a triad of skin hyperpigmentation, nail dystrophy, and mucosal leukoplakia, but every organ system of the body can be affected [4, 5]. The primary cause of death is from bone marrow failure (~70–80 %), which is followed by pulmonary disease (~10–15 %) and malignancy (~10 %) [5, 6]. The pulmonary involvement is typically a rapidly progressive interstitial fibrosis with restrictive physiology [6].

Telomeres are specialized structures at the end of chromosomes [7, 8]. The enzyme telomerase catalyzes the addition of repetitive DNA sequences to telomeres, which counteracts the progressive shortening of the chromosome with each cell division [7, 9]. The most common form of DC is due to an X-linked recessive mutation in *DKC1* that encodes the protein dyskerin [4]. Dyskerin binds to telomerase RNA, TERC, and is an important component of the RNA complex needed for telomerase assembly and translocation to telomeres [4]. Through unclear mechanisms, those with dyskerin mutations have insufficient TERC levels and reduced telomerase activity [4]. This lack of telomerase activity reduces stem cell proliferation capacity over time; this is supported by the fact that DC worsens with age and that the most severely affected tissues are those that require constant stem cell renewal [4].

Heterozygous mutations in three genes (*TERC, TERT,* and *TINF2*) have been recognized in the autosomal dominant forms of DC [5]. Telomerase reverse transcriptase enzyme, TERT, is another core component of telomerase. TERC contains the template that TERT uses to add TTAGGG repeats to telomeres [4]. Mutations in *TERC* and *TERT,* in addition to causing autosomal dominant DC, have been linked to familial pulmonary fibrosis cases [7, 10]. Generally, DC related to *TERC* mutations tends to be milder than the X-linked disease [4]. Families with *TERC* mutations also demonstrate genetic anticipation with subsequent generations developing more severe disease at younger ages [4]. *TERT* mutations tend to have lower penetrance and, therefore, result in milder and more heterogeneous DC than *TERC* mutations [4].

Mutations in the TIN2 gene, *TINF2*, a component of the shelterin complex, are also a cause of autosomal dominant DC. Shelterin proteins determine the structure of the telomere terminus and cap the telomere, which prevents cellular DNA repair mechanisms from mistaking the telomere as double-stranded DNA breaks [5, 11]. Absent shelterin activity results in short telomeres and triggers a sequence of activities that leads to apoptosis [11]. Autosomal recessive forms of DC have been described but are not associated with pulmonary involvement [5, 6].

## Familial Hypocalciuric Hypercalcemia

Familial hypocalciuric hypercalcemia (FHH) is an autosomal dominant disorder with asymptomatic hypercalcemia, mild hypomagnesemia, and low urinary calcium excretion [12, 13]. It is caused by a heterozygous mutation in the extracellular calcium-sensing receptor gene (*CaSR*) found on chromosome 3 that results in altered calcium metabolism [13]. FHH is generally an asymptomatic condition but can be associated with pulmonary fibrosis and recurrent respiratory tract infections [12–14].

## Familial Pulmonary Fibrosis

Familial pulmonary fibrosis (FPF) is defined by the presence of confirmed pulmonary fibrosis in at least two first-degree relatives. The exact prevalence is unknown but FPF is estimated to represent only 0.5–3.7 % of IPF cases [15]. The clinical presentation of FPF is identical to sporadic IPF, except the age of onset is typically earlier [6]. FPF is discussed in more detail in section "Genes Implicated in Familial Pulmonary Fibrosis."

## Gaucher Disease

Gaucher disease (GD) is an autosomal recessive lysosomal storage disease that causes glucosylceramide accumulation from β-glucosidase deficiency [16].

β-Glucosidase deficiency is the result of a mutation in *GBA,* the only gene known to be associated with GD [16]. The prevalence is highest among Ashkenazi Jews, but GD can be found with all ethnic backgrounds [16]. GD patients present with a large variety of symptoms that typically include hepatosplenomegaly, anemia, thrombocytopenia, and long bone erosions. Three major clinical types of GD have been described [16, 17]. Type 1 GD is rarely complicated by pulmonary hypertension or hepatopulmonary syndrome (HPS) [17]. Type 2 GD causes alveolar consolidation from accumulated Gaucher cells [17]. Type 3 GD can cause either alveolar or interstitial Gaucher cell accumulation associated with pulmonary fibrosis [17].

## Hermansky-Pudlak Syndrome

Hermansky-Pudlak syndrome (HPS) is a rare, autosomal recessive disorder characterized by a triad of oculocutaneous albinism, storage pool deficiency, and lysosomal ceroid accumulation [12, 18]. The majority of cases arise in Northwest Puerto Rico due to founder effect, but affected individuals are found worldwide [12, 18]. Seven subtypes have been described (HPS-1–7), but only HPS-1 and HPS-4 are associated with pulmonary fibrosis [18, 19]. HPS-1 and HPS-4 are caused by mutations in the genes *HPS-1* and *HPS-4*, respectively [12, 18]. Pulmonary fibrosis develops early (second to third decade) and usually results in death by the fourth to fifth decade of life [12]. HPS has a similar radiographic, physiological, and clinical picture to IPF.

## Hyper-Immunoglobulin E Syndrome

Hyper-immunoglobulin E (hyper-IgE) syndrome (HEIS) is a rare primary immune deficiency disorder characterized by elevated IgE levels, eczema, and recurrent staphylococcal skin and lung infections [1, 20]. Nearly all (95 %) patients have a mutation in the signal transducer and activator of transcription 3 (*STAT3*) gene that is primarily sporadic, but autosomal dominant transmission in families has also been described [1]. Affected individuals have impaired interleukin-17-producing T-helper cell (TH17) function, which results in impaired cellular immunity [20]. Pulmonary involvement (Table 9.2) includes pneumatoceles and bronchiectasis from recurrent pneumonia [1]. A National Institute of Health (NIH) diagnostic scoring system based on characteristic features has been established [1, 20, 21] and will likely be modified to include *STAT3* mutation genetic testing in the future [20].

## Lysinuric Protein Intolerance

Lysinuric protein intolerance (LPI) is an autosomal recessive multisystem disorder of cationic amino acid (lysine, arginine, and ornithine) transport [1, 22]. Mutations

**Table 9.2** Hyper-IgE syndrome scoring system features

| Immunologic features | Nonimmune features |
|---|---|
| Elevated IgE | Retained primary teeth |
| Eosinophilia | Scoliosis |
| Decreased TH17 cells | Joint hyperextensibility |
| Recurrent infections | Bone fractures following minimal trauma |
| Eczema | Characteristic facial features |
| Candidiasis | Vascular abnormalities |

*TH17* interleukin-17-producing T-helper cells

in the y+ LAT1 protein gene, *SLC7A7*, are associated with the condition [22]. Pulmonary involvement is varied including life-threatening respiratory failure due to endogenous lipid pneumonia, mild asymptomatic ILD, or pulmonary alveolar proteinosis [1, 22].

## Niemann-Pick Disease

Niemann-Pick disease (NPD) is an autosomal recessive neurovisceral lipid storage disease where sphingomyelin accumulates in cells due to sphingomyelinase deficiency [23]. Six variants, A–F, of NPD have been described; pulmonary fibrosis is a rare manifestation of types B and C [12, 24]. The age of onset and clinical presentation of pulmonary disease in NPD is highly variable [24]. Radiographic features include diffuse nodular infiltrates at the lung bases with honeycombing [24].

## Neurofibromatosis Type I

Neurofibromatosis type I (NF1) is an autosomal dominant condition characterized by café au lait spots, neurofibromas, axillary and groin freckling, optic gliomas, melanotic iris hamartomas, and bony dysplasia [25, 26]. NF1 is due to a mutation in the tumor suppressor protein neurofibromin gene, *NF1,* on chromosome 17 [12, 26]. Approximately 7–25 % of patients with NF1 develop pulmonary manifestations that include pulmonary fibrosis, cystic lung disease, chest wall abnormalities, thoracic neural tumors, and pulmonary hypertension [25, 26].

## Tuberous Sclerosis/Lymphangioleiomyomatosis

Tuberous sclerosis is an autosomal dominant multisystem disorder characterized by the development of benign tumors (hamartomas) and malformations (hamartias) that can involve the brain, skin, kidneys, and lungs [1, 12, 27]. Affected individuals have mutations in the tumor suppressor genes harmatin (*TSC1*) or tuberin (*TSC2*) [12, 28]. Patients with pulmonary involvement generally present with spontaneous pneumothorax, chest pain, hemoptysis, or exertional dyspnea [27]. The most common radiographic findings are diffuse pulmonary fibrosis with honeycombing [27]. Histopathologic examination of the lungs reveals multiple subpleural cysts [27].

Lymphangioleiomyomatosis (LAM) is rare disease found exclusively in women. LAM can occur in isolation as a spontaneous non-germline somatic mutation in *TSC2* or as a component of the tuberous sclerosis complex (TSC) [1, 28]. It is caused by the proliferation of smooth muscle-like cells in the small airways, vasculature, or lymphatic structures [1]. LAM cell proliferation results in airway narrowing, air trapping, and the formation of cystic lung lesions or lymphangioleiomyomas [28]. The ILD of LAM is indistinguishable from that of tuberous sclerosis [1]. Patient radiographs show numerous thin-walled cysts. As in tuberous sclerosis, pneumothorax is common, occurring in up to 80 % of the affected individuals [1, 28].

## Genes Implicated in Familial Pulmonary Fibrosis

The genetics of familial pulmonary fibrosis (FPF) is heterogeneous and complex. Multiple genetic variations have been described in association with FPF, but each individually only confers moderate overall risk [7, 15, 29–39]. Additionally, not all families display the same mutation, and within families not all persons with the same mutation develop pulmonary fibrosis or the same phenotype [29, 34, 37, 40]. This suggests that FPF is the result of multiple genetic, host, and environmental risk factors.

### *Mucin 5B*

Previously, large-scale linkage analyses have failed to show genetic linkage across multiple families [40]. This paradigm shifted after a genome-wide linkage scan detected linkage between pulmonary fibrosis and a single-nucleotide polymorphism (SNP) on chromosome 11 in over 80 families [33]. The *MUC5B* variant (rs35705950) T allele was found to be present in approximately 34 % of FPF subjects compared to 9 % of healthy controls [33, 38]. *MUC5B* is a gel-forming mucin gene expressed by bronchial epithelial cells that is expressed in higher levels among patients with FPF and sporadic IPF and unaffected subjects who express the *MUC5B* minor allele [33, 38]. The relationship between *MUC5B* expression and the pathogenesis of pulmonary fibrosis remains unknown [33, 38].

## Telomerase

Mutations in the genes encoding core telomerase components, *TERT* and *TERC*, can result in progressive telomere length shortening [7, 10]. Unlike the X-linked form of ILD seen in patients with DC related to a mutation in the dyskerin component of telomerase, autosomal dominant forms of FPF without features of DC are seen with mutations in the *TERT* and *TERC* [7, 40]. TERC mutations are rare, while heterozygous TERT mutations are found in approximately 18 % of FPF and 3 % of sporadic IPF cases [10]. Pulmonary fibrosis as the result of telomerase mutations is discussed in more detail in section "Links to Aging."

## Genetic Disorders of Surfactant Proteins

Mutations in the genes encoding surfactant proteins A2, C, and the ATP-binding cassette transporter have been described in association with familial and sporadic pulmonary fibrosis. ILD as the result of genetic disorders of surfactant proteins is discussed in more detail in section "Other Associations."

## Links to Aging

IPF has long been recognized as a disease of aging with the median age at diagnosis being 66 years old [41]. Prevalence studies of IPF have demonstrated a strong age dependence in the development of disease, and a study using a large US insurance database and strictly defined criteria for the diagnosis of IPF showed an increased incidence and prevalence of IPF in each decade of life, with a peak prevalence of 87.9 per 100,000 individuals of age 75+ for men and 48.4 per 100,000 in women [42]. One potential mechanism for the relationship between aging and IPF has emerged from genetic studies of familial IPF in which individuals in affected families present at significantly earlier ages. Independent studies by Armanios [7] and Garcia [43] identified mutations in the telomerase genes, TERT and TERC, in a subset of pedigrees with FPF. The consequence of these mutations is premature telomere shortening. Telomere length is known to decline with age, and the effect of telomere shortening is accelerated cellular aging. As decreasing telomere length reaches a critical level, cellular apoptosis occurs. Hence, telomere length functions as a cellular aging clock that regulates and times cell death, but the exact mechanism leading to pulmonary fibrosis is not known. However, one potential mechanism is that when type I alveolar epithelial cells die, they are initially replaced by division of type II cells. However, this reservoir of type II epithelial cells can ultimately be depleted, and subsequent epithelial loss must be resolved by the influx of fibroblasts.

Other data supporting the link between IPF susceptibility and telomere length come from several studies that evaluated telomere length independent of genetic mutations in the telomere genes. These studies showed shortened telomeres (below the first percentile for age) in patients with sporadic IPF [44, 45]. Interestingly, mouse studies indicate that telomere length is heritable but independent of telomere gene sequence [46]. Thus, the term "short telomere syndrome" has been coined to encompass the disease entity associated with premature telomere shortening [46]. While other features of aging including environmental and occupational exposures may contribute to the age association in IPF, telomere length-associated cellular apoptosis provides a cogent mechanism linking aging to the development of fibrosis.

## Other Associations

### Genetic Disorders of Surfactant Proteins

Surfactant is crucial for reducing alveolar surface tension and preventing end-expiratory atelectasis. Surfactant proteins are synthesized exclusively by type II alveolar epithelial cells (type II AECs). Surfactant metabolism dysfunction is associated with a variety of pulmonary manifestations including neonatal respiratory failure and pulmonary alveolar proteinosis [1]. Inherited and de novo mutations of surfactant-associated protein genes are also associated with the development of pulmonary fibrosis in children and adults (Table 9.3) [15, 32, 34, 37, 47].

**Table 9.3** Surfactant-associated protein mutations and pulmonary fibrosis[a]

| Protein | Gene | Mutation(s)[b] | Inheritance pattern | Proposed pathogenesis | Presentation |
|---------|------|----------------|---------------------|------------------------|--------------|
| SP-A2 | SFTPA2 | G231V F198S | AD | ER stress | FPF, lung cancer |
| SP-C | SFTPC | I73T c.435+1G>A L188Q | AD, sporadic | SP-C deficiency/ER stress | FPF, IPF |
| ABCA3 | ABCA3 | E292V | AR | Defective phospho-lipid transport | PAP, ILD |

SP-A2 surfactant protein A2, SP-C surfactant protein C, ABCA3 ATP-binding cassette protein A3, AD autosomal dominant, AR autosomal recessive, ER endoplasmic reticulum
[a]Adapted from [1]
[b]Only the most common listed

## Surfactant Protein A2

Surfactant protein A2 (SP-A2) is a hydrophilic protein that plays a primary role in the innate cellular immunity of the lung [31]. Two mutations in the SP-A2 gene, *SFTPA2*, have been identified in two unrelated families with pulmonary fibrosis [37]. The first results in a transposition of glycine to valine at position 231 (G231V); the second is a substitution of phenylalanine to serine at position 198 (F198S) [6, 37]. Both mutations result in a SP-A2 protein that is retained in the endoplasmic reticulum (ER) resulting in reduced protein stability and increased ER stress [15, 31, 37, 40]. This ER stress results in type II alveolar epithelial cell injury and eventually apoptosis [47].

## Surfactant Protein C

Surfactant protein C, SP-C, is a hydrophobic protein encoded by a single gene on chromosome 8, *SFTPC* [30]. Unlike SP-A2, which plays a role in host defense, SP-C contributes to the surface tension-lowering activity of surfactant [47, 48]. Over 35 SP-C gene sequence variations have been identified (see Table 9.3) [15, 47]. The most common mutation, substitution of threonine (T) for isoleucine (I) on codon 73 (I73T), is present in 25 % of the SP-C-associated cases [47]. *SFTPC* mutations show an autosomal dominant inheritance pattern with variable penetrance or can arise de novo in sporadic IPF cases [15, 30]. Overall, *SFTPC* mutations are rare, appearing in less than 1 % of patients with pulmonary fibrosis [15, 30].

The phenotype associated with SFTPC mutations is highly variable. The age of onset ranges from infancy to late adulthood, and histopathologic patterns include NSIP and UIP [30]. This histologic variability is also exhibited within families carrying the same mutation [47]. The mechanism of this variability is unknown but, once again, suggests host and environmental modifiers [48, 49].

Two mechanisms of lung injury related to SFTPC mutation have been described. The first is related to expression and/or mistrafficking of abnormal SP-C [48]. Similar to SFTPA2 mutations, this results in endoplasmic stress on type II alveolar epithelial cells and ultimately leads to cell injury and death [6]. The second is related to SP-C deficiency. Patients with certain SFTPC mutations lack mature SP-C in the lung tissue and bronchoalveolar lavage (BAL) fluid [18]. Absent or deficient SP-C could result in lung injury from mechanical injury due to unopposed shear forces [18].

## Adenosine Triphosphate-Binding Cassette Transporter A3

Adenosine triphosphate (ATP)-binding cassette transporter A3 (*ABCA3*) mutations alter the translocation of phospholipids into lamellar bodies during the production of surfactant in type II AEC [1]. The disorder is inherited in an autosomal recessive pattern with over 100 distinct mutations identified to date [1]. Disease phenotype is highly variable and ranges from neonatal respiratory failure and death to chronic mild ILD [1].

## Variability of ILD Manifestations in Family Studies

### Telomerase Families with Variable Disease Manifestations

The description of multiple pedigrees with mutations in the telomerase genes, TERT and TERC, provides evidence that even patients with the same mutation may display differing lung involvement that ranges from seemingly normal to classic IPF [7]. A recent study documented histopathology from open lung biopsies on patients with telomerase mutations and showed nonspecific fibrosis and discordant pathology in 33 % of mutation carriers [45].

### Familial Clusterings of Non-UIP and Mixed Pathology

Familial clusterings of fatal desquamative interstitial pneumonia (DIP) in infants have been reported by a number of groups [50, 51]. Some of these early-onset DIP patients have been shown to have mutations in the SPC gene [32]. A number of unique family mutations in SPC have been described that associate with early-onset ILD. Interestingly, individuals in one family cohort with a unique SPC mutation that was characterized as a leu188-to-gln (L188Q) substitution in a highly conserved region of the C-terminal domain displayed UIP in adults and cellular NSIP in children, suggesting that a single genetic variant may result in a different pathology over time [34].

## New Directions

The findings in ILD genetics to date represent only the beginning of what is sure to be a rapidly developing resource for clinicians seeking to provide earlier diagnosis and improved approaches to ILD therapy. Many questions remain including whether there are common genetic variants that contribute risk in diverse forms of ILD such as medication-associated, autoimmune and hypersensitivity pneumonitis. Can disease be limited through by treating patients with known ILD genetic risk factors prior to the onset of symptoms? Also, what can be learned about common mechanisms of lung injury from rare Mendelian forms of ILD?

Thus, the strategies for discovery moving forward will include the combination of studies of unique families with FPF as well as more broad evaluation of unrelated patients with similar forms of ILD using genome-wide association studies. A feature that will inform further success in GWAS studies is the enhanced phenotyping that genomics and proteomic evaluations can add to clinical, radiologic, and pathologic evaluations. In addition, the large patient populations required for such studies will necessitate multi-institution and multinational cooperation for the assembly and characterization of patient samples.

One additional area for exploration is the epigenetics of disease risk. A recent study has implicated a micro-RNA processing defect in rapidly progressive IPF [52]. Although not classically considered epigenetics, telomere length has also been strongly associated with IPF risk. Thus, even with the potential insights of classic genetics, further exploration is required to fully understand the genetics of ILD susceptibility. The goal of all of these investigations is to ultimately develop approaches that facilitate presymptomatic diagnosis and the identification of "prophylactic" agents to prevent overt disease development as well as to better match diagnosis to therapeutic agent. The potential benefits to patients of these advances cannot be overstated.

# References

1. Devine MS, Garcia CK. Genetic interstitial lung disease. Clin Chest Med. 2012;33(1):95–110.
2. Tomassetti S, Carloni A, Chilosi M, Maffè A, Ungari S, Sverzellati N, et al. Pulmonary features of Birt-Hogg-Dube syndrome: cystic lesions and pulmonary histiocytoma. Respir Med. 2011;105(5):768–74.
3. Furuya M, Tanaka R, Koga S, Yatabe Y, Gotoda H, Takagi S, et al. Pulmonary cysts of Birt-Hogg-Dube syndrome: a clinicopathologic and immunohistochemical study of 9 families. Am J Surg Pathol. 2012;36(4):589–600.
4. Mason PJ, Bessler M. The genetics of dyskeratosis congenita. Cancer Genet. 2011;204(12):635–45.
5. Dokal I. Dyskeratosis congenita. Hematology Am Soc Hematol Educ Program. 2011;2011: 480–6.
6. Garcia CK. Idiopathic pulmonary fibrosis: update on genetic discoveries. Proc Am Thorac Soc. 2011;8(2):158–62.
7. Armanios MY, Chen JJ, Cogan JD, Alder JK, Ingersoll RG, Markin C, et al. Telomerase mutations in families with idiopathic pulmonary fibrosis. N Engl J Med. 2007;356(13):1317–26.
8. Moyzis RK, Buckingham JM, Cram LS, Dani M, Deaven LL, Jones MD, et al. A highly conserved repetitive DNA sequence, (TTAGGG)n, present at the telomeres of human chromosomes. Proc Natl Acad Sci USA. 1988;85(18):6622–6.
9. Morin GB. The human telomere terminal transferase enzyme is a ribonucleoprotein that synthesizes TTAGGG repeats. Cell. 1989;59(3):521–9.
10. Diaz de Leon A, Cronkhite JT, Yilmaz C, Brewington C, Wang R, Xing C, et al. Subclinical lung disease, macrocytosis, and premature graying in kindreds with telomerase (TERT) mutations. Chest. 2011;140(3):753–63.
11. Calado RT, Young NS. Telomere diseases. N Engl J Med. 2009;361(24):2353–65.
12. Wurfel MM, Raghu G. Genetics of pulmonary fibrosis. Semin Respir Crit Care Med. 2002;23(2):177–87.

13. Ward BK, Magno AL, Walsh JP, Ratajczak T. The role of the calcium-sensing receptor in human disease. Clin Biochem. 2012;45(12):943–53.
14. Demedts M, Lissens W, Wuyts W, Matthijs G, Thomeer M, Bouillon R. A new missense mutation in the CASR gene in familial interstitial lung disease with hypocalciuric hypercalcemia and defective granulocyte function. Am J Respir Crit Care Med. 2008;177(5):558–9.
15. Lawson WE, Grant SW, Ambrosini V, Womble KE, Dawson EP, Lane KB, et al. Genetic mutations in surfactant protein C are a rare cause of sporadic cases of IPF. Thorax. 2004;59(11): 977–80.
16. Pastores GM, Hughes DA. Gaucher disease. In: Pagon RA, Bird TD, Dolan CR, Stephens K, Adam MP, editors. GeneReviews. Seattle, WA: University of Washington; 1993.
17. Lo SM, Liu J, Chen F, Pastores GM, Knowles J, Boxer M, et al. Pulmonary vascular disease in Gaucher disease: clinical spectrum, determinants of phenotype and long-term outcomes of therapy. J Inherit Metab Dis. 2011;34(3):643–50.
18. Grutters JC, du Bois RM. Genetics of fibrosing lung diseases. Eur Respir J. 2005;25(5): 915–27.
19. Pierson DM, Ionescu D, Qing G, Yonan AM, Parkinson K, Colby TC, et al. Pulmonary fibrosis in hermansky-pudlak syndrome. A case report and review. Respiration. 2006;73(3):382–95.
20. Woellner C, Gertz EM, Schaffer AA, Lagos M, Perro M, Glocker EO, et al. Mutations in STAT3 and diagnostic guidelines for hyper-IgE syndrome. J Allergy Clin Immunol. 2010;125(2):424–32.e8.
21. Grimbacher B, Schaffer AA, Holland SM, Davis J, Gallin JI, Malech HL, et al. Genetic linkage of hyper-IgE syndrome to chromosome 4. Am J Hum Genet. 1999;65(3):735–44.
22. Ogier de Baulny H, Schiff M, Dionisi-Vici C. Lysinuric protein intolerance (LPI): a multi organ disease by far more complex than a classic urea cycle disorder. Mol Genet Metab. 2012;106(1):12–7.
23. Palmeri S, Tarugi P, Sicurelli F, Buccoliero R, Malandrini A, De Santi MM, et al. Lung involvement in Niemann-Pick disease type C1: improvement with bronchoalveolar lavage. Neurol Sci. 2005;26(3):171–3.
24. Minai OA, Sullivan EJ, Stoller JK. Pulmonary involvement in Niemann-Pick disease: case report and literature review. Respir Med. 2000;94(12):1241–51.
25. Katsenos S, Nikolopoulou M, Rallis E, Constantopoulos SH. Chronic eosinophilic pneumonia associated with neurofibromatosis type 1: an unusual complication. J Med Invest. 2009;56(1–2):64–9.
26. Hirsch NP, Murphy A, Radcliffe JJ. Neurofibromatosis: clinical presentations and anaesthetic implications. Br J Anaesth. 2001;86(4):555–64.
27. Malik SK, Pardee N, Martin CJ. Involvement of the lungs in tuberous sclerosis. Chest. 1970;58(5):538–40.
28. Hohman DW, Noghrehkar D, Ratnayake S. Lymphangioleiomyomatosis: a review. Eur J Intern Med. 2008;19(5):319–24.
29. Chibbar R, Shih F, Baga M, Torlakovic E, Ramlall K, Skomro R, et al. Nonspecific interstitial pneumonia and usual interstitial pneumonia with mutation in surfactant protein C in familial pulmonary fibrosis. Mod Pathol. 2004;17(8):973–80.
30. Guillot L, Epaud R, Thouvenin G, Jonard L, Mohsni A, Couderc R, et al. New surfactant protein C gene mutations associated with diffuse lung disease. J Med Genet. 2009;46(7):490–4.
31. Maitra M, Wang Y, Gerard RD, Mendelson CR, Garcia CK. Surfactant protein A2 mutations associated with pulmonary fibrosis lead to protein instability and endoplasmic reticulum stress. J Biol Chem. 2010;285(29):22103–13.
32. Nogee LM, Dunbar 3rd AE, Wert SE, Askin F, Hamvas A, Whitsett JA. A mutation in the surfactant protein C gene associated with familial interstitial lung disease. N Engl J Med. 2001;344(8):573–9.
33. Seibold MA, Wise AL, Speer MC, Brown KK, Loyd JE, et al. A common MUC5B promoter polymorphism and pulmonary fibrosis. N Engl J Med. 2011;364(16):1503–12.
34. Thomas AQ, Lane K, Phillips 3rd J, et al. Heterozygosity for a surfactant protein C gene mutation associated with usual interstitial pneumonitis and cellular nonspecific interstitial pneumonitis in one kindred. Am J Respir Crit Care Med. 2002;165(9):1322–8.

35. van Moorsel CH, van Oosterhout MF, Barlo NP, de Jong PA, van der Vis JJ, Ruven HJ, et al. Surfactant protein C mutations are the basis of a significant portion of adult familial pulmonary fibrosis in a dutch cohort. Am J Respir Crit Care Med. 2010;182(11):1419–25.
36. Verleden GM, du Bois RM, Bouros D, Drent M, Millar A, Müller-Quernheim J, et al. Genetic predisposition and pathogenetic mechanisms of interstitial lung diseases of unknown origin. Eur Respir J Suppl. 2001;32:17s–29.
37. Wang Y, Kuan PJ, Xing C, Cronkhite JT, Torres F, Rosenblatt RL, et al. Genetic defects in surfactant protein A2 are associated with pulmonary fibrosis and lung cancer. Am J Hum Genet. 2009;84(1):52–9.
38. Zhang Y, Noth I, Garcia JG, Kaminski N. A variant in the promoter of MUC5B and idiopathic pulmonary fibrosis. N Engl J Med. 2011;364(16):1576–7.
39. Ono S, Tanaka T, Ishida M, Kinoshita A, Fukuoka J, Takaki M, et al. Surfactant protein C G100S mutation causes familial pulmonary fibrosis in Japanese kindred. Eur Respir J. 2011;38(4):861–9.
40. Lawson WE, Loyd JE, Degryse AL. Genetics in pulmonary fibrosis–familial cases provide clues to the pathogenesis of idiopathic pulmonary fibrosis. Am J Med Sci. 2011;341(6):439–43.
41. King Jr TE, Pardo A, Selman M. Idiopathic pulmonary fibrosis. Lancet. 2011;378(9807):1949–61.
42. Raghu G, Weycker D, Edelsberg J, Bradford WZ, Oster G. Incidence and prevalence of idiopathic pulmonary fibrosis. Am J Respir Crit Care Med. 2006;174(7):810–6.
43. Tsakiri KD, Cronkhite JT, Kuan PJ, Xing C, Raghu G, Weissler JC, et al. Adult-onset pulmonary fibrosis caused by mutations in telomerase. Proc Natl Acad Sci USA. 2007;104(18):7552–7.
44. Alder JK, Chen JJ, Lancaster L, Danoff S, Su SC, Cogan JD, et al. Short telomeres are a risk factor for idiopathic pulmonary fibrosis. Proc Natl Acad Sci USA. 2008;105(35):13051–6.
45. Cronkhite JT, Xing C, Raghu G, Chin KM, Torres F, Rosenblatt RL, et al. Telomere shortening in familial and sporadic pulmonary fibrosis. Am J Respir Crit Care Med. 2008;178(7):729–37.
46. Armanios M, Alder JK, Parry EM, Karim B, Strong MA, Greider CW. Short telomeres are sufficient to cause the degenerative defects associated with aging. Am J Hum Genet. 2009;85(6):823–32.
47. Hamvas A, Cole FS, Nogee LM. Genetic disorders of surfactant proteins. Neonatology. 2007;91(4):311–7.
48. Beers MF, Mulugeta S. Surfactant protein C biosynthesis and its emerging role in conformational lung disease. Annu Rev Physiol. 2005;67:663–96.
49. Bullard JE, Nogee LM. Heterozygosity for ABCA3 mutations modifies the severity of lung disease associated with a surfactant protein C gene (SFTPC) mutation. Pediatr Res. 2007;62(2):176–9.
50. Tal A, Maor E, Bar-Ziv J, Gorodischer R. Fatal desquamative interstitial pneumonia in three infants siblings. J Pediatr. 1984;104(6):873–6.
51. Tsukahara M, Yoshii H, Imamura T, Kamei T, Koga M, Furukawa S. Desquamative interstitial pneumonia in sibs. Am J Med Genet. 1995;59(4):431–4.
52. Oak SR, Murray L, Herath A, Sleeman M, Anderson I, Joshi AD, et al. A micro RNA processing defect in rapidly progressing idiopathic pulmonary fibrosis. PLoS One. 2011;6(6):e21253.

# Chapter 10
# Idiopathic Pulmonary Fibrosis Phenotypes

**Steven D. Nathan**

**Abstract** Idiopathic pulmonary fibrosis is a distinct progressive fibrotic disorder that is characterized by heterogeneity in its presentation, clinical course, pathology, and other nuanced features. This has resulted in the recognition of distinct clinical phenotypes within the rubric of this disorder. Phenotypes may be recognized based on clinical features, physiologic testing, radiographic appearance, or patients' subsequent disease course. This chapter will discuss the various IPF phenotypes and their unique distinguishing features.

**Keywords** Pulmonary fibrosis • Phenotype • Hypertension • Pulmonary • Pulmonary disease, chronic obstructive • Connective tissue diseases • Radiographic image interpretation • Computer assisted

## Introduction

In the late 1970s and early 1980s, idiopathic pulmonary fibrosis (IPF) was a wastebasket term for many forms of idiopathic lung disease that had a component of fibrosis as a hallmark of their pathologic picture. In the latter part of the last century, distinct clinico-pathologic entities were described and carved out from this broad term, ultimately culminating in the description and categorization of the idiopathic interstitial pneumonias [1]. IPF was retained as a distinct, more homogeneous clinical entity characterized by a histopathologic pattern of usual interstitial pneumonia (UIP) with its defining pathologic feature of microscopic heterogeneity. This theme of heterogeneity in IPF is not, however, confined to its pathologic fingerprint but also pertains to many other aspects of

S.D. Nathan, M.D. (✉)
Advanced Lung Disease and Lung Transplant Program, Department of Medicine,
Inova Fairfax Hospital, 3300 Gallows Road, Falls Church, VA 22042, USA
e-mail: steven.nathan@inova.org

K.C. Meyer and S.D. Nathan (eds.), *Idiopathic Pulmonary Fibrosis: A Comprehensive Clinical Guide*, Respiratory Medicine 9, DOI 10.1007/978-1-62703-682-5_10,
© Springer Science+Business Media New York 2014

the disease. The perplexing, unpredictable nature of disease progression is likely related to this clinical heterogeneity. Similarly, the mixed (or muted) signals from many of the clinical studies that have been undertaken could be related to heterogeneity in treatment response. These differences in presentation, course, and outcomes have provided a foundation for the concept of distinct IPF phenotypes.

The term phenotype has been broadly defined as the entire physical, physiologic, and biochemical makeup of an individual as determined both genetically and environmentally. The physical makeup of an individual with any disease might include features on physical examination. However, IPF patients have no unique, clinically distinctive features that characterize or influence the disease course or management, apart from digital clubbing, which has been associated with worse outcomes. In the context of IPF, the physical constituent of the disease may include not only the clinical presentation and features on physical examination but also the radiographic and histologic appearance of the disease. The appearance of the disease as assessed by high-resolution computed tomography (HRCT) may be regarded as a physical feature, and, therefore, radiographic variants might be regarded as specific disease phenotypes. In this regard, typical and atypical appearing HRCTs, the extent of the disease, the presence of traction bronchiectasis, and asymmetric disease have been reported to be associated with different outcomes or possibly distinct etiologies (in the case of asymmetric disease) [2–4] (Fig. 10.1).

The clinical course of the disease may help delineate distinct phenotypes, albeit in a reflective fashion. The disease course is likely determined by the physical characteristics of the disease and is undoubtedly influenced by the patient's genotype and, possibly, the environment. Environmental factors may be extrinsic, such as air pollution and cigarette smoking, or intrinsic, such as gastroesophageal disease and obstructive sleep apnea [5–7]. With regard to the latter, these are generally regarded as IPF comorbidities rather than distinct phenotypes.

The physiologic component of the phenotype might include characteristics of lung function studies and pulmonary hemodynamics. Pulmonary function tests (PFTs) alone do not define distinct phenotypes, but certain PFT characteristics may be associated with clinical phenotypes; for example, evidence of obstruction might be seen in association with the combined pulmonary fibrosis/emphysema phenotype. On the other hand, pulmonary hypertension (PH), a physiologic marker of compromised pulmonary vasculature, appears to be a distinct phenotype that is associated with greater functional impairment and an accelerated disease course [8–11]. Distinct phenotypes based on biochemical profiling remain to be determined and warrant further study in the context of IPF.

The definition of a phenotype also raises the further question of how much variation within each phenotype is permissible before it can or should be regarded as a separate entity. The degree to which nuanced phenotypes should be explored and differentiated ultimately depends on whether such distinctions make any substantive difference to the patient and their outcomes or to the clinician and their management of the case.

For environmental exposures or genetic modifiers to be regarded as defining distinct IPF phenotypes, they must be associated with distinct manifestations or

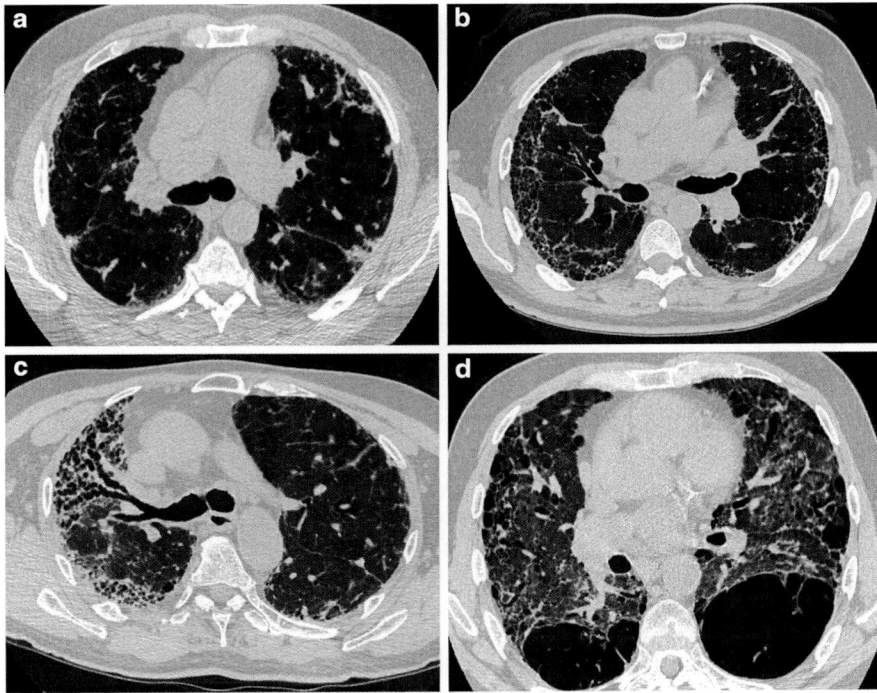

**Fig. 10.1** Radiographic phenotypes (**a**) HRCT demonstrating subpleural patchy infiltrates, but no distinct honeycombing. This appearance represents a possible UIP pattern. (**b**) HRCT that is typical for IPF with extensive subpleural reticulation and honeycombing. (**c**) Asymmetric IPF with right-sided predominance. (**d**) Combined pulmonary fibrosis/emphysema with diffuse fibrotic changes and extensive bullous disease (posterior)

constellations of features. Therefore, familial IPF would qualify as a distinct phenotype, because there are unique characteristics of its presentation and course [12]. However, IPF patients with an environmental exposure history, such as cigarette smoke and extraneous environmental ambient pollution, do not have distinctive clinical features and, therefore, would not be defined as a specific disease phenotype. On the other hand, cigarette smoking may predispose patients to combined IPF/COPD, which does indeed appear to be a distinct clinical phenotype [13–17]. A schematic of the various phenotypes and their overlap is shown in Fig. 10.2.

## Familial IPF

There is wide variation in the percentage of IPF patients who are believed to have the familial variant that is recognized when two or more individuals from the same family have pulmonary fibrosis consistent with an idiopathic interstitial pneumonia

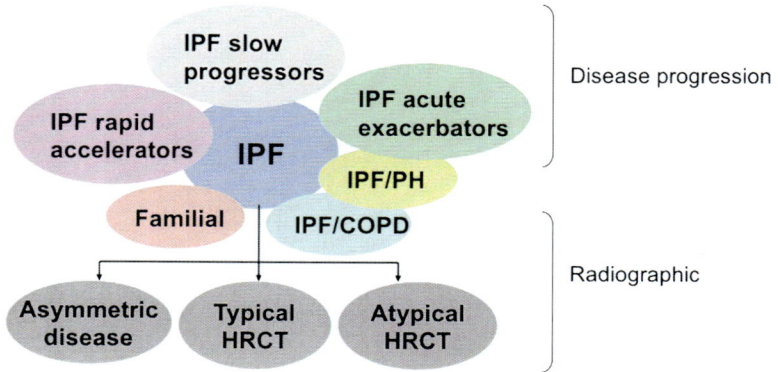

**Fig. 10.2** Diagrammatic representation of the various IPF phenotypes and their overlap

(IIP) [18]. Familial IPF is covered in more detail in a dedicated chapter. Whether this patient subgroup has a disease course that is sufficiently different to be regarded as a distinct phenotype is uncertain. However, what is known is that those with a familial predisposition can develop not only IPF but other forms of IIP, which suggests that genetic mutations predispose patients to a number of IIP pathologies other than UIP.

A number of genetic mutations have been shown to predispose to IPF. These include telomerase mutations, surfactant protein C, surfactant protein A2, and ELMOD2 [18]. Patients with familial IPF, including those with telomerase mutations, tend to be diagnosed and die at an earlier age. However, their clinical presentation and disease course appear similar to that of sporadic IPF patients with a mean life expectancy after diagnosis of 2.4–3 years [12, 19].

## IPF Combined with COPD

It has been recognized for about two decades that IPF can occur in combination with emphysema [13, 14]. However, with the advent of HRCT, there is a growing appreciation of this as a distinct clinical entity [15–17]. It has been described as occurring in 28 % of patients with IPF [16]. It is not surprising given the high prevalence of prior cigarette smoking among IPF patients that the most common of the obstructive and interstitial diseases should, on occasion, occur together.

Combined IPF/emphysema (CPFE) is diagnosed with HRCT by the presence of fibrotic changes seen in conjunction with emphysematous changes, which can manifest as overt bullous disease in ~50 % of cases, or with more subtle but distinct areas of decreased attenuation and a paucity of vascular markings [15] (see Fig. 10.1). The emphysematous component tends to be more upper lung zone in its distribution with both panacinar and paraseptal emphysema being described [15]. The fibrotic changes retain their predilection for the lower lobes, and typical IPF findings are commonly seen that include reticular changes, honeycombing, and traction bronchiectasis. Although the emphysema and fibrotic changes have a predilection to occur in different areas of the lung, the two processes frequently may be found adjacent to one another [16]. Subtle ground-glass attenuation has also been described in two-thirds of patients, which may suggest the additional presence of smoking-related ILD such as respiratory bronchiolitis-associated ILD or desquamative interstitial pneumonia [15].

As opposed to IPF, in which the prevalence of prior or current cigarette smoking is seen ~70 % of cases, in combined IPF/emphysema (CPFE), almost all patients have a history of cigarette smoking with a greater pack-year exposure [15, 16]. Additionally, there appears to be a greater male predominance of this specific phenotype. In one series of patients in whom previous radiographic studies were available, the evidence of emphysema was noted prior to the appearance of fibrotic changes in 32 %; however, the fibrosis predated the emphysema in 6 %, and the two entities were diagnosed concomitantly in 62 % of the cases [15]. Although the two entities might be pathophysiologically distinct, the observation that the fibrosis can occur prior to the emphysematous changes in a small subset of patients raises the possibility that in some cases, the fibrosis may influence the subsequent development of emphysema. Conceivably, this might occur through mechanical traction or other mechanisms such as the release of cytokines, including tumor necrosis factor-α (alpha) and platelet-derived growth factor [20]. Additional shared pathogenic processes include apoptosis of alveolar epithelial cells, increased oxidative stress, and abnormalities of telomerase activity [19].

There are no distinctive clinical features of CPFE, and patients present with a similar constellation of symptoms and physical findings to others with IPF. A clue to the presence of CPFE can frequently be found in patients' pulmonary function tests. Due to the counterbalancing effects of coexistent restrictive and obstructive processes, the two opposing forces tend to "mask" one another with patients frequently presenting with normal lung volumes. An obstructive ventilatory defect is seen in ~50 % of patients, while there is evidence of restriction in only 21 % of cases, and "pseudonormalization" of spirometry is seen in approximately one-third of cases [15].

Although pathologically distinct, emphysema and fibrosis do share a propensity for destruction of the pulmonary parenchyma. Therefore, there are mutual pathophysiologic consequences that in summation tend to be more profound. In this regard, another important clue to the presence of CPFE is the single breath diffusing capacity for carbon monoxide (DLCO), which is frequently reduced disproportionately to any lung volume abnormalities. Similarly, most of these patients tend to be hypoxemic at rest and have evidence of exercise desaturation [15].

The pulmonary vasculature may be involved by both processes with evidence for the presence of PH reported in many patients [15, 16]. Those patients whose CPFE is complicated by PH have shortened median survivals of 4.8 years compared to those without PH, whose median survivals have been reported at just over 9 years [15]. Additionally, patients with CPFE appear to be at heightened risk for lung cancer.

There are conflicting reports of outcomes in those patients with CPFE compared to others with IPF. One study reported a 5-year survival after the diagnosis of CPFE of 54.6 % with a median survival of just over 6 years [15]. This is significantly better than recent reports on IPF survival [21, 22]. However, patients with CPFE have also been reported to have worse outcomes compared to those with IPF, which might be accounted for by the greater propensity for the CPFE group to also have PH [16].

There are no specific treatment recommendations for CPFE. In the absence of universally accepted therapies for IPF, it might be reasonable to treat the emphysematous component of the disease in those patients with obstructive physiology. In this regard, treatment guidelines for COPD can help direct therapy.

## IPF with Pulmonary Hypertension

PH can complicate the course of many different forms of parenchymal lung disease, including IPF [8–10, 23]. It is clear that the presence of PH is associated with a worse prognosis and increased functional impairment [8]. Whether PH should be regarded as a complication, comorbidity, or distinct clinical phenotype is uncertain. Some patients may have PH at their initial presentation while others might develop it with progression of their disease [24, 25]. It is difficult to predict which patients will develop PH over time, although those who are so inclined might have a distinct genomic fingerprint [26–28]. Because the course of disease appears to be modified by the presence of PH, it seems reasonable to regard it as its own IPF phenotype.

Some patients do appear to have a greater propensity for PH and may develop it in the context of well-preserved lung function [11] (Fig. 10.3). In addition to a poor correlation between the severity of restrictive physiology and PH, there is also a lack of correlation between the extent of fibrosis on HRCT and PH (Fig. 10.4). This suggests that factors other than the fibrosis are involved in the genesis of PH. Destruction of the alveolar capillary bed by the fibrotic process certainly does play a role, while the presence of two pathologically distinct causes of alveolar capillary destruction with counterbalancing effects on lung volumes might explain the lack of correlation between lung volumes and PH in those patients with coexistent emphysema. There are multiple other contributory factors including hypoxemia, which may be intermittent or nocturnal. It is also conceivable that due to the heterogeneous nature of the disease, regional hypoxia may be present which cannot be detected on standard clinical testing. Additionally, in the context of the complex pathogenic sequence that leads to progressive fibrosis, it is possible that dysregulated cytokines might have effects on angiostasis, angiogenesis, and vessel remodeling, resulting in or contributing to the development of PH [29]. Some of the cytokines implicated in this regard include endothelin-1, vascular endothelial growth factor, pigment epithelium-derived factor, transforming growth factor-beta, platelet-derived growth factor, endostatin, angiostatin, fibroblast growth factor-2, and angiotensin-II [29]. The role of comorbidities in the development of PH should not be overlooked, especially in the more elderly in whom there may be coexistent diastolic heart failure,

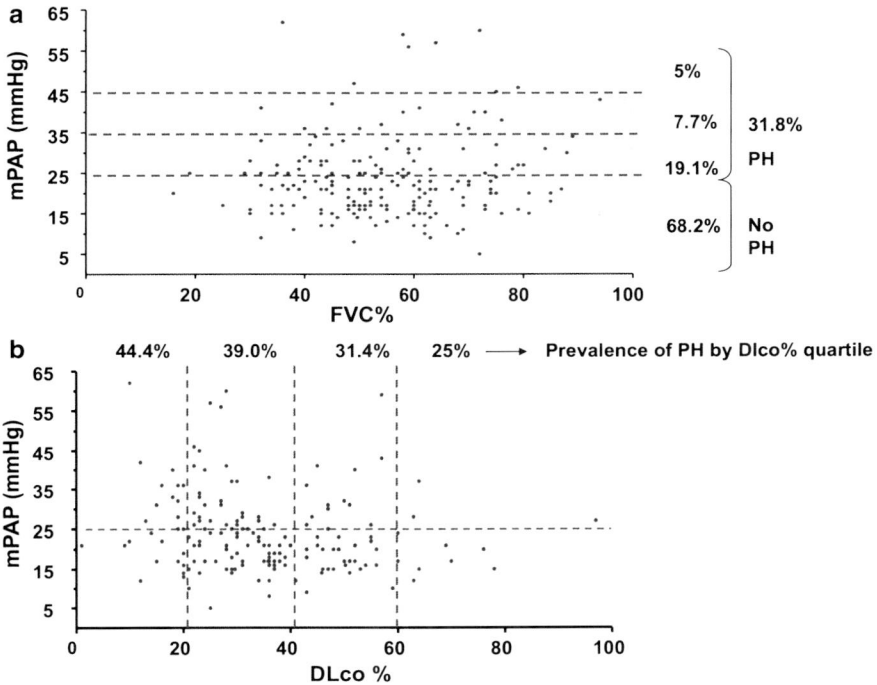

**Fig. 10.3** (a) Graph of the mean pulmonary artery pressures versus the FVC% predicted showing a lack of correlation between these two variables. The prevalence of PH is demonstrated on the right y-axis, which also depicts the relative proportion of patients with various degrees of PH. (b) Plot of the mean pulmonary artery pressure to DLCO%, also demonstrating the prevalence of pulmonary hypertension by DLCO% predicted range on the top y-axis (Inova Fairfax data)

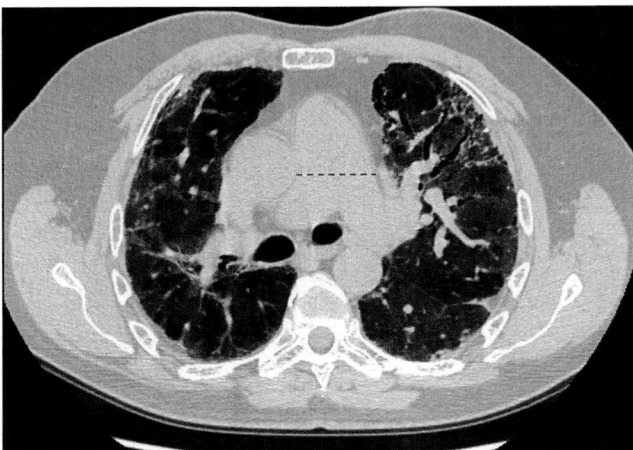

**Fig. 10.4** HRCT of patient with IPF and an FVC of 50 % predicted with a mean pulmonary artery pressure of 52 mmHg. Note the enlarged pulmonary artery segment (*dashed line*)

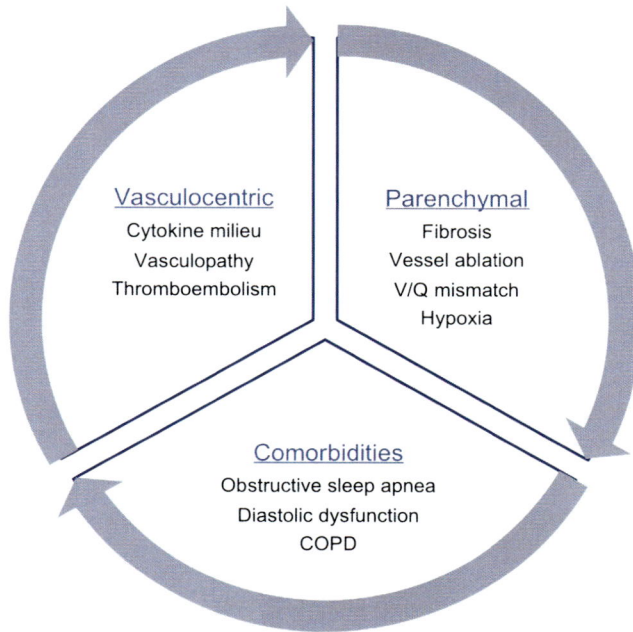

**Fig. 10.5** Factors that may contribute to the pathogenesis of PH in IPF

obstructive sleep apnea, and coronary artery disease. All of these entities have been demonstrated to have a higher prevalence in IPF patients [7, 30–35]. The various factors that may contribute to the pathogenesis of PH in IPF are depicted in Fig. 10.5.

When present, PH is usually mild to moderate; therefore, the clinical findings of PH may be subtle or absent. In approximately half of the cases, the mean pulmonary artery pressure (mPAP) is in the range of 25–30 mmHg, while more severe PH (mPAP>40 mmHg) has been described in only ~9 % of IPF patients listed for lung transplantation [8, 10]. Therefore, clinical signs are frequently absent, although the presence of an increased $P_2$ component to the second heart sound may be the first sign and should raise suspicion for underlying PH. Other findings, including jugular venous distension and peripheral edema, are typically rare, as patients will usually succumb to their disease prior to the development of overt right-sided heart failure. Important clues to the presence of underlying PH are dyspnea or desaturation that is out of proportion to the impairment in lung function.

Although lung volumes do not predict PH, a markedly reduced DLCO (typically <40 % of predicted) does have a correlation with PH, and the lower the DLCO, the more likely that coexistent PH will be present [11] (see Fig. 10.3b). A reduced FVC% to DLCO% may also be a useful screen; specifically those patients with a ratio of 1.0–1.4 have an associated prevalence of PH of 22.6 % compared to those with a ratio >3.0 in whom the prevalence is 50 % [11]. A shorter distance, lower oxygen saturation nadir, and diminished pulse rate response obtained during and after a 6-min walk test are all associated with underlying PH [8, 36]. On cardiopulmonary testing, IPF patients with PH demonstrate lower maximum work rates, peak oxygen updates, anaerobic thresholds, and peak oxygen pulses, but with higher ventilatory equivalents for $CO_2$ elimination [37]. Biomarkers in the form of brain natriuretic peptide or pro-N terminal brain natriuretic peptide, which can also be elevated in heart failure, may similarly be useful screening tools for PH in IPF, but these require further validation [25, 38].

As with all forms of PH, echocardiography is a good screening tool, but it should not be relied upon to make the diagnosis, because it is frequently inaccurate, especially in patients with IPF and other forms of advanced lung disease [39, 40]. Additionally, echocardiography only provides an estimate of the right ventricular systolic pressure (RVSP), which in the absence of pulmonic stenosis approximates the pulmonary artery systolic pressure. The higher this pressure, the more likely the patient has PH. Specifically, an estimated RVSP >60 mmHg is 92 % specific for underlying PH, but the sensitivity of this threshold is unacceptably low at only 27 % [40]. Conversely, a threshold of 35 mmHg has a sensitivity for PH of 86 %, but this is at the expense of a specificity of only 29 %. Echocardiography may overestimate the RVSP in ~50 % but may also provide an underestimation in ~10 % of IPF patients [40]. Therefore, the gold standard for a definitive diagnosis remains right heart catheterization. The ability of differing pressure estimates by echocardiography to predict prognosis does, however, raise the issue of whether it is the systolic pressure that has a closer link to prognosis than the mPAP [9, 25].

As opposed to IPF for which there are no universally recognized or accepted medical therapies, there are now multiple therapies available for the treatment of pulmonary arterial hypertension. This has raised ongoing interest in targeting the PH of IPF with these same medications. Although there are a number of case series attesting to the benefits of this approach, the prospective trials to date have not borne this out [41, 42]. The most robust of these studies was the STEP-IPF study of sildenafil for patients with advanced IPF, which was undertaken by the NIH-sponsored IPF Network. This study was enriched for IPF patients with PH by virtue of the inclusion criteria of a DLCO <35 % of the normal predicted value. Although the study failed to meet its primary endpoint of a 20 % change in the 6-min walk test distance, there were a number of secondary endpoints that were met, suggesting a salutary effect [42]. A subsequent subgroup analysis of those patients with right ventricular dysfunction on echocardiogram did indeed demonstrate a benefit in the 6-min walk test distance for the treatment arm [43]. Therefore, it does appear that there may be a subgroup of patients with IPF and complicating PH who may benefit from pulmonary vasoactive therapies, but this requires further validation in appropriately designed prospective studies.

# Disease Course Variants

The course of patients with IPF is very difficult to predict. Although the median survival is approximately 3 years from the time of diagnosis, there is wide temporal variation in disease progression and outcomes. Whether there are distinct clinical phenotypes within this spectrum of outcomes is uncertain.

## *Rapid Progressors*

There appears to be a subgroup of patients with a more accelerated course who are at greater risk of succumbing within the first year from the time of diagnosis [44–46]. These patients tend to present earlier after the onset of symptoms than those who have a more protracted course [44]. This might be due to the rapidity of progression of their symptoms. At-risk patients are more likely to be males and smokers [44]. However, they remain a difficult group to discern at baseline due to a lack of specific demographic, radiographic, physiologic, or characteristic pathologic features [44, 45]. However, rapid progressors appear to have a distinct genomic fingerprint with a propensity for the overexpression of genes involved in morphogenesis, oxidative stress, migration/proliferation, and genes from fibroblasts/smooth muscle cells [44]. Toll-like receptor 9, an innate immune sensor that is released in response to certain infections, has also been shown to be upregulated in IPF patients with a more accelerated course [45]. It appears that Toll-like receptor 9 can also drive the fibrotic process, raising the interesting possibility that occult infection may play a role, which is consistent with the multiple hit theory that is commonly invoked in IPF pathogenesis. This may also help to explain the unpredictable course seen in most patients.

## *Slow Progressors*

On the other end of the spectrum are those patients who survive 5 years and beyond from their initial diagnosis and whose disease course appears to follow a more attenuated trajectory [46]. These patients are also difficult to distinguish at presentation, but as a group they have higher body mass indices, FVC%, $FEV_1$%, TLC%, and DLCO% predicted, as well as lower $FEV_1$/FVC ratios and mPAPs [46]. Rather than being a distinct subgroup of patients, these patients likely represent the protracted extreme of a continuous spectrum of outcomes. There are data to suggest that ongoing survival portends a better prognosis and that "the longer IPF patients live, the more likely they will live longer" [46].

## *Acute Exacerbators*

Acute exacerbations (AEs) of IPF are the topic of a dedicated chapter (Chap. 17), and readers are encouraged to refer to this. Whether those patients who develop AEs should be regarded as a distinct phenotype or whether this should be regarded as an IPF complication is uncertain. The idiopathic nature of AEs makes this distinction difficult. Specifically, if occult aspiration, viral infections, or any other intercurrent insults were the precipitating factor, then this would qualify AEs as a complication. Elevated pepsin levels have been described in one-third of cases of IPF AEs, attesting to aspiration as possibly playing a role in at least some cases [47]. However, if a specific milieu or genomic phenotype that predisposes some patients to develop an AE is eventually identified, this patient subset would be more appropriately classified as a distinct IPF phenotype. Indeed, it has been shown that IPF-AE lung tissues have a distinct genomic profile with upregulation of stress response genes such as heat shock proteins, alpha-defensins, and mitosis-related genes including histones and CCNA2 [48]. This gene dysregulation is localized mostly to the alveolar epithelial cells, rather than fibroblasts. Interestingly, from the same gene analysis of IPF-AE lung tissue, there did not appear to be upregulation of genes that are typically associated with infection or inflammation. Although the epithelial cell has been shown to be a potential precursor cell for fibroblasts through epithelial-mesenchymal transition, why these cells should alter their expression to that of a more acute lung injury phenotype remains uncertain.

There do not appear to be any distinct clinical features that can reliably identify those patients at risk for an acute exacerbation. However, it has been reported that patients with lower FVCs and nonsmokers are at higher risk. Additionally, male gender and undergoing a surgical lung biopsy may also represent risk factors [49, 50].

## IPF Sine CTD (Connective Tissue Disease)

There appears to be a spectrum of connective tissue disease (CTD) manifestations that may be seen in association with a UIP pattern of injury (Fig. 10.6). It remains unclear whether a distinct IPF phenotype exists within the spectrum of possible CTD manifestations. It is possible that an occult CTD or predisposition to develop a CTD (as manifest by positive serologies) sets the stage and predisposes patients to an injurious process that can be considered similar to the effects of an occupational exposure in a predisposed patient. Alternatively, autoimmune activation in response to the injurious process may also be possible. Indeed, evolving evidence suggests that autoimmunity may play a significant role in the initiation or perpetuation of IPF [51, 52].

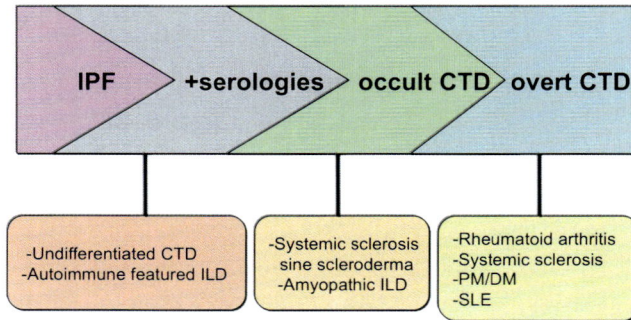

**Fig. 10.6** Diagram depicting the spectrum of connective tissue disease features from IPF to overt autoimmune disease

It has been recognized from the earliest descriptions of IPF that some cases may be associated with low-grade positive autoantibodies, most notably low-titer antinuclear antibodies (ANA). It has been proposed that patients with positive serologies and at least one symptom of a CTD who do not otherwise fulfill criteria for a specific CTD should be regarded as having a distinct entity termed "autoimmune-featured ILD" or to have an undifferentiated CTD, which has been described in 13 % of IPF patients [53, 54]. It is not clear that these patients should be regarded as representing a distinct IPF phenotype, since their outcomes appear to be similar to that of IPF patients who lack findings suggestive of CTD. Whether these patients can be differentiated by a different treatment response profile remains to be determined. It has been estimated that 15–20 % of patients with ILD may have an occult CTD or subsequently develop one [55]. These patients may be difficult to identify at the outset, even in the presence of autoantibodies (which do not necessarily predict the subsequent development of a CTD) [56]. Therefore, patients might be diagnosed with apparent IPF at the outset, but this diagnosis might require modification when the autoimmune process manifests, which can be months to many years after the initial diagnosis of IPF is made [57, 58].

In polymyositis/dermatomyositis (PM/DM), ILD may occur before the onset of systemic disease in up to 20–38 % of cases, and ILD may be the sole manifestation of the disease in 30 % of patients [58–61]. Within the spectrum of PM/DM is the antisynthetase syndrome, which is a specific subgroup of patients who have autoantibodies against aminoacyl-tRNA synthetases. The aminoacyl-tRNA synthetases are cytoplasmic enzymes that facilitate the attachment of amino acids to their respective transfer RNAs [58]. Of these, the anti-Jo1 antibody is most commonly measured and is seen in 30 % of cases [59]. However, routine commercial testing for the other antisynthetase antibodies is not readily available. Clinical manifestations of the associated myositis may be subtle or absent, making this diagnosis difficult to attain. Seropositive amyopathic ILD falls within the spectrum of the antisynthetase syndrome, but this variant occurs without associated muscle weakness or abnormal muscle enzymes. Nonetheless, these patients may still have myopathic findings on electromyogram or muscle biopsy.

Another CTD that may be subtle in its manifestations is systemic sclerosis sine scleroderma, which is a rare form of scleroderma in which patients may manifest with systemic disease but lack skin thickening or sclerodactyly. They will usually have scattered telangiectasias, abnormal nailfolds on capillaroscopy, Raynaud's phenomenon, or esophageal dysmotility [62]. A nucleolar staining pattern to the ANA should also raise the suspicion for underlying scleroderma, especially since both the anti-centromere and anti-Scl 70 antibodies are not usually found in the sine scleroderma variant [62].

On one end of the CTD spectrum, there are the clinically overt CTDs with their inherent systemic manifestations that are seen in association with ILD. Indeed, the UIP pattern of injury that characterizes IPF is well described in many of the CTDs, including rheumatoid arthritis, in which UIP is the major pathologic manifestation of complicating ILD. Although a nonspecific interstitial pneumonia pattern of injury tends to predominate in the other CTDs, a UIP pattern can still be seen in many cases.

## Radiographic Phenotypes

The most pertinent study for the diagnosis of IPF is the HRCT. The value of HRCT has gained increased recognition and importance, and it is central to the diagnostic algorithm provided in the most recent 2011 IPF consensus statement [63]. When the HRCT displays a pattern that is typical for the presence of UIP, this is sufficient to make the diagnosis of IPF without the need for a confirmatory lung biopsy. A typical HRCT for IPF includes the following: (1) subpleural, basal predominant reticular abnormalities, (2) honeycombing with or without traction bronchiectasis, and (3) the absence of inconsistent features. If only honeycombing is lacking, the HRCT is regarded as consistent with a "possible UIP pattern," while the presence of atypical features on HRCT is regarded as "inconsistent with a UIP pattern" (Fig. 10.7). Atypical radiographic features include upper or mid-lung predominance, peribronchovascular predominance, extensive ground-glass abnormalities, profuse micronodules, discrete cysts, diffuse mosaic attenuation/air trapping, or consolidation. Prior to the most recent consensus statement, patients with atypical HRCT findings and UIP histopathology had been described as having better outcomes [2]. Most of these patients were regarded as having atypical scans based on a lack of honeycombing. Whether the absence or presence of this feature defines different clinical phenotypes or patients at different stages of their disease course (or both) has not yet been determined.

The recent consensus guidelines clearly delineate the diagnostic criteria for IPF. There are numerous permutations of radiographic and histologic pattern combinations with which the diagnosis can be attained (see Fig. 10.7). It is unclear if the specific diagnostic combinations will eventually emerge as disease conditions that are in other ways distinct. In the context of a full evaluation that includes a HRCT and surgical lung biopsy, some patients may still not qualify as having IPF and are labeled as "probable IPF" (see Fig. 10.7). This entity probably does include some patients with and others

| HRCT / Histopathology | UIP Pattern ❶Subpleural, basal predominance ❷Reticular abnormality ❸Honeycombing+/- traction bronchiectasis ❹Absence of inconsistent features | Possible UIP Pattern ❶Subpleural, basal predominance ❷Reticular abnormality ❸Absence of inconsistent features | Inconsistent with UIP Pattern ❶Upper or mid-lung predominance ❷Peribronchovascular predominance ❸Extensive ground glass abnorm ❹Profuse micronodules ❺Discrete cysts ❻Diffuse mosaic attenuation/air-trapping ❼Consolidation |
|---|---|---|---|
| UIP Pattern ❶Marked fibrosis/architectural distortion +/- honeycombing, subpleural/paraseptal ❷ Patchy fibrosis ❸ Fibroblastic foci ❹Absence of features suggesting alternate diagnosis | IPF Yes | IPF Yes | IPF Probable |
| Probable UIP Pattern ❶ and ❸ As above ❷ Absence of either patchy fibrosis or fibroblastic foci ❹Honeycomb changes only | IPF Yes | IPF Yes | IPF No |
| Possible UIP Pattern ❶Patchy or diffuse fibrosis +/-interstitial inflammation ❷ Absence of other criteria for UIP ❸As above Nonclassifiable fibrosis | IPF Yes | IPF Probable | IPF No |
| Not UIP Pattern (any of 6) ❶Hyaline membranes ❷Organizing pneumonia ❸Granulomas ❹Marked interstitial inflammation ❺Predominant airway centered changes ❻Features suggestive of other diagnosis | IPF No | IPF No | IPF No |

**Fig. 10.7** Permutations of HRCT and histologic pattern combinations for the diagnosis of IPF

without IPF. As a group, whether or not they have a differing pathogenesis, disease course, or response to therapy remains to be determined. If patients with "probable IPF" are indeed shown to have distinctive characteristics in future studies, these patients may be redefined as constituting another IPF phenotype, if not another disease.

## Hybrid (Crossover) Phenotypes

There are patients who can manifest features of more than one IPF phenotype (see Fig. 10.2). For example, patients with CPFE have a higher prevalence of PH and may demonstrate a nonspecific ANA in approximately one-third of cases [15]. Additionally, IPF/PH patients have been described to be at greater risk for AEs [64]. There is obvious overlap between those patients who develop AEs and those who have an accelerated disease course; indeed, patients may occasionally have clinical features that make it difficult to identify them as having one or the other phenotype. Fresh collagen deposition can result in a ground-glass appearance on HRCT, which may be indistinguishable from the infiltrates of diffuse alveolar damage that characterize AEs. Whether patients with any of the radiographic variants are more inclined to develop other phenotypic manifestations including an AE or PH/IPF remains to be determined.

# Summary

The concept and identification of IPF phenotypes continue to evolve with a number of distinct entities now identified. However, as yet, there are no clear definitions or classifications of these phenotypes. A greater understanding of IPF phenotypes is needed in order to better discern the course of the disease and to appropriately stratify patients in treatment trials. Indeed, it is possible that distinct phenotypes might have different responses to therapy. An area for future study is the further genomic profiling of IPF phenotypes to better understand the genetic component of each entity's unique expression.

# References

1. American Thoracic Society, European Respiratory Society. American Thoracic Society/ European Respiratory Society International Multidisciplinary Consensus Classification of the Idiopathic Interstitial Pneumonias. Joint statement of the American Thoracic Society (ATS) and the European Respiratory Society (ERS) adopted by the ATS board of directors and by the ERS Executive Committee, June 2001. Am J Respir Crit Care Med. 2002;165:277–304.
2. Flaherty KR, Thwaite EL, Kazerooni EA, Gross BH, Toews GB, Colby TV, et al. Radiological versus histological diagnosis in UIP and NSIP: survival implications. Thorax. 2003;58:143–8.
3. Sumikawa H, Johkoh T, Colby TV, Ichikado K, Suga M, Taniguchi H, et al. Computed tomography findings in pathological usual interstitial pneumonia: relationship to survival. Am J Respir Crit Care Med. 2008;177:433–9.
4. Tcherakian C, Cottin V, Brillet PV, Freynet O, Naggara N, Carton Z, et al. Progression of idiopathic pulmonary fibrosis: lessons from asymmetrical disease. Thorax. 2011;66:226–31.
5. Tobin RW, Pope CE, Pellegrini CA, Emond MJ, Sillery J, Raghu G. Increase prevalence of gastroesophageal reflux in patients with idiopathic pulmonary fibrosis. Am J Respir Crit Care Med. 1998;158:1804–8.
6. Raghu G, Yang ST, Spada C, Hayes J, Pellegrini CA. Sole treatment of acid gastroesophageal reflux in idiopathic pulmonary fibrosis: a case series. Chest. 2006;129:794–800.
7. Lancaster LH, Mason WR, Parnell JA, Rice TW, Loyd JE, Milstone AP, et al. Obstructive sleep apnea is common in idiopathic pulmonary fibrosis. Chest. 2009;136:772–8.
8. Lettieri CJ, Nathan SD, Barnett S, Ahmad S, Shorr AF. Prevalence and outcomes of pulmonary arterial hypertension in idiopathic pulmonary fibrosis. Chest. 2006;129:746–52.
9. Nadrous HF, Pellikka PA, Krowka MJ, Swanson KL, Chaowalit N, Decker PA, et al. Pulmonary hypertension in patients with idiopathic pulmonary fibrosis. Chest. 2005;128:2393–9.
10. Shorr AF, Wainright JL, Cors CS, Letteri CJ, Nathan SD. Pulmonary hypertension in patients with pulmonary fibrosis awaiting transplant. Eur Respir J. 2007;30:715–21.
11. Nathan SD, Shlobin OA, Ahmad S, Urbanek S, Barnett SD. Pulmonary hypertension and pulmonary function testing in idiopathic pulmonary fibrosis. Chest. 2007;131:657–63.
12. Lee HL, Ryu JH, Wittmer MH, Hartman TE, Lymp JF, Tazelaar HD, et al. Familial idiopathic pulmonary fibrosis: clinical features and outcomes. Chest. 2005;127:2034–41.
13. Wiggins J, Strickland B, Turner-Warwick M. Combined cryptogenic fibrosing alveolitis and emphysema: the value of high resolution computed tomography in assessment. Respir Med. 1990;84:365–9.
14. Hiwatari N, Shimura S, Takishima T. Pulmonary emphysema followed by pulmonary fibrosis of undetermined cause. Respiration. 1993;60:354–8.

15. Cottin V, Nunes H, Brillet PY, Delaval P, Devouassoux G, Tillie-Leblond I, et al. Combined pulmonary fibrosis and emphysema: a distinct underrecognized entity. Eur Respir J. 2005;26:586–93.

16. Mejia M, Carrillo G, Rojas-Serrano J, Estrada A, Suarez T, Alonso D, et al. Idiopathic pulmonary fibrosis and emphysema: decreased survival associated with severe pulmonary hypertension. Chest. 2009;136:10–5.

17. Akagi T, Matsumoto T, Harada T, Tanaka M, Kuraki T, Fujita M, et al. Coexistent emphysema delays the decrease of vital capacity in idiopathic pulmonary fibrosis. Respir Med. 2009;103:1209–15.

18. Lawson WE, Loyd JE, Degryse AL. Genetics in pulmonary fibrosis-familial cases provide clues to the pathogenesis of idiopathic pulmonary fibrosis. Am J Med Sci. 2011;341:439–43.

19. De Leon AD, Cronkhite JT, Katzenstein AA, Godwin JD, Raghu G, Glazer CS, et al. Telomere lengths, pulmonary fibrosis and telomerase (TERT) mutations. PLoS One. 2010;5:e10680.

20. Lundblad LK, Thompson-Figueroa J, Leclair T, Sullivan MJ, Poynter ME, Irvin CG, et al. Tumor necrosis factor-alpha overexpression in lung disease: a single cause behind a complex phenotype. Am J Respir Crit Care Med. 2005;171:1363–70.

21. Nathan SD, Shlobin OA, Weir N, Ahmad S, Kaldjob JM, Battle E, et al. Long-term course and prognosis of idiopathic pulmonary fibrosis in the modern era. Chest. 2011;140:221–9.

22. Fernandez Perez ER, Daniels CE, Schroeder DR, Sauver JS, Hartman TE, Bartholmai BJ, et al. Incidence, prevalence, and clinical course of idiopathic pulmonary fibrosis. Chest. 2010;137:129–37.

23. Nathan SD, Noble P, Tuder R. Idiopathic pulmonary fibrosis and pulmonary hypertension: connecting the dots. Am J Respir Crit Care Med. 2007;175:875–80.

24. Nathan SD, Shlobin OA, Ahmad S, Kraus T, Koch J, Barnett SD, et al. Serial development of pulmonary hypertension in patients with advanced idiopathic pulmonary fibrosis. Respiration. 2008;76:288–94.

25. Song JW, Song JK, Kim DS. Echocardiography and brain natriuretic peptide as prognostic indicators in idiopathic pulmonary fibrosis. Respir Med. 2009;103:180–6.

26. Rajkumar R, Konishi K, Richards TJ, Ishizawar DC, Wiechert AC, Kaminski N, et al. Genomewide RNA expression profiling in lung identifies distinct signatures in idiopathic pulmonary arterial hypertension and secondary pulmonary hypertension. Am J Physiol Heart Circ Physiol. 2010;298:H1235–48.

27. Gagermeier J, Dauber J, Yousem S, Gibson K, Kaminiski N. Abnormal vascular phenotypes in patients with idiopathic pulmonary fibrosis and secondary pulmonary hypertension. Chest. 2005;128:601S.

28. Mura M, Anraku M, Yun Z, McRae K, Liu M, Waddell TK, et al. Gene expression profiling in the lungs of patients with pulmonary hypertension associated with pulmonary fibrosis. Chest. 2012;141:661–73.

29. Farkas L, Gauldie J, Voelkel NF, Kolb M. Pulmonary hypertension and idiopathic pulmonary fibrosis: a tale of angiogenesis, apoptosis, and growth factors. Am J Respir Cell Mol Biol. 2011;45:1–15.

30. Papadopoulos CE, Pitsiou G, Karamitsos TD, Karvounis HI, Kontakiotis T, Giannakoulas G, et al. left ventricular diastolic dysfunction in idiopathic pulmonary fibrosis: a tissue Doppler ECG study. Eur Respir J. 2008;31:701–6.

31. Nathan SD, Basavaraj A, Reichner C, Shlobin OA, Ahmad S, Kiernan J, et al. Prevalence and impact of coronary artery disease in idiopathic pulmonary fibrosis. Respir Med. 2010;104:1035–41.

32. Kizer JR, Zisman DA, Blumenthal NP, Kotloff RM, Kimmel SE, Strieter RM, et al. Association between pulmonary fibrosis and coronary artery disease. Arch Intern Med. 2004;164:551–6.

33. Hubbard RB, Smith C, Le Jeune I, Gribbin J, Fogarty AW. The association between idiopathic pulmonary fibrosis and vascular disease. Am J Respir Crit Care Med. 2008;178:1257–61.

34. Ponnuswamy A, Manikandan R, Sabetpour A, Keeping IM, Finnerty JP. Association between ischaemic heart disease and interstitial lung disease: a case-control study. Respir Med. 2009;103:503–7.

35. Izbicki G, Ben-Dor I, Shitrit D, Bendayan D, Aldrich TK, Kornowski R, et al. The prevalence of coronary artery disease in end-stage pulmonary disease: is pulmonary fibrosis a risk factor? Respir Med. 2009;103:1346–9.
36. Swigris JJ, Olson A, Shlobin OA, Ahmad S, Brown KK, Nathan SD. Heart rate recovery after 6MWT predicts pulmonary hypertension in patients with IPF. Respirology. 2011;16:439–45.
37. Boutou A, Pitsiou GG, Trigonis I, Papakosta D, Kontou PK, Chavouzis N, et al. Exercise capacity in idiopathic pulmonary fibrosis: the effect of pulmonary hypertension. Respirology. 2011;16:451–8.
38. Leuchte HH, Baumgartner RA, Nounou ME, Vogeser M, Neurohr C, Trautnitz M. Brain natriuretic peptide is a prognostic parameter in chronic lung disease. Am J Respir Crit Care Med. 2006;173:744–50.
39. Arcasoy SM, Christie JD, Ferrari VA, Sutton MS, Zisman DA, Blumenthal NP, et al. Echocardiographic assessment of pulmonary hypertension in patients with advanced lung disease. Am J Respir Crit Care Med. 2003;167:735–40.
40. Nathan SD, Barnett SD, Saggar R, Belperio JA, Shlobin OA, Ross DJ, et al. Right ventricular systolic pressure by echocardiography as a predictor of pulmonary hypertension in patients with idiopathic pulmonary fibrosis. Respir Med. 2008;102:1305–10.
41. Krowka MJ, Ahmad S, de Andrade JA, Frost A, Glassberg M, Lancaster LH, et al. A randomized, double-blind, placebo-controlled study to evaluate the safety and efficacy of iloprost inhalation in adults with abnormal pulmonary arterial pressure and exercise limitation associated with idiopathic pulmonary fibrosis (abstract). Chest. 2007;132:633S.
42. The Idiopathic Pulmonary Fibrosis Clinical Research Network, Zisman DA, Schwarz M, Anstrom KJ, Collard HR, Flaherty KR, Hunninghake GW. A controlled trial of sildenafil in advanced idiopathic pulmonary fibrosis. N Engl J Med. 2010;363:620–8.
43. Han MK, Bach D, Hagan P, Schmidt SL, Flaherty KR, Toews GB, et al. Presence of right ventricular dysfunction modifies treatment response to sildenafil in the Step-IPF Trial [abstract]. Am J Respir Crit Care Med. 2011;183:A5301.
44. Selman M, Carrillo G, Estrada A, Mejia M, Becerril C, Cisneros J, et al. Accelerated variant of idiopathic pulmonary fibrosis: clinical behaviours and gene expression pattern. PLoS One. 2007;2(5):e482.
45. Trujillo G, Meneghin A, Flaherty KR, Sholl LM, Myers JL, Kazerooni EA, et al. TLR9 differentiates rapidly from slowly progressing forms of idiopathic pulmonary fibrosis. Sci Transl Med. 2010;2(57):57ra82.
46. Brown AW, Shlobin OA, Weir N, Albano MC, Ahmad S, Smith M, et al. Dynamic patient counseling: A novel concept in idiopathic pulmonary fibrosis. Chest. 2012;142:1005–10.
47. Lee JS, Song JW, Wolters PJ, Elicker BM, Ling TE, Kim DS, et al. Bronchoalveolar lavage pepsin in acute exacerbation of idiopathic pulmonary fibrosis. Eur Respir J. 2012;39:352–8.
48. Konishi K, Gibson KF, Lindell KO, Richards TJ, Zhang Y, Dhir R, et al. Gene expression profiles of acute exacerbations of idiopathic pulmonary fibrosis. Am J Respir Crit Care Med. 2009;180:167–75.
49. Song JW, Hong S-B, Lim C-M, Koh Y, Kim DS. Acute exacerbation of idiopathic pulmonary fibrosis: incidence, risk factors and outcomes. Eur Respir J. 2011;37:356–63.
50. Collard HR, Moore BB, Flaherty KR, Brown KK, Kaner RJ, King Jr TE, et al. Acute exacerbations of idiopathic pulmonary fibrosis. Am J Respir Crit Care Med. 2007;176:636–43.
51. Taillé C, Grootenboer-Mignot S, Boursier C, Michel L, Debray MP, Fagart J, et al. Identification of periplakin as a new target for autoreactivity in idiopathic pulmonary fibrosis. Am J Respir Crit Care Med. 2011;183:759–66.
52. Feghali-Bostwick CA, Tsai CG, Valentine VG, Kantrow S, Stoner MW, Pilewski JM, et al. Cellular and humoral autoreactivity in idiopathic pulmonary fibrosis. J Immunol. 2007;179:2592–9.
53. Vij R, Noth I, Strek ME. Autoimmune-featured interstitial lung disease: a distinct entity. Chest. 2011;140:1292–9.

54. Corte TJ, Copley SJ, Desai SR, Zappala CJ, Hansell DM, Nicholson AG, et al. Significance of connective tissue disease features in idiopathic interstitial pneumonia. Eur Respir J. 2012;39:661–8.
55. Strange C, Highland KB. Interstitial lung disease in the patient who has connective tissue disease. Clin Chest Med. 2004;25:549–59.
56. Homma Y, Ohtsuka Y, Tanimura K, Kusaka H, Munakata M, Kawakami Y, et al. Can interstitial pneumonia as the sole presentation of collagen vascular diseases be differentiated from idiopathic interstitial pneumonia? Respiration. 1995;62:248–51.
57. Tzelepis GE, Toya SP, Moutsopoulos HM. Occult connective tissue diseases mimicking idiopathic interstitial pneumonias. Eur Respir J. 2008;31:11–20.
58. Yoshifuji H, Fujii T, Kobayashi S, Imura Y, Fujita Y, Kawabata D, et al. Anti-aminoacyl-tRNA synthetase antibodies in clinical course prediction of interstitial lung disease complicated with idiopathic inflammatory myopathies. Autoimmunity. 2006;39:233–41.
59. Marie I, Hachulla E, Cherin P, Dominique S, Hatron PY, Hellot MF, et al. Interstitial lung disease in polymyositis and dermatomyositis. Arthritis Rheum. 2002;47:614–22.
60. Tansey D, Wells AU, Colby TV, Ip S, Nikolakoupolou A, du Bois RM, et al. Variations in histological patterns of interstitial pneumonia between connective tissue disorders and their relationship to prognosis. Histopathology. 2004;44:585–96.
61. Douglas WW, Tazelaar HD, Hartman TE, Hartman RP, Decker PA, Schroeder DR, et al. Polymyositis–dermatomyositis-associated interstitial lung disease. Am J Respir Crit Care Med. 2001;164:1182–5.
62. Fischer A, Mehan RT, Feghali-Bostwick CA, West SG, Brown KK. Unique characteristics of systemic sclerosis sine scleroderma-associated interstitial lung disease. Chest. 2006;130:976–81.
63. Raghu G, Collard HR, Egan JJ, Martinez FJ, Behr J, Brown KK, et al. An official ATS/ERS/JRS/ALAT statement: idiopathic pulmonary fibrosis: evidence-based guidelines for diagnosis and management. Am J Respir Crit Care Med. 2011;183:788–824.
64. Judge EP, Fabre A, Adamali HI, Egan JJ. Acute exacerbations and pulmonary hypertension in advanced idiopathic pulmonary fibrosis. Eur Respir J. 2012;40(1):93–100.

# Chapter 11
# Idiopathic Interstitial Pneumonia and Connective Tissue Disease-Associated Interstitial Lung Disease: Similarities and Differences

**Joshua J. Solomon and Aryeh Fischer**

**Abstract**  Determining whether an "idiopathic" interstitial pneumonia (IP) is actually a manifestation of an underlying connective tissue disease (CTD) is important, because this knowledge often has a significant impact on management and prognosis. The detection of occult CTD (and distinguishing these cases from idiopathic disease) is challenging and can be optimized by a thorough and multidisciplinary evaluation. In this chapter, we discuss the complex intersection that exists between CTD and interstitial lung disease (ILD) and highlight specific clinical, laboratory, radiologic, and histopathologic features that are useful in distinguishing CTD-associated ILD from idiopathic interstitial pneumonia (IIP).

**Keywords**  Connective tissue disease • Interstitial lung disease • Idiopathic interstitial pneumonia • Collagen vascular disease

## Introduction

The idiopathic interstitial pneumonias (IIP) are a group of diffuse parenchymal lung disorders that are grouped together based on similar clinical, radiologic, and histopathologic features [1]. Usual interstitial pneumonia (UIP) is the most common subtype of the IIPs, and when identified in the absence of an associated cause or

J.J. Solomon, M.D.
Department of Medicine, Autoimmune and Interstitial Lung Disease Program, National Jewish Health, Denver, CO, USA

A. Fischer, M.D. (✉)
Division of Rheumatology, Department of Medicine, Autoimmune and Interstitial Lung Disease Program, National Jewish Health, 1400 Jackson Street, Denver, CO 80206, USA
e-mail: fischera@njhealth.org

K.C. Meyer and S.D. Nathan (eds.), *Idiopathic Pulmonary Fibrosis: A Comprehensive Clinical Guide*, Respiratory Medicine 9, DOI 10.1007/978-1-62703-682-5_11,
© Springer Science+Business Media New York 2014

**Table 11.1** List of connective tissue diseases

| |
|---|
| Rheumatoid arthritis |
| Systemic lupus erythematosus |
| Systemic sclerosis (scleroderma) |
| Primary Sjögren's syndrome |
| Polymyositis/dermatomyositis/anti-synthetase syndrome |
| Mixed connective tissue disease |
| Undifferentiated connective tissue disease |

**Table 11.2** Pulmonary manifestations of connective tissue disease

- Pleural disease
  - Pleurisy
  - Effusion/thickening
- Airways
  - Upper
    - Cricoarytenoid disease
    - Tracheal disease
  - Lower
    - Bronchiectasis
    - Bronchiolitis
- Parenchymal
  - Interstitial lung disease
    - NSIP, UIP, OP, LIP, DAD, DIP
  - Diffuse alveolar hemorrhage
  - Acute pneumonitis
- Vascular
  - Pulmonary arterial hypertension
  - Vasculitis
- Rheumatoid nodules

underlying disease, a clinical diagnosis of idiopathic pulmonary fibrosis (IPF) is rendered [1, 2]. IPF is a devastating chronic progressive fibrotic interstitial lung disease (ILD) that is typically encountered in older adults and is associated with a very poor prognosis. Before determining that an interstitial pneumonia (IP) is truly "idiopathic" in nature, the clinician must exclude an exhaustive list of known etiologies, including underlying connective tissue disease (CTD) [1, 2].

The CTDs comprise a spectrum of systemic autoimmune diseases characterized by autoimmune phenomena (e.g., circulating autoantibodies) and autoimmune-mediated organ damage (Table 11.1). Although grouped together, there is significant heterogeneity of clinical features that are associated with the CTDs. Furthermore, many patients have an incomplete presentation, with clinical features that fall short of meeting existing classification criteria for a specific CTD, resulting in a clinical diagnosis of "undifferentiated CTD" [3].

Many pulmonary manifestations are associated with the CTDs; essentially every component of the respiratory tract is at risk (Table 11.2) [4, 5]. Furthermore, there is a wide spectrum of lung involvement among the CTDs, and certain ones are associated with specific forms of lung involvement. As an example, certain CTDs are more likely to be associated with ILD (e.g., systemic sclerosis [SSc], poly-/

dermatomyositis [PM/DM], and rheumatoid arthritis [RA]), but all CTD patients are at risk, and there is an expanding appreciation that ILD may be the first or only manifestation of a CTD [6–8]. Complicating matters further, nearly all of the histopathologic patterns characteristic of "idiopathic" forms of IP may be seen with any of the CTDs.

Thus, the intersection of ILD and CTD is quite complex and may include any of the following scenarios:

1. The identification of IP in patients that have a preexisting CTD (e.g., rheumatoid arthritis).
2. The identification of an occult CTD in patients that present with a so-called "idiopathic" IP.
3. The most controversial scenario, whereby patients with ILD have suggestive forms of CTD.

In this chapter, we review the clinical aspects of these intersecting conditions and focus especially on clinical features that distinguish CTD-associated ILD (CTD-ILD) from that of IIP.


# The Clinical Landscape of CTD-ILD

## *ILD Within Preexisting CTD*

ILD is commonly identified in patients with preexisting CTD. In fact, recent studies have shown radiographic prevalence rates of subclinical ILD of 33–57 % in various CTD cohorts [9]. ILD is particularly common in patients with SSc, PM/DM, RA, primary Sjögren's syndrome, and mixed CTD (MCTD). However, just because a patient with CTD is identified as having parenchymal lung disease does not mean the two are necessarily related. For example, the presence of preexisting SSc may be associated with the development of lung injury due to other causes (e.g., aspiration-associated pneumonitis). Furthermore, because CTD patients are often on immunosuppressive medications, the finding of new pulmonary infiltrates in these patients should raise strong suspicions for respiratory infection with either typical or atypical pathogens. Moreover, consideration for medication-induced lung toxicity is warranted, because many of the immunomodulatory and anti-inflammatory therapies, especially methotrexate, are associated with drug-induced pneumonitis [10]. In this regard, just as with any other patient that presents with an IP, a comprehensive evaluation is needed to explore all potential etiologies (e.g., infection, medication toxicity, environmental and occupational exposures, familial disease, smoking-related lung disease, and malignancy). Certainly, the possibility of CTD-ILD warrants consideration, but determining that the ILD is truly associated with the preexisting CTD is usually decided through a process of elimination [5, 11, 12].

## *ILD as the Presenting Feature of CTD*

Considering the possibility of underlying CTD is an important aspect of the evaluation of patients presenting with a so-called "idiopathic" IP [6]. Within this scenario, the identification of occult CTD is common. In fact, Mittoo and colleagues reported that of 114 consecutive ILD patients evaluated at a tertiary referral center, 17 (15 %) were confirmed to have a new CTD diagnosis [13].

There is no standardized approach to the assessment of underlying CTD. Current practice includes a thorough history and physical examination and testing for circulating autoantibodies. Many centers have found that a multidisciplinary approach that includes rheumatologic consultation may also be useful [14]. In practice, it is both unrealistic and impractical to have a rheumatologic evaluation for all cases of IIP, but certain proposed guidelines for deciding when to seek a rheumatologic consultation may be more realistic (Table 11.3) [5].

Because the extrathoracic features of occult CTD can be subtle, confirming the presence of an underlying CTD can be challenging. Homma and colleagues evaluated whether IP as the sole presentation of CTD can be differentiated from an IIP [15]. They described 68 patients who presented with an IIP and were followed prospectively over 11 years. Thirteen patients (19 %) eventually developed a classifiable CTD. The prevalence of a positive rheumatoid factor (RF) or antinuclear antibody (ANA) was no different in the group that developed CTD compared with those that did not. The authors concluded that patients defined as having an IIP cannot be distinguished from those with CTD-ILD before the systematic manifestations appear [15].

As the following select studies demonstrate, a thorough evaluation with heightened surveillance for subtle extrathoracic features of CTD, assessing a broader array of autoantibodies (Table 11.4), and consideration of radiographic and histopathologic features are all important components of the ILD evaluation and make the detection of occult CTD more likely.

Fischer and colleagues retrospectively identified a cohort of 285 patients with biopsy-proven UIP considered to have IPF [16]. Twenty-five subjects (9 %) were found to have ANA positivity with a nucleolar-staining pattern, and of these, 13 also had a positive Th/To (a nucleolar antibody highly specific for SSc) antibody. Retrospectively, most of those with nucleolar ANA positivity, and especially those with the SSc-specific Th/To antibody, had subtle extrathoracic features of SSc that included digital edema, Raynaud's phenomenon, telangiectasia, and esophageal hypomotility. Since these individuals had autoantibody positivity known to be highly specific for SSc, extrathoracic features suggestive of SSc, and an IP pattern common for SSc, the authors concluded that they likely had occult presentation of SSc rather than IPF [16]. This same group also described six patients evaluated over a 12-month period for "idiopathic" NSIP or UIP [17]. All had a positive nucleolar-pattern ANA, along with either an anti-Th/To or anti-Scl-70 antibody, and all had subtle extrathoracic features of SSc that included telangiectasia, Raynaud's phenomenon, digital edema, or esophageal hypomotility. This small cohort further

**Table 11.3** Suggested categories of ILD patients that require further rheumatologic evaluation[a]

1. Women, particularly those younger than 50
2. Any patient with extrathoracic manifestations highly suggestive of CTD (i.e., Raynaud's phenomenon, esophageal hypomotility, inflammatory arthritis of the metacarpal-phalangeal joints or wrists, digital edema, or symptomatic keratoconjunctivitis sicca)
3. All cases of NSIP, LIP, or any ILD pattern with secondary histopathology features that might suggest CTD (i.e., extensive pleuritis, dense perivascular collagen, lymphoid aggregates with germinal center formation, prominent plasmacytic infiltration)
4. Patients with a positive ANA or RF in high titer (generally considered to be ANA > 1:320 or RF > 60 IU/mL), a nucleolar-staining ANA at any titer, or any positive autoantibody specific as to a particular CTD (i.e., anti-CCP, anti-Scl-70, anti-Ro, anti-La, anti-dsDNA, anti-Smith, anti-RNP, anti-tRNA synthetase)

[a]Reprinted with permission from Fischer A, du Bois RM. A practical approach to connective tissue disease-associated lung disease. In: Baughman RP, duBois RM, eds. Diffuse lung disease: a practical approach. 2nd ed. New York: Springer; 2012:217–237

**Table 11.4** Useful antibodies for CTD-ILD assessment

| Autoantibody | Associated CTD |
| --- | --- |
| High-titer ANA (>1:320 titer) | Many |
| High-titer RF (>60 IU/mL) | RA, Sjögren's disease, SLE |
| Anti-CCP | RA |
| Anti-centromere | Systemic sclerosis |
| Anti-nucleolar ANA | Systemic sclerosis |
| Anti-Ro (SS-A) | Many |
| Anti-La (SS-B) | SLE, Sjögren's disease |
| Anti-Smith | SLE |
| Anti-ribonucleoprotein | SLE, MCTD |
| Anti-dsDNA | SLE |
| Anti-topoisomerase (Scl-70) | Systemic sclerosis |
| Anti-tRNA synthetase antibodies | Poly-/dermatomyositis (anti-synthetase syndrome) |
| Anti-PM-Scl | Systemic sclerosis/myositis overlap |
| Anti-Th/To | Systemic sclerosis |
| Anti-U3 ribonucleoprotein | Systemic sclerosis |
| Anti-tRNA synthetase antibodies | Poly-/dermatomyositis (anti-synthetase syndrome) |
| ANCA panel | Systemic vasculitis |

reinforced the concept that IP may be the presenting manifestation of SSc and that strong suspicions for SSc are warranted in patients with a nucleolar-pattern ANA and NSIP or UIP patterns of lung injury [16, 17].

Mittoo and colleagues retrospectively evaluated a cohort of 114 consecutive patients referred to a tertiary referral center for ILD evaluation [13]. Thirty-four subjects (30 %) were found to have CTD-ILD, and of these, only half had presented with preexisting CTD. Of the 17 cases with the so-called "idiopathic" disease that were identified to have occult CTD, ten had PM/DM, three had systemic lupus erythematosus (SLE), two had undifferentiated CTD, and one patient each with SSc and systemic vasculitis, respectively. They argued that when confronted with an IIP, the presence of younger age, high-titer ANA, and elevated muscle enzymes was associated with an underlying CTD [13]. In another study, Castellino and colleagues described a cohort of 50 ILD patients that underwent multidisciplinary evaluation at a tertiary referral center. Of the 25 patients confirmed to have a diagnosis of CTD-ILD, 28 % had been initially referred with a diagnosis of IPF [14].

Fischer and colleagues described a cohort of nine patients evaluated over a 2-year period with idiopathic NSIP that were ANA negative but found to have the anti-synthetase syndrome based on the presence of a tRNA synthetase antibody, the presence of NSIP, and subtle extrathoracic features that included "mechanic's hands," Raynaud's phenomenon, inflammatory arthritis, myositis, or esophageal hypomotility [18]. Interestingly (and characteristic of the anti-synthetase syndrome), these individuals were all ANA and RF negative. The authors emphasized the importance of cross-specialty evaluation of IIP and that heightened suspicions for underlying CTD are warranted in cases of NSIP, even when the ANA and RF are negative. Additional assessment for tRNA synthetase antibodies may help identify occult presentations of anti-synthetase syndrome [18]. Similarly, Watanabe and colleagues screened 198 consecutive cases of IIP with a panel of anti-tRNA synthetase antibodies and identified positive anti-synthetase antibodies in 13 cases (7 %) [19], and they reported that patients with positive antibodies were younger and more likely to have NSIP or UIP with lymphoid follicles. Furthermore, among the 13 with a positive tRNA synthetase antibody, extrathoracic manifestations of anti-synthetase syndrome were retrospectively identified in only seven cases (54 %) [19].

Finally, two recent series have shown that ILD may also be the presenting manifestation of RA and that assessing for RA-specific autoantibodies in patients with IIP may identify an at-risk phenotype for later RA development. Gizinski and colleagues described a series of four patients with ILD, RF, and anti-cyclic-citrullinated peptide (CCP) positivity and no articular findings of RA [20]. All were male, former smokers, and the average age at the time of diagnosis of the ILD was 70 years. Three patients died within 2 years of the diagnosis from progressive lung fibrosis and never developed articular symptoms consistent with RA, but one case met full criteria for the articular aspects of RA several months after stopping immunosuppressive treatment for ILD. In a larger series, Fischer and colleagues described 74 subjects evaluated over a 2-year period with anti-CCP antibody positivity, lung disease, and no evidence of RA or other CTD. Most were women and former cigarette smokers [21]. Four distinct radiographic phenotypes were identified: isolated airways disease (54 %), isolated parenchymal lung disease (14 %), mixed airways and parenchymal lung disease (26 %), and combined pulmonary fibrosis with emphysema (7 %). Among subjects with high-titer anti-CCP positivity (45 %), three developed the articular manifestations of RA within 2 years of surveillance: only one of the three ever smoked, two had isolated inflammatory airways disease, and one had combined airways and parenchymal lung disease. The authors highlighted their observations that (1) the lung disease in this cohort resembled that seen in established

RA, (2) lung disease may be the presenting manifestation of RA, and (3) anti-CCP positivity in inflammatory airways or parenchymal lung disease may be considered a pre-RA phenotype [21].

## Suggestive Forms of CTD-ILD (Table 11.5)

There is a growing appreciation that many patients with an IIP have subtle features suggestive of an autoimmune etiology and yet often do not meet established classification criteria for a specific CTD [4, 5, 7]. In some of these individuals, an auto-antibody known to be highly specific for a well-defined CTD (such as anti-Scl-70 with SSc) may be present, despite the absence of overt systemic features.

These patients, in whom it appears that the lung disease is either the lone or the most clinically significant manifestation of an occult CTD, are suspected of having a systemic autoimmune disease based on the presence of circulating autoantibodies, specific histopathologic features on surgical lung biopsy, or subtle extrathoracic manifestations. Such patients could be considered to have a *"lung-dominant CTD"* rather than "idiopathic" disease [7]. Although there is an expanding appreciation that incomplete forms of CTD-ILD exist, we do not know whether these cases behave in a fashion that is similar to definite forms of CTD-ILD or IIP.

## Undifferentiated CTD (See Table 11.5)

In 2007, Kinder and colleagues proposed a broad set of undifferentiated CTD (UCTD) criteria and applied these criteria to a cohort of patients with IIP [22]. Retrospectively, they identified 28 subjects with an IIP that met their criteria for UCTD and compared these subjects with a control group of 47 subjects with an IIP that did not meet their criteria. Interestingly, those with UCTD were more likely to be female, younger, and nonsmokers and were more likely to have ground-glass opacities on HRCT and NSIP on surgical lung biopsy. In all, 88 % of those with idiopathic NSIP had UCTD, which led the authors to conclude that most patients previously classified as having idiopathic NSIP have clinical, serologic, radiographic, and pathologic characteristics of autoimmune disease. They therefore proposed that idiopathic NSIP is the lung manifestation of UCTD [22]. More recently, Corte and colleagues have called into question the clinical relevance of defining ILD patients as having UCTD and specifically challenged the applicability of the broader, less specific UCTD criteria proposed by Kinder and colleagues [23]. They retrospectively studied 45 patients with biopsy-proven NSIP and 56 patients with biopsy-proven UIP. They reported that CTD features are common in patients with IIP, with 31 % of NSIP and 13 % of IPF patients fulfilling the stricter, more traditional criteria for UCTD. However, when the broader criteria were applied, an astounding 71 % of NSIP and 36 % of IPF patients could be reclassified as having UCTD. Because of its lack of specificity, the authors argued against further

**Table 11.5** Proposed criteria for various suggestive forms of CTD-ILD[a]

| Proposed category | Clinical features | Laboratory or histopathology findings |
|---|---|---|
| Undifferentiated CTD (stricter definition) (requires at least one clinical feature and one laboratory finding) | One or more of the following symptoms<br>Dry eyes or dry mouth, joint pain, or swelling<br>Raynaud's phenomenon<br>Proximal muscle weakness<br>Morning stiffness | One or more of these autoantibodies<br>ANA (<u>high</u> titer)<br>RF (high titer)<br>Anti-Smith<br>Anti-ribonucleoprotein<br>Anti-dsDNA<br>Anti-Ro<br>Anti-La<br>Anti-Jo-1<br>Anti-topoisomerase (Scl-70)<br>Anti-centromere |
| Undifferentiated CTD (broader definition) (requires at least one clinical feature and one laboratory finding) | One or more of the following symptoms<br>Dry eyes or dry mouth<br>Gastroesophageal reflux disease<br>Weight loss<br>Recurrent unexplained fever<br>Joint pain or swelling<br>Rash<br>Photosensitivity<br>Dysphagia<br>Nonandrogenic alopecia<br>Mouth ulcers<br>Raynaud's phenomenon<br>Morning stiffness<br>Proximal muscle weakness | One or more of these laboratory abnormalities<br>ANA (<u>any</u> titer)<br>RF<br>Anti-Ro<br>Anti-La<br>Anti-Jo-1<br>Anti-topoisomerase (Scl-70)<br>Erythrocyte sedimentation rate (two times normal)<br>C-reactive protein elevation |
| Lung-dominant CTD (requires all three listed clinical features and either 4a or 4b) | *All* of the following features<br>1. NSIP, UIP, LIP, OP, DAD (or DIP if no smoking history), as determined by surgical lung biopsy or suggested by HRCT <u>and</u><br>2. Insufficient extrathoracic features of a definite CTD <u>and</u><br>3. No identifiable alternative etiology for IP <u>and</u> | 4a. Any *one* of these autoantibodies<br>ANA > 1:320 titer<br>RF > 60 IU/mL<br>Anti-nucleolar ANA (any titer)<br>Anti-centromere<br>Anti-CCP<br>Anti-Ro<br>Anti-La<br>Anti-dsDNA<br>Anti-ribonucleoprotein<br>Anti-Smith<br>Anti-topoisomerase (Scl-70)<br>Anti-tRNA synthetase<br>Anti-PM-Scl<br>4b. *Or at least two* of these histopathology features<br>Lymphoid aggregates with germinal centers<br>Extensive pleuritis<br>Prominent plasmacytic infiltration<br>Dense perivascular collagen |

(continued)

**Table 11.5**  (continued)

| Proposed category | Clinical features | Laboratory or histopathology findings |
|---|---|---|
| Autoimmune-featured ILD (requires at least one clinical feature and one laboratory finding) | One or more of the following symptoms<br>Dry eyes or dry mouth<br>Gastroesophageal reflux disease<br>Weight loss<br>Foot or leg swelling<br>Joint pain or swelling<br>Rash<br>Photosensitivity<br>Dysphagia<br>Hand ulcers<br>Mouth ulcers<br>Raynaud's phenomenon<br>Morning stiffness<br>Proximal muscle weakness | One or more of these laboratory abnormalities<br>ANA ≥ 1:160 titer<br>RF<br>Anti-Ro<br>Anti-La<br>Anti-Smith<br>Anti-ribonucleoprotein<br>Anti-dsDNA<br>Anti-topoisomerase (Scl-70)<br>Anti-CCP<br>Anti-Jo-1<br>Aldolase<br>Creatine phosphokinase |

[a]Reprinted from The Lancet, 380, Aryeh Fischer, Roland du Bois, Interstitial lung disease in connective tissue disorders, 689–698, Copyright 2012, with permission from Elsevier

implementation of the Kinder criteria to define UCTD in patients with ILD. Furthermore, the identification of UCTD by either the more traditional or the broader criteria did not impact survival. Instead, Corte and colleagues devised an algorithm that was predictive of the presence of NSIP and improved survival consisting of the absence of typical HRCT features of IPF, a compatible demographic profile (women < 50), or the presence of Raynaud's phenomenon [23].

## *Autoimmune-Featured ILD (See Table 11.5)*

Vij and colleagues have described a cohort of UIP-predominant ILD patients that was retrospectively identified as having a possible form of CTD-ILD [24]. Among 200 patients that presented to an ILD referral center, 63 were considered to have "autoimmune-featured ILD" if they had a sign or symptom suggestive of a CTD with a serologic test reflective of an autoimmune process but with insufficient features to label as definite CTD. The cohort that met their case definition of autoimmune-featured ILD had a similar demographic profile as IPF: most were older (average age of 66 years) and male. The most common clinical symptoms in the autoimmune-featured ILD cohort were symptoms of dry eyes or dry mouth (57 %) and gastroesophageal reflux disease (44 %). Seventy-five percent of those that met their case definition for autoimmune-featured ILD had a lung injury pattern of UIP. Finally, the survival of those with autoimmune-featured ILD was similar to that of IPF and worse compared to CTD-ILD [24]. Interestingly, and arguing against the inclusion of nonspecific symptoms in the proposed criteria, only the presence of an ANA at >1:1280 titer was associated with improved survival.

## *Lung-Dominant CTD (See Table 11.5)*

Fischer and colleagues have proposed a set of provisional classification criteria to define the cohort of individuals with suggestive forms of CTD-ILD as having "lung-dominant CTD" (LD-CTD) [7]. A classification of LD-CTD would be reserved for those cases in which the ILD has a *"rheumatologic flavor"* as supported by specific autoantibodies or histopathologic features and yet do not meet criteria for a defined CTD based on the lack of adequate extrapulmonary features. The authors argued that the concept of LD-CTD implies that one must recognize that specific autoantibodies and/or histopathologic features alone can be enough to classify a patient as having CTD-ILD. The presence of objective extrapulmonary features highly suggestive of CTD (e.g., Raynaud's phenomenon, inflammatory arthritis) is important and will lend further support for an underlying CTD, but their absence should not preclude a classification of LD-CTD [7].

A number of advantages to the introduction of this novel classification were suggested and include the following: (1) the criteria offered are objective and measurable; (2) nonspecific symptoms (such as dry eyes, myalgias, arthralgias, or gastroesophageal reflux disease), nonspecific inflammatory markers (such as erythrocyte sedimentation rate or C-reactive protein), and low-titer ANA or RF are not included, because all occur commonly in patients without CTD; (3) individuals with LD-CTD require surveillance for evolution to characterizable forms of CTD; (4) conferring a diagnosis of LD-CTD will isolate them from the (default) category of IIP, yet allow their distinction from well-characterized forms of CTD. Additionally, this concept does not attempt to redefine existing CTD categories (such as UCTD) and provides a framework by which questions regarding this subset's natural history, pathobiology, treatment, and prognosis can be answered [7].

## *Autoantibody-Positive IPF*

Nonspecific autoantibody positivity (such as with low-titer ANA or RF) is known to occur in "healthy" individuals and is also commonly identified among patients with an IIP. It remains to be determined whether the presence of these nonspecific autoantibodies impacts the natural history of IIP. Song and colleagues compared secondary histopathologic features among three groups of patients with biopsy-proven UIP (Group 1 [$n=39$] comprised CTD-UIP, Group 2 [$n=27$] antibody-positive (ANA or RF) idiopathic UIP [i.e., antibody-positive IPF], and Group 3 [$n=34$] antibody-negative idiopathic UIP [i.e., antibody-negative IPF]) and showed that the presence of circulating autoantibodies is associated with specific "autoimmune" histopathologic features, even in the absence of a CTD [25]. Among those with CTD-UIP there were more germinal centers, plasma cells, and fewer fibroblastic foci when compared with all subjects who had IPF. Interestingly, histopathologic features differed between subgroups 2 and 3 depending on autoantibody status.

Although none of the antibody-positive IPF subjects (Group 2) had extrapulmonary features of CTD, they had higher germinal center scores and more plasma cells than antibody-negative IPF subjects (Group 3). Notably, no histopathologic features distinguished CTD-UIP (Group 1) from antibody-positive IPF (Group 2). Among those with IPF (Groups 2 and 3), antibody status did not predict survival, and these cohorts of antibody-positive or negative IPF had a worse prognosis than CTD-UIP (Group 1) [25]. The significance of these findings is not known, but we believe they merit further investigation [5].

# Clues to Distinguishing IIP from CTD-ILD

## Demographics and Clinical Features

Demographic features can help distinguish the patient with an underlying CTD. In comparison to IPF, patients with CTD-ILD are more likely to be younger and female [8, 23, 26–28]. Indeed, current guidelines for an IPF diagnosis encourage a high index of suspicion for an underlying CTD in young patients with an IIP [2].

A detailed review of systems and thorough physical examination can be very helpful when assessing for an underlying CTD. Certain specific clinical features lend more support for underlying CTD than others. Of the CTD symptoms encountered in patients with IIP, perhaps none is as important as Raynaud's phenomenon. The presence of Raynaud's phenomenon is associated with a pattern of NSIP [23]. When Raynaud's phenomenon is identified in a patient with ILD, this finding should raise a strong suspicion for an underlying CTD in general and SSc (with or without overt skin thickening) in particular [8, 16, 17, 23]. Indeed, Raynaud's phenomenon is encountered in nearly all patients with SSc and is a common finding in patients with PM/DM, anti-synthetase syndrome, primary Sjögren's syndrome, MCTD, SLE, and UCTD. Performing nailfold capillary microscopy is useful when assessing a patient with Raynaud's phenomenon. In particular, the presence of dilated or tortuous capillary loops or significant areas lacking capillary loops (i.e., capillary dropout) may be suggestive of SSc or PM/DM (Fig. 11.1).

The reporting of symmetric joint swelling or stiffness, or the identification of synovitis, on physical examination is very useful and suggests an underlying CTD. Because inflammatory arthritis is encountered in all of the CTDs, autoantibody profiles may be needed to clarify which specific CTD is present. In contrast, nonspecific symptoms such as gastroesophageal reflux, pain, fatigue, dry eyes, dry mouth, alopecia, and weight loss are not nearly as helpful because they are ubiquitous and not specific for CTD.

The cutaneous manifestations of SSc and anti-synthetase syndrome are worthy of special mention since these two disorders are so commonly associated with ILD and their extrathoracic features are very specific and yet often quite subtle. It is important to recognize that the "mechanic's hands" sign of anti-synthetase

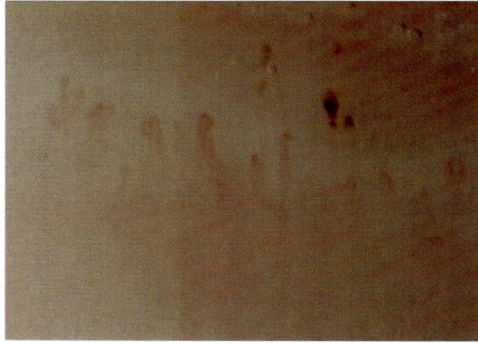

**Fig. 11.1** Nailfold capillary microscopic image in a patient with systemic sclerosis demonstrating capillary loop tortuosity, dilation, and areas of dropout. Reprinted with permission from Fischer A, du Bois RM. A practical approach to connective tissue disease-associated lung disease. In: Baughman RP, duBois RM, eds. Diffuse lung disease: a practical approach. 2nd ed. New York: Springer; 2012:217–237

syndrome can be as subtle as only mild distal digital fissuring (Fig. 11.2) and that palmar telangiectasia (Fig. 11.3) may be limited to the finding of only a single or scattered few dilated capillaries. Nonetheless, when such findings are present in a patient with an IIP, they are highly suggestive of an underlying CTD.

## Autoantibodies

Since autoantibody positivity is a hallmark of CTD, autoantibody assessment is a fundamental part of the evaluation of patients with IIP. In the most recent guidelines for the diagnosis of IPF, a panel of screening serologies that includes ANA, RF, and anti-CCP antibody testing is recommended [2]. In addition to these autoantibodies, we would recommend a broader panel of screening serologies (see Table 11.5) [5]. It is also important to take note of the pattern of immunofluorescence when the ANA is positive, as the nucleolar-staining ANA pattern in patients with ILD suggests the SSc spectrum of disease [16, 17].

Importantly, we highlight that the ANA and RF are poor screening tests: they have low specificity—particularly when present at low titer—and can be seen in healthy individuals. In addition, given that a negative ANA and RF may dissuade some clinicians from pursuing further evaluation, cases of occult CTD that may be ANA and RF negative (e.g., anti-synthetase syndrome) are missed.

## Radiologic Features

Thoracic HRCT imaging plays a central role in the evaluation of ILD by providing detailed information on the pattern, distribution, and extent of the ILD, assessing

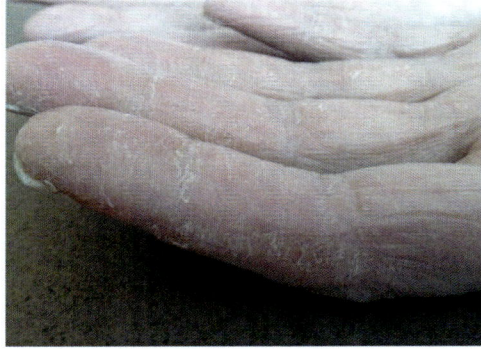

Fig. 11.2 "Mechanic's hands" (distal digital fissuring) in a patient with anti-PL12 synthetase syndrome

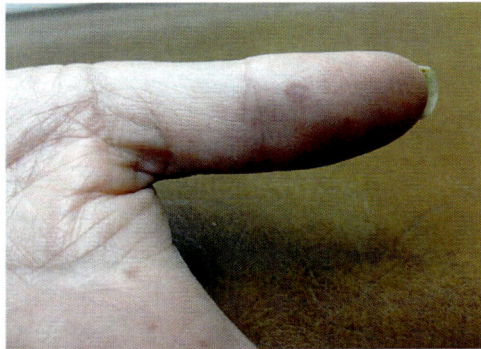

Fig. 11.3 Scattered palmar telangiectasia in a patient with systemic sclerosis sine scleroderma

disease severity and detecting the presence of extraparenchymal abnormalities including pleural disease and lymphadenopathy [29–31]. In contrast to IIP, patients with CTD-ILD are more likely to have ground-glass abnormalities, pleural effusions, pericardial effusions, pericardial thickening, and esophageal dilatation and less likely to have honeycombing [29–31] (Fig. 11.4). Patients with CTD are also more likely to have a HRCT pattern suggestive of NSIP when compared to patients without CTD, and a UIP pattern in this group as a whole is rare [29–31]. HRCT has varying degrees of correlation with histopathologic patterns. For example, in one series of patients with Sjögren's syndrome, a HRCT pattern of NSIP has a 94 % positive predictive value for a histopathologic diagnosis of NSIP [32]. Furthermore, among CTD-ILD patients with a typical HRCT pattern for UIP, the histopathology almost always correlates [24]. The converse, however, does not hold true; CTD patients with histopathologic patterns of UIP may have HRCT patterns suggestive of NSIP. In a recent study, Song and colleagues found that patients with CTD-UIP had a lower emphysema score, less honeycombing, and were more likely to have an atypical UIP pattern [25].

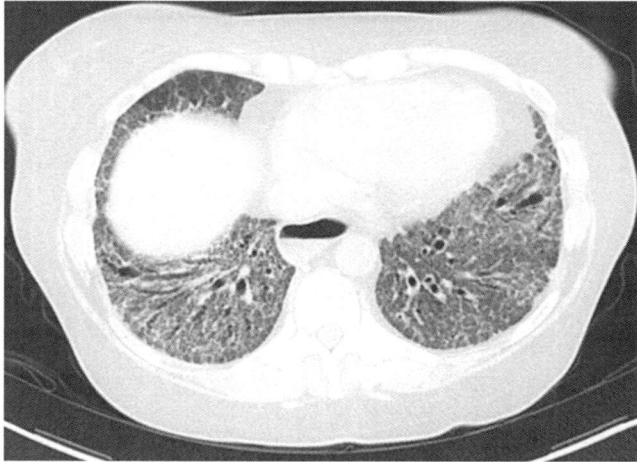

**Fig. 11.4** High-resolution computed tomographic image in a patient with systemic sclerosis demonstrating moderate bibasilar-predominant ground-glass opacifications, reticulation, and traction bronchiectasis without honeycombing suggestive of fibrotic NSIP. Note the markedly dilated, fluid-filled esophagus

## Histopathologic Features

Several histopathologic features may be useful when trying to distinguish an IIP from CTD-ILD. An initial clue to an underlying CTD is the presence of multi-compartment involvement on the biopsy; in addition to parenchymal lung injury, there may be components of airways, vascular, or pleural disease [33]. When compared to IPF, CTD-UIP is characterized by fewer fibroblastic foci, lower fibrosis scores, less honeycombing, and less alveolar cellularity [25, 34, 35]. Flaherty and colleagues compared the histopathologic features of nine patients with CTD-UIP to that of 99 patients with IPF [26]. Those with CTD-UIP were younger, had better lung function, and shorter duration of symptoms. They found that those with IPF had significantly higher fibroblast focus scores than CTD-UIP and that the fibroblast focus score was the most discriminative feature between these groups. Song and colleagues compared histopathologic features in 39 patients with CTD-UIP to 61 patients with IPF and found that CTD-UIP patients had fewer fibroblastic foci and smaller honeycombing spaces with higher germinal centers and total inflammation scores than IPF patients [25]. Furthermore, the germinal center score was the best distinguishing feature between CTD-UIP and IPF [25]. Additional histopathologic features that lend support for the presence of underlying CTD include the presence of lymphoid aggregates, germinal centers, increased perivascular collagen, lymphoplasmacytic inflammation, eosinophil infiltration, or pleuritis [33].

## Impact of Histopathology on Survival

UIP is the most common pattern among cohorts of patients with IIP [1]. In contrast, nonspecific interstitial pneumonia (NSIP) is the most common lung injury pattern encountered in those with CTD [28]. The only exception is RA, with recent data suggesting that the UIP pattern is more common than NSIP [28, 40–42]. It is well established that for IIP, a histopathologic pattern of UIP is associated with worse survival than an NSIP pattern [28, 43–45]. Interestingly, for CTD-ILD, the impact of the underlying histopathologic pattern on survival is less certain. In the largest series of biopsied SSc-associated ILD (SSc-ILD) subjects ($n=80$), Bouros and colleagues showed that changes in the diffusing capacity (DLCO) over time, but not histopathologic distinction between NSIP and UIP, predicted prognosis [46]. Similarly, Park and colleagues analyzed prognostic features in a cohort of 93 patients with a variety of types of CTD-ILD [28]. They demonstrated that age, pulmonary function, and degree of dyspnea were of prognostic importance, but that differences in histopathologic pattern did not have a significant impact on survival. Subset analyses of the cohort with RA-ILD suggested that survival in RA-UIP may be similar to that of IPF and worse than that of CTD-associated NSIP (CTD-NSIP) or non-RA-CTD-UIP. However, with adjustments for age, gender, and lung function, these differences did not persist [28]. In another series of RA-ILD ($n=18$), Lee and colleagues found that RA-UIP ($n=10$) was associated with a worse survival compared with RA-NSIP ($n=6$) [41]. More recently, Kim and colleagues assessed whether a high-resolution computed tomography (HRCT) diagnosis of UIP predicted prognosis in RA-ILD. The median survival time for all RA-ILD subjects ($n=82$) was 5 years [40]. However, RA-UIP had a worse median survival time than RA-non-UIP (3.2 versus 6.6 years, respectively; $p=0.04$). Median survival time did not differ between RA-UIP and IPF ($p=0.66$). In addition to male gender, lower baseline forced vital capacity (FVC), lower DLCO, and a definite UIP pattern on HRCT were all associated with worse survival in RA-ILD [40]. In light of these data, these investigators suggested that incorporating knowledge of underlying histopathology in RA-ILD should inform the management approach. Patients with RA-NSIP should be treated with immunosuppression, but those with RA-UIP should be informed of their worse prognosis and counselled to consider lung transplantation [40, 42].

The relatively small cohort sizes of existing studies and the impact of treatment, selection, and referral bias cannot be discounted; therefore, the predictive power of different patterns of lung histopathology remains uncertain in CTD-ILD.

## Management Considerations

A general rule for CTD-ILD is that not all patients require treatment. Therapy for CTD-ILD is typically comprised of immunosuppressive medications (such as cyclophosphamide, azathioprine, cyclosporine, mycophenolate mofetil, or tacrolimus) and is usually reserved for those patients with clinically significant, progressive disease. The decision to offer immunosuppressive therapy is based upon a constellation of clinical assessment tools that include both subjective and objective measures of respiratory impairment [36]. Furthermore, when considering immunomodulatory therapy options for CTD-ILD, both intrathoracic and extrathoracic disease aspects and degrees of activity need to be considered. Disease monitoring, choice of therapy, and ongoing longitudinal assessment and reassessment of treatment response are complex and not evidence based. Efforts should be made to tailor any treatment recommendation to the individual, fully considering the numerous factors apart from the CTD-ILD itself, including the specific underlying CTD, medical comorbidities, patient preferences and compliance, insurance coverage, and access to care. Unfortunately, we are left with few data to guide choice of specific therapeutic agents, because there are no controlled clinical trial data (other than for using cyclophosphamide to treat SSc-ILD) to provide an evidence base to guide management decisions [37, 38]. Other challenges relate to the paucity of available therapeutic options, the risk of potentially significant toxicity that currently available therapies carry, the heterogeneity of disease within the CTD-ILD spectrum, and the lack of well-defined outcome measures.

Defining a patient as having CTD-ILD rather than an IIP may impact therapeutic decisions [4]. In particular, the defining of ILD as CTD associated, rather than idiopathic, may significantly impact decisions of choice and duration of immunosuppressive therapy. For example, when idiopathic (i.e., cryptogenic) organizing pneumonia (OP) is diagnosed, high-dose corticosteroids may only be indicated for a short period of time (~6 months) followed by a taper and ultimate discontinuation of immunosuppression. In contrast, when OP occurs within the context of an underlying CTD, such as with PM/DM, a course of high-dose corticosteroids is often followed by the addition of a steroid-sparing agent (such as azathioprine) due to knowledge that long-term immunosuppression will be needed due to the chronic, autoimmune nature of the systemic illness.

The pattern of UIP is associated with more uncertainty and controversy. For IPF, current guidelines do not recommend immunosuppressive therapy, and recent data suggest that immunosuppressive treatment may even be harmful [2, 39]. In contrast, for CTD-associated UIP (CTD-UIP) that is significant and clinically progressive, treatment with immunosuppression is often indicated. The arena of RA-associated UIP (RA-UIP) is more controversial in this regard. Because recent data suggest that RA-UIP may have a poor prognosis that is similar to that for IPF [28, 40–42], some have argued that immunosuppression may not be warranted and have instead suggested that management should be similar to that recommended for patients with IPF [42]. It also remains to be determined how to manage a patient with UIP and a suggestive form of CTD. If such an individual is considered to have IPF, immunosuppression is not indicated and may be harmful. But if that patient is, in fact, considered to have CTD-UIP, immunosuppression may be helpful and provide clinical benefit. Furthermore, when considering enrollment into an IPF clinical trial, how should those individuals who have suggestive forms of CTD be regarded? Should a patient with UIP and a positive specific autoantibody without evidence of a CTD be allowed to enroll in an IPF trial? Should a potentially beneficial IPF therapy be withheld from a patient with UIP when only a suggestive form of CTD has been identified?

## Summary

ILD is commonly encountered in patients with preexisting CTD or can be the presenting manifestation of a CTD. Furthermore, ILD frequently arises within the context of a suggestive form of CTD. Determining that ILD is associated with CTD and distinguishing these cases from non-CTD-ILD are clinically important, because this knowledge often has a significant impact on management and prognosis. The detection of occult CTD within the setting of a so-called "idiopathic" IP is challenging and often optimized by a multidisciplinary, thorough evaluation. When confronted with a patient with an IIP, clinicians should pay careful attention to a number of variables that include the demographic profile, historical clues, subtle physical examination findings, specific autoantibody positivity, radiologic findings, and histopathologic features in order to determine whether the ILD is CTD associated rather than "idiopathic."

## References

1. ATS/ERS. American Thoracic Society/European Respiratory Society International Multidisciplinary Consensus Classification of the Idiopathic Interstitial Pneumonias. This joint statement of the American Thoracic Society (ATS), and the European Respiratory Society (ERS) was adopted by the ATS board of directors, June 2001 and by the ERS Executive Committee, June 2001. Am J Respir Crit Care Med. 2002;165(2):277–304.
2. Raghu G, Collard HR, Egan JJ, Martinez FJ, Behr J, Brown KK, et al. An official ATS/ERS/JRS/ALAT statement: idiopathic pulmonary fibrosis: evidence-based guidelines for diagnosis and management. Am J Respir Crit Care Med. 2011;183(6):788–824.
3. Mosca M, Tani C, Carli L, Bombardieri S. Undifferentiated CTD: a wide spectrum of autoimmune diseases. Best Pract Res Clin Rheumatol. 2012;26(1):73–7.
4. Fischer A, du Bois R. Interstitial lung disease in connective tissue disorders. Lancet. 2012;380(9842):689–98.
5. Fischer A, du Bois RM. A practical approach to connective tissue disease-associated lung disease. In: Baughman RP, du Bois RM, editors. Diffuse lung disease: a practical approach. 2nd ed. New York: Springer; 2012. p. 217–37.
6. Cottin V. Interstitial lung disease: are we missing formes frustes of connective tissue disease? Eur Respir J. 2006;28(5):893–6.
7. Fischer A, West SG, Swigris JJ, Brown KK, du Bois RM. Connective tissue disease-associated interstitial lung disease: a call for clarification. Chest. 2010;138(2):251–6.
8. Tzelepis GE, Toya SP, Moutsopoulos HM. Occult connective tissue diseases mimicking idiopathic interstitial pneumonias. Eur Respir J. 2008;31(1):11–20.
9. Doyle TJ, Hunninghake GM, Rosas IO. Subclinical interstitial lung disease: why you should care. Am J Respir Crit Care Med. 2012;185(11):1147–53.
10. Camus P. Drug-induced infiltrative lung diseases. 4th ed. Hamilton: BC Decker, Inc.; 2003.

11. Frankel SK, Brown KK. Collagen vascular diseases of the lung. Clin Pulm Med. 2006; 13(1):25–36.
12. Olson AL, Brown KK. Connective tissue disease-associated lung disorders. Eur Respir Mongr. 2009;46:225–50.
13. Mittoo S, Gelber AC, Christopher-Stine L, Horton MR, Lechtzin N, Danoff SK. Ascertainment of collagen vascular disease in patients presenting with interstitial lung disease. Respir Med. 2009;103(8):1152–8.
14. Castelino FV, Goldberg H, Dellaripa PF. The impact of rheumatological evaluation in the management of patients with interstitial lung disease. Rheumatology (Oxford). 2011; 50(3):489–93.
15. Homma Y, Ohtsuka Y, Tanimura K, Kusaka H, Munakata M, Kawakami Y, et al. Can interstitial pneumonia as the sole presentation of collagen vascular diseases be differentiated from idiopathic interstitial pneumonia? Respiration. 1995;62(5):248–51.
16. Fischer A, Pfalzgraf FJ, Feghali-Bostwick CA, Wright TM, Curran-Everett D, West SG, et al. Anti-th/to-positivity in a cohort of patients with idiopathic pulmonary fibrosis. J Rheumatol. 2006;33(8):1600–5.
17. Fischer A, Meehan RT, Feghali-Bostwick CA, West SG, Brown KK. Unique characteristics of systemic sclerosis sine scleroderma-associated interstitial lung disease. Chest. 2006;130(4):976–81.
18. Fischer A, Swigris JJ, du Bois RM, Lynch DA, Downey GP, Cosgrove GP, et al. Anti-synthetase syndrome in ANA and anti-Jo-1 negative patients presenting with idiopathic interstitial pneumonia. Respir Med. 2009;103(11):1719–24.
19. Watanabe K, Handa T, Tanizawa K, Hosono Y, Taguchi Y, Noma S, et al. Detection of antisynthetase syndrome in patients with idiopathic interstitial pneumonias. Respir Med. 2011;105(8):1238–47.
20. Gizinski AM, Mascolo M, Loucks JL, Kervitsky A, Meehan RT, Brown KK, et al. Rheumatoid arthritis (RA)-specific autoantibodies in patients with interstitial lung disease and absence of clinically apparent articular RA. Clin Rheumatol. 2009;28(5):611–3.
21. Fischer A, Solomon JJ, du Bois RM, Deane KD, Olson AL, Fernandez-Perez ER, et al. Lung disease with anti-CCP antibodies but not rheumatoid arthritis or connective tissue disease. Respir Med. 2012;106(7):1040–7.
22. Kinder BW, Collard HR, Koth L, Daikh DI, Wolters PJ, Elicker B, et al. Idiopathic nonspecific interstitial pneumonia: lung manifestation of undifferentiated connective tissue disease? Am J Respir Crit Care Med. 2007;176(7):691–7.
23. Corte TJ, Copley SJ, Desai SR, Zappala CJ, Hansell DM, Nicholson AG, et al. Significance of connective tissue disease features in idiopathic interstitial pneumonia. Eur Respir J. 2012;39(3):661–8.
24. Vij R, Noth I, Strek ME. Autoimmune-featured interstitial lung disease: a distinct entity. Chest. 2011;140(5):1292–9.
25. Song JW, Do KH, Kim MY, Jang SJ, Colby TV, Kim DS. Pathologic and radiologic differences between idiopathic and collagen vascular disease-related usual interstitial pneumonia. Chest. 2009;136(1):23–30.
26. Flaherty KR, Colby TV, Travis WD, Toews GB, Mumford J, Murray S, et al. Fibroblastic foci in usual interstitial pneumonia: idiopathic versus collagen vascular disease. Am J Respir Crit Care Med. 2003;167(10):1410–5.
27. Papiris SA, Vlachoyiannopoulos PG, Maniati MA, Karakostas KX, Constantopoulos SH, Moutsopoulos HH. Idiopathic pulmonary fibrosis and pulmonary fibrosis in diffuse systemic sclerosis: two fibroses with different prognoses. Respiration. 1997;64(1):81–5.
28. Park JH, Kim DS, Park IN, Jang SJ, Kitaichi M, Nicholson AG, et al. Prognosis of fibrotic interstitial pneumonia: idiopathic versus collagen vascular disease-related subtypes. Am J Respir Crit Care Med. 2007;175(7):705–11.
29. Hwang JH, Misumi S, Sahin H, Brown KK, Newell JD, Lynch DA. Computed tomographic features of idiopathic fibrosing interstitial pneumonia: comparison with pulmonary fibrosis related to collagen vascular disease. J Comput Assist Tomogr. 2009;33(3):410–5.

30. Lynch DA. Quantitative CT, of fibrotic interstitial lung disease. Chest. 2007;131(3):643–4.
31. Lynch DA, Travis WD, Muller NL, Galvin JR, Hansell DM, Grenier PA, et al. Idiopathic inter-stitial pneumonias: CT features. Radiology. 2005;236(1):10–21.
32. Ito I, Nagai S, Kitaichi M, Nicholson AG, Johkoh T, Noma S, et al. Pulmonary manifestations of primary Sjogren's syndrome: a clinical, radiologic, and pathologic study. Am J Respir Crit Care Med. 2005;171(6):632–8.
33. Leslie KO, Trahan S, Gruden J. Pulmonary pathology of the rheumatic diseases. Semin Respir Crit Care Med. 2007;28(4):369–78.
34. Enomoto N, Suda T, Kato M, Kaida Y, Nakamura Y, Imokawa S, et al. Quantitative analysis of fibroblastic foci in usual interstitial pneumonia. Chest. 2006;130(1):22–9.
35. Flaherty KR, Mumford JA, Murray S, Kazerooni EA, Gross BH, Colby TV, et al. Prognostic implications of physiologic and radiographic changes in idiopathic interstitial pneumonia. Am J Respir Crit Care Med. 2003;168(5):543–8.
36. Fischer A, Brown KK, Frankel SK. Treatment of connective tissue disease related interstitial lung disease. Clin Pulm Med. 2009;16(2):74–80.
37. Hoyles RK, Ellis RW, Wellsbury J, Lees B, Newlands P, Goh NS, et al. A multicenter, prospec-tive, randomized, double-blind, placebo-controlled trial of corticosteroids and intravenous cyclophosphamide followed by oral azathioprine for the treatment of pulmonary fibrosis in scleroderma. Arthritis Rheum. 2006;54(12):3962–70.
38. Tashkin DP, Elashoff R, Clements PJ, Goldin J, Roth MD, Furst DE, et al. Cyclophosphamide versus placebo in scleroderma lung disease. N Engl J Med. 2006;354(25):2655–66.
39. Raghu G, Anstrom KJ, King Jr TE, Lasky JA, Martinez FJ. Prednisone, azathioprine, and N-acetylcysteine for pulmonary fibrosis. N Engl J Med. 2012;366(21):1968–77.
40. Kim EJ, Elicker BM, Maldonado F, Webb WR, Ryu JH, Van Uden JH, et al. Usual interstitial pneumonia in rheumatoid arthritis-associated interstitial lung disease. Eur Respir J. 2010;35(6):1322–8.
41. Lee HK, Kim DS, Yoo B, Seo JB, Rho JY, Colby TV, et al. Histopathologic pattern and clinical features of rheumatoid arthritis-associated interstitial lung disease. Chest. 2005;127(6):2019–27.
42. Kim EJ, Collard HR, King Jr TE. Rheumatoid arthritis-associated interstitial lung disease: the relevance of histopathologic and radiographic pattern. Chest. 2009;136(5):1397–405.
43. Bjoraker JA, Ryu JH, Edwin MK, Myers JL, Tazelaar HD, Schroeder DR, et al. Prognostic significance of histopathologic subsets in idiopathic pulmonary fibrosis. Am J Respir Crit Care Med. 1998;157(1):199–203.
44. Daniil ZD, Gilchrist FC, Nicholson AG, Hansell DM, Harris J, Colby TV, et al. A histologic pattern of nonspecific interstitial pneumonia is associated with a better prognosis than usual interstitial pneumonia in patients with cryptogenic fibrosing alveolitis. Am J Respir Crit Care Med. 1999;160(3):899–905.
45. Nicholson AG, Colby TV, du Bois RM, Hansell DM, Wells AU. The prognostic significance of the histologic pattern of interstitial pneumonia in patients presenting with the clinical entity of cryptogenic fibrosing alveolitis. Am J Respir Crit Care Med. 2000;162(6):2213–7.
46. Bouros D, Wells AU, Nicholson AG, Colby TV, Polychronopoulos V, Pantelidis P, et al. Histopathologic subsets of fibrosing alveolitis in patients with systemic sclerosis and their relationship to outcome. Am J Respir Crit Care Med. 2002;165(12):1581–6.

# Chapter 12
# Aging and IPF: What Is the Link?

Moisés Selman, Yair Romero, and Annie Pardo

**Abstract** Idiopathic pulmonary fibrosis (IPF) is a progressive and usually lethal interstitial lung disease of unknown etiology that is characterized by epithelial cell injury and aberrant activation, expansion of the mesenchymal cell population with the formation of fibroblast/myofibroblast foci, and exaggerated extracellular matrix accumulation. IPF is an aging-related disease, and most patients are over 60 years of age at the time of clinical presentation and diagnosis. Age also influences mortality, and the median survival time is significantly shorter in older individuals compared with younger patients. However, the fundamental mechanisms linking aging to IPF remain unclear. In this chapter, we will discuss some of the modifications naturally occurring in the elderly that may be implicated in the pathogenesis of IPF, including endoplasmic reticulum stress, oxidative stress, mitochondrial dysfunction, dysregulated autophagy, telomere attrition, and a number of epigenetic changes.

**Keywords** Pulmonary fibrosis • Aging • Alveolar epithelial cells • Epigenetic • Autophagy

M. Selman, M.D. (✉)
Dirección de Investigación, Instituto Nacional de Enfermedades Respiratorias,
Ismael Cosio Villegas, Tlalpan 4502, México D.F 14080, Mexico
e-mail: mselmanl@yahoo.com.mx; moises.selma@salud.gob.mx

Y. Romero, M.Sc. • A. Pardo, Ph.D.
Facultad de Ciencias, Laboratorio de Bioquímica, Universidad Nacional
Autónoma de México, México D.F., Mexico

K.C. Meyer and S.D. Nathan (eds.), *Idiopathic Pulmonary Fibrosis: A Comprehensive Clinical Guide*, Respiratory Medicine 9, DOI 10.1007/978-1-62703-682-5_12,
© Springer Science+Business Media New York 2014

# Introduction

## *Aging*

Aging is a complex process that is characterized by the progressive decline of the capacity to properly resolve the interaction between injury and repair, leading to progressive multi-organ deterioration and an elevated risk of disease. Aging is associated with the accumulation of damage to molecules, cells, and tissues over a lifetime, which leads to frailty and malfunction [1]. Two theories prevail regarding the aging process; specifically these include the programmed and the damage theories. The programmed concept holds the notion that cells or systems have a biological clock that is responsible for switching on deterioration (programmed longevity, telomere shortening, and immunological changes). The damage theory includes the cumulative effects of oxidative stress caused by free radicals, DNA damage, and other perpetuators. However, no single universal theory fully explains the aging process [2].

### Molecular Mechanisms of Aging

Currently, there are multiple modifications that appear to be involved in aging. These include oxidative stress, telomere shortening, heterochromatin loss, autophagy, senescence, and epigenetic changes. Multilevel combinations and interactions of these processes may participate in the normal aging process and explain the development of age-related diseases.

### Epigenetic Changes

Epigenetic modifications, including DNA methylation, histone modifications, noncoding RNA, nucleosome positioning, and chromatin arrangement, play central roles in controlling changes in gene expression and genome instability during aging [3].

### DNA Methylation

DNA methylation is the epigenetic change most frequently studied. In this process, DNA methyltransferases transfer a methyl group from $S$-adenosyl-methionine to the C5 position of the pyrimidine ring of cytosine residues in genomic CpG dinucleotides [4]. Hypermethylation in gene promoter or CpG island regions has been shown to repress, while hypomethylation enhances, gene expression [5, 6]. Importantly, DNA methylation does not occur exclusively at CpG islands but also in the so-called CpG island shores (regions of lower CpG density that lie in close proximity (~2 kb) of CpG islands), which are also closely associated with transcriptional inactivation.

Different methylation patterns have far-reaching implications for human biology and age-related diseases. With aging, a global hypomethylation process together with hypermethylation of a number of specific loci has been described. Loss of global DNA methylation over time has also been reported in cancer, but this loss is in repetitive sequences, and its effects on aging are unclear [7]. Likewise, multiple genes from tumor suppressor factors, DNA-binding factors, and transcription factors are increasingly methylated with age [8, 9]. In general, cancer cells are characterized by a massive global loss of DNA methylation, while specific patterns of hypermethylation at the CpG islands of certain promoters are often acquired [10].

**Histone Modifications**

Histones are basic proteins that interact with DNA, and their posttranslational modifications affect accessibility of diverse transcription factors to the genome. Normally, the nucleosome is composed of a histone octamer with two groups of H2A, H2B, H3, and H4. Histone H1 is located between each nucleosome, which is subject to many types of posttranslational modifications (e.g., methylation, acetylation, phosphorylation, ubiquitination, SUMOylation), especially on their flexible amino-terminal tails [11].

The main histone modifications are acetylation and methylation. Histone hyperacetylation is characterized by a relaxed chromatin structure and active gene transcription, while deacetylation is linked with a compact and inactive chromatin structure. Histones can become mono-, di-, or trimethylated, and the functional consequences depend on the number of methyl groups, the residue itself, and its location within the histone tail. Repression marks could play a pivotal role in aging. Loss of H3K27 trimethylation via downregulation of the histone methyltransferase, EzH2, in humans could be associated with aging [12]. Likewise, H4K16 hypoacetylation, which is caused by the reduced association of a histone acetyltransferase, leads to early onset of cellular senescence [13].

**Nucleosome Positioning and Chromatin Arrangement in the Nucleus**

Chromatin involves DNA and all associated proteins, but their configuration and distribution along the nucleus are still poorly characterized. The fundamental unit of chromatin is the nucleosome, and ATP-dependent chromatin-remodeling complexes, which alter nucleosome composition and positioning, are necessary to increase DNA accessibility and to carry out transcription as well as DNA repair [14]. In terms of its transcriptional state, euchromatin is transcriptionally active and is characterized by high levels of acetylation and trimethylated H3K4, H3K36, and H3K79. In contrast, heterochromatin contains low levels of acetylation and high levels of H3K9, H3K27, and H4K20 methylation and is related to transcriptional repression.

A heterochromatin loss model of aging has been proposed, which suggests that heterochromatin domains that were established during embryogenesis decline with the aging process [15]. Recent observations indicate a significant interdependence between heterochromatin, epigenetic landscape, and aging [16]. Evidence indicates that epigenetics have a fundamental role in aging; mainly, H3K27me3 and acetylation on H4K16, which are both repressive marks, decline over time [17]. However, detection of numerous noncoding RNAs from heterochromatic regions challenges the concept of heterochromatin as a transcriptionally inactive region [18].

## Noncoding RNA

Recent evidence supports the notion that noncoding RNAs play a critical and dynamic role in transcriptional regulation and epigenetic signaling [19]. Based on its length, noncoding RNAs can be divided into at least three groups: short ncRNA, including microRNA (miRNA; 22–23 nts) and piwi-interacting RNA (piRNA; 26–31 nts); medium ncRNA (50–200 nts); and long ncRNA (>200 nts). miRNAs are the best characterized and are primarily involved in posttranscriptional regulation of mRNA [20].

Recent studies demonstrate that diverse miRNAs are differentially expressed during aging. In general, the patterns of miRNA expression during aging appear to be tissue specific. For example, miR-669c and miR-709 levels are increased in mid-age (18-month to 33-month) murine liver tissue, whereas miR-93 and miR-214 are increased in extremely old (33-month) mice compared with 4- or 10-month-old mice [21]. Likewise, upregulation of miR-143 induces senescence in human fibroblasts [22]. Actually, many miRNAs seem to be key modulators of cellular senescence and influence specific senescence-regulatory proteins [23].

## Oxidative Stress, Autophagy, and Caloric Restriction

Accumulation of damage contributes to the aging phenotype and to age-related diseases. Three key processes, oxidative stress, autophagy, and caloric restriction, can increase, reduce, or prevent damage that causes cellular dysfunction.

## Oxidative Stress

Reactive oxygen species (ROS) are mainly produced in the mitochondria and affect cell function when an imbalance occurs between the production of ROS and the activity of detoxification enzymes such as superoxide dismutases, catalases, glutathione peroxidases, and peroxiredoxins. Strong evidence supports that the average life span is inversely correlated with the rate of mitochondrial superoxide anions and hydrogen peroxide generation. Moreover, the rates of ROS production from mitochondria increase with age in the brain, heart, and kidney of mice [24]. In addition, a wide spectrum of alterations in mitochondria and mitochondrial DNA have been observed with aging, including disorganization of mitochondrial structure, decline in mitochondrial oxidative phosphorylation function, and accumulation of mtDNA mutations [24].

## Autophagy

Autophagy is a homeostatic process of self-degradation of cellular components. There are three general types of autophagy: microautophagy, chaperone-mediated autophagy (CMA), and macroautophagy. Macroautophagy is the most widely studied process and represents the major pathway of degradation under basal cellular activity. It is usually upregulated by several stimuli that include starvation, hypoxia, microbial infection, endoplasmic reticulum (ER) stress, and oxidative stress [25]. Damaged, superfluous macromolecules or organelles must be isolated from cytosol by autophagosomes. The formation of phagophores requires generation of phospholipid "PtdIns3p" and involvement of two ubiquitin-like systems: LC3 and ATG5-12-16. Phagophores expand to form complete autophagosomes with a double membrane, and the external membrane merges with the lysosome membrane to degrade internal vesicles. CMA is a selective autophagy of soluble proteins that requires unfolding of the cargo protein before entering lysosomes and interacting with a receptor protein, lysosome-associated protein type 2A (LAMP-2A). In microautophagy, the lysosomal membrane itself invaginates to trap the cargo.

Importantly, autophagy declines with age and causes accumulation of toxic metabolites in the cell, which may be due to a specific CMA failure and to an unsatisfactory degradation of lysosomes [26, 27].

Microautophagy represents the specific degradation of mitochondria, which are very susceptible to damage in aging, and it is involved with the unfolding protein response (UPR) in the endoplasmic reticulum that can activate apoptosis [28, 29].

Defects in the cellular machinery that mediate autophagy are present in almost all age-related diseases, including cancer, metabolic disorders, and neurodegenerative diseases. Evidence shows that autophagy activity must be maintained in order to extend life span in various genetically modified organisms, and autophagy-related proteins have been shown to directly mediate longevity pathways [30].

## Senescence and Telomere Shortening

Cellular senescence is synonymous with an irreversible arrest of cell growth. In normal replicative senescence, the cell simply enters senescence after a certain number of replications, which is primarily related to a progressive shortening of telomeres [31]. In addition, differential expression of p53 isoforms and of the retinoblastoma tumor suppressor protein and its signaling partners including p16INK4A (a cyclin-dependent kinase inhibitor) has been linked to replicative senescence [32]. However, premature senescence can be induced in the absence of any detectable telomere loss or dysfunction by a variety of stresses. In general, if DNA damage exceeds a certain threshold, cells are destined to undergo either apoptosis or senescence.

**Telomere Shortening**

Telomeres are tandem arrays of duplex 5′-TTAGGG-3′ repeats located at the ends of eukaryotic chromosomes that protect them from degradation and DNA repair activities. The maintenance of telomeres depends on a specialized ribonucleoprotein, telomerase, which is an RNA-dependent DNA polymerase that can synthesize telomeric repeats and extend telomeres de novo during cell division [33]. Telomerases have two essential components: telomerase reverse transcriptase (TERT) and RNA template (TR). After birth, telomerase is silenced in most somatic cells, and telomeres progressively shorten with aging [31, 34]. Critically short telomeres cannot be repaired by any of the known DNA repair mechanisms, and shortened telomeres consequently trigger a persistent DNA damage response that leads to cellular senescence and/or apoptosis that eventually compromises tissue regenerative capacity and function, which contributes to organismal aging [34].

# Aging Lung

Most of the age-related functional changes in the respiratory system involve alterations in the lung itself as well as a decrease in compliance of the chest wall and a decrease in the strength of the respiratory muscles, which affects control of breathing. However, the rate of progression of these changes can differ greatly from person to person.

The aging lung is characterized by decreased static elastic recoil, dilatation of alveolar ducts and alveoli with a loss of gas exchange surface area, and a decline in the number of capillaries per alveolus, which is often referred to as "senile emphysema." This goes along with a decrease in the diameter of small airways that increases their tendency to close at a given lung volume, which leads to a decrease in expiratory flows and elicits an increase in residual volume at the expense of vital capacity [35]. Concomitantly, there is an increase in lung compliance while chest wall compliance progressively declines, which is presumably related to calcification and other structural changes within the rib cage and its articulations [36].

**Extracellular Matrix**

The decrease in the lung elastic recoil has been associated with structural and functional alterations in the extracellular matrix (ECM) of the lung parenchyma. Collagens and elastin are the main proteins in the ECM that comprise the scaffold of the alveolar structures and are central in determining the mechanical properties of lung parenchyma. In general, elastic fibers primarily influence lung compliance at the lower pressure range, while collagen fibrils become more important at high lung volumes where inflation becomes limited. Several studies have demonstrated that changes in lung mechanics are associated with structural modifications of the lung ECM. Collagens are the most abundant proteins of the ECM, and collagens represent 15 % to 20 % of the total dry weight of lung tissue. The collagen family is constituted by 28 different types of collagen proteins that together with other ECM components organize a complex network in the lung tissue. Fibrillar types I and III collagens are the most abundant and represent 90 % of the total lung collagen.

Many age-associated alterations of organs and tissues are associated with changes of the ECM proteins. Such changes include differences in posttranslational modifications of glycoproteins such as advanced glycation end-products (AGEs), which in turn influence the turnover of other glycoproteins [37].

Glycation, glycoxidation, and cross-linking of collagens are increased in many aged tissues, which cause changes of physical properties that include fiber stiffness and higher resistance to degradation [37, 38]. Studies in mice have shown that the process of aging contributes to an altered lung ECM, including fibrillar collagens and the AGE load [39].

It is unclear how the total collagen lung content changes with aging. Some bio-chemical studies in experimental models describe no changes, an increase, or a decrease in collagen proteins in response to lung aging [40–43]. The different results might be related to differences in the methodological procedures used to measure lung collagen content.

Although there is also some debate about the total elastin content in old lung tis-sue, it appears that functionally intact elastin is reduced with aging, which could also be influenced by an increased modification with AGEs [44, 45].

## Immune Response

The aging lung exhibits an increased susceptibility to infections and inflammation, and alterations in both the innate and adaptive arms of the immune system have been implicated.

During the aging process, the lungs usually exhibit some degree of inflammation, even in healthy individuals. Thus, there is evidence for an augmented proinflamma-tory milieu, with increased levels of cytokines and acute-phase molecules in associa-tion with functional decline, a phenomenon that has been termed the "inflamm-aging" [46]. Furthermore, increased levels of interleukin (IL)-1, IL-6, IL-8, IL-18, IL-1 receptor antagonist, and tumor necrosis factor (TNF)-alpha are found in plasma, serum, and mononuclear blood cell culture from elderly subjects [47].

Additionally, a number of alterations in the T-cell-mediated immune response that affect the function and proportions of T-cell subsets are associated with advanc-ing age. Immunosenescence, characterized by a reduction of naive T-cells and a shrinking T-cell repertoire, is a well-recognized phenomenon in humans and ani-mals and is likely responsible for the increased susceptibility to infections and can-cer in older individuals [48]. Numerous studies indicate that aging is associated with impaired influenza virus-specific T-cell responses that may be related to a decreased frequency of naive T-cells as well as diminished function of memory and effector T-cells [49]. A decreased memory CD4+ T-cell response to the influenza vaccine has been reported in the elderly, and the CD8+ T-cell response to the influenza virus also diminishes with advancing age [50, 51].

Specifically relevant to the fibrotic response, normal aging is associated with a shift in T lymphocytes from a predominantly Th1 phenotype to a predominantly Th2 phenotype, which is especially evident in frail older people. The Th2-like response promotes the expression of profibrotic factors, and Th2-biased animals are more susceptible to lung injury and fibrosis [52]. Humans with chronic fibrotic lung disease also demonstrate a Th2-biased phenotype [52].

Toll-like receptors (TLRs), initially described as pattern-recognition receptors that identify and protect against microbes, can display impaired function with aging. Specifically, TLR4 function declines with age or cigarette smoke exposure in humans. Furthermore, mice deficient in TLR4 exhibit age-related lung enlargement that is similar, both histologically and functionally, to human lung emphysema. Additionally, TLR4 deficiency is associated with increased reactive oxygen species generation, collectively referred to as oxidant stress, via the upregulation of the NADPH oxidase, Nox3 [53].

## Oxidative Stress

Increased oxidative stress, resulting from an imbalance of pro-oxidants and antioxidants, occurs with aging, and the excessive, destructive presence of reactive oxygen species can adversely affect the lung. Senescence of the pulmonary endothelium is implicated in susceptibility to oxidative stress, impaired nitric oxide signaling, and insufficient tissue repair and regeneration [54]. In general, enzymes implicated in the cytoprotective reduction of ROS, such as Cu/Zn superoxide dismutase and NADPH oxidase (among others), tend to have decreased levels in aged pulmonary endothelial cells [55].

## Epigenetic Changes in the Aging Lung

Age-related changes in DNA methylation, as described above, have been implicated in cellular senescence and longevity, although the causes and functional consequences in the lungs remain unclear. Lepeule et al. examined the relationships between DNA methylation in nine genes related to inflammation and lung function in a cohort of 756 elderly men (73.3 ± 6.7 years old) [55]. They found that older people had decreased DNA methylation in the carnitine O-acetyltransferase (CRAT), coagulation factor-3 (F3), and Toll-like receptor-2 (TLR2) genes that was significantly associated with lower values for forced vital capacity (FVC) and forced expiratory volume in 1 s (FEV1). This decline in lung function is considered to be related to changes in the large airways. By contrast, decreased methylation in interferon-gamma (IFNγ) and IL-6 genes was paradoxically associated with better lung function. This finding might be explained by the varying roles of IFNγ and IL-6, which may display pro- and anti-inflammatory activities [55].

In summary, the cellular and molecular mechanisms of physiological aging and their association with various lung diseases are still not well understood. Oxidative stress, telomere length regulation, cellular immunosenescence, epigenetic changes, and ECM modifications probably represent some of the key mechanisms that account for declining lung function with advanced age.

## Aging in the Pathogenesis of Idiopathic Pulmonary Fibrosis (IPF)

IPF is a progressive and lethal lung disease of unclear etiology that primarily affects older patients. Symptoms usually occur between ages 50 and 70, and most patients are older than 60 years at the time of clinical presentation and diagnosis. Both the prevalence and incidence of IPF increase markedly with advancing age, particularly after the sixth decade, with a prevalence that has been estimated to exceed 175 cases per 100,000 individuals over 75 years of age [56]. Age also influences mortality, and the median survival time is significantly shorter in older individuals compared with younger patients [57].

Interestingly, predominantly subpleural basal reticular abnormalities on high-resolution computed tomography (HRCT) have been identified in a large number of asymptomatic individuals over 75 years of age, whereas these findings are virtually absent in those under 55 years old [58]. In addition, cysts can be seen in 25 % of subjects in the older age group. Bronchial dilation and wall thickening are also seen significantly more often in older individuals compared to a those in a younger age group. Importantly, all these findings have been demonstrated as independent of pack-year smoking history and indicate that some older individuals may develop interstitial lung abnormalities suggestive of possible UIP without apparent clinical significance. However, uncertainty still remains regarding the relevance of these findings to lung health and whether there are any long-term prognostic implications. In the same context, it has been demonstrated that subclinical interstitial lung disease (ILD) with subpleural distribution is present in a significant proportion of older smokers (56–72 years) screened for the development of COPD [59]. In this study, as compared with participants without interstitial changes on HRCT, those with abnormalities were more likely to have a restrictive lung deficit, suggesting that subclinical ILD may represent an early disease stage for a subset of individuals who will progress to clinically significant ILD.

## Mechanisms Linking IPF to Aging

The fundamental molecular mechanism linking aging to IPF is unknown, but several modifications naturally occurring in the elderly may be implicated including oxidative stress, mitochondrial dysfunction, deregulated autophagy, telomere attrition, and others (Fig. 12.1).

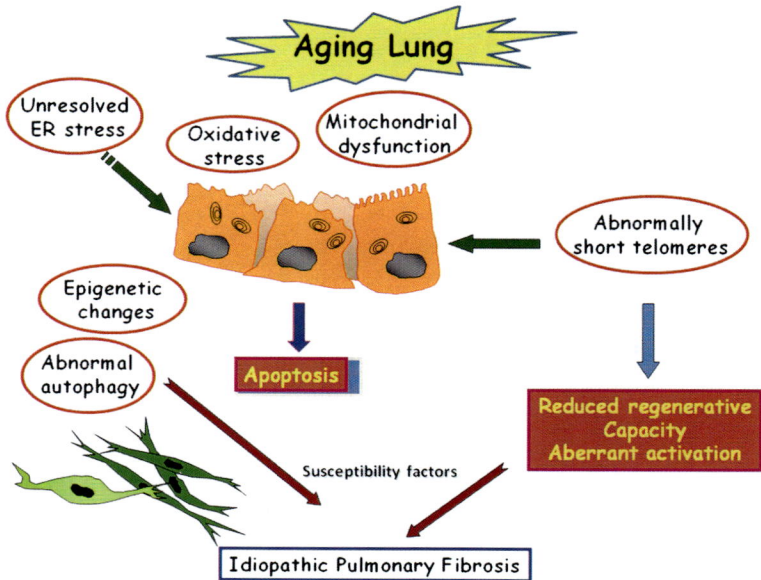

**Fig. 12.1** Putative mechanisms linking aging to the development of IPF. A variety of modifications naturally occurring in the elderly may affect the behavior of alveolar epithelial cells (in *yellow*) or fibroblasts (in *green*), increasing the susceptibility to develop IPF

## Oxidative Stress

Reactive oxygen species (ROS) induce cellular dysfunction (such as stress-induced premature senescence), which is believed to contribute to normal aging and play a role in age-related diseases. In aging, systemic imbalance between the antioxidant system (e.g., superoxide dismutases, glutathione) and ROS results in the generation of excess free radicals that can overwhelm cellular antioxidant defenses. Several studies have associated excessive oxidative stress with IPF. Thus, for example, mitochondrial generation of ROS has been suggested to be linked to increased cellular oxidative stress and apoptosis of alveolar epithelial cells [60]. Moreover, there is evidence suggesting that ROS can increase the release of TGF-β from alveolar epithelial cells [61] and can directly activate TGF-β in cell-free systems by disrupting its interaction with latency-associated peptide [62].

Strong evidence has shown that the transcription factor called nuclear factor (erythroid-derived 2)-like 2, or Nrf2, is a "master regulator" in the antioxidant response through the coordinated induction of antioxidant and phase II detoxifying enzymes that are under the regulatory influence of the antioxidant response mechanism [63]. Importantly, however, Nrf2 modulates the expression of hundreds of genes including not only antioxidant enzymes but a large number of genes that control tissue remodeling and fibrosis [63]. Mice that lack Nrf2 are highly susceptible to bleomycin-induced pulmonary inflammation and fibrosis, likely by inducing a Th1 to Th2 switch [64]. However, the expression of Nrf2 has been found to be increased in IPF lungs, which may represent an unsuccessful adaptive attempt to compensate for the increased oxidant burden [65]. Of particular interest, the increased expression of Nrf2 in IPF lungs was localized to alveolar epithelial cells whose chronic injury/activation is a crucial pathogenic event in IPF. More recently, however, decreased expression of nuclear Nrf2 was demonstrated in lung fibroblasts from patients with IPF, which was associated with the appearance of a myofibroblast phenotype [66]. Moreover, Nrf2 inhibition with siRNA induced myofibroblastic differentiation that was associated with increased oxidative stress, while conversely, Nrf2 activation with Keap1 knockdown restored the oxidant/antioxidant balance and reversed the myofibroblastic differentiation [66].

**Endoplasmic Reticulum (ER) Stress**

Several recent reports have demonstrated that ER stress and apoptosis occur frequently in alveolar epithelial cells (AECs) from IPF lungs [67, 68]. To better understand the putative implication of ER stress in the pathogenesis of lung fibrosis, Lawson et al. developed a transgenic mouse model in which the inducible mutant, L188Q SFTPC, was expressed in type II AECs in the adult mouse. Interestingly, the expression of L188Q SFTPC in type II AECs resulted in ER stress and unfolded protein response (UPR) activation but did not result in fibrotic remodeling. However, after a second profibrotic stimulus (bleomycin) was administered, increased epithelial cell death and fibroblast accumulation with an enhanced lung fibrotic response was found [69]. Similar findings were observed in mice treated with the ER stress-inducing agent tunicamycin. These findings indicate that dysfunctional type II AECs predispose the lung to excessive and dysregulated remodeling after injury.

Importantly, the cell has evolved an adaptive coordinated response to limit accumulation of unfolded proteins in the ER through a series of cell protective responses known collectively as the UPR. With advanced age, however, many of the key components of the UPR (such as the chaperones and enzymes) display reduced expression and activity resulting in ER dysfunction. Moreover, those proteins that remain are more vulnerable to oxidation by ROS [70]. In fact, several recent studies examining the effect of age on the ER stress response support the notion of a diminished protective response and more robust proapoptotic signaling with aging [71].

Therefore, it is possible to speculate that older individuals may have ER stress induced by multiple environmental injuries. Furthermore, because the UP is less efficient in AECs, these cells may respond with apoptotic pathway activation or induced changes in cell phenotype that can occur through epithelial to mesenchymal transition, which may increase the risk to develop IPF.

**Autophagy**

Autophagy, one mechanism by which the cell rids itself of misfolded proteins, declines with age and contributes to cellular senescence. The role of autophagy in fibrosis has recently being examined, but results from different models have given contradictory results. Therefore, the role of autophagy in disease pathogenesis remains unclear and may involve either impaired or accelerated autophagic activity or imbalances in the activation of autophagic proteins. For example, recent findings suggest that autophagy represents a cytoprotective mechanism that negatively regulates and limits excess collagen accumulation in the kidney, thereby mitigating experimental renal fibrosis [72]. Thus, reduced beclin-1 expression in primary mouse mesangial cells results in increased levels of type I collagen (Col-I). Inhibition of autolysosomal protein degradation by bafilomycin A(1) also increased Col-I protein levels, whereas treatment with trifluoperazine, an inducer of autophagy, results in decreased induction of Col-I levels by TGF-β1 (without alterations in Col-I α1 mRNA). By contrast, autophagy of activated stellate cells has been found to be a necessary requirement for hepatic fibrogenesis in mice [73]. In this case, loss of autophagic function in cultured mouse stellate cells and in mice following hepatic injury was associated with reduced fibrogenesis and matrix accumulation. According to these results, autophagy provides energy that is essential to support stellate cell activation and maintain energy homeostasis in the face of increasing cellular energy demands conferred by fibrogenesis and cell proliferation [73].

It has been shown that genetic or pharmacologic inhibition of Toll-like receptor 4 (TLR4) exacerbates bleomycin-induced pulmonary inflammation and fibrosis by attenuating autophagy-associated degradation of collagen and cell death in fibrotic lung tissues [74]. Moreover, rapamycin, an autophagy activator, reverses the effects of TLR4 antagonism, while attenuation of autophagy by 3-methyladenine reverses the pro-resolving and antifibrotic roles of TLR4 agonists and was associated with reduced survival.

Similarly, lung tissues from patients with IPF demonstrate evidence of decreased autophagic activity as assessed by LC3, p62 protein expression and immunofluorescence, and numbers of autophagosomes [75]. In addition, this report provided evidence that autophagy is not activated in the setting of IPF despite well-described elevations in ER stress, oxidative stress, and (HIF)-1α, which are all known to induce autophagy. Moreover, in vitro experiments demonstrate that the profibrotic mediator, TGF-β1, is likely responsible for the decreased autophagy [75].

Recent evidence has described a potential role of autophagy in aging-associated organ deterioration. Thus, cardiac hypertrophy and fibrosis have been found in aged mice compared with young mice. Levels of beclin-1, Atg5, and the LC3-II/LC3-I ratio were decreased in aged hearts. The involvement of autophagy in cardiac aging was further substantiated by the induction of in vitro autophagy with rapamycin alleviating aging-induced cardiomyocyte mechanical and intracellular Ca2+ derangements [76].

The above findings in various models indicate that the function of autophagy in fibrotic processes remains unclear and may involve either impaired or accelerated autophagic activity. In chronic obstructive pulmonary disease (COPD), another aging-related disease, there is an increase of several autophagic proteins in the lung tissue, while ultrastructural analysis of COPD tissue reveals an increased abundance of autophagosomes relative to normal lung tissue [77]. By contrast, in the case of IPF, the autophagic response seems to be impaired.

## Telomere Shortening

A number of age-related pathologies (including that found in the IPF lung and in premature aging syndromes) have been associated with an accelerated rate of telomere shortening. The speed at which telomeres shorten with aging can be influenced by factors considered to accelerate aging and increase the risk of premature death, such as socioeconomic status, perceived stress, smoking, and obesity (all of which have been proposed to negatively affect telomere length) [78]. Studies in patients with familial forms of pulmonary fibrosis have found that the disease appears to be associated with telomere shortening in a subset of patients. This disease susceptibility is provoked by mutations in hTERT or hTR, which underlie the inheritance in 8–15 % of familial cases [79, 80]. In contrast, telomerase mutations are uncommon in patients with sporadic IPF. However, patients with IPF may show telomere lengths below the first percentile for their age in circulating leukocytes, and, importantly, telomeres have been shown to be shortened in alveolar epithelial cells from IPF lungs [81].

However, shortening of telomeres is also observed in COPD [82]. Moreover, telomerase-deficient mice that have sequential shortening of telomeres spontaneously develop emphysema-like lung lesions [83]. Curiously, telomerase deficiency in a murine model leads to telomere shortening, but this does not predispose these animals to enhanced bleomycin-induced lung fibrosis [84].

## Epigenetic Changes

As mentioned, environmental factors may contribute to aging-associated diseases through the induction of epigenetic modifications, such as DNA methylation and chromatin remodeling, which may induce alterations in gene expression programs. The definitive corroboration on intraindividual epigenetic variation over time in humans was recently provided in a longitudinal study of DNA methylation patterns in which successive DNA samples were collected more than 10 years apart in more than 100 individuals [7]. Time-dependent changes in global DNA methylation of greater than 20 % were observed within the same individual over an 11- to 16-year span within 8–10 % of individuals in two separate study populations that resided in two widely separated geographic locations. In this study, both losses and gains of DNA methylation were observed over time in different individuals.

In a recent study in IPF, the global methylation pattern was evaluated using human CpG island microarrays [85]. Differential methylation in 625 CpG islands was found in IPF lung tissue samples when compared to control lung tissue samples. Most of these methylation changes were located in intronic, exonic, or intergenic areas, but only 8.8 % were found in gene promoters, where hypomethylation of CpG islands was generally found. The genes with differentially methylated CpG islands in their promoters were associated with biological processes such as cellular assembly and organization, cellular growth and proliferation, cell morphology, cancer, cell signaling, gene expression, and cell death. Interestingly, this study also revealed that the methylation pattern observed in IPF shows great similarity to the methylation pattern of lung cancer.

In another recent study, genome-wide DNA methylation and RNA expression were also examined in IPF and normal control lung tissue [86]. No differences were observed in global DNA methylation, but higher DNMT3a and 3b expression levels were noticed in the IPF lung tissue. Several interesting genes were found to be hyper- or hypomethylated (e.g., TP53INP1, a p53-inducible cell stress response protein that can upregulate genes, and claudin 5 and ZNF167, which are zinc finger proteins that enhance nuclear retention and transactivation of STAT3 that can down-regulate genes) [86].

Hypo- or hypermethylation of some specific genes has been reported in IPF [86]. Thus, for example, hypomethylated DNA seems to contribute to the rapid progression of IPF through a Toll-like receptor (TLR) 9-dependent process [87]. Under this mechanism, surgical lung biopsies from rapidly progressive IPF patients clinically exhibit elevated levels of TLR9 gene transcript expression compared to those from stable IPF patients.

Thy-1(CD90) is a cell-surface glycoprotein expressed in normal lung fibroblasts that modulates the profibrotic phenotype of fibroblasts by several mechanisms [88, 89]. In fibroblastic foci of IPF lungs, epigenetic silencing of Thy-1 by promoter region hypermethylation has been demonstrated [90]. After this first report, it was found that treatment with the histone deacetylase inhibitor, trichostatin A, restored Thy-1 expression in Thy-1(−) cells in a time-dependent and concentration-dependent fashion, which was associated with enrichment of histone acetylation [91]. Importantly, restoration of the expression of Thy-1 was associated with both changes in chromatin marks and demethylation of the Thy-1 promoter region. This supports the concept that histone modifications and DNA methylation are coordinately regulated to change the biological behavior of fibrotic lung fibroblasts.

More recently, it has been demonstrated that IPF fibroblasts have reduced expression of the proapoptotic p14ARF due to promoter hypermethylation of CpG islands, which may explain, at least partially, their likely resistance to apoptosis [92]. P14ARF gene expression was restored by treatment with the DNA methyltransferase inhibitor, 5-aza, and this result was further corroborated by using restriction digestion with McrBc, which showed a high level of methylation of the p14ARF promoter in IPF fibroblast primary lines.

## Chromatin Structural Changes

Defective histone acetylation is responsible for the repression of COX2 expression, a gene that is likely involved in the antifibrotic response [93]. Using a chromatin immunoprecipitation assay, it was revealed that transcription factor binding to the COX-2 promoter was reduced in IPF fibroblasts compared to that in normal fibroblasts. This effect was dynamically linked to reduced histone H3 and H4 acetylation due to decreased recruitment of histone acetyltransferases and recruitment of the NCoR, CoREST, and mSin3a transcriptional corepressor complexes to the COX-2 promoter [93].

### Epigenetic Control of Epithelial to Mesenchymal Transition (EMT)

EMT is a fundamental developmental process that involves actin cytoskeleton reorganization with loss of apical-basal polarity and cell-to-cell contact, resulting in the conversion of epithelial cells to mesenchymal cells [94]. Although there is still some controversy, several studies suggest that an EMT-like process occurs in IPF [95–98]. Recently, global epigenetic reprogramming was observed during TGF-β(beta)-induced EMT in mouse hepatocytes [99]. In this study, the dynamic nature of genome-scale epigenetic reprogramming during EMT induced by this growth factor was demonstrated. Specifically, genome-wide reprogramming of large heterochromatin domains (LOCKs) to a state of reduced H3K9Me2, new LOCK-wide modifications of H3K4Me3 at specific GC-rich LOCKs, and enrichment of H3K36Me3 at LOCK boundaries and numerous EMT-related genes was demonstrated across the genome. This reprogramming appeared to be critical for the EMT induction by TGF-β, because inhibition of bulk chromatin changes by Lsd1 loss of function had marked effects on cell migration and chemoresistance [99].

However, it is unclear if aging affects EMT of alveolar epithelial cells. Interestingly, aging-associated cellular senescence may be involved. Thus, accumulating evidence shows that senescent fibroblasts that acquire a senescence-associated secretory phenotype have the ability to promote tumor progression, in part by inducing EMT in nearby epithelial cells [100]. Moreover, increasing evidence suggests that EMT and senescence, two processes that seem to operate independently, are in fact intertwined [101].

### MicroRNAs

As mentioned, miRNAs form a particular class of 21- to 24-nucleotide RNAs that can regulate gene expression posttranscriptionally by affecting the translation and stability of target messenger RNAs. Importantly, some miRNAs have emerged as key regulators during cellular senescence.

A growing body of evidence indicates that dysregulated expression of miRNAs is linked to fibrotic diseases in different organs [102–108]. Recent evidence also supports the notion that miRNAs can regulate cellular plasticity. For example, miR-145 expression facilitates the differentiation of fibroblasts to myofibroblasts suggesting that miRNAs may regulate the plasticity of mesenchymal cells [109].

Regarding lung fibrotic remodeling, several studies have reported disturbed expression of a number of miRNAs. For example, downregulation of mir-29 has been found in bleomycin-induced lung fibrosis in mice. In addition, miR-29 is suppressed by TGF-β1 in lung fibroblasts, and miR-29 levels are inversely correlated with the expression of several profibrotic target genes and with the severity of the fibrosis [110]. By contrast, lungs of mice with bleomycin-induced fibrosis as well as IPF lungs show an upregulation of miR-21 primarily localized to myofibroblasts [105]. Increasing miR-21 levels promote, while reduced levels attenuate, the profibrogenic activity of TGF-β1 in fibroblasts, while miR-21 antisense probes attenuate bleomycin-induced lung fibrosis. Likewise, miR-155 (targeting the angiotensin II type 1 receptor) and keratinocyte growth factor are upregulated in the lungs of mice with bleomycin-induced lung fibrosis [111, 112].

The extent of changes of miRNAs in IPF lungs was recently demonstrated when RNA from IPF and control lungs was extracted and hybridized to miRNA arrays that contained probes for ~450 miRNAs. In this work, 10 % of the miRNAs on the array were significantly different between IPF and control lungs [104]. One of the downregulated miRNAs, let-7d, was primarily localized in epithelial cells and was directly inhibited by TGF-β. Let-7d regulates EMT in alveolar epithelial cells (at least partially) due to the overexpression of the high-mobility group, AT-hook 2 (HMGA2), a member of the nonhistone chromosomal high-mobility group (HMG) protein family.

## Summary

Recent research into the mechanisms of aging and IPF has suggested that they share several common molecular pathways including mitochondrial dysfunction, dysregulated autophagy, telomere attrition, epigenetic changes, and others. However, many studies are still necessary to verify the existing findings in larger cohorts and to establish the mechanisms underlying the putative association between aging and IPF. Identification of the aging-affected signaling pathways that are implicated in the pathogenesis of the pulmonary fibrosis also holds promise in furthering our understanding of IPF. A better knowledge of the age-related changes in lung cells will also help to elucidate the lung aging process itself and eventually to recognize which of these modifications are truly involved in the pathogenesis of IPF.

**Acknowledgment** Our research was partially supported by PAPIIT IN214612.

## References

1. Heemels MT. Ageing. Nature. 2010;464:503.
2. Berdasco M, Esteller M. Hot topics in epigenetic mechanisms of aging: 2011. Aging Cell. 2012;11:181–6.

3. Rando TA, Chang HY. Aging, rejuvenation, and epigenetic reprogramming: resetting the aging clock. Cell. 2012;148:46–57.
4. Lister R, Ecker JR. Finding the fifth base: genome-wide sequencing of cytosine methylation. Genome Res. 2009;19:959–66.
5. Weber M, Hellmann I, Stadler MB, Ramos L, Pääbo S, Rebhan M, et al. Distribution, silencing potential and evolutionary impact of promoter DNA methylation in the human genome. Nat Genet. 2007;39:457–66.
6. Irizarry RA, Ladd-Acosta C, Wen B, Wu Z, Montano C, Onyango P, et al. The human colon cancer methylome shows similar hypo- and hypermethylation at conserved tissue-specific CpG island shores. Nat Genet. 2009;41:178–86.
7. Bjornsson HT, Sigurdsson MI, Fallin MD, Irizarry RA, Aspelund T, Cui H, et al. Intra-individual change over time in DNA methylation with familial clustering. JAMA. 2008;299:2877–83.
8. So K, Tamura G, Honda T, Homma N, Waki T, Togawa N, et al. Multiple tumor suppressor genes are increasingly methylated with age in non-neoplastic gastric epithelia. Cancer Sci. 2006;97:1155–58.
9. Hernandez DG, Nalls MA, Gibbs JR, Arepalli S, van der Brug M, Chong S, et al. Distinct DNA methylation changes highly correlated with chronological age in the human brain. Hum Mol Genet. 2011;20:1164–72.
10. Portela A, Esteller M. Epigenetic modifications and human disease. Nat Biotechnol. 2010;28:1057–68.
11. Lachner M, Jenuwein T. The many faces of histone lysine methylation. Curr Opin Cell Biol. 2002;14:286–98.
12. Shumaker DK, Dechat T, Kohlmaier A, Adam SA, Bozovsky MR, Erdos MR, et al. Mutant nuclear lamin A leads to progressive alterations of epigenetic control in premature aging. Proc Natl Acad Sci USA. 2006;103:8703–8.
13. Krishnan V, Chow MZ, Wang Z, Zhang L, Liu B, Liu X, et al. Histone H4 lysine 16 hypo-acetylation is associated with defective DNA repair and premature senescence in Zmpste24-deficient mice. Proc Natl Acad Sci USA. 2011;108:12325–30.
14. Wang GG, Allis CD, Chi P. Chromatin remodeling and cancer, Part II: ATP dependent chromatin remodeling. Trends Mol Med. 2007;13:373–80.
15. Villeponteau B. The heterochromatin loss model of aging. Exp Gerontol. 1997;32:383–94.
16. Koch CM, Suschek CV, Lin Q, Bork S, Goergens M, Joussen S, et al. Specific age-associated DNA methylation changes in human dermal fibroblasts. PLoS One. 2011;6(2):e16679.
17. Fraga MF, Esteller M. Epigenetics and aging: the targets and the marks. Trends Genet. 2007;23:413–18.
18. Zaratiegui M, Irvine DV, Martienssen RA. Noncoding RNAs and gene silencing. Cell. 2007;128:763–76.
19. Guttman M, Rinn JL. Modular regulatory principles of large non-coding RNAs. Nature. 2012;482:339–46.
20. Krol J, Krol J, Loedige I, Filipowicz W. The widespread regulation of microRNA biogenesis, function and decay. Nat Rev Genet. 2010;11:597–610.
21. Smith-Vikos T, Slack FJ. MicroRNAs and their roles in aging. J Cell Sci. 2012;125(Pt 1):7–17.
22. Bonifacio LN, Jarstfer MB. MiRNA profile associated with replicative senescence, extended cell culture, and ectopic telomerase expression in human foreskin fibroblasts. PLoS One. 2010;5(9):e12519.
23. Gorospe M, Abdelmohsen K. MicroRegulators come of age in senescence. Trends Genet. 2011;27:233–41.
24. Lee HC, Wei YH. Mitochondria and aging. Adv Exp Med Biol. 2012;942:311–27.
25. Hara T, Nakamura K, Matsui M, Yamamoto A, Nakahara Y, Suzuki-Migishima R, et al. Suppression of basal autophagy in neural cells causes neurodegenerative disease in mice. Nature. 2006;441:885–9.
26. Cuervo AM, Dice JF. Age-related decline in chaperone-mediated autophagy. J Biol Chem. 2000;275:31505–13.

27. Martinez-Vicente M, Sovak G, Cuervo AM. Protein degradation and aging. Exp Gerontol. 2005;40:622–33.
28. Kim I, Rodriguez-Enriquez S, Lemasters JJ. Selective degradation of mitochondria by mitophagy. Arch Biochem Biophys. 2007;462:245–53.
29. Woehlbier U, Hetz C. Modulating stress responses by the UPRosome: a matter of life and death. Trends Biochem Sci. 2011;36:329–37.
30. Cuervo AM. Autophagy and aging: keeping that old broom working. Trends Genet. 2008;24:604–12.
31. Harley CB, Futcher AB, Greider CW. Telomeres shorten during ageing of human fibroblasts. Nature. 1990;345:458–60.
32. Kuilman T, Michaloglou C, Mooi WJ, Peeper DS. The essence of senescence. Genes Dev. 2010;24:2463–79.
33. Londoño-Vallejo JA, Wellinger RJ. Telomeres and telomerase dance to the rhythm of the cell cycle. Trends Biochem Sci. 2012;37(9):391–9.
34. Vera E, Blasco MA. Beyond average: potential for measurement of short telomeres. Aging (Albany NY). 2012;4:379–92.
35. Janssens JP, Pache JC, Nicod LP. Physiological changes in respiratory function associated with ageing. Eur Respir J. 1999;13:197–205.
36. Meyer KC. Aging. Proc Am Thorac Soc. 2005;2:433–9.
37. Reddy GK. AGE-related cross-linking of collagen is associated with aortic wall matrix stiffness in the pathogenesis of drug-induced diabetes in rats. Microvasc Res. 2004;68:132–42.
38. DeGroot J, Verzijl N, Budde M, Bijlsma JW, Lafeber FP, TeKoppele JM. Accumulation of advanced glycation end products decreases collagen turnover by bovine chondrocytes. Exp Cell Res. 2001;266:303–10.
39. Rolewska P, Al-Robaiy S, Navarrete Santos A, Simm A, Silber RE, Bartling B. Age-related expression, enzymatic solubility and modification with advanced glycation end-products of fibrillar collagens in mouse lung. Exp Gerontol. 2013;48:29–37.
40. Calabresi C, Arosio B, Galimberti L, Scanziani E, Bergottini R, Annoni G, et al. Natural aging, expression of fibrosis-related genes and collagen deposition in rat lung. Exp Gerontol. 2007;42:1003–11.
41. Huang K, Rabold R, Schofield B, Mitzner W, Tankersley CG. Age-dependent changes of airway and lung parenchyma in C57BL/6J mice. J Appl Physiol. 2007;102:200–6.
42. Paxson JA, Gruntman A, Parkin CD, Mazan MR, Davis A, Ingenito EP, et al. Age-dependent decline in mouse lung regeneration with loss of lung fibroblast clonogenicity and increased myofibroblastic differentiation. PLoS One. 2012;6:e23232.
43. Takubo Y, Hirai T, Muro S, Kogishi K, Hosokawa M, Mishima M. Age-associated changes in elastin and collagen content and the proportion of types I and III collagen in the lungs of mice. Exp Gerontol. 1999;34:353–64.
44. Sherratt MJ. Tissue elasticity and the ageing elastic fibre. Age (Dordr). 2009;31:305–25.
45. Konova E, Baydanoff S, Atanasova M, Velkova A. Age-related changes in the glycation of human aortic elastin. Exp Gerontol. 2004;39:249–54.
46. Franceschi C, Capri M, Monti D, Giunta S, Olivieri F, Sevini F, et al. Inflammaging and anti-inflammaging: a systemic perspective on aging and longevity emerged from studies in humans. Mech Ageing Dev. 2007;128:92–105.
47. Ito K. Does lung aging have an impact on chronic obstructive pulmonary disease? J Organ Dysfunction. 2007;3:204–20.
48. Pawelec G, Larbi A. Immunity and ageing in man: annual review 2006/2007. Exp Gerontol. 2008;43:34–8.
49. Lee N, Shin MS, Kang I. T-Cell biology in aging, with a focus on lung disease. J Gerontol A Biol Sci Med Sci. 2012;67A:254–63.
50. Kang I, Hong MS, Nolasco H, Park SH, Dan JM, Choi JY, et al. Age-associated change in the frequency of memory CD4+ T cells impairs long term CD4+ T cell responses to influenza vaccine. J Immunol. 2004;173:673–81.

51. Mora AL, Woods CR, Garcia A, Xu J, Rojas M, Speck SH, et al. Lung infection with gamma-herpesvirus induces progressive pulmonary fibrosis in Th2-biased mice. Am J Physiol Lung Cell Mol Physiol. 2005;289:L711–21.
52. Selman M, Rojas M, Mora AL, Pardo A. Aging and interstitial lung diseases: unraveling an old forgotten player in the pathogenesis of lung fibrosis. Semin Respir Crit Care Med. 2010;31:607–17.
53. Volkova M, Zhang Y, Shaw AC, Lee PJ. The role of Toll-like receptors in age-associated lung diseases. J Gerontol A Biol Sci Med Sci. 2012;67A:247–53.
54. Jane-Wit D, Chun HJ. Mechanisms of dysfunction in senescent pulmonary endothelium. J Gerontol A Biol Sci Med Sci. 2012;67:236–41.
55. Lepeule J, Baccarelli A, Motta V, Cantone L, Litonjua AA, Sparrow D, et al. Gene promoter methylation is associated with lung function in the elderly: the normative aging study. Epigenetics. 2012;7:261–9.
56. Raghu G, Weycker D, Edelsberg J, Bradford WZ, Oster G. Incidence and prevalence of idiopathic pulmonary fibrosis. Am J Respi Crit Care Med. 2006;174:810–16.
57. Noth I, Martinez FJ. Recent advances in idiopathic pulmonary fibrosis. Chest. 2007;132:637–50.
58. Copley SJ, Wells AU, Hawtin KE, Gibson DJ, Hodson JM, Jacques AE, et al. Lung morphology in the elderly: comparative CT study of subjects over 75 years old versus those under 55 years old. Radiology. 2009;251:566–73.
59. Washko GR, Hunninghake GM, Fernandez IE, Nishino M, Okajima Y, Yamashiro T, et al. COPDGene investigators. Lung volumes and emphysema in smokers with interstitial lung abnormalities. N Engl J Med. 2011;364:897–906.
60. Kuwano K, Hagimoto N, Maeyama T, Fujita M, Yoshimi M, Inoshima I, et al. Mitochondria-mediated apoptosis of lung epithelial cells in idiopathic interstitial pneumonias. Lab Invest. 2002;82:1695–706.
61. Bellocq A, Azoulay E, Marullo S, Flahault A, Fouqueray B, Philippe C, et al. Reactive oxygen and nitrogen intermediates increase transforming growth factor-beta1 release from human epithelial alveolar cells through two different mechanisms. Am J Respir Cell Mol Biol. 1999;21:128–36.
62. Barcellos-Hoff MH, Dix TA. Redox-mediated activation of latent transforming growth factor-beta 1. Mol Endocrinol. 1996;10:1077–83.
63. Hybertson BM, Gao B, Bose SK, McCord JM. Oxidative stress in health and disease: the therapeutic potential of Nrf2 activation. Mol Aspects Med. 2011;32:234–46.
64. Kikuchi N, Ishii Y, Morishima Y, Yageta Y, Haraguchi N, Itoh K, et al. Nrf2 protects against pulmonary fibrosis by regulating the lung oxidant level and Th1/Th2 balance. Respir Res. 2010;11:31.
65. Markart P, Luboeinski T, Korfei M, Schmidt R, Wygrecka M, Mahavadi P, et al. Alveolar oxidative stress is associated with elevated levels of nonenzymatic low-molecular-weight antioxidants in patients with different forms of chronic fibrosing interstitial lung diseases. Antioxid Redox Signal. 2009;11:227–40.
66. Artaud-Macari E, Goven D, Brayer S, Hamimi A, Besnard V, Marchal-Somme J, et al. Nrf2 nuclear translocation induces myofibroblastic dedifferentiation in idiopathic pulmonary fibrosis. Antioxid Redox Signal. 2013;18(1):66–79.
67. Korfei M, Ruppert C, Mahavadi P, Henneke I, Markart P, Koch M, et al. Epithelial endoplasmic reticulum stress and apoptosis in sporadic idiopathic pulmonary fibrosis. Am J Respir Crit Care Med. 2008;178:838–46.
68. Lawson WE, Crossno PF, Polosukhin VV, Roldan J, Cheng DS, Lane KB, et al. Endoplasmic reticulum stress in alveolar epithelial cells is prominent in IPF: association with altered surfactant protein processing and herpesvirus infection. Am J Physiol Lung Cell Mol Physiol. 2008;294:L1119–26.
69. Lawson WE, Cheng DS, Degryse AL, Tanjore H, Polosukhin VV, Xu XC, et al. Endoplasmic reticulum stress enhances fibrotic remodeling in the lungs. Proc Natl Acad Sci USA. 2011;108:10562–67.

70. Naidoo N. ER and aging-protein folding and the ER stress response. Ageing Res Rev. 2009;8:150–9.
71. Hussain SG, Ramaiah KV. Reduced eIF2alpha phosphorylation and increased proapoptotic proteins in aging. Biochem Biophys Res Commun. 2007;355:365–70.
72. Kim SI, Na HJ, Ding Y, Wang Z, Lee SJ, Choi ME. Autophagy promotes intracellular degradation of type I collagen induced by transforming growth factor (TGF)-β1. J Biol Chem. 2012;287:11677–88.
73. Hernández-Gea V, Ghiassi-Nejad Z, Rozenfeld R, Gordon R, Fiel MI, Yue Z, et al. Autophagy releases lipid that promotes fibrogenesis by activated hepatic stellate cells in mice and in human tissues. Gastroenterology. 2012;142:938–46.
74. Yang HZ, Wang JP, Mi S, Liu HZ, Cui B, Yan HM, et al. TLR4 activity is required in the resolution of pulmonary inflammation and fibrosis after acute and chronic lung injury. Am J Pathol. 2012;180:275–92.
75. Patel AS, Lin L, Geyer A, Haspel JA, An CH, Cao J, et al. Autophagy in idiopathic pulmonary fibrosis. PLoS One. 2012;7(7):e41394.
76. Hua Y, Zhang Y, Ceylan-Isik AF, Wold LE, Nunn JM, Ren J. Chronic Akt activation accentuates aging-induced cardiac hypertrophy and myocardial contractile dysfunction: role of autophagy. Basic Res Cardiol. 2011;106:1173–91.
77. Chen ZH, Kim HP, Sciurba FC, Lee SJ, Feghali-Bostwick C, Stolz DB, et al. Egr-1 regulates autophagy in cigarette smoke-induced chronic obstructive pulmonary disease. PLoS One. 2008;3(10):e3316.
78. Blasco MA. Telomere length, stem cells and aging. Nat Chem Biol. 2007;3:640–9.
79. Armanios MY, Chen JJ, Cogan JD, Alder JK, Ingersoll RG, Markin C, et al. Telomerase mutations in families with idiopathic pulmonary fibrosis. N Engl J Med. 2007;356:1317–26.
80. Tsakiri KD, Cronkhite JT, Kuan PJ, Xing C, Raghu G, Weissler JC, et al. Adult-onset pulmonary fibrosis caused by mutations in telomerase. Proc Natl Acad Sci USA. 2007;104:7552–7.
81. Alder JK, Chen JJ, Lancaster L, Danoff S, Su SC, Cogan JD, et al. Short telomeres are a risk factor for idiopathic pulmonary fibrosis. Proc Natl Acad Sci USA. 2008;105:13051–6.
82. Savale L, Chaouat A, Bastuji-Garin S, Marcos E, Boyer L, Maitre B, et al. Shortened telomeres in circulating leukocytes of patients with chronic obstructive pulmonary disease. Am J Respir Crit Care Med. 2009;179:566–71.
83. Lee J, Reddy R, Barsky L, Scholes J, Chen H, Shi W, et al. Lung alveolar integrity is compromised by telomere shortening in telomerase-null mice. Am J Physiol. 2009;296:L57–70.
84. Degryse AL, Xu XC, Newman JL, Mitchell DB, Tanjore H, Polosukhin VV, et al. Telomerase deficiency does not alter bleomycin-induced fibrosis in mice. Exp Lung Res. 2012;38:124–34.
85. Rabinovich EI, Kapetanaki MG, Steinfeld I, Gibson KF, Pandit KV, Yu G, et al. Global methylation patterns in idiopathic pulmonary fibrosis. PLoS One. 2012;7(4):e33770.
86. Sanders YY, Ambalavanan N, Halloran B, Zhang X, Liu H, Crossman DK, et al. Altered DNA methylation profile in idiopathic pulmonary fibrosis. Am J Respir Crit Care Med. 2012;186(6):525–35.
87. Trujillo G, Meneghin A, Flaherty KR, Sholl LM, Myers JL, Kazerooni EA, et al. TLR9 differentiates rapidly from slowly progressing forms of idiopathic pulmonary fibrosis. Sci Transl Med. 2010;2:57ra82.
88. Rege TA, Hagood JS. Thy-1, a versatile modulator of signaling affecting cellular adhesion, proliferation, survival, and cytokine/growth factor responses. Biochim Biophys Acta. 2006;1763:991–9.
89. Ramírez G, Hagood JS, Sanders Y, Ramírez R, Becerril C, Segura L, et al. Absence of Thy-1 results in TGF-β induced MMP-9 expression and confers a profibrotic phenotype to human lung fibroblasts. Lab Invest. 2011;91:1206–18.
90. Sanders YY, Pardo A, Selman M, Nuovo GJ, Tollefsbol TO, Siegal GP, et al. Thy-1 promoter hypermethylation: a novel epigenetic pathogenic mechanism in pulmonary fibrosis. Am J Respir Cell Mol Biol. 2008;39:610–18.
91. Sanders YY, Tollefsbol TO, Varisco BM, Hagood JS. Epigenetic regulation of thy-1 by histone deacetylase inhibitor in rat lung fibroblasts. Am J Respir Cell Mol Biol. 2011;45:16–23.

92. Cisneros J, Hagood J, Checa M, Ortiz-Quintero B, Negreros M, Herrera I, et al. Hypermethylation-mediated silencing of p14ARF in fibroblasts from idiopathic pulmonary fibrosis. Am J Physiol Lung Cell Mol Physiol. 2012;303(4):L295–303.
93. Coward WR, Watts K, Feghali-Bostwick CA, Knox A, Pang L. Defective histone acetylation is responsible for the diminished expression of cyclooxygenase 2 in idiopathic pulmonary fibrosis. Mol Cell Biol. 2009;29:4325–39.
94. Thiery JP, Acloque H, Huang RY, Nieto MA. Epithelial-mesenchymal transitions in development and disease. Cell. 2009;139:871–90.
95. King Jr TE, Pardo A, Selman M. Idiopathic pulmonary fibrosis. Lancet. 2011;378:1949–61.
96. Willis BC, Liebler JM, Luby-Phelps K, Nicholson AG, Crandall ED, du Bois RM, et al. Induction of epithelial-mesenchymal transition in alveolar epithelial cells by transforming growth factor-beta1: potential role in idiopathic pulmonary fibrosis. Am J Pathol. 2005;166:1321–32.
97. Kim KK, Kugler MC, Wolters PJ, Robillard L, Galvez MG, Brumwell AN, et al. Alveolar epithelial cell mesenchymal transition develops in vivo during pulmonary fibrosis and is regulated by the extracellular matrix. Proc Natl Acad Sci USA. 2006;103:13180–85.
98. Rock JR, Barkauskas CE, Cronce MJ, Xue Y, Harris JR, Liang J, et al. Multiple stromal populations contribute to pulmonary fibrosis without evidence for epithelial to mesenchymal transition. Proc Natl Acad Sci USA. 2011;108:E1475–83.
99. McDonald OG, Wu H, Timp W, Doi A, Feinberg AP. Genome-scale epigenetic reprogramming during epithelial-to-mesenchymal transition. Nat Struct Mol Biol. 2011;18:867–74.
100. Laberge RM, Awad P, Campisi J, Desprez PY. Epithelial-mesenchymal transition induced by senescent fibroblasts. Cancer Microenviron. 2012;5:39–44.
101. Smit MA, Peeper DS. Epithelial-mesenchymal transition and senescence: two cancer-related processes are crossing paths. Aging (Albany NY). 2010;2:735–41.
102. van Rooij E, Sutherland LB, Thatcher JE, DiMaio JM, Naseem RH, Marshall WS, et al. Dysregulation of microRNAs after myocardial infarction reveals a role of miR-29 in cardiac fibrosis. Proc Natl Acad Sci USA. 2008;105:13027–32.
103. Thum T, Gross C, Fiedler J, Fischer T, Kissler S, Bussen M, et al. MicroRNA-21 contributes to myocardial disease by stimulating MAP kinase signalling in fibroblasts. Nature. 2008;456:980–4.
104. Pandit KV, Corcoran D, Yousef H, Yarlagadda M, Tzouvelekis A, Gibson KF, et al. Inhibition and role of let-7d in idiopathic pulmonary fibrosis. Am J Respir Crit Care Med. 2010;182:220–9.
105. Liu G, Friggeri A, Yang Y, Milosevic J, Ding Q, Thannickal VJ, et al. miR-21 mediates fibrogenic activation of pulmonary fibroblasts and lung fibrosis. J Exp Med. 2010;207:1589–97.
106. Kato M, Zhang J, Wang M, Lanting L, Yuan H, Rossi JJ, Natarajan R. MicroRNA-192 in diabetic kidney glomeruli and its function in TGF-beta-induced collagen expression via inhibition of E-box repressors. Proc Natl Acad Sci USA. 2007;104:3432–37.
107. Shan H, Zhang Y, Lu Y, Zhang Y, Pan Z, Cai B, et al. Downregulation of miR-133 and miR-590 contributes to nicotine-induced atrial remodelling in canines. Cardiovasc Res. 2009;83:465–72.
108. Duisters RF, Tijsen AJ, Schroen B, Leenders JJ, Lentink V, van der Made I, et al. miR-133 and miR-30 regulate connective tissue growth factor: implications for a role of microRNAs in myocardial matrix remodeling. Circ Res. 2009;104:170–8.
109. Cordes KR, Sheehy NT, White MP, Berry EC, Morton SU, Muth AN, et al. miR-145 and miR-143 regulate smooth muscle cell fate and plasticity. Nature. 2009;460:705–10.
110. Cushing L, Kuang PP, Qian J, Shao F, Wu J, Little F, et al. MIR-29 is a major regulator of genes associated with pulmonary fibrosis. Am J Respir Cell Mol Biol. 2011;45:287–94.
111. Pottier N, Maurin T, Chevalier B, Puisségur MP, Lebrigand K, Robbe-Sermesant K, et al. Identification of keratinocyte growth factor as a target of microRNA-155 in lung fibroblasts: implication in epithelial-mesenchymal interactions. PLoS One. 2009;4(8):e6718.
112. Martin MM, Lee EJ, Buckenberger JA, Schmittgen TD, Elton TS. MicroRNA-155 regulates human angiotensin II type 1 receptor expression in fibroblasts. J Biol Chem. 2006;281: 18277–84.

# Chapter 13
# Gastroesophageal Reflux and IPF

Stephenie M. Takahashi, Karen C. Patterson, and Imre Noth

**Abstract** Idiopathic pulmonary fibrosis (IPF) is a chronic fibrosing disease of the lung and the most common of the idiopathic interstitial pneumonias. The pathophysiology of IPF involves recurrent epithelial cell injury, abnormal wound repair responses, and aberrant fibroblast proliferation. Recent studies have shed light upon the potential role of gastroesophageal reflux (GER) and microaspiration as a possible etiology or trigger for the suspected recurrent epithelial injury and fibrosis that characterize IPF. Although acid aspiration has been linked to IPF, the mechanism and relationship of abnormal GER to the cause or progression of IPF have not been adequately addressed. This association is of great interest to the scientific and clinical communities, and active investigations are ongoing. Herein, we review what is currently understood about the relationship between GER and IPF and explore the evidence supporting this relationship.

**Keywords** Gastroesophageal reflux • Gastroesophageal reflux disease • Idiopathic pulmonary fibrosis • Microaspiration • Bile acid • Hiatal hernia • Interstitial lung disease

S.M. Takahashi, B.A., M.D. (✉)
Department of Medicine, Section of Pulmonary and Critical Care,
University of Chicago Medical Center, 5841 S. Maryland Avenue,
MC 6076, Chicago, IL 60637, USA

1949 W. Argyle Street #2, Chicago, IL 60640, USA
e-mail: stephenie.takahashi@uchospitals.edu

K.C. Patterson, M.D. • I. Noth, M.D.
Department of Medicine, Section of Pulmonary and Critical Care,
University of Chicago Medical Center, 5841 S. Maryland Avenue,
MC 6076, Chicago, IL 60637, USA

K.C. Meyer and S.D. Nathan (eds.), *Idiopathic Pulmonary Fibrosis: A Comprehensive Clinical Guide*, Respiratory Medicine 9, DOI 10.1007/978-1-62703-682-5_13,
© Springer Science+Business Media New York 2014

# Introduction

Idiopathic pulmonary fibrosis (IPF) is a chronic fibrosing disease of the lung and the most common of the IIPs. To date, there are no approved therapies in the United States for this disease, which carries 50 % mortality at 2–5 years from diagnosis [1]. The pathophysiology of IPF is thought to revolve around recurrent epithelial cell injury and abnormal wound repair responses that include aberrant fibroblast activity [2]. The cause of epithelial injury remains unknown, but cigarette smoking, chronic viral infections, exposure to wood and dust particles, and drug toxicities have been associated with IPF [3]. In addition to such exposures, recent studies have shed light on the potential role of GER and microaspiration as a possible cause of recurrent epithelial injury [4]. GER includes reflux of both acidic and nonacidic foregut contents, and although GER is frequently symptomatic, asymptomatic reflux events often occur. However, while a high incidence of acid aspiration in IPF has been detected in several case series, the role of GER in either the cause or the progression of IPF is not well understood [5]. Therefore, the association of GER and IPF is an intense area of active, ongoing investigation. Herein, we review the data on GER in IPF, and we discuss the implications of this association for the screening and treatment of GER in patients with IPF.

# Pathophysiology and Diagnosis of Gastroesophageal Reflux Disease

Gastroesophageal reflux disease (GERD) is defined as the reflux of gastric contents into the esophagus that leads to symptomatic esophagitis, symptoms sufficient to impair quality of life, or an increased risk of long-term complications [6]. This definition, created by an international working group, emphasizes that GER should be regarded as a disease (GERD) when it affects quality of life or causes macroscopic damage to the esophagus [7]. GERD, when defined by weekly symptoms and/or acid regurgitation, is very common, affecting 10–20 % of people in the Western world [8]. The cause of GER is variable, with multiple studies having attempted to elucidate the genetic, demographic, and lifestyle risk factors for this disorder. The association between age and the development of reflux or the presence of symptoms remains unclear. Coffee, alcohol, smoking, and chocolate can inappropriately relax the lower esophageal sphincter (LES), and are, therefore, thought to be associated with GER [7].

GER is thought to occur when normal protective physiologic mechanisms fail to prevent reflux. These protective mechanisms include the combined actions of the LES, a segment of smooth muscle that contracts to generate a pressure greater than that in the stomach, and the crural diaphragm, which provides extrinsic pressure and a barrier to separate the esophageal and gastric compartments [9]. The pathophysiology of reflux is thought to be due to impaired function of the LES in particular, because contraction of this smooth muscle creates a barrier that prevents gastric contents refluxing into the lower esophagus [10]. Dysfunction of the LES can be mechanical from loss of tone or functional, where the frequency of LES relaxations is increased. While temporary relaxations of the LES are normal, these episodes are thought to occur more frequently in individuals with GERD and can result in prolonged periods of esophageal exposure to refluxed gastric contents [11].

Additionally, the pressure gradient between the abdomen and thorax can influence the development of GER. It has been postulated that patients with chronic obstructive pulmonary disease (COPD), who have increased negative intrathoracic pressure, increased lung compliance, and decreased elastic recoil, may be predisposed to reflux [12, 13]. An abnormal pressure gradient may also be a contributing factor in patients with IPF, who have decreased compliance and increased elastic recoil as a result of lung fibrosis. However, the role of intrathoracic pressure and lung compliance in GER is complicated. Obstructive lung diseases, such as asthma and COPD, are marked by air trapping and increased intrathoracic pressures, which can lead to defects in the diaphragm and predispose to the development of a hiatal hernia. Indeed, a higher prevalence of diaphragmatic defects and hiatal hernias has been documented in patients with emphysema [14]. Similarly, it has been postulated that restrictive lung disease can influence the pressure in the intrathoracic space by reducing the overall lung volume, which can lead to disruption to the diaphragm and potentially increase the predisposition for reflux. Additionally, it is well known that increased abdominal pressure from obesity can lead to a weakened LES, and obesity is, therefore, a significant risk factor for GER.

The presence of a hiatal hernia increases the time of LES relaxation and increases the risk of esophagitis, GER, and GERD [15]. Hiatal hernias also alter the crux of the diaphragm, which can structurally affect the lower esophageal sphincter and thereby provide a further predisposition to reflux. Additionally, the degree of a hiatal hernia and the effect on GER are interrelated. A sliding hiatal hernia (type I hernia) has a small effect, whereas a large hiatal hernia (type IV hernia), where part of the stomach resides in the chest cavity, will have a larger effect [16]. Given this, hiatal hernias have been associated with diminished pressure of the LES, episodes of microaspiration, and an increased risk of erosive esophagitis [17].

Because GER can occur without causing GERD, the presence of symptoms has been shown to be a poor indicator of underlying reflux and aspiration, and this may be particularly true in patients with IPF [4]. Therefore, diagnostic studies are often necessary to adequately assess for presence of GER and aspiration. Commonly employed diagnostic approaches for GER include 24-h pH monitoring with or without esophageal manometry, a modified barium swallow, or endoscopy [7]. Less common diagnostic tests include gastroesophageal-pulmonary scintigraphy, testing for pepsin and bile salts in bronchoalveolar lavage (BAL) fluid, and exhaled breath condensate (EBC) [4]. All of these studies have important limitations to consider. Endoscopy can only indirectly assess for regurgitation via the identification of esophageal mucosal injury, and modified barium swallow evaluations are limited by a low sensitivity for reflux and aspiration. Ambulatory pH monitoring does not directly assess for aspiration and cannot identify nonacidic gastric refluxate [4].

However, because ambulatory pH monitoring measures the pH at two different esophageal sites, a composite pH score (the DeMeester score) can be generated, and pH monitoring is considered more sensitive and specific for regurgitation [18]. Most specialists consider this test, with the composite score, as the gold standard test. Overall, given the strengths and weaknesses of any given individual test, clinicians frequently employ a combination of these tests in diagnosing GER.

Given the above barriers to reaching a confident diagnosis, biomarkers for GER and microaspiration are greatly needed. Historically, an alkalemic esophageal aspirate suggested the presence of duodenogastric reflux. However, the poor sensitivity and specificity of an increased pH (typically >7.0) make this an unreliable tool to accurately assess for significant duodenogastric reflux. In contrast, gastric and esophageal bilirubin concentrations in most patients parallel the severity of duodenogastric reflux. The recent development of a fiber-optic probe (the Bilitec 2000), which measures the concentration of esophageal bilirubin, is a more reliable and generally well-tolerated test for duodenogastric reflux [4]. Bilirubin testing by this method could be useful to study the role of refluxed biliary secretions in IPF. The diagnosis of GER is also complicated given that many patients are asymptomatic. Therefore, a number of issues hinder diagnosing GER and GERD, especially in the absence of a gold standard diagnostic test.

## Animal Models of Aspiration

Animal models of aspiration have contributed substantially to our understanding of the role of the reflux and aspiration of acid in lung disease. Some of the earliest investigations of the effects of acid aspiration into the lungs were performed on rabbits using hydrochloric acid. Induced aspiration of agents that mimic the acidity of stomach contents was shown to cause pulmonary edema and hemorrhage, infiltration of neutrophils, and de-epithelialization of the bronchial mucosa [19]. After this initial response, the host forms a granulomatous reaction to the aspirated material. Similarly, in a model of aspiration in intubated dogs, the degree of lung injury was proportional to the acidity of the aspirate. In dog studies, the acute histopathology changes revealed damaged type II epithelial cells and capillaries, while at 48 h, the lungs evolved to a pattern of interstitial edema and hyaline membrane formation [20].

These earlier studies suggest multiple different pathologic outcomes from acid aspiration with variations of acute lung injury. However, other groups have subsequently developed animal models of chronic aspiration and discovered a profibrotic response. In a murine model of aspiration, the mice developed evidence of fibrosis with collagen deposition 2 weeks after the aspiration injury [21]. Profibrotic mechanisms have also been implicated in a rat model of chronic aspiration, with increased levels of transforming growth factor beta 1 (TGF-beta) in the BAL fluid as well as increased collagen and fibronectin in the lung parenchyma of the rodents in response to aspiration [22]. The inflammatory response in a chronic aspiration model was found to have increased macrophages and an increased CD4+/CD8+ T lymphocyte ratio with evidence of a lymphocytic and obliterative bronchiolitis lasting up to 16 weeks. In addition, TGF-beta and other inflammatory cytokines were increased along with fibrosis in the lung. These studies suggest the potential for different histological patterns of injury, including the development or worsening of lung fibrosis from acid aspiration events of varying intensity and duration.

## Pulmonary Manifestations of GER

If a patient suffers from symptomatic or asymptomatic GER, they may or may not have pulmonary manifestations of their disease, and not all patients with GER or GERD have aspiration. However, if the gastric contents travel as high as the cricopharyngeal region, esophageal contents can enter the airway. The inhalation of oropharyngeal or gastric contents into the larynx or lower respiratory tract is defined as aspiration [23] (Fig. 13.1). The resulting pulmonary syndrome due to an aspiration event depends on the contents of the material, the volume of aspirate, and the host's response to the aspiration event. When patients have asymptomatic aspiration of oropharyngeal secretions or gastric fluid into their lungs, it is called silent microaspiration. It has been demonstrated that approximately one-half of healthy adults

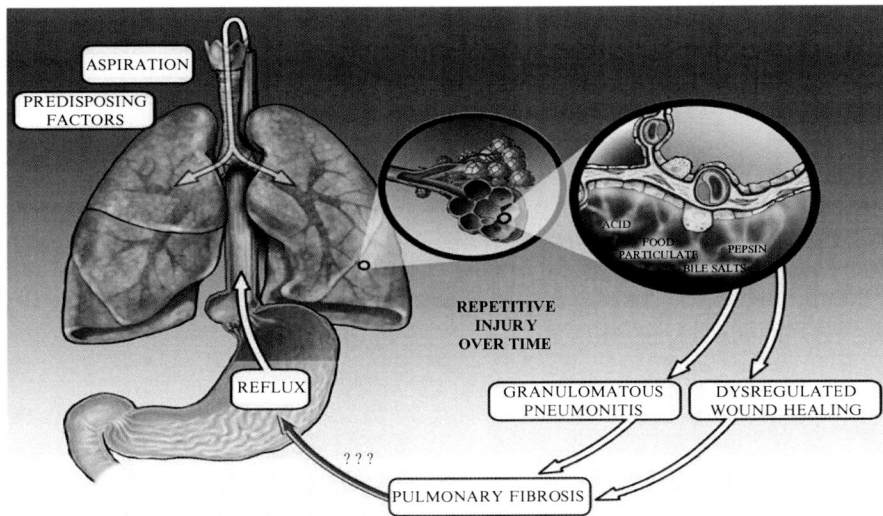

**Fig. 13.1** Potential mechanism of chronic aspiration in IPF. Gastric contents can travel through a weakened lower esophageal sphincter up into the esophagus. If the gastric contents travel as high as the cricopharyngeal region, esophageal contents can enter the airway. Chronic microaspiration may cause repeated injury leading to dysregulated wound healing, granulomatous pneumonitis, and lung fibrosis. Reprinted from the American Journal of Medicine, 123/4, Lee JS, Collard HR, Raghu G, Sweet MP, Hays SR, Campos GM, et al., Chronic microaspiration and idiopathic pulmonary fibrosis, 304–11, Copyright 2010, with permission from Elsevier

may experience mild, silent microaspiration during sleep [24]. Normally, natural defenses, including coughing and epiglottic closing, are protective of microaspiration, but these defenses may occasionally become impaired, and wheezing and coughing may occur [25].

In addition to the aspiration of gastric contents, aspirated biliary contents may also contribute to lung injury. Biliary contents include bile acids, pancreatic enzymes, and bicarbonate. The regurgitation of biliary contents occurs in the setting of duodenogastric reflux. While small amounts of duodenogastric reflux can be common in the postprandial period, a substantial amount of reflux is not normal. In human studies, the severity of duodenogastric reflux has been associated with the severity of esophageal inflammation, and abnormal duodenogastric reflux is common among patients with refractory, symptomatic heartburn [26, 27]. In animal models, excessive biliary secretions have been demonstrated to directly damage the esophageal mucosa [24]. Furthermore, bile acids may be directly injurious to the lung. The finding of elevated bile acids in the bronchoalveolar lavage fluid of lung transplant recipients who developed bronchiolitis obliterans syndrome versus recipients with good graft function supports the concept that bile acids can injure the lung [28, 29]. Proposed mechanisms of injury include alterations of cellular cationic permeability, disruption of type II pneumocyte cell membranes, and the creation of a "barrier breaker" for pulmonary surfactant through the detergent properties of bile salts [30]. Bile acids may also alter local immune functions [31]. The prevalence and role of duodenogastric reflux and biliary secretions in pulmonary fibrosis are unknown, but these are of great interest in the ongoing evaluation of the pathological role of reflux in lung injury. It has been suggested that acid reflux and nonacid reflux, including the reflux of biliary contents, may act synergistically in damaging the esophageal mucosa [24], and such synergistic action may be important in reflux-induced pulmonary damage as well.

There is increasing recognition that gastric refluxate, either acidic or nonacidic, can be a risk factor for many respiratory symptoms including chronic cough [32, 33] and hoarseness [34]. In both animal and clinical data, GER may evoke bronchospasm and/or potentiate the bronchomotor response to additional triggers [35]. Therefore, it is hypothesized that acid GER may trigger asthmatic symptoms. The correlation between GER and asthma has been shown in a prospective study where the prevalence of abnormal 24-h pH monitoring was 62 % in asthmatic patients without GER symptoms [36]. A large systematic review examined 28 studies that assessed the incidence of GERD in patients with asthma and found that the average prevalence of reflux symptoms in asthma patients was 59.2 %, which was significantly higher than the control group's prevalence of 38.1 %. They also noted an increased prevalence of esophagitis and hiatal hernia in asthma patients when compared to controls [37]. Additionally, asthmatics with reflux had a significant dose–response association between breathlessness and reflux symptoms [38]. The prevalence of GER in chronic bronchitis patients as measured by pH monitoring has been shown to be slightly more than half, which is comparable to asthma patients at [39].

The treatment of GERD to alleviate respiratory symptoms has been studied more extensively in asthmatic patients than in patients with other pulmonary disorders.

It has been shown that 71 % of asthmatic patients with symptoms of reflux benefited from medical therapy or lifestyle modification, as demonstrated by an improvement in their pulmonary symptoms [40]. In a study that selected patients whose respiratory symptoms were likely due to untreated GER (i.e., nonallergic asthmatics), surgical therapy in addition to medical therapy was shown to be effective [41]. In patients with GERD and asthma who were treated with Nissen fundoplication, there was an immediate and sustained reduction in nocturnal symptoms for 24 months [42]. By the end of the 2-year time point, a marked improvement was observed in 75 % of the surgical group versus 9 % of the medically treated group. Although no difference in pulmonary function was detected, the authors suggest that anti-reflux surgery may significantly improve the pulmonary symptoms and clinical status of patients with significant GERD.

Although the relationship of asthma to GERD has been studied more than other respiratory disorders, many other disorders have also been linked to GERD. In a large population-based study that examined over 100,000 military veterans, patients with reflux esophagitis were found to be at an increased risk for a large variety of laryngeal, sinus, and respiratory diseases including COPD, bronchiectasis, chronic bronchitis, and pneumonia [43]. Furthermore, several studies have implicated GER exposure to recurrent pneumonias [44, 45].

The association of cystic fibrosis (CF) with GER has also furthered the understanding of the pulmonary manifestations of GER. A significantly higher prevalence of abnormal esophageal acid exposure, as evidenced by elevated DeMeester scores and symptoms, has been demonstrated for patients with cystic fibrosis prior to transplantation (while on the lung transplant wait list) and following lung transplantation [46]. Cystic fibrosis patients who are not listed for lung transplant also have evidence of significant GER that has been associated with more cough and poorer lung function. Additionally, these patients have been shown to have bile acids in their saliva, lower airways, and in BAL fluid, which may be regarded as evidence of GER with microaspiration events [47, 48].

Although many associations between reflux disease and respiratory disorders have been established, it is difficult to establish a definitive causal relationship of GER and lung disease. Given this, many hypothesize that repetitive injury from either acidic or nonacidic reflux into the lungs can lead to epithelial cell injury and subsequent fibrosis. The potential relevance of GER in pulmonary fibrosis is highlighted by outcomes in scleroderma. Over 50 % of patients with scleroderma develop interstitial lung disease (ILD), where fibrotic nonspecific interstitial pneumonia (NSIP) is the most commonly observed histopathologic pattern [49, 50]. Esophageal dysfunction is very common in scleroderma. Esophageal dysfunction is marked by reduced lower esophageal sphincter pressure, a strong risk factor for reflux events, and reduced peristalsis, which leads to prolonged refluxate exposure. Both of these esophageal alterations contribute to GER. GER in scleroderma is often asymptomatic, but esophageal damage from silent events is well documented.

In scleroderma, the relationship between esophageal dysfunction and ILD has been an intense area of investigation, but whether esophageal dysfunction and ILD pathogenesis are tightly linked remains an unresolved issue, because currently available evidence is conflicting. In earlier studies, no definite association was observed between GER and pulmonary function test (PFT) parameters that are commonly assessed in ILD [51, 52]. More recently, prospective studies, including some with radiographic assessments, have added to our understanding of the relationship between GER and ILD in scleroderma. Marie et al. found that esophageal dysfunction (determined by manometry) was associated with a higher prevalence of ILD on computed tomographic (CT) imaging. Additionally, the prevalence of ILD was positively correlated with increasing severity of esophageal dysfunction [53]. Furthermore, at a 2-year follow-up time point, patients with severe esophageal dysfunction demonstrated a significant decrease in diffusing capacity of the lung for carbon monoxide (DLCO) when compared to those with no or mild esophageal dysfunction, although there was no significant change in either the total lung capacity (TLC) or forced vital capacity (FVC). More recently, Savarino et al. found that patients with scleroderma complicated by ILD had reduced LES pressures, reduced esophageal contraction amplitudes, and an increased frequency of proximal reflux events compared to scleroderma patients without ILD [54], and they demonstrated a dose–response association between GER and ILD with reflux frequency correlating with thoracic CT fibrosis scores. Additionally, both acid and nonacid reflux were demonstrated, and both types of reflux were more common in scleroderma patients with ILD compared to those without. The demonstration of proximal esophageal reflux suggests that GER in scleroderma may indeed lead to microaspiration and ILD, but while the results from these studies suggest an association between GER and ILD, causality remains to be demonstrated.

In an attempt to address this, Gilson et al. did not find an independent association between esophageal dysfunction and PFT decline [55]. In their prospective evaluation of a large cohort of patients, esophageal dysfunction (as determined by manometry) was not found to be a significant, independent predictor of PFT decline after multivariate analysis was performed. While GER was not directly assessed, and radiographic imaging with CT provides a more sensitive assessment of ILD than pulmonary function, their results do not support either an association or a causative role of GER in scleroderma-associated ILD. In short, while several studies suggest an association between esophageal dysfunction and ILD in scleroderma, varying methodologies have lead to some conflicting reports such that further clinical investigation is needed.

It is reasonable to conclude that esophageal dysfunction may play a role in scleroderma lung disease and that esophageal dysfunction may lead to gastrointestinal harm if it remains undiagnosed. Therefore, evaluating for the presence of GER seems reasonable for all patients with scleroderma including those with ILD. Impedance monitoring or manometry testing is a recommended as diagnostic tests. As GER is often asymptomatic in scleroderma, screening by symptoms alone is insensitive. Furthermore, as nonacid reflux may contribute to GER, pH monitoring alone may not capture the extent of the underlying disease. However, once diagnosed, it remains unclear if treating GER affects the development or the course of pulmonary fibrosis. Further research on the effect of treatments that target both acid and nonacid GER is certainly needed, and such research will further inform our understanding of the role of GER in the pathogenesis of ILD in scleroderma.

## GER in Patients with IPF

There is long-standing interest in the role of GER and repetitive microaspiration in the development of IPF that dates back over 50 years. A number of studies have more recently investigated the prevalence, incidence, and treatment effects of GER in patients with IPF over the last two decades. In this section, we review the landmark studies that have been performed that have contributed to our understanding of the role of GER in IPF.

In one of the first clinical reports on GER and lung injury, Tobin and colleagues evaluated the prevalence of acid reflux in patients with IPF and in control patients with other forms of ILD. In this prospective study, ambulatory pH monitoring to diagnose GER was performed on 17 consecutive, newly diagnosed IPF patients and in 8 control patients with non-IPF ILD. GER was significantly more prevalent in the IPF group [56]. Specifically, 16 of the 17 (94 %) IPF patients had abnormal distal or proximal esophageal acid exposure compared to four of the eight (50 %) patients with ILD. Interestingly, most of the IPF patients with abnormal esophageal reflux were asymptomatic, and there was no correlation between the DLCO and acid exposure. Of note, the IPF patients had a particularly high incidence of proximal acid exposure in the supine or nocturnal position, which is very uncommon in healthy individuals. The authors hypothesized that there are increased GER events during sleep when the upper esophageal sphincter pressure is greatly reduced and cough reflexes are suppressed. This increase in GER event frequency may lead to recurrent microaspiration events that may be a source of repetitive injury to the lungs of IPF patients.

In the largest prospective study to date, investigators examined 65 IPF patients and 133 asthma patients where the prevalence of abnormal acid reflux in IPF patients was shown to be 87 %, which was significantly higher than that for the asthmatic patients. They found that half of the IPF patients were asymptomatic and found no correlation of GER severity with pulmonary function [57]. In addition to using asthmatics as controls, 65 % of the IPF patients were taking PPIs at the time, and therefore, the true prevalence of GER might have been even higher. The high prevalence of abnormal acid exposure in patients on PPIs also suggests that standard doses of this class of agents may not be effective in the management of GER in IPF.

Bandeira and colleagues also attempted to quantify the prevalence of abnormal acid reflux in IPF. In a prospective study, 28 IPF patients underwent esophageal manometry, ambulatory 24-h pH probe testing, PFTs, and a symptom survey [58]. In agreement with Tobin's study, they also confirmed a significantly high proportion (80 %) of patients with reflux events in the supine position. Similarly, there was no association between pulmonary function and the presence of GER. Similar to non-ILD patients, the diagnosis of GERD in IPF is often made using a combination of diagnostic tools. In a recent study, GER was evaluated in IPF patients by a reflux cough questionnaire, measurement of pepsin in the exhaled breath condensate (EBC), and *Helicobacter pylori* antibody detection by ELISA [59]. EBC measurement of pepsin is thought to be a reliable technique to measure pepsin as a surrogate for GER in the upper airways. Additionally, the relationship between pulmonary microaspiration and pepsin concentration in BAL fluid in animal and human studies has been demonstrated. In this study, patients with IPF had significantly higher reflux questionnaire scores (19.6 %) vs. controls (3 %). Pepsin was detected via EBC in 2 out of 17 IPF patients but none of the controls, while there was no difference in *H. pylori* serologies between the two groups. The reflex cough questionnaire scores, a validated measure of nonacidic airway reflux, were significantly higher in the IPF patients, suggesting the potential importance of nonacidic reflux disease in these patients.

The investigation of GER in IPF patients referred for lung transplantation represents an opportunity to gain further insight from a more severe group of patients. In a study by Sweet and colleagues, 67 % of IPF patients referred for lung transplantation had abnormal esophageal reflux, while 65 % of these patients had a hypotensive LES. Furthermore, 50 % of patients with reflux had abnormal esophageal peristalsis [60]. The authors note that distal reflux and markers of microaspiration have been associated with early chronic allograft rejection after transplantation, which suggest that microaspiration may cause direct lung injury [28, 61]. In addition to verifying a high prevalence of GER in IPF, this study also confirmed the findings that symptoms do not significantly correlate with reflux severity.

Elevated pepsin in BAL samples has proven to be a useful biomarker for aspiration in lung transplant recipients [62], and BAL pepsin levels were recently evaluated in a cohort of patients with IPF. It has been previously hypothesized that acute exacerbations of IPF may be caused by microaspiration [63]. Indeed, significantly elevated pepsin levels were detected in a significant percentage of IPF patients experiencing exacerbations compared to control IPF patients with stable disease [64]. However, it remains to be determined if there is any difference in pepsin levels for patients with stable or early IPF as compared to healthy controls without lung disease.

It has been hypothesized that an asymmetric fibrotic pattern (one lung vs. the other) may be a potential indicator of GER with microaspiration as a risk factor. Among 32 IPF patients with more than 20 % asymmetrical fibrosis by CT scan, the prevalence of symptomatic reflux and GER on objective testing was higher than in those who lacked an asymmetric fibrosis pattern (62.5 % vs. 31.3 %) [65]. Additionally, patients with asymmetric disease had a higher incidence of acute exacerbations of their IPF (46.9 % vs. 17.2 %), with the right lung being more commonly involved. These results not only support the potential role of GER in the etiology of acute exacerbations of IPF, but they also serve to underscore the notion that an asymmetric pattern on CT scan should raise the suspicion that underlying GER and microaspiration are present.

Hiatal hernia has been shown to have a known association with GER and may contribute to the development and/or severity of IPF. It is thought that the presence of a hiatal hernia contributes to weakness of the LES and is, therefore, associated with GER and esophagitis [17, 66]. In respiratory disorders, it is unclear how the presence of a hiatal hernia may affect or contribute to the nature of pressure variations in the thorax. We speculate that obstructive lung disorders, such as asthma or COPD, may cause increased intrathoracic pressures that push the hemidiaphragms downward and thereby promote the development of a hiatal hernia. In contrast, the volume loss and increased elastic recoil of the lung that is associated with fibrotic

ILD may lead to cranially directed forces being exerted on the diaphragm that may also potentially disrupt the integrity of the LES. Noth and colleagues demonstrated that the prevalence of hiatal hernia, which was diagnosed on CT scans, was significantly higher in IPF patients (39 %), compared to the controls with asthma or COPD (16.7 % and 13.3 %, respectively) [5]. Although there were no differences in pulmonary function or composite physiologic index (CPI) in IPF patients with and without hiatal hernia, IPF patients with hiatal hernia on anti-reflux therapy had significantly higher DLCOs compared to those not on therapy (58 % vs. 50 %). Furthermore, in a small subset of these patients who underwent esophageal pH monitoring and manometry, those with hiatal hernias were demonstrated to have significantly higher DeMeester scores (22.8 vs. 10.2). Although previous studies were unable to demonstrate an association between a decline in lung function with the presence of reflux, this study suggests that the treatment of reflux in IPF patients with hiatal hernias may have a protective role on lung function.

In summary, a multitude of clinical studies have been reported that show an increased prevalence of GER in IPF, and a variety of diagnostic modalities have been utilized, often in combination, to establish the presence of GER in patients with IPF. These include screening for the presence of reflux symptoms, ambulatory esophageal pH monitoring, esophageal manometry, EBC, and detecting the presence of a hiatal hernia. Because many studies suggest that GER in IPF patients may be asymptomatic, clinicians are encouraged to have a low threshold to initiate an evaluation to detect the presence of GER.

## Treatment of GERD in IPF

IPF is a relentless, progressive disease that is nearly uniformly fatal. Currently, there are no approved medications for patients with this disease. Historically, antifibrotic or anti-inflammatory therapies have been proven ineffective in altering the progression of disease or survival. Therefore, the notion of treating reflux disease in IPF has obvious appeal to both clinicians and investigators alike. However, how aggressive GERD should be addressed with medical or surgical interventions remains poorly defined, and no specific guidelines have been published.

Several studies have examined whether treating GERD, either medically or surgically, can affect pulmonary symptoms and the progression of fibrosis. Raghu et al. [13] retrospectively reviewed the clinical course of four newly diagnosed IPF patients with documented abnormal GER to determine whether therapeutic intervention to adequately suppress acid reflux could have an impact on disease progression. These patients were treated with PPIs and Nissen fundoplication for repair of a hiatal hernia (if present), and the patients were followed regularly over 2–4 years with serial pulmonary function testing. Two out of the four patients showed deterioration with non-adherence to antiacid therapy, but subsequently stabilized when acid suppression therapy was resumed. Although the clinical courses of these four patients were variable, the authors concluded that treatment of GER was associated with stabilization or improvement in respiratory status as measured by FVC and DLCO. During the follow-up period, none of the patients required treatment for respiratory decompensation or experienced an acute exacerbation of IPF. Although the numbers were small, the authors suggested that suppression of acid and preventing GER (in the case of those who underwent surgery for hiatal hernia) halted the progression of fibrosis. Although limited by the small number of subjects and the retrospective nature of the study, it was the first report to suggest that aggressive treatment of GER may be beneficial in the natural history of pulmonary fibrosis, and these observations were thought to support the hypothesis that repetitive parenchymal injury is mediated by the chronic microaspiration of refluxed gastric acid.

As mentioned previously, the presence of reflux in the setting of lung transplantation might predispose individuals to the development of bronchiolitis obliterans. Linden and colleagues compared 14 IPF patients awaiting lung transplant who underwent laparoscopic Nissen fundoplication to IPF patients who did not undergo surgery [67]. There were no complications from surgery and the authors concluded that such laparoscopic procedures could be performed safely in patients with advanced IPF. Postsurgery, no patients had recurrent heartburn or regurgitation symptoms, although some experienced superficial wound infections and esophageal strictures. Furthermore, surgery was associated with a reduction in supplemental oxygen from 3.0 to 2.5 L/min, whereas those who did not undergo surgery had an average increase from 2.0 to 3.0 L/min. In addition, over a mean follow-up of 15 months, exercise capacity and lung function remained stable in the surgical treatment group. While these results are encouraging, this was a relatively small retrospective study, and larger randomized trials of surgical intervention in IPF patients with reflux will be informative.

A recent large study of over 200 IPF patients that examined the survival of patients with GERD demonstrated that the use of GERD medications was an independent indicator or predictor of longer survival [68], and the use of GERD medications was associated with a lower radiographic fibrosis score. While these results suggest that treatment of GERD may confer a survival benefit, it is possible that nonrandomized patients receiving GERD therapy may also receive other valuable interventions such as pulmonary rehabilitation and pneumonia vaccinations. Moreover, patients who have GERD and are on medications may have been diagnosed with IPF sooner than others, resulting in a lead-time survival bias.

Cumulatively, these studies suggest that medical and/or surgical therapies for GER may have a positive effect on important clinical parameters in IPF including supplemental oxygen requirements, the trajectory of pulmonary function change over time, and perhaps even survival. Given the current lack of approved antifibrotic therapies in IPF and the relative ease of treating acid reflux, many clinicians attempt empiric GER treatment. Further investigation is clearly needed to definitively clarify the role of GER treatment in the care of IPF patients. In addition, the results of studies to evaluate anti-reflux surgical interventions in IPF will inform our understanding of the pathogenic role of duodenogastric reflux. Because the production of biliary secretions may not be affected by PPI therapy, the distinction between duodenogastric reflux and gastric reflux has both pathogenic and therapeutic implications.

# Summary

Multiple investigations have established an association between GER and IPF, and a potential role of reflux and microaspiration in the development and natural history of IPF has been suggested. However, while abnormal GER may be highly prevalent among IPF patients, it is unknown how many patients have attributable microaspiration events that contribute to their lung function decline. There is no gold standard test to diagnose microaspiration, but the detection of pepsin and bile salts in the BAL fluid of IPF patients may represent a promising diagnostic tool. Until a good diagnostic test is established, acid reflux disease will likely continue to serve as a surrogate diagnosis for microaspiration in these patients. More accurate diagnostic measures for microaspiration are needed to advance our understanding of the role of aspiration in causing pulmonary fibrosis. In particular, the question still remains whether GER causes fibrosis or, on the other hand, whether fibrosis causes reflux. The former implies that repetitive injury, via aspiration of either acidic or nonacidic gastric or duodenogastric secretions, may cause epithelial damage and inflammation that can lead to poor wound healing and an exaggerated fibroproliferative response in the genetically susceptible host. Additionally, we hypothesize that the presence of severe pulmonary fibrosis may alter respiratory mechanics, which may cause and perpetuate associated reflux disease. In particular, the decrease in lung compliance may lead to increased negative intrapleural pressures that can be transmitted to other mediastinal structures, including the esophagus [41]. This relayed pressure can ultimately lead to a weakened LES, which may be a major etiology of GERD in patients with IPF. While this hypothesis is plausible, multiple studies have failed to demonstrate a relationship between the degree of lung function decline and the presence of GERD. Finally, it is unknown if treating or preventing GER and microaspiration will affect the course of IPF. Until a causal relationship is established and an effective therapy is demonstrated, clinicians will continue to question the utility of treating IPF patients with significant but asymptomatic GER. Further research into the pathophysiology of IPF and the response to therapeutic interventions, including ones that target reflux disease, is ongoing. These efforts will hopefully enhance our care of patients with this devastating disease.

# References

1. Raghu G, Collard HR, Egan JJ, Martinez FJ, Behr J, Brown KK, et al. An official ATS/ERS/JRS/ALAT statement: idiopathic pulmonary fibrosis: evidence-based guidelines for diagnosis and management. Am J Respir Crit Care Med. 2011;183(6):788–824.
2. Harari S, Caminati A. Idiopathic pulmonary fibrosis. Allergy. 2005;60(4):421–35.
3. American Thoracic Society. Idiopathic pulmonary fibrosis: diagnosis and treatment. International consensus statement. American Thoracic Society (ATS), and the European Respiratory Society (ERS). Am J Respir Crit Care Med. 2000;161(2 Pt 1):646–64.
4. Lee JS, Collard HR, Raghu G, Sweet MP, Hays SR, Campos GM, et al. Does chronic micro-aspiration cause idiopathic pulmonary fibrosis? Am J Med. 2010;123(4):304–11.

5. Noth I, Zangan SM, Soares RV, Forsythe A, Demchuk C, Takahashi SM, et al. Prevalence of hiatal hernia by blinded multidetector CT in patients with idiopathic pulmonary fibrosis. Eur Respir J. 2012;39(2):344–51.
6. Dent J, Armstrong D, Delaney B, Moayyedi P, Talley NJ, Vakil N. Symptom evaluation in reflux disease: workshop background, processes, terminology, recommendations, and discussion outputs. Gut. 2004;53 Suppl 4:iv1–24.
7. Moayyedi P, Talley NJ. Gastro-oesophageal reflux disease. Lancet. 2006;367(9528):2086–100.
8. Dent J, El-Serag HB, Wallander MA, Johansson S. Epidemiology of gastro-oesophageal reflux disease: a systematic review. Gut. 2005;54(5):710–7.
9. Fahim A, Crooks M, Hart SP. Gastroesophageal reflux and idiopathic pulmonary fibrosis: a review. Pulm Med. 2011;2011:634613.
10. Kahrilas PJ. GERD pathogenesis, pathophysiology, and clinical manifestations. Cleve Clin J Med. 2003;70 Suppl 5:S4–19.
11. Dent J. Patterns of lower esophageal sphincter function associated with gastroesophageal reflux. Am J Med. 1997;103(5A):29S–32.
12. Demeter P, Pap A. The relationship between gastroesophageal reflux disease and obstructive sleep apnea. J Gastroenterol. 2004;39(9):815–20.
13. Raghu G, Yang ST, Spada C, Hayes J, Pellegrini CA. Sole treatment of acid gastroesophageal reflux in idiopathic pulmonary fibrosis: a case series. Chest. 2006;129(3):794–800.
14. Caskey CI, Zerhouni EA, Fishman EK, Rahmouni AD. Aging of the diaphragm: a CT study. Radiology. 1989;171(2):385–9.
15. Jones MP, Sloan SS, Rabine JC, Ebert CC, Huang CF, Kahrilas PJ. Hiatal hernia size is the dominant determinant of esophagitis presence and severity in gastroesophageal reflux disease. Am J Gastroenterol. 2001;96(6):1711–7.
16. Skinner D. Hernias (hiatal, traumatic, and congenital). In: Berk J, editor. Gastroenterology. 4th ed. Philadelphia, PA: WB Saunders; 1985.
17. Lord RV, DeMeester SR, Peters JH, Hagen JA, Elyssnia D, Sheth CT, et al. Hiatal hernia, lower esophageal sphincter incompetence, and effectiveness of Nissen fundoplication in the spectrum of gastroesophageal reflux disease. J Gastrointest Surg. 2009;13(4):602–10.
18. Johnson LF, Demeester TR. Twenty-four-hour pH monitoring of the distal esophagus. A quantitative measure of gastroesophageal reflux. Am J Gastroenterol. 1974;62(4):325–32.
19. Teabeaut 2nd JR. Aspiration of gastric contents; an experimental study. Am J Pathol. 1952;28(1):51–67.
20. Greenfield LJ, Singleton RP, McCaffree DR, Coalson JJ. Pulmonary effects of experimental graded aspiration of hydrochloric acid. Ann Surg. 1969;170(1):74–86.
21. Amigoni M, Bellani G, Scanziani M, Masson S, Bertoli E, Radaelli E, et al. Lung injury and recovery in a murine model of unilateral acid aspiration: functional, biochemical, and morphologic characterization. Anesthesiology. 2008;108(6):1037–46.
22. Kwan M, Xu YD, Raghu G, Khalil N. Acid treatment of normal rat lungs releases transforming growth factor-beta1 (TGF-beta1) and increases connective tissue synthesis. Proceedings of the American Thoracic Society (PATS). Am J Respir Crit Care Med. 2007;175:A967.
23. Marik PE. Aspiration pneumonitis and aspiration pneumonia. N Engl J Med. 2001;344(9):665–71.
24. Vaezi MF, Singh S, Richter JE. Role of acid and duodenogastric reflux in esophageal mucosal injury: a review of animal and human studies. Gastroenterology. 1995;108(6):1897–907.
25. Warner MA, Warner ME, Weber JG. Clinical significance of pulmonary aspiration during the perioperative period. Anesthesiology. 1993;78(1):56–62.
26. Vaezi MF, Richter JE. Role of acid and duodenogastroesophageal reflux in gastroesophageal reflux disease. Gastroenterology. 1996;111(5):1192–9.
27. Ours TM, Fackler WK, Richter JE, Vaezi MF. Nocturnal acid breakthrough: clinical significance and correlation with esophageal acid exposure. Am J Gastroenterol. 2003;98(3):545–50.
28. D'Ovidio F, Mura M, Tsang M, Waddell TK, Hutcheon MA, Singer LG, et al. Bile acid aspiration and the development of bronchiolitis obliterans after lung transplantation. J Thorac Cardiovasc Surg. 2005;129(5):1144–52.

29. Blondeau K, Mertens V, Vanaudenaerde BA, Verleden GM, Van Raemdonck DE, Sifrim D, et al. Gastro-oesophageal reflux and gastric aspiration in lung transplant patients with or without chronic rejection. Eur Respir J. 2008;31(4):707–13.
30. D'Ovidio F, Mura M, Ridsdale R, Takahashi H, Waddell TK, Hutcheon M, et al. The effect of reflux and bile acid aspiration on the lung allograft and its surfactant and innate immunity molecules SP-A and SP-D. Am J Transplant. 2006;6(8):1930–8.
31. Chang KO, Sosnovtsev SV, Belliot G, Kim Y, Saif LJ, Green KY. Bile acids are essential for porcine enteric calicivirus replication in association with down-regulation of signal transducer and activator of transcription 1. Proc Natl Acad Sci USA. 2004;101(23):8733–8.
32. Kastelik JA, Redington AE, Aziz I, Buckton GK, Smith CM, Dakkak M, et al. Abnormal oesophageal motility in patients with chronic cough. Thorax. 2003;58(8):699–702.
33. Ford AC, Forman D, Moayyedi P, Morice AH. Cough in the community: a cross sectional survey and the relationship to gastrointestinal symptoms. Thorax. 2006;61(11):975–9.
34. Wiener GJ, Koufman JA, Wu WC, Cooper JB, Richter JE, Castell DO. Chronic hoarseness secondary to gastroesophageal reflux disease: documentation with 24-h ambulatory pH monitoring. Am J Gastroenterol. 1989;84(12):1503–8.
35. Simpson WG. Gastroesophageal reflux disease and asthma. Diagnosis and management. Arch Intern Med. 1995;155(8):798–803.
36. Harding SM, Guzzo MR, Richter JE. The prevalence of gastroesophageal reflux in asthma patients without reflux symptoms. Am J Respir Crit Care Med. 2000;162(1):34–9.
37. Havemann BD, Henderson CA, El-Serag HB. The association between gastro-oesophageal reflux disease and asthma: a systematic review. Gut. 2007;56(12):1654–64.
38. Nordenstedt H, Nilsson M, Johansson S, Wallander MA, Johnsen R, Hveem K, et al. The relation between gastroesophageal reflux and respiratory symptoms in a population-based study: the Nord-Trondelag health survey. Chest. 2006;129(4):1051–6.
39. Ducolone A, Vandevenne A, Jouin H, Grob JC, Coumaros D, Meyer C, et al. Gastroesophageal reflux in patients with asthma and chronic bronchitis. Am Rev Respir Dis. 1987;135(2): 327–32.
40. Schnatz PF, Castell JA, Castell DO. Pulmonary symptoms associated with gastroesophageal reflux: use of ambulatory pH monitoring to diagnose and to direct therapy. Am J Gastroenterol. 1996;91(9):1715–8.
41. Larrain A, Carrasco E, Galleguillos F, Sepulveda R, Pope 2nd CE. Medical and surgical treatment of nonallergic asthma associated with gastroesophageal reflux. Chest. 1991;99(6):1330–5.
42. Sontag SJ, O'Connell S, Khandelwal S, Greenlee H, Schnell T, Nemchausky B, et al. Asthmatics with gastroesophageal reflux: long term results of a randomized trial of medical and surgical antireflux therapies. Am J Gastroenterol. 2003;98(5):987–99.
43. el-Serag HB, Sonnenberg A. Comorbid occurrence of laryngeal or pulmonary disease with esophagitis in United States military veterans. Gastroenterology. 1997;113(3):755–60.
44. Perrin-Fayolle M. Gastroesophageal reflux and chronic respiratory disease in adults. Influence and results of surgical therapy. Clin Rev Allergy. 1990;8(4):457–69.
45. Barish CF, Wu WC, Castell DO. Respiratory complications of gastroesophageal reflux. Arch Intern Med. 1985;145(10):1882–8.
46. Button BM, Roberts S, Kotsimbos TC, Levvey BJ, Williams TJ, Bailey M, et al. Gastroesophageal reflux (symptomatic and silent): a potentially significant problem in patients with cystic fibrosis before and after lung transplantation. J Heart Lung Transplant. 2005;24(10): 1522–9.
47. Blondeau K, Dupont LJ, Mertens V, Verleden G, Malfroot A, Vandenplas Y, et al. Gastro-oesophageal reflux and aspiration of gastric contents in adult patients with cystic fibrosis. Gut. 2008;57(8):1049–55.
48. Aseeri A, Brodlie M, Lordan J, Corris P, Pearson J, Ward C, et al. Bile acids are present in the lower airways of people with cystic fibrosis. Am J Respir Crit Care Med. 2012;185(4):463.
49. McCarthy DS, Baragar FD, Dhingra S, Sigurdson M, Sutherland JB, Rigby M, et al. The lungs in systemic sclerosis (scleroderma): a review and new information. Semin Arthritis Rheum. 1988;17(4):271–83.

50. Bouros D, Wells AU, Nicholson AG, Colby TV, Polychronopoulos V, Pantelidis P, et al. Histopathologic subsets of fibrosing alveolitis in patients with systemic sclerosis and their relationship to outcome. Am J Respir Crit Care Med. 2002;165(12):1581–6.
51. Troshinsky MB, Kane GC, Varga J, Cater JR, Fish JE, Jimenez SA, et al. Pulmonary function and gastroesophageal reflux in systemic sclerosis. Ann Intern Med. 1994;121(1):6–10.
52. Denis P, Ducrotte P, Pasquis P, Lefrancois R. Esophageal motility and pulmonary function in progressive systemic sclerosis. Respiration. 1981;42(1):21–4.
53. Marie I, Dominique S, Levesque H, Ducrotte P, Denis P, Hellot MF, et al. Esophageal involvement and pulmonary manifestations in systemic sclerosis. Arthritis Rheum. 2001;45(4):346–54.
54. Savarino E, Bazzica M, Zentilin P, Pohl D, Parodi A, Cittadini G, et al. Gastroesophageal reflux and pulmonary fibrosis in scleroderma: a study using pH-impedance monitoring. Am J Respir Crit Care Med. 2009;179(5):408–13.
55. Gilson M, Zerkak D, Wipff J, Dusser D, Dinh-Xuan AT, Abitbol V, et al. Prognostic factors for lung function in systemic sclerosis: prospective study of 105 cases. Eur Respir J. 2010;35(1):112–7.
56. Tobin RW, Pope 2nd CE, Pellegrini CA, Emond MJ, Sillery J, Raghu G. Increased prevalence of gastroesophageal reflux in patients with idiopathic pulmonary fibrosis. Am J Respir Crit Care Med. 1998;158(6):1804–8.
57. Raghu G, Freudenberger TD, Yang S, Curtis JR, Spada C, Hayes J, et al. High prevalence of abnormal acid gastro-oesophageal reflux in idiopathic pulmonary fibrosis. Eur Respir J. 2006;27(1):136–42.
58. Bandeira CD, Rubin AS, Cardoso PF, Moreira Jda S, Machado Mda M. Prevalence of gastroesophageal reflux disease in patients with idiopathic pulmonary fibrosis. J Bras Pneumol. 2009;35(12):1182–9.
59. Fahim A, Dettmar PW, Morice AH, Hart SP. Gastroesophageal reflux and idiopathic pulmonary fibrosis: a prospective study. Medicina (Kaunas). 2011;47(4):200–5.
60. Sweet MP, Patti MG, Leard LE, Golden JA, Hays SR, Hoopes C, et al. Gastroesophageal reflux in patients with idiopathic pulmonary fibrosis referred for lung transplantation. J Thorac Cardiovasc Surg. 2007;133(4):1078–84.
61. Cantu 3rd E, Appel 3rd JZ, Hartwig MG, Woreta H, Green C, Messier R, et al. J. Maxwell Chamberlain Memorial Paper. Early fundoplication prevents chronic allograft dysfunction in patients with gastroesophageal reflux disease. Ann Thorac Surg. 2004;78(4):1142–51. discussion-51.
62. Stovold R, Forrest IA, Corris PA, Murphy DM, Smith JA, Decalmer S, et al. Pepsin, a biomarker of gastric aspiration in lung allografts: a putative association with rejection. Am J Respir Crit Care Med. 2007;175(12):1298–303.
63. Collard HR, Moore BB, Flaherty KR, Brown KK, Kaner RJ, King Jr TE, et al. Acute exacerbations of idiopathic pulmonary fibrosis. Am J Respir Crit Care Med. 2007;176(7):636–43.
64. Lee JS, Song JW, Wolters PJ, Elicker BM, King Jr TE, Kim DS, et al. Bronchoalveolar lavage pepsin in acute exacerbation of idiopathic pulmonary fibrosis. Eur Respir J. 2012;39(2):352–8.
65. Tcherakian C, Cottin V, Brillet PY, Freynet O, Naggara N, Carton Z, et al. Progression of idiopathic pulmonary fibrosis: lessons from asymmetrical disease. Thorax. 2011;66(3):226–31.
66. Fein M, Ritter MP, DeMeester TR, Oberg S, Peters JH, Hagen JA, et al. Role of the lower esophageal sphincter and hiatal hernia in the pathogenesis of gastroesophageal reflux disease. J Gastrointest Surg. 1999;3(4):405–10.
67. Linden PA, Gilbert RJ, Yeap BY, Boyle K, Deykin A, Jaklitsch MT, et al. Laparoscopic fundoplication in patients with end-stage lung disease awaiting transplantation. J Thorac Cardiovasc Surg. 2006;131(2):438–46.
68. Lee JS, Ryu JH, Elicker BM, Lydell CP, Jones KD, Wolters PJ, et al. Gastroesophageal reflux therapy is associated with longer survival in patients with idiopathic pulmonary fibrosis. Am J Respir Crit Care Med. 2011;184(12):1390–4.

# Chapter 14
# Pharmacological Treatment of Idiopathic Pulmonary Fibrosis

Paolo Spagnolo, Fabrizio Luppi, Gloria Montanari, and Luca Richeldi

**Abstract**  Idiopathic pulmonary fibrosis (IPF) is the most common and most lethal diffuse fibrosing lung disease, with a mortality rate that exceeds that of many types of cancer. At present there is no effective standard treatment recommended by guideline documents. However, several high-quality clinical trials evaluating a number of novel therapies have recently been concluded. The results have mostly been disappointing, although some compounds have shown promising results. In particular, pirfenidone seems to be the most advanced agent for IPF treatment, having been approved in Europe, Japan, and India. In general, due to the complexity and the uncertainties intrinsic to IPF, it is essential that each therapeutic strategy be tailored to the individual patient after discussing the potential benefits and pitfalls. Randomized controlled trials still represent a valid choice for IPF patients, and their completion is critically important to achieving the ultimate goal of curing IPF.

**Keywords**  Idiopathic pulmonary fibrosis • Clinical trials • Pirfenidone • Treatment • Endpoints

## Introduction

In the last decade, the pharmacological approach to the management of idiopathic pulmonary fibrosis (IPF) has changed considerably, thus mirroring the evolving understanding in the disease pathogenesis. The initial thinking was that a persistent

P. Spagnolo, M.D., Ph.D. • F. Luppi, M.D., Ph.D. • G. Montanari, M.D.
Center for Rare Lung Diseases, University Hospital Policlinico of Modena, Modena, Italy

L. Richeldi, M.D., Ph.D. (✉)
Chair of Interstitial Lung Disease, University Hospital Southampton, Tremona Road, Southampton SO16 6YD, United Kingdom
e-mail: L.Richeldi@soton.ac.uk

K.C. Meyer and S.D. Nathan (eds.), *Idiopathic Pulmonary Fibrosis: A Comprehensive Clinical Guide*, Respiratory Medicine 9, DOI 10.1007/978-1-62703-682-5_14,
© Springer Science+Business Media New York 2014

**Table 14.1** Summary of the current evidence-based recommendations on pharmacological treatment of patients with IPF[a]

|  | Recommendation | | | |
|---|---|---|---|---|
|  | For | | Against | |
|  | Weak | Strong | Strong | Weak |
| Corticosteroids alone |  |  | × |  |
| Colchicine |  |  | × |  |
| Cyclosporin A |  |  | × |  |
| Cyclophosphamide + corticosteroids |  |  | × |  |
| Azathioprine + corticosteroids |  |  | × |  |
| Azathioprine + corticosteroids + NAC[b] |  |  |  | × |
| NAC alone |  |  |  | × |
| Interferon-γ-1b |  |  | × |  |
| Bosentan |  |  | × |  |
| Etanercept |  |  | × |  |
| Warfarin[b] |  |  |  | × |
| Pirfenidone |  |  |  | × |

NAC N-acetylcysteine

Note: Official recommendations are not available for sildenafil and imatinib, as the results of clinical trials evaluating these drugs have been published after the publication of the ATS/ERS/JRS/ALAT 2011 guideline document [2]. See text for details

[a]Adapted from [2]

[b]Recommendations on these drugs are likely to change in the near future based on the results from recently published clinical trials

inflammatory process triggered fibrosis and scarring of the lung. As such, trials did evaluate the efficacy of drugs that primarily exert their functions by suppressing inflammatory or immune responses, such as corticosteroids and immunomodulatory agents: the results of these trials have all been uniformly disappointing. Over the last decade, the perspective on IPF pathogenesis has profoundly changed, and nowadays the disease is thought to result from an aberrant reparative mechanism with excessive deposition of extracellular matrix, following an injury that primarily affects the lung epithelium [1]. Accordingly, more recent randomized, controlled trials have shifted their focus to molecules with antifibrotic and antiproliferative properties. Nonetheless, because the pathogenesis of IPF remains incompletely understood, the rationale of some trials evaluating the efficacy of specific compounds has been derived from post hoc analyses of previous studies. Several drugs approved for the treatment of different diseases, but with some background for being effective in fibrotic disorders, have also been evaluated in IPF clinical trials.

Available therapeutic options for IPF have recently been systematically assessed in keeping with current approaches to "evidence-based medicine" and according to the GRADE methodology (Table 14.1) [2, 3]. Thus, for the very first time, clinicians confronted with an IPF patient can base their clinical decisions on the evidence derived from data obtained from randomized controlled trials.

## Anti-inflammatory and Immunomodulatory Drugs

Early therapeutic studies in IPF focused largely on the effects of corticosteroids, because of their anti-inflammatory effects and wide use in clinical practice for a number of fibrotic lung disorder. Generally, these studies were conducted prior to the international guidelines published in 2000 [4], thus resulting in a more heterogeneous patient cohort than those currently defined as having IPF. The majority of these studies were anecdotal and noncontrolled and likely included patients with other idiopathic interstitial pneumonias (such as nonspecific interstitial pneumonia) that are more likely to respond to anti-inflammatory therapies. A 2003 Cochrane systematic review of the results available for efficacy of corticosteroids in IPF surprisingly did not identify any randomized controlled trial addressing this important clinical issue [5]. An update of that same systematic review published in 2010 [6] once again did not identify any properly designed trial, thus confirming the absolute lack of evidence for the use of corticosteroids in IPF. On the other hand, long-term corticosteroid therapy is associated with significant treatment-related morbidity and various potentially severe side effects. As a result, current evidence-based guidelines [2] provide a strong recommendation against the use of corticosteroid monotherapy in IPF, albeit in the absence of any randomized placebo-controlled trial. Similarly, low-quality evidence is available for the use of nonsteroid immunomodulatory drugs, such as colchicine, cyclosporin A, cyclophosphamide, or azathioprine, either alone or in combination with corticosteroids [7]. As such, current guidelines [2] recommend against the use of immunomodulatory agents in the treatment of IPF patients. Nevertheless, azathioprine, which in combination with low-dose steroids has long represented the suggested *standard of care* in IPF [4], warrants more extensive discussion.

Azathioprine, which is an antimetabolite, blocks most T-cell functions, inhibits primary antibody synthesis, and decreases the number of circulating monocytes and granulocytes [8]. In a prospective, double-blind, placebo-controlled trial, 27 newly diagnosed patients with IPF were randomized in a 1:1 ratio to prednisone [1.5 mg/(kg day) for 2 weeks, with a biweekly taper until a maintenance dose of 20 mg/day] plus either placebo or azathioprine [3 mg/(kg day) to a maximum of 200 mg/day] [9]. After 1 year, changes in lung function, as measured by resting $P[A-a]O_2$, forced vital capacity (FVC), and diffusing capacity of the lung for carbon monoxide (DLCO), were all somewhat better in the azathioprine/prednisone group than in the prednisone/placebo arm, although none of these comparisons were statistically significant. The number of adverse events did not differ between groups.

## Antioxidants

The IFIGENIA (Idiopathic Pulmonary Fibrosis International Group Exploring N-Acetylcysteine) was a double-blind, randomized, placebo-controlled multicenter study that assessed the effectiveness over 1 year of a high oral dose (600 mg three times daily) of *N*-acetylcysteine (NAC), a precursor of the antioxidant glutathione, which has been shown to be reduced in the lungs of patients with IPF [10], added to *standard therapy* (i.e., a combination of prednisone and azathioprine) [11]. As compared to prednisone plus azathioprine (the "placebo" arm), the use of this so-called triple therapy slowed the rate of deterioration of vital capacity (VC) and DLCO (the primary endpoints), by 9 % and 24 %, respectively. Weaknesses of this study related mainly to the lack of a true placebo arm, the fact that the reduction in the decline of VC and DLCO in the *N*-acetylcysteine arm did not translate into a survival benefit, and the high drop-out rate with the consequent impact on the statistics that were utilized for data analysis. Specifically, the least squared last observation carried forward imputations approach tends to preserve the sample size despite a high drop-out rate but may make unwarranted assumptions about the missing data, thus potentially resulting in either underestimating or overestimating the treatment effects. Due to these drawbacks, and in spite of the positive results of the study, recent evidence-based guidelines made a weak recommendation against the use of this combination therapy. The inference of a weak recommendation is that the majority of patients with IPF should not be treated with this form of *triple therapy*, but that this therapeutic approach may be a reasonable choice in a minority [2].

To further investigate the possible efficacy of *N*-acetylcysteine in patients with IPF, the National Heart, Lung, and Blood Institute (NHLBI)-sponsored IPFnet consortium designed a placebo-controlled, randomized three-arm trial, the PANTHER-IPF (Prednisone, Azathioprine, and *N*-acetylcysteine: A Study That Evaluates Response in IPF) study in which patients with mild-to-moderate lung function impairment were randomized in a 1:1:1 ratio to prednisone, azathioprine plus NAC (combination therapy), NAC alone, or placebo. The primary outcome was the change in longitudinal FVC measurements over a 60-week time period. Secondary outcomes included mortality, time to death, frequency of acute exacerbations, and time to disease progression as defined by the composite end point of death or a relative drop in FVC $\geq 10$ %. A prespecified efficacy and safety interim analysis (planned to occur at approximately 50 % of the data collection) unexpectedly showed that the combination therapy was associated with a statistically significant increase in all-cause mortality (11 % vs. 1 %), all-cause hospitalizations (29 % vs. 8 %), and treatment-related severe adverse events (31 % vs. 9 %) as compared to placebo [12]. These observations, coupled with no evidence of physiological or clinical benefit for combination therapy, prompted the independent Data and Safety Monitoring Board to recommend termination of the combination therapy group at a mean follow-up of 32 weeks. The NAC alone and the placebo arms continue to enroll patients. These largely unexpected results not only provide evidence against the use of this combination of drugs in patients with IPF but also underscore the importance of placebo-controlled trials in areas where the effects of treatment are largely based on limited evidence or low-quality data.

## Interferon Gamma-1b

Interferon gamma-1b (IFN-$\gamma$-1b), a naturally occurring human protein secreted primarily by T cells (CD4 T cells, CD8 T cells, and natural killer cells), is thought to play a key role in downregulating expression of TGF-$\beta$, thus limiting fibroblast proliferation and collagen synthesis. A pilot study by Ziesche and coworkers showed significantly better lung function at 12 months in IPF patients treated with both IFN-$\gamma$-1b and prednisolone as compared to prednisolone alone [13]. In a large randomized, double-blind, placebo-controlled phase III trial, 330 IPF patients were assigned to receive subcutaneous IFN-$\gamma$-1b 200 $\mu$g three times weekly ($n = 162$) or placebo ($n = 168$) [14]. The primary endpoint of progression-free survival, which was defined by time to disease progression or death, was not achieved. Similarly, no significant treatment effect was observed on lung function, gas exchange, extent of fibrosis on HRCT, or quality of life. However, secondary analyses suggested that patients with mild-to-moderate impairment in lung function at study entry might be more likely to benefit from IFN-$\gamma$-1b treatment. In addition, 10 % of patients in the IFN-$\gamma$-1b arm died as compared with 17 % of patients in the placebo group, although this difference did not reach statistical significance ($p = 0.08$). While IFN-$\gamma$-1b was generally well tolerated with few discontinuations due to adverse events, there was an unexplained excess of nonfatal pneumonias in the IFN-$\gamma$-1b-treated group versus placebo. A subsequent meta-analysis involving 390 patients suggested that treatment with IFN-$\gamma$-1b was associated with a significant reduction in mortality when compared with the control group [15]. Based on these findings, a larger randomized, controlled trial of over 800 patients with mild-to-moderate IPF (International Study of Survival Outcomes in Idiopathic Pulmonary Fibrosis with Interferon Gamma-1b, the INSPIRE trial) was specifically designed to assess the efficacy of IFN-$\gamma$-1b on survival time in IPF patients with mild-to-moderate impairment in baseline pulmonary function [16]. A protocol-defined interim analysis revealed that the hazard ratio for mortality among patients randomized to treatment with IFN-$\gamma$-1b crossed the predefined stopping boundary for lack of minimal benefit. After a median duration of 77 weeks on therapy, 14.5 % of patients in the IFN-$\gamma$-1b group had died compared to 12.7 % of patients in the placebo group ($p = 0.497$). As such, current evidence-based guidelines recommend that patients with IPF should not be treated with IFN-$\gamma$ (strong recommendation, high-quality evidence) [2].

## Drugs Acting on the Pulmonary Vasculature

Data from basic science, animal, and translational studies lend support to the hypothesis that the endothelin system, and endothelin (ET)-1 in particular, is a potentially important contributor to the pathobiology of several fibrotic disorders including IPF [17]. In fact, ET-1 has been shown to modulate matrix production and turnover, leading to increased collagen synthesis and decreased interstitial collagenase production [18].

## Bosentan

In a randomized, double-blind, placebo-controlled study (Bosentan Use in Interstitial Lung Disease, BUILD-1), 158 IPF patients received either bosentan, a dual ET receptor antagonist ($ET_A$ and $ET_B$), or placebo for 12 months [19]. Bosentan was not superior to placebo in affecting exercise capacity, as measured by a modified 6-min walking test (6MWT). However, a post hoc analysis revealed a trend in favor of bosentan in time to death or disease progression in a subset of patients who had undergone a confirmatory surgical lung biopsy and who exhibited very limited honeycombing on HRCT of the chest. This secondary analysis prompted a second, prospective, randomized (2:1), double-blind, placebo-controlled trial (BUILD-3) in patients with IPF ($n=616$) of less than 3 years' duration, confirmed by surgical lung biopsy, and without extensive honeycombing (<5 %) on HRCT [20]. The primary endpoint was time to IPF worsening (a decrease from baseline in FVC $\geq$10 % and DLCO $\geq$15 %, or acute exacerbation of IPF) or death. However, despite the efficacy signal from the subgroup analysis of BUILD-1, the primary objective of the BUILD-3 trial was not met ($p=0.2110$). Similarly, no differences were observed between treatment groups with respect to changes from baseline to 1 year in health-related quality of life or dyspnea. A small and nonsignificant delay in the time to IPF worsening (excluding death) was observed, as were small differences favoring the bosentan treatment group in changes in absolute FVC and DLCO values from baseline to 1 year.

## Ambrisentan

Ambrisentan is a selective antagonist of the $ET_A$ receptor approved for the treatment of pulmonary arterial hypertension [21]. The $ET_A$ receptor also exerts pro-fibrotic activities through the stimulation of transforming growth factor-$\beta$ and by promoting epithelial-to-mesenchymal transition [22]. Importantly, evidence from preclinical models shows that the phenotypic and transcriptional responses to ambrisentan are different from bosentan, thus suggesting that clinical effects in IPF may also be different [23]. The ARTEMIS-IPF (Randomized, Placebo-Controlled Study to Evaluate Safety and Effectiveness of Ambrisentan in IPF) trial was a randomized, double-blind, placebo-controlled, multinational trial evaluating the effectiveness of ambrisentan in reducing the rate of progression of IPF. The results of this study have not yet been published in full; however, the trial was halted prematurely following an interim analysis that indicated a very low likelihood of efficacy for the primary endpoint and a likely increase in disease progression for patients in the active treatment arm [24].

## Sildenafil

Sildenafil, a phosphodiesterase-5 inhibitor that induces pulmonary vasodilatation by stabilizing the second messenger of nitric oxide, cyclic guanosine monophosphate, has been shown to induce pulmonary vasodilation in patients with pulmonary fibrosis [25]. Collard and colleagues evaluated the 6-min walk test distance (6MWD) before and after 3 months of sildenafil therapy in an open-label study of patients with IPF and associated pulmonary hypertension [26]. The study included 14 patients, although only 11 completed both 6MWTs. Sildenafil treatment was associated with a significant improvement in the 6MWD with more than half of the patients (57 %) improving their 6MWD by $\geq$20 %. These observations prompted a phase III, randomized controlled trial of sildenafil in patients with IPF (Sildenafil Trial of Exercise Performance in Idiopathic Pulmonary Fibrosis, STEP-IPF). One hundred and eighty subjects were randomized to sildenafil (20 mg three times daily) or placebo for 12 weeks with a subsequent 12-week open-label phase in which all patients received active drug [27]. The difference in the primary outcome was not significant, with 9 of 89 patients (10 %) in the sildenafil group and 6 of 91 (7 %) in the placebo group having an improvement of $\geq$20 in the 6MWD ($p$=0.39). On the other hand, significant differences favor sildenafil in a number of secondary outcomes, including the $PaO_2$, DLCO, the degree of dyspnea, and quality of life. While the primary endpoint of this study was not met, the presence of some positive secondary outcomes creates clinical equipoise for further research.

## Etanercept

Etanercept is a recombinant, soluble monoclonal antibody directed against the human tumor necrosis factor-alpha (TNF-$\alpha$) receptor and neutralizes TNF-$\alpha$ activity. The rationale for its use in IPF comes from the observations that TNF-$\alpha$ has inflammatory and fibrogenic properties, and elevated levels of this cytokine have been detected in the lungs of patients with IPF [28, 29]. Additionally, TNF antagonists inhibit pulmonary inflammation and fibrosis in animal models of pulmonary fibrosis [30], suggesting that such agents could potentially diminish the fibrotic response in the lungs of patients with IPF. In a very carefully designed and conducted phase II, randomized, prospective, double-blind, placebo-controlled multicenter trial, IPF patients were randomly assigned to either placebo ($n$=41) subcutaneous etanercept (25 mg; $n$=46), which was given twice weekly [31]. At 48 weeks, no significant differences in efficacy endpoints [changes in the % predicted FVC, % predicted DLCO, or the P(A–a)$O_2$ from baseline values] were observed between the groups. On the other hand, using rate of disease progression (death or absolute reduction in FVC) in a post hoc analysis, the authors observed a trend favoring etanercept that was statistically insignificant.

## Pirfenidone

Pirfenidone is a pyridone compound with antifibrotic, anti-inflammatory, and antioxidant activity, although its precise mode of action is largely unknown. The first report of its possible efficacy in IPF was revealed in a phase II trial in patients with advanced disease. In this open-label study, 54 consecutive patients with IPF who had deteriorating lung function despite conventional therapy or who were unable to tolerate or unwilling to try conventional therapy were treated with oral pirfenidone and followed for mortality, change in lung function, and adverse effects [32]. Pirfenidone appeared to slow the decline in lung function and enabled corticosteroid dosage to be reduced to discontinuation in the majority of patients. In addition, the drug was well tolerated. In a subsequent multicenter, randomized, double-blind, placebo-controlled phase II trial, 107 Japanese patients were randomly assigned to receive an escalating dosage of either pirfenidone or placebo [33]. There was no significant difference between the pirfenidone and placebo groups in the primary endpoint measure, which was the change in the lowest blood oxygen saturation ($SpO_2$) during a 6-min steady-state exercise test. However, in a prespecified subset of patients who maintained a $SpO_2$ greater than 80 % during the baseline 6-min exercise test, an improvement was noted in the lowest $SpO_2$ at 6 and 9 months in the pirfenidone group. Positive treatment effects were also observed in change in VC at 9 months and rate of acute exacerbations, and acute exacerbations occurred exclusively in the placebo group. Significant adverse events were associated with pirfenidone; skin photosensitivity, gastrointestinal symptoms, and liver function test abnormalities were the most common ones, although there was no significant difference in the treatment discontinuation rate between the two groups at 9 months.

In a subsequent larger, multicenter, double-blind, placebo-controlled, randomized phase III clinical trial of pirfenidone, 275 Japanese patients with IPF were randomly assigned in a 2:1:2 ratio to high dose (1,800 mg/day), low dose (1,200 mg/day), or placebo [34]. Significant differences were observed in terms of decline in the VC (the primary endpoint) from baseline to week 52 between the placebo group (−0.16 L) and both the high- (−0.09 L; $p=0.042$) and the low-dose groups (−0.08 L; $p=0.039$). Further, significant differences were observed in progression-free survival (PFS) time between the high-dose and the placebo arms ($p=0.028$) and in the difference of mean changes in total lung capacity (TLC) between the low-dose and the placebo arms ($p=0.040$). Similarly to the previous study, photosensitivity was the most common adverse event in the pirfenidone arm, but it was not a major reason for discontinuation from the study. Overall, the drug-related adverse events were mild and disappeared with a decrease in dose or temporary withholding of the medication.

Finally, in two concurrent international, multicenter, randomized, double-blinded, placebo-controlled trials (PIPF 006: CAPACITY 1 and PIPF 004: CAPACITY 2), patients with IPF were randomly assigned to oral pirfenidone or placebo for a minimum of 72 weeks [35]. In study 004, patients were assigned in a 2:1:2 ratio to pirfenidone 2,403 mg/day, pirfenidone 1,197 mg/day, or placebo, while in study 006, patients were assigned in a 1:1 ratio to pirfenidone 2,403 mg/day or placebo. The primary endpoint was change in percentage predicted FVC at week 72. In study 004, the mean FVC change at week 72 was −8.0 % in the pirfenidone 2,403 mg/day arm and −12.4 % in the placebo group ($p=0.001$), while mean change in percentage FVC in the pirfenidone 1,197 mg/day group was intermediate to that in the pirfenidone 2,403 mg/day and placebo groups. Conversely, in study 006, the difference between groups in FVC change at week 72 was not significant

($p = 0.501$). Intrinsic IPF heterogeneity, different prevalence of comorbidities (such as pulmonary hypertension), and the effect of genetic variations might explain the discrepancies in the results of these two parallel, otherwise identical, large trials.

All these trials have had sufficient methodological quality to allow their inclusion in a recent Cochrane systematic review [7]. Based on the results of this meta-analysis, it was concluded that pirfenidone appears to significantly reduce the risk of disease progression (as measured by progression-free survival) by 30 % and to ameliorate the loss of lung function. Some limitations to the interpretation of these data still apply, mostly related to a certain degree of methodological heterogeneity across studies with regard to reporting of lung function data.

The recent approval in Europe of pirfenidone (already approved in Japan and India) for mild-to-moderate IPF patients further corroborates the potential relevance of this drug in IPF. Conversely, the US Food and Drug Administration (FDA) has declined approval of pirfenidone for treatment of IPF and asked for additional evidence. As a result, a further phase III randomized, double-blinded, placebo-controlled trial (Assessment of Pirfenidone to Confirm Efficacy and Safety in IPF, the ASCEND trial) is currently enrolling patients in the USA. Current IPF guidelines, considering the cost of therapy and the potentially relevant side effects, expressed a weak recommendation against the use of this drug. However, it has to be noted that the majority of panel experts abstained in this voting. Whether pirfenidone should be given to all IPF patients is still a matter of debate. In any event, patients willing to receive pirfenidone should be fully informed of the available evidence attesting to the efficacy of the drug as well as to its possible side effects.

# Anticoagulants

Inflammation and vascular injury have been proposed to contribute to a prothrombotic state in IPF [36]. Based on this pathogenetic hypothesis, 56 Japanese patients with IPF were randomly assigned to prednisolone alone or prednisolone plus anticoagulation (unfractionated or low-molecular-weight heparin during follow-up when rehospitalized and warfarin during outpatient treatment) in an unblinded study [37]. While the incidence of acute exacerbations did not differ between the groups, the mortality associated with acute exacerbation was significantly reduced in the anticoagulant group compared to that in the non-anticoagulant group (18 % vs. 71 %, respectively; $p = 0.008$). In turn, this translated to a significant improvement in survival at 3 years (63 % in the anticoagulant group compared with 35 % in the non-anticoagulant one). Several methodological issues raise concerns regarding this study. These include absence of blinding, incidence of acute exacerbation higher than what is usually observed (64 % in the placebo group), patient recruitment on initial hospitalization that may have caused a selection bias toward patients with more advanced and rapidly progressive disease, substantial withdrawals of patients in the anticoagulant group after randomization but before initiating treatment (which makes it difficult to exclude the possibility that patients who withdrew were more ill and would have had higher mortality), and failure to exclude pulmonary embolism as a potential cause of acute deterioration. Therefore, treatment with anticoagulants was not recommended for routine use in patients with IPF (weak recommendation, very low-quality evidence) [2].

More recently, the Anticoagulant Effectiveness in Idiopathic Pulmonary Fibrosis (ACE-IPF) trial (sponsored by the IPFnet in the USA) was specifically designed to test the hypothesis that warfarin would reduce rates of mortality, hospitalization, and decline in FVC [38]. In this double-blind, placebo-controlled trial patients were randomly assigned in a 1:1 ratio to warfarin or matching placebo for a planned treatment period of 48 weeks. Due to a low probability of benefit and an increase in mortality observed in the subjects randomized to warfarin (14 warfarin vs. 3 placebo deaths; $p = 0.005$), the independent Data and Safety Monitoring Board recommended stopping the study after 145 of the planned 256 subjects were enrolled (72 warfarin, 73 placebo). Similar trends in the warfarin arm were observed in all-cause hospitalization, respiratory-related hospitalization, and acute exacerbation of IPF. In partial accordance with the current guideline recommendations, the results of this study strongly argue against the routine use of warfarin for the treatment of IPF. As such, recommendations on this drug are very likely to change in the near future.

# Tyrosine Kinase Inhibitors

Tyrosine kinases regulate a variety of physiological cell processes that include metabolism, growth, differentiation, and apoptosis, and aberrant tyrosine kinase activity has been shown to promote the development and progression of both neoplastic and non-neoplastic diseases [39, 40]. Signaling pathways activated by tyrosine kinases have also been suggested to be involved in lung fibrosis [41]. This, in turn, has prompted clinical trials evaluating the efficacy of tyrosine kinase inhibitors in IPF.

## Nintedanib (BIBF 1120)

The TOMORROW (To Improve Pulmonary Fibrosis With BIBF 1120) study (a 12-month, randomized, double-blind, placebo-controlled trial) evaluated the safety and efficacy of Nintedanib [42], which is an intracellular inhibitor of various tyrosine kinase receptors including platelet-derived growth factor receptors (PDGFR) α and β; vascular endothelial growth factor receptors (VEGFR) 1, 2, and 3; and fibroblast growth factor receptors (FGFR) 1, 2, and 3 [43].

Four different oral doses of Nintedanib (50 mg once a day, 50 mg, 100 mg, or 150 mg all twice a day) were tested. The primary endpoint was the annual rate of decline in FVC. Secondary endpoints included acute exacerbations, quality of life (measured with the SGRQ), and total lung capacity. Nintedanib at a dose of 150 mg twice daily showed a trend toward a reduction in the decline in lung function (along with fewer acute exacerbations and preserved quality of life) as compared with placebo. Specifically, in the group receiving 150 mg of Nintedanib twice a day, FVC declined by 0.06 L per year, as compared with 0.19 L per year in the placebo group, a 68.4 % reduction in the rate of loss of lung function. In addition, patients treated with 150 mg of Nintedanib twice daily had a lower incidence of acute exacerbations and a small decrease in SGRQ score (as compared with an increase with placebo). Additionally, Nintedanib showed an acceptable safety profile. In fact, while gastrointestinal side effects (diarrhea, nausea, and vomiting) and increases in levels of liver aminotransferases were more frequent in the high-dose group than in the placebo arm, severe adverse events occurred with similar frequency in all groups. These results warrant the further investigation of Nintedanib in a phase III clinical study, which is underway with results expected to become available in 2014.

## *Imatinib*

Imatinib is a tyrosine kinase inhibitor with activity against several fibrogenic factors (including PDGFR-$\alpha$ and $\beta$). It has been investigated in IPF based on encouraging data from animal models of lung fibrosis, and imatinib has been shown to inhibit lung fibroblast-myofibroblast transformation and proliferation as well as extracellular matrix production through inhibition of PDGF and TGF-$\beta$ signaling [44].

In a phase II, randomized, double-blind, placebo-controlled study, 119 IPF patients collected from 13 centers in the USA and Mexico were randomly assigned to receive imatinib (600 mg orally once daily; $n = 59$) or placebo ($n = 60$) for 96 weeks [45]. Patients were eligible if they had had clinical worsening within the past year as demonstrated by any one of the following: $\geq 10$ % decrease in FVC% predicted, worsening chest X-ray, or worsening dyspnea at rest or on exertion. This trial specifically sought to study patients with "mild-or-moderate" IPF. The primary outcome was a combined measure of disease progression defined as a $\geq 10$ % decline in FVC from baseline or death. Secondary endpoints included change from baseline in DLCO% predicted, change from baseline in the resting arterial blood gas assessment of A–a gradient, change in the distance walked in a 6MWT, change from baseline in SGRQ assessments, and overall mortality, and all endpoints were evaluated after 96 weeks. No differences in the predefined primary or secondary endpoints were observed between the imatinib and the placebo groups, and serious adverse events occurred at similar rates in the two study groups.

## Summary

The last decade has been extraordinarily fruitful for the study of IPF with a steadily increasing number of high-quality clinical studies being designed, undertaken, and completed. This massive effort of both the medical community and pharmaceutical/

biotechnology industry has led to the approval (in Japan, Europe, and India) of the first drug (pirfenidone) for clinical use in IPF. In addition, the well-characterized patient datasets of these studies have provided valuable insights about the natural history of the disease. Crucial information has also been gained about the lack of efficacy of specific drugs that had showed preclinical promise as potential inhibitors of fibrosis. The failure of both anticoagulants and endothelin receptor antagonists to show any benefit in patients with IPF suggests that pathways involving the coagulation cascade or the endothelin system are not as critical in disease pathogenesis as was previously thought. This serves to underscore the fact that our understanding of the intricate interaction of the diverse pathways involved in the development and progression of pulmonary fibrosis remains incomplete. These negative phase III study findings should also encourage the development of new animal models (or the refinement of existing ones) that are able to better recapitulate the complex pathobiology of pulmonary fibrosis in humans [46].

The growth in IPF clinical trials in the past few years has highlighted the challenge of identifying the appropriate patient population for enrollment. Thus far, clinical trials in IPF have enrolled patients with mild-to-moderate disease, as assessed by FVC. However, the identification and inclusion of individuals at highest risk of disease progression, who are the ones more likely to respond to any given treatment, would permit enrichment in study populations and potentially allow a corresponding reduction in required sample sizes. In this regard, a recently developed multidimensional prediction model that combines individual variables (gender [G], age [A], and two lung physiology variables [P] [FVC and DLCO]) could facilitate future research in IPF by identifying patients at high risk for clinically significant outcomes, thus maximizing the efficiency and power of future clinical trials [47].

Considerable debate continues concerning the most appropriate, clinically meaningful outcome measures that should be used in future clinical trials in IPF [48, 49]. Although enhanced survival is undoubtedly the most robust primary endpoint, the number of patients and study duration required for adequate power (particularly, for patients with "early" IPF) to be attained may be prohibitive, unless patients with advanced disease were also enrolled. On the other hand, such patients are likely to behave quite differently from those with mild-to-moderate disease and may frequently die of pulmonary vascular complications rather than progressive fibrosis. As such, a number of surrogate markers for survival benefit have been proposed. Of these, change in FVC (either *absolute* or *relative*) has been the most commonly employed measure of disease progression, because it closely fulfills the ideal characteristics of being reliable, reproducible, easy to measure, and applicable to all IPF patients [50, 51]. Nevertheless, progression-free survival, which is usually employed in lung cancer patients, or composite endpoints, may also represent meaningful outcomes in clinical trials of IPF. Improvement of the standard of care for patients with IPF requires the continued commitment and efforts of patients, expert clinicians, the pharmaceutical industry, and regulatory agencies. Thus, clinicians and patients alike need to be fully aware of all available clinical trials and urged to participate in the global effort to find efficacious treatment regimens for patients with IPF.

A drug or drug regimen that provides a universally agreed upon standard of care for patients with IPF has yet to emerge. In addition, owing to the plethora of potential disease pathways, the future treatment of IPF will likely require a multi-agent strategy that targets all components of disease pathogenesis (injury, inflammation, if any, and fibrosis). Nonetheless, the current momentum in this area of research, together with experience gained and emerging insights from more refined studies of genetic susceptibility, provides hope for future success in the treatment of this devastating disease.

# References

1. King Jr TE, Pardo A, Selman M. Idiopathic pulmonary fibrosis. Lancet. 2011;378:1949–61.
2. Raghu G, Collard HR, Egan JJ, Martinez FJ, Behr J, Brown KK, et al. An official ATS/ERS/ JRS/ALAT statement: idiopathic pulmonary fibrosis: evidence-based guidelines for diagnosis and management. Am J Respir Crit Care Med. 2011;183:788–824.
3. Schünemann HJ, Jaeschke R, Cook DJ, Bria WF, El-Solh AA, Ernst A, et al. An official ATS statement: grading the quality of evidence and strength of recommendations in ATS guidelines and recommendations. Am J Respir Crit Care Med. 2006;174:605–14.
4. American Thoracic Society. Idiopathic pulmonary fibrosis: diagnosis and treatment. International consensus statement. American Thoracic Society (ATS), and the European Respiratory Society (ERS). Am J Respir Crit Care Med. 2000;161:646–64.
5. Richeldi L, Davies HR, Ferrara G, Franco F. Corticosteroids for idiopathic pulmonary fibrosis. Cochrane Database Syst Rev. 2003;(3):CD002880.
6. Richeldi L, Davies HR, Spagnolo P, Luppi F. Corticosteroids for idiopathic pulmonary fibrosis. Cochrane Database Syst Rev. 2010;(2):CD002880.
7. Spagnolo P, Del Giovane C, Luppi F, Cerri S, Balduzzi S, Walters EH, et al. Non-steroid agents for idiopathic pulmonary fibrosis. Cochrane Database Syst Rev. 2010;(9):CD003134.
8. Mueller XM. Drug immunosuppression therapy for adult heart transplantation. Part 1: immune response to allograft and mechanism of action of immunosuppressants. Ann Thorac Surg. 2004;77:354–62.
9. Raghu G, Depaso WJ, Cain K, Hammar SP, Wetzel CE, Dreis DF, et al. Azathioprine combined with prednisone in the treatment of idiopathic pulmonary fibrosis: a prospective double-blind, randomized, placebo-controlled clinical trial. Am Rev Respir Dis. 1991;144:291–6.
10. Cantin AM, Hubbard RC, Crystal RG. Glutathione deficiency in the epithelial lining fluid of the lower respiratory tract in idiopathic pulmonary fibrosis. Am Rev Respir Dis. 1989;139: 370–2.
11. Demedts M, Behr J, Buhl R, Costabel U, Dekhuijzen R, Jansen HM, et al. High-dose acetylcysteine in idiopathic pulmonary fibrosis. N Engl J Med. 2005;353:2229–42.
12. The Idiopathic Pulmonary Fibrosis Clinical Research Network. Prednisone, azathioprine, and N-acetylcysteine for pulmonary fibrosis. N Engl J Med. 2012;366:1968–77.
13. Ziesche R, Hofbauer E, Wittmann K, Petkov V, Block LH. A preliminary study of long-term treatment with interferon gamma-1b and low-dose prednisolone in patients with idiopathic pulmonary fibrosis. N Engl J Med. 1999;341:1264–9.
14. Raghu G, Brown KK, Bradford WZ, Starko K, Noble PW, Schwartz DA, et al. A placebo-controlled trial of interferon gamma-1b in patients with idiopathic pulmonary fibrosis. N Engl J Med. 2004;350:125–33.
15. Bajwa EK, Ayas NT, Schulzer M, Mak E, Ryu JH, Malhotra A. Interferon-gamma1b therapy in idiopathic pulmonary fibrosis: a metaanalysis. Chest. 2005;128:203–6.

16. King Jr TE, Albera C, Bradford WZ, Costabel U, Hormel P, Lancaster L, et al. Effect of inter-feron gamma-1b on survival in patients with idiopathic pulmonary fibrosis (INSPIRE): a multicentre, randomised, placebo-controlled trial. Lancet. 2009;374:222–8.
17. Swigris JJ, Brown KK. The role of endothelin-1 in the pathogenesis of idiopathic pulmonary fibrosis. BioDrugs. 2010;24:49–54.
18. Shi-Wen X, Denton CP, Dashwood MR, Holmes AM, Bou-Gharios G, Pearson JD, et al. Fibroblast matrix gene expression and connective tissue remodeling: role of endothelin-1. J Invest Dermatol. 2001;116:417–25.
19. King Jr TE, Behr J, Brown KK, du Bois RM, Lancaster L, de Andrade JA, et al. BUILD-1: a randomized placebo-controlled trial of bosentan in idiopathic pulmonary fibrosis. Am J Respir Crit Care Med. 2008;177:75–81.
20. King Jr TE, Brown KK, Raghu G, du Bois RM, Lynch DA, Martinez F, et al. BUILD-3: a randomized, controlled trial of bosentan in idiopathic pulmonary fibrosis. Am J Respir Crit Care Med. 2011;184(1):92–9.
21. Galié N, Olschewski H, Oudiz RJ, Torres F, Frost A, Ghofrani HA, et al. Ambrisentan for the treatment of pulmonary arterial hypertension: results of the ambrisentan in pulmonary arterial hypertension, randomized, double blind, placebo-controlled, multicenter, efficacy (ARIES) study 1 and 2. Circulation. 2008;117:3010–9.
22. Jain R, Shaul PW, Borok Z, Willis BC. Endothelin-1 induces alveolar epithelial-mesenchymal transition through endothelin type A receptor-mediated production of TGF-beta1. Am J Respir Cell Mol Biol. 2007;37:38–47.
23. Henderson WR, Bammler TK, Beyer RP, Farin FM, Xue J, Ye X, et al. Effect of endothelin A (ETA) and endothelin B (ETB) receptor antagonists on gene expression in lungs with established fibrosis from a mouse pulmonary fibrosis model. Am J Respir Crit Care Med. 2011;183:A6043.
24. Raghu G, Behr J, Brown KK, Egan JJ, Kawut SM, Flaherty KR, et al. Treatment of idiopathic pulmonary fibrosis with ambrisentan: a parallel, randomized trial. Ann Intern Med. 2013;158(9):641–9.
25. Ghofrani HA, Wiedemann R, Rose F, Schermuly RT, Olschewski H, Weissmann N, et al. Sildenafil for treatment of lung fibrosis and pulmonary hypertension: a randomised controlled trial. Lancet. 2002;360:895–900.
26. Collard HR, Anstrom KJ, Schwarz MI, Zisman DA. Sildenafil improves walk distance in idiopathic pulmonary fibrosis. Chest. 2007;131:897–9.
27. Idiopathic Pulmonary Fibrosis Clinical Research Network, Zisman DA, Schwarz M, Anstrom KJ, Collard HR, Flaherty KR, Hunninghake GW. A controlled trial of sildenafil in advanced idiopathic pulmonary fibrosis. N Engl J Med. 2010;363:620–8.
28. Piguet PF, Ribaux C, Karpuz V, Grau GE, Capanci Y. Expression and localization of tumor necrosis factor-alpha and its mRNA in idiopathic pulmonary fibrosis. Am J Pathol. 1993;143:651–5.
29. Kapanci Y, Desmouliere A, Pache JC, Redard M, Gabbiani G. Cytoskeletal protein modulation in pulmonary alveolar myofibroblasts during idiopathic pulmonary fibrosis: possible role of transforming growth factor beta and tumor necrosis factor alpha. Am J Respir Crit Care Med. 1995;152:2163–9.
30. Piguet PF, Vesin C. Treatment by human recombinant soluble TNF receptor of pulmonary fibrosis induced by bleomycin or silica in mice. Eur Respir J. 1994;7:515–8.
31. Raghu G, Brown KK, Costabel U, Cottin V, du Bois RM, Lasky JA, et al. Treatment of idiopathic pulmonary fibrosis with etanercept: an exploratory, placebo-controlled trial. Am J Respir Crit Care Med. 2008;178:948–55.
32. Raghu G, Johnson WC, Lockhart D, Mageto Y. Treatment of idiopathic pulmonary fibrosis with a new antifibrotic agent, pirfenidone: results of a prospective, open-label Phase II study. Am J Respir Crit Care Med. 1999;159:1061–9.

33. Azuma A, Nukiwa T, Tsuboi E, Suga M, Abe S, Nakata K, et al. Double-blind, placebo-controlled trial of pirfenidone in patients with idiopathic pulmonary fibrosis. Am J Respir Crit Care Med. 2005;171:1040–7.

34. Taniguchi H, Ebina M, Kondoh Y, Ogura T, Azuma A, Suga M, et al. Pirfenidone in idiopathic pulmonary fibrosis. Eur Respir J. 2010;35:821–9.

35. Noble PW, Albera C, Bradford WZ, Costabel U, Glassberg MK, Kardatzke D, et al. Pirfenidone in patients with idiopathic pulmonary fibrosis (CAPACITY): two randomised trials. Lancet. 2011;377:1760–9.

36. Walter N, Collard HR, King Jr TE. Current perspectives on the treatment of idiopathic pulmonary fibrosis. Proc Am Thorac Soc. 2006;3:330–8.

37. Kubo H, Nakayama K, Yanai M, Suzuki T, Yamaya M, Watanabe M, et al. Anticoagulant therapy for idiopathic pulmonary fibrosis. Chest. 2005;128:1475–82.

38. Noth I, Anstrom KJ, Calvert SB, de Andrade J, Flaherty KR, Glazer C, et al. A placebo-controlled randomized trial of warfarin in idiopathic pulmonary fibrosis. Am J Respir Crit Care Med. 2012;186:88–95.

39. Grimminger F, Schermuly RT, Ghofrani HA. Targeting non-malignant disorders with tyrosine kinase inhibitors. Nat Rev Drug Discov. 2010;9:956–70.

40. Ciardiello F, Tortora G. EGFR antagonists in cancer treatment. N Engl J Med. 2008;358:1160–74.

41. Beyer C, Distler JH. Tyrosine kinase signaling in fibrotic disorders: translation of basic research to human disease. Biochim Biophys Acta. 1832;2013:897–904.

42. Richeldi L, Costabel U, Selman M, Kim DS, Hansell DM, Nicholson AG, et al. Efficacy of a tyrosine kinase inhibitor in idiopathic pulmonary fibrosis. N Engl J Med. 2011;365:1079–87.

43. Hilberg F, Roth GJ, Krssak M, Kautschitsch S, Sommergruber W, Tontsch-Grunt U, et al. BIBF 1120: triple angiokinase inhibitor with sustained receptor blockade and good antitumor efficacy. Cancer Res. 2008;68:4774–82.

44. Daniels CE, Wilkes MC, Edens M, Kottom TJ, Murphy SJ, Limper AH, et al. Imatinib mesylate inhibits the profibrogenic activity of TGF-beta and prevents bleomycin-mediated lung fibrosis. J Clin Invest. 2004;114:1308–16.

45. Daniels CE, Lasky JA, Limper AH, Mieras K, Gabor E, Schroeder DR, Imatinib-IPF Study Investigators. Imatinib treatment for IPF: randomised placebo controlled trial results. Am J Respir Crit Care Med. 2010;181:604–10.

46. Moeller A, Ask K, Warburton D, Gauldie J, Kolb M. The bleomycin animal model: a useful tool to investigate treatment options for idiopathic pulmonary fibrosis? Int J Biochem Cell Biol. 2008;40:362–82.

47. Ley B, Ryerson CJ, Vittinghoff E, Ryu JH, Tomassetti S, Lee JS, et al. A multidimensional index and staging system for idiopathic pulmonary fibrosis. Ann Intern Med. 2012;156:684–91.

48. Raghu G, Collard HR, Anstrom KJ, Flaherty KR, Fleming TR, King Jr TE, et al. Idiopathic pulmonary fibrosis: clinically meaningful primary endpoints in phase 3 clinical trials. Am J Respir Crit Care Med. 2012;185:1044–8.

49. du Bois RM, Nathan SD, Richeldi L, Schwarz MI, Noble PW. Idiopathic pulmonary fibrosis: lung function is a clinically meaningful endpoint for phase 3 trials. Am J Respir Crit Care Med. 2012;186:712–5.

50. du Bois RM, Weycker D, Albera C, Bradford WZ, Costabel U, Kartashov A, et al. Forced vital capacity in patients with idiopathic pulmonary fibrosis: test properties and minimal clinically important difference. Am J Respir Crit Care Med. 2011;184:1382–9.

51. Richeldi L, Ryerson CJ, Lee JS, Wolters PJ, Koth LL, Ley B, et al. Relative versus absolute change in forced vital capacity in idiopathic pulmonary fibrosis. Thorax. 2012;67:407–11.

# Chapter 15
# Recognizing and Treating Comorbidities of IPF

Teng Moua and Jay H. Ryu

**Abstract** Idiopathic pulmonary fibrosis (IPF) is a progressive and unrelenting disease whose natural history may be complicated by multiple comorbidities. Among these, this chapter will highlight the prevalence, clinical approach, and management of the following: acute exacerbation (AE), combined pulmonary fibrosis and emphysema (CPFE), pulmonary hypertension (PH), gastroesophageal reflux disease (GERD), thromboembolic disease, cardiovascular disease, lung cancer, and end-of-life care.

**Keywords** Idiopathic pulmonary fibrosis comorbidities • Acute exacerbation • Combined pulmonary fibrosis and emphysema • Pulmonary hypertension • Gastroesophageal reflux disease • Cardiovascular disease • Thromboembolic disease • Dyspnea • Palliative care

## Introduction

The clinical course of patients with idiopathic pulmonary fibrosis (IPF) is often unpredictable but progressive and unrelenting. While many experience gradual decline in respiratory status due to progressive pulmonary fibrosis, some encounter unexpected acute illnesses, complications related to progressive respiratory insufficiency, and the added burden of coexisting medical conditions. Eventual cause of death for the majority of patients is IPF itself though others may die from pneumonia, aspiration, myocardial infarction, stroke, and other non-pulmonary causes [1, 2].

T. Moua, M.D. (✉)
Division of Pulmonary and Critical Care Medicine, Mayo Clinic, Gonda 18 South,
200 First Street, SW, Rochester, MN 55902, USA
e-mail: Moua.Teng@mayo.edu

J.H. Ryu, M.D.
Division of Pulmonary and Critical Care Medicine, Mayo Clinic, Rochester, MN, USA

K.C. Meyer and S.D. Nathan (eds.), *Idiopathic Pulmonary Fibrosis: A Comprehensive Clinical Guide*, Respiratory Medicine 9, DOI 10.1007/978-1-62703-682-5_15,
© Springer Science+Business Media New York 2014

**Table 15.1** Comorbidities with associated frequency, risk of morbidity or mortality, and current therapies

| Comorbidity | Frequency | Associated morbidity/mortality | Current therapy |
|---|---|---|---|
| AE | 9.6–57 % over 2–3 years [4, 8] | 22–86 % mortality at the time of AE [14, 22] | High-dose steroids, supportive management |
| CPFE | 5–28 % [38, 39] | Median survival 25 months [38]; 40 % mortality at 1 year [42] | Directed PH management (vasoactive drug, diuretic, etc.), unproven |
| PH | 31.6–84 % [49, 50] | 28 % mortality at 1 year [49] | Directed PH management |
| GERD | 67–94 % [69, 70, 72] | Apparent longer survival with empiric treatment [76] | PPI, H2-blocker, behavioral modifications (head-of-bed elevation, diet) |
| VTE | 1.5 % incidence [83], risk 34 % higher than in background population [85] | Increased risk of death and death at a younger age [85] | Directed anticoagulation if discovered, no evidence for prophylaxis |
| CV disease | 28.6–65.8 % with CAD on heart cath [92, 94], twice the risk of CV disease than the general population followed over 3 years [83] | Unknown in terms of additional risk of morbidity or death | Directed therapy if known, no evidence for screening or improvement in outcomes with treatment |
| Lung cancer | 4.2–22 % of IPF patients [102, 107] | Varied mortality at 2 and 5 years less than the general population, increased perioperative morbidity due to pulmonary complications | Surgical resection if feasible in stage IA disease |

*AE* acute exacerbation, *CAD* coronary artery disease, *CPFE* combined pulmonary fibrosis with emphysema, *CV* cardiovascula, *GERD* gastroesophageal reflux disease, *IPF* idiopathic pulmonary fibrosis, *PH* pulmonary hypertension, *PPI* proton pump inhibitor, *VTE* venous thromboembolism

In this chapter, we highlight issues of acute exacerbation (AE), combined pulmonary fibrosis and emphysema (CPFE), pulmonary hypertension (PH), gastroesophageal reflux disease (GERD), venous thromboembolism (VTE), cardiovascular disease, lung cancer, and end-of-life care (Table 15.1).

## Acute Exacerbation

Although IPF is generally progressive and unrelenting, its natural history may be punctuated by single or multiple deteriorations resulting in periods of rapid clinical decline and sometimes death. Prior studies have described the phenomenon of acute exacerbation (AE) associated with chronic lung fibrosis and defined it by varied clinical and physiological parameters [3–5]. Kondoh et al. first described acute respiratory failure without a definable precipitating cause in three patients with pulmonary fibrosis [6]. A recent international consensus statement defines acute exacerbation in IPF by the following criteria (1) previous or concurrent diagnosis of fibrotic lung disease, (2) unexplained worsening of dyspnea within 30 days, (3) computed tomography (CT) findings of increased ground glass or opacification superimposed on underlying features of usual interstitial pneumonia, (4) exclusion of infection by bronchoscopic assessment, and finally, (5) the clinical exclusion of other known etiologies of acute respiratory failure including heart failure, pulmonary embolism, or other causes of lung injury (aspiration, sepsis, drug toxicity, etc.) [7]. Room is provided in this definition for "suspected AE" where a complete work up may not be feasible in fully meeting the above criteria.

Prior studies [4, 8, 9] are limited in their assessment of the exact incidence and prevalence of AE, notably because of varied definitions prior to the 2007 international consensus statement. Commonly referenced prevalences range from 9.6 to 57 % at 2–3 years after diagnosis [4, 7, 8, 10]. A recent randomized controlled trial assessing the antifibrotic agent pirfenidone found an IPF-related death rate representing AE or rapid decline of 8 % in the control arm [11]. Most recently, Song et al. presented the largest retrospective cohort of patients with IPF to date describing both acute exacerbation and "rapid deterioration" and found a 1- and 2-year incidence of 14.2 % and 20.7 %, respectively [12]. Nearly one-third of patients experienced rapid deterioration requiring hospitalization with either AE or infection as the most common underlying etiologies. Longitudinally, AE was also associated with a greater risk of death and morbidity even in survivors (15.5 months vs. 60.6 months in those without AE) [12]. AE may also be the presenting manifestation of undiagnosed pulmonary fibrosis in some patients [12–14]. It has also been recognized to occur in fibrotic lung diseases other than IPF, such as the connective tissue disease-related ILDs and chronic hypersensitivity pneumonitis [14–16].

The exact pathophysiology of AE remains elusive, with recent hypotheses suggesting AE as a rapid progression of underlying fibrosis, manifestation of a biologically unique form of lung injury, or manifestation of an occult secondary injury unrelated to the fibrotic process [7, 17]. Recent work suggests the mechanism of AE may be dependent on Type II alveolar epithelial cell dysfunction along with endothelial cell injury and coagulation abnormalities, with little evidence of Type I alveolar epithelial cell response or inflammation [18, 19]. This hypothesis proposes rapid inappropriate cellular repair and fibrosis perhaps triggered by an unknown acute injury such as infection or aspiration [20, 21].

Histopathologically, AE manifests as diffuse alveolar damage indistinguishable from the lung injury of acute respiratory distress syndrome (ARDS) or acute interstitial pneumonia (AIP) [22]. Underlying usual interstitial pneumonia (UIP) delineates AE of IPF from these other disease entities. AE has also been reported in patients with underlying histological nonspecific interstitial pneumonia (NSIP) and may pose similar risks of morbidity and mortality as seen in UIP or IPF [23]. Although AE most commonly manifests as diffuse alveolar damage, organizing pneumonia has also been reported as the histopathologic pattern underlying AE [14, 24]. The current consensus statement does not require histopathological confirmation for the diagnosis AE in IPF [7].

Risk factors delineated from the largest retrospective cohort study to date note more severe baseline disease (lower forced vital capacity [FVC] and forced expiratory volume in one second [$FEV_1$]), nonsmoking history, and use of corticosteroids or cytotoxic agents as associated with increased risk of exacerbation [12]. A recent study investigating the risk of AE in patients with advanced IPF awaiting lung transplant found an increased risk in those with pulmonary hypertension but no association with other baseline characteristics [25]. Similarly, no definable baseline risk factors were consistently found in other cohort studies [3, 4, 14]. The presence of GERD and aspiration is believed to be associated with progression of fibrotic lung disease with a recent report finding increased pepsin levels in the bronchoalveolar lavage (BAL) fluid of patients with AE compared to those with stable disease [21]. Reports also suggest an increased risk of AE in patients undergoing invasive diagnostic procedures [26–38].

The approach to assessing and managing AE involves the diagnostic evaluation for known or secondary etiologies, including infection, heart failure, and pulmonary embolism. Patients usually present with rapid or acute increase in dyspnea and cough over several weeks. Fever or flu-like symptoms without significant productive sputum are commonly reported [3, 4, 14]. Physical exam is generally nonspecific, and laboratory testing reveals mild to moderate leukocytosis and elevated serum lactate dehydrogenase (LDH) levels [3, 4]. As noted, AE may be associated with invasive procedures such as surgical lung biopsy or bronchoscopy [26, 29]. One recent report found increased 30-day risk of exacerbation associated with bronchoalveolar lavage [30]. Radiologic features are nonspecific and commonly consist of ground-glass opacities superimposed on pulmonary fibrosis (peripheral honeycombing and reticular opacities) at the time of exacerbation. Computed tomography findings of diffuse or multifocal opacities have been reported to be associated with worse outcome compared to peripherally distributed disease [5], though this observation was not confirmed on a subsequent radiological study [15]. CT quantitative scoring and comparison of pre-exacerbation severity of ground glass have been shown to be prognostically useful [31]. In general, bronchoalveolar lavage is recommended to delineate an infectious etiology with neutrophilia the most commonly seen BAL differential cell count at the time of exacerbation [3, 4, 14].

Once identifiable causes of acute deterioration have been excluded, management remains primarily supportive. Evidence for intravenous high-dose corticosteroids (e.g., 1 g of methylprednisolone daily) remains inconclusive and, although commonly practiced, is of unproven benefit with survival remaining dismal. Prior studies have reported anecdotal success with the use of cyclosporine and other anti-inflammatory agents [32, 33]. Short-term mortality associated with AE has ranged from 22 [22] to 86 % [14], with additional deaths occurring over the ensuing year [12]. The need for mechanical ventilation in the setting of AE portends a poor outcome, and despite lung-protective strategies, mortality remains high in those requiring intensive care unit admission [34–37]. The prognosis associated with mechanical ventilation in the management of AE needs to be discussed with patients and their families prior to intubation. No particular prophylactic approach to decrease the incidence of AE is known, and continued research is needed to identify risk factors for AE and effective strategies to manage the underlying disease progression such that consensus can be reached regarding prevention and treatment of AE episodes.

## Combined Pulmonary Fibrosis and Emphysema

Although believed to occur by separate pathophysiological mechanisms, recent reports have focused on the association of pulmonary fibrosis and emphysema (Fig. 15.1). Termed combined pulmonary fibrosis and emphysema (CPFE), debate continues as to whether this represents a distinct entity with unique features or simply the development of lung fibrosis in patients with preexisting emphysema related to smoking. Characteristic features of this syndrome include its predominantly male prevalence, association with pulmonary hypertension, and increased morbidity when compared to pulmonary fibrosis without emphysema.

In 2009, Mejía et al. reported in a single-center retrospective review of IPF patients over a 10-year span a concomitant emphysema prevalence of 28 %, suggesting a higher frequency than previously thought [38]. Similar to prior reports, there was a preponderance of male smokers, and combined disease was highly associated with pulmonary hypertension. Cottin et al. estimated a concomitant emphysema prevalence of around 5–10 % of patients with pulmonary fibrosis in their multicenter survey-based assessment of 61 cases defined by radiological appearance of combined disease [39]. Predominant CT features were upper lobe emphysema and lower

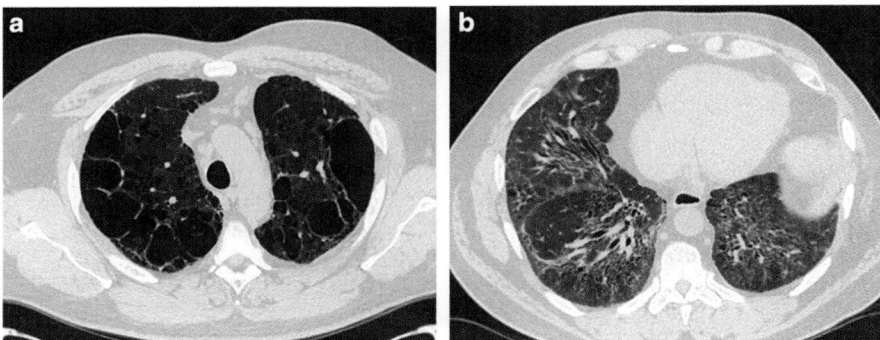

**Fig. 15.1** A 51-year-old male with combined lung fibrosis and emphysema. Note predominant *upper lobe* bullous emphysema and *lower lobe* interstitial fibrosis (patient reported 40 pack-years smoking history)

lobe fibrosis [40]. This study specifically excluded patients with secondary interstitial lung disease and followed the progression of radiologic disease over time; combined fibrosis and emphysema was discovered at the initial presentation in
approximately half of the cases [39]. The median smoking history by pack-years
was 5 (range of 0–60 pack-years) in the cohort reported by Mejía et al. [38] and a
mean of $46 \pm 27$ years in the report by Cottin et al. [39], though no association of
CPFE with pack-years was found. A majority were active smokers in one study [38],
while only a third were active in another [39]. Pulmonary function findings in CPFE
have ranged from restrictive to a mixed obstructive restrictive pattern, with a consistently low diffusing capacity for carbon monoxide (DLCO) [38, 39, 41, 42].

Remarkably, all cohort studies reported the association of CPFE with advanced
pulmonary hypertension (PH) [38, 39, 41]. Mejía et al. and Cottin et al. found a
prevalence of 100 % [38] and 47 % [39], respectively, and noted increased morbidity
and mortality associated with PH in combined disease compared with pulmonary
fibrosis or emphysema alone. A reported delay of $16.5 \pm 25$ months between respiratory symptoms and right heart catheterization (RHC) confirmation of pulmonary
hypertension was noted in one report [42]. The mean right ventricular systolic pressure (RVSP) as reported in one cohort [38] was notably severe at 82.3 mmHg, with
right heart catheterization revealing a mean pulmonary artery pressure range from 24
to 56 mmHg [42] in a second study. The majority of patients with CPFE progressed
or presented with moderate to severe disease and appear to be at greater risk of death
and cor pulmonale versus patients with lone idiopathic pulmonary artery hypertension or pulmonary hypertension associated with lone emphysema or lone pulmonary
fibrosis [42]. It is theorized that smoking-related vascular injury may occur in a
unique fashion in those patients with combined fibrotic and emphysematous disease,
allowing more rapid progression and decline [43]. Hypoxemia may also be contributory to pulmonary hypertension with gas exchange being more impaired than in
those with lone emphysema or fibrosis. No particular study exists regarding the specific management of pulmonary hypertension in CPFE and its effect on survival.

Notably, the appearance of lone emphysema prior to pulmonary fibrosis was
seen in approximately one-fourth of the cohort reported by Cottin et al. with a
median of approximately 5 years between imaging studies [39]. Understanding the
role of emphysema in the modification of fibrosis or vice versa remains elusive.
Prior reports suggest clinically occult fibrosis may be common in patients with
advanced emphysema, the so-called smoking-related interstitial fibrosis (SRIF)
whose pathology is distinctive from the idiopathic interstitial pneumonias [44, 45].
Katzenstein et al. described theses features as thickened alveolar interstitium filled
by eosinophilic collagenous fibrosis, with occasional fibroblast foci, but without the
typical architectural features of UIP or the other idiopathic or secondary interstitial
lung diseases [45]. Of this reported cohort, none had radiographic or pulmonary
function features of fibrosis or restriction. Such findings suggest the presence of
fibrosis to be more common than clinically suspected in patients with emphysema,
but whether such fibrosis has any bearing on the progression of emphysema is
unknown. Recent work suggests the role of matrix metalloproteases (MMP), a family of structurally related enzymes involved in the degradation and formation of

extracellular matrix and basement membranes, in both IPF and emphysema. Members of this enzyme family are upregulated in both diseases and share overlapping profiles at the histological level [46]. Rogliani et al. assessed the enzyme profile of patients with lone fibrosis, lone emphysema, and combined fibrosis and emphysema and found a similar MMP profile between those with IPF and combined disease, suggesting similarity in the underlying fibrotic process of CPFE and IPF, though CPFE may represent a more rapid or aggressive form of fibrotic progression [46]. This finding supports CPFE as perhaps a predominantly fibrotic process that may concomitantly drive emphysema.

The clinical implications of recognizing and identifying CPFE include the increased morbidity of the syndrome when compared to lone fibrosis, its increased association with severe pulmonary hypertension and cor pulmonale, and the difficulty of following progression or response to therapy as pulmonary function testing may not fully reflect the severity of respiratory impairment, with relatively well-preserved airflow and lung volumes. Inclusion of patients with CPFE in clinical trials may confound pulmonary function endpoints, and indeed in clinical practice, the longitudinal assessment of pulmonary function in such patients may not be prognostically relevant. A proposed composite physiological index score adjusting for fibrosis and inclusive of pulmonary function values was recently reported as predictive of mortality in a cohort of patients of which approximately half were diagnosed with CPFE [47]. No other markers of disease progression or response to therapy have been studied in this regard. Management remains difficult as no specific effect on survival from the management of pulmonary hypertension in patients with CPFE was found by Cottin et al. in their review, with treatments ranging from diuretics to bosentan and sildenafil [42]. Caution was suggested by the authors based on the retrospective and uncontrolled nature of their study along with heterogeneity of the study population and treatment modalities.

## Pulmonary Hypertension

Pulmonary hypertension (PH) secondary to ILD was included in the most recent international classification [48] under section 3.2, which encompasses secondary lung disease and hypoxemia. Previous studies of PH associated with IPF have defined it as mean pulmonary artery pressure (mPAP) >25 mmHg on right heart catheterization (RHC) [49] without LV dysfunction or systolic pulmonary artery pressure (which is essentially equivalent to the right ventricular systolic pressure) greater than 35 mmHg as seen on transthoracic echocardiography (TTE) [50]. The practice of obtaining RHC is often reserved until the time of lung transplant evaluation. However, a systematic approach to predicting and obtaining diagnosis of PH has been the subject of several reports, as it contributes significantly to morbidity and mortality [51–54].

The prevalence of PH in IPF ranges from approximately a third to nearly 85 % of patients with end-stage or advanced disease [49, 50, 55, 56]. Its prevalence is nearly

100 % in those with CPFE and portends an increase in morbidity and mortality [38, 41, 42]. Given the overlap of clinical presentation between pulmonary fibrosis and PH, the presence of pulmonary vascular disease may easily be overlooked in patients with IPF. Studies evaluating CT features, pulmonary function testing, and echocardiographic findings as predictors of PH have found these modalities to be relatively inaccurate in diagnosing underlying PH [54, 56–58]. Zisman et al. proposed a clinical prediction tool based on oxygen saturation and percent-predicted FVC and DLCO which reported good sensitivity and negative predictive value at a specified cutoff [53]. Others have evaluated functional parameters such as 6-min walk and return to resting heart rate after activity as correlating with the presence of PH [52].

Clinical risk factors for the development of PH in IPF are not entirely clear. While pulmonary hypertension is well defined in patients with advanced fibrosis, its frequency in patients with early disease is not well established, but is known to occur. Letteri et al. reported a linear correlation between mPAP and mortality in their single-center study of patients undergoing RHC [49]. Even after exclusion of left ventricular dysfunction, over half who died had PH as compared to only a third of survivors. Nadrous et al. reported a similar correlation with increasing systolic pulmonary artery pressures as measured by echocardiography and worse survival [50].

Predominant theories on the pathophysiology of PH in fibrotic lung disease include hypoxemic vascular remodeling and reduction in the total vascular bed by fibrotic obliteration. As the pulmonary vasculature develops in close proximity to airways and alveoli, it is theorized that lung destruction from fibrosis results in decreased vascular cross-sectional area and increased precapillary pressures [59]. Pathological examination of explanted lungs from IPF patients has noted increased neovascularization in areas of cellular fibrosis but absent vascularity in end-stage fibrotic or honeycomb regions [25]. This pathological feature suggests difficulty in treating lung fibrosis as decreased blood flow to fibrotic regions makes advanced fibrosis likely irreversible. Presumably, regions of active fibrogenesis may be more amenable to therapeutic agents. Unfortunately local epithelial injury responsible for acute fibrotic processes also promotes vascular and endothelial cell injury and apoptosis, with increased production of vasoconstrictors and recruitment of fibroblasts and vascular smooth muscle cells leading to eventual vessel remodeling and further worsening of vascular resistance [60]. Histological examination of pulmonary arteries and arterioles from explanted fibrotic lungs reveals broad structural alterations including increased intimal and smooth muscle wall thickening as well as plexiform lesions [61]. More severe vascular abnormalities are seen in regions of greater parenchymal fibrosis. Although such mechanisms support fibrosis over hypoxemic vasoconstriction as the primary contributor to IPF-associated PH, the severity of fibrosis as found on radiologist CT scoring was not predictive of presence or severity of PH [54].

IPF-associated PH has not been specifically studied as an endpoint in treatment trials, though 6-min walk distance and secondary markers of health-associated quality of life and delayed time to death or disease progression were evaluated in two randomized controlled trials of the endothelin receptor antagonist, bosentan [62, 63]. A trend towards improved quality of life and delay in clinical disease progression was found in a subset of patients with atypical CT features and biopsy-proven UIP, likely representing early disease [62], although this finding was not confirmed when disease progression (FVC) was used as the primary endpoint in a subsequent study [63]. Sildenafil was shown to improve walking distance by a mean of 49 m after 3 months of use in patients with IPF in an open-label study [64] with a prior study of 16 patients with varied secondary fibrotic lung diseases also demonstrating physiological improvements in cardiac index, mPAP, and pulmonary vascular resistance [65]. One report suggested inhaled iloprost as helpful in decreasing vascular resistance in IPF-associated PH with effects comparable to that of inhaled nitric oxide or IV prostacyclin [66]. Treprostinil was reported as possibly helpful in bridging end-stage disease to transplant in the setting of severe and advanced fibrosis-associated PH [67]. As PH contributes significantly to increased morbidity and mortality in IPF, it is hoped that directed management may extend life, though definitive improvements in survival with current treatments have yet to be established.

## Gastroesophageal Reflux Disease

Gastroesophageal reflux disease (GERD) is frequently seen in patients with IPF, ranging from 67 to 94 % [68–70]. Defined by an elevated DeMeester score on 24-h pH monitoring [71] as well as clinical reflux symptoms, the prevalence of GERD appears to be increased in patients with IPF as compared to those with other lung diseases including asthma and non-IPF interstitial lung diseases [69, 72]. Approximately 67 % of patients awaiting lung transplant who underwent esophageal manometry and 24-h pH monitoring had GERD [70]. An increased association of symptomatic reflux with occult lung fibrosis and scarring has also been reported [73, 74]. Patients reporting symptomatic GERD range from approximately a third to nearly half [70, 72, 75, 76], with most investigators proposing that symptoms are unreliable as predictors of reflux and possible reflux-associated fibrosis.

Although there is a notable increased association of IPF with gastroesophageal reflux, the exact relationship between reflux and fibrosis is unclear, particularly as GERD is commonly present in the general population while IPF is an uncommon disorder. Microaspiration of acidic gastric content has been demonstrated to increase fibrotic lung injury in experimental animal studies [77]. Increased pepsin seen in the BAL of patients with acute exacerbation suggests gastric content aspiration may be a possible trigger of this acute deterioration [21]. Interestingly, pathological identification of aspirated foreign bodies associated with acute exacerbation, early disease, or end-stage disease with explant or autopsy is uncommon. Both acidic and nonacidic microaspiration are likely contributory to lung injury based on the observation that proton pump inhibitor (PPI) or histamine-2 (H2) blocker usage does not decrease mechanical reflux, and lung fibrosis progresses despite empiric medical therapy in many patients [78]. Changes in chest wall anatomy with perturbations of the esophagus as lung disease progresses have been proposed as contributory to abnormal lower and upper esophageal sphincter tone [75]. In that regard, increased GERD may be indicative of progressive lung disease rather than a direct cause of lung injury itself. Some have proposed microaspiration as perhaps one among other triggers in the setting of a genetically susceptible patient, whose response to recurrent aspiration injury may be that of exuberant fibrosis and dysfunctional repair [79].

A recent retrospective review found empiric treatment with PPI or H2 blockers was associated with a decreased CT fibrosis score and was an independent predictor of better survival [76], though others have found no association between the severity of GERD and the severity of radiologic manifestations of disease in IPF [68, 69]. Some propose that the decision to empirically treat may be appropriate, given the relatively safe profile of current therapies, while also recognizing that mechanical reflux is not affected by medical management. IPF patients with symptomatic GERD undergoing Nissen fundoplication while awaiting lung transplant were found to have stabilized oxygen needs in comparison to those without surgical intervention, though lung function remained similar between the two groups [80]. In post-transplant patients, fundoplication was shown to stabilize progression of bronchiolitis obliterans in those with demonstrated mechanical reflux or symptomatic GERD [81, 82]. Unfortunately, Nissen fundoplication or other surgical interventions may not guarantee cure of mechanical reflux and may only reduce or ameliorate the severity of disease. As microaspiration may simply be a trigger for fibrosis and not directly result in fibrotic injury, the morbidity of such a procedure has not been justified for pretransplant IPF patients. If symptomatic GERD is present, the combination of both empiric PPI therapy and behavioral changes such as head-of-bed elevation, diet modification, and weight reduction seems prudent, and it is not clear that a need for confirmatory invasive esophageal testing to confirm disease is necessary [78]. Therefore, diagnostic testing for GERD in patients with IPF should be individualized.

## Venous Thromboembolic Disease

Three prior population-based reports suggest an increased risk and incidence of venous thromboembolic disease (VTE) in patients with IPF (Fig. 15.2). In a British study, 920 incident cases of IPF were compared to 3,593 matched controls assessing the frequency of underlying cardiovascular and thromboembolic disease, and found patients with IPF had twice the incident risk of deep vein thrombosis (DVT) prior to diagnosis, and one and a half to seven times the risk after the diagnosis of IPF had been made [83]. Follow-up of incident usage of cardioprotective drugs in patients with or without IPF found increased usage of warfarin and ACE inhibitors. Sode et al. conducted a study of the Danish population examining the association of ever-diagnosed DVT and the risk of interstitial lung disease [84] and found increased ILD with diagnoses of both pulmonary embolism (PE) and DVT as compared to controls, particularly in those never treated with anticoagulation. Finally, a US population-based study using death records of patients from 1998 to 2007 found an increased risk of VTE at the time of death for IPF patients (34 %) and death at a younger age in IPF patients with VTE compared to those without [85]. The authors suggest higher epidemiological risk of thromboembolic disease in

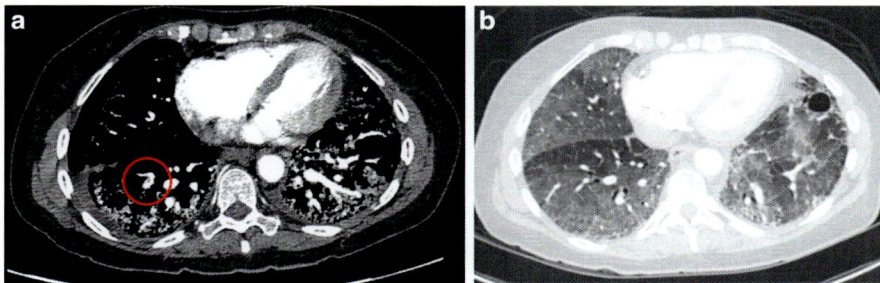

**Fig. 15.2** Concomitant pulmonary embolism in a 58-year-old female presenting with acute exacerbation of IPF when the initial diagnosis of underlying fibrotic lung disease was made (confirmed on biopsy as DAD superimposed on UIP)

those with IPF compared to that seen in COPD and lung cancer. Clinically, PE is of concern during acute exacerbations and patients are commonly evaluated with CT angiography. The incidence of underlying or associated PE in IPF patients experiencing acute deterioration is unknown. In a review of patients with IPF admitted with respiratory failure to an ICU, 2 of 32 (6 %) patients were diagnosed with pulmonary embolism [86].

Decreased mobility associated with progressive pulmonary fibrosis is a risk factor for venous thromboembolism. In addition, a procoagulant state has been hypothesized to contribute to the fibrotic process in IPF and perhaps to thromboembolic disease as well. Mechanisms for an association between fibrosis and venous thromboembolism have been proposed based on study of acute and chronic interstitial lung processes. Excessive fibrin turnover and deposition in the lung is believed to be secondary to tissue factor initiation and responsible for the abnormal coagulative state in the injured lung [87]. Proinflammatory and profibrotic cytokines from acute injury promote alveolar deposition of fibrin through increased alveolar wall permeability and promotion of antifibrinolytic pathways [88]. The deposition of fibrin incorporates and reduces surfactant availability, resulting in further atelectasis with fibrin itself serving as a supportive matrix for recruitment and accumulation of fibroblasts and the initiation of fibrosis [87]. In COPD, clinical risk factors associated with thromboembolic disease include increased sedentary state, low-grade chronic inflammation, and recurrent infection, with pulmonary embolism, perhaps the underlying etiology of acute respiratory failure in one-fifth to a quarter of so-called COPD exacerbations [89, 90]. Similar clinical risk factors for the development of VTE may be relevant in advanced or end-stage IPF. Sprunger et al., in their US population study, noted an increased risk of VTE in older female patients (>65) as compared to younger females with IPF and no risk difference across all ages in men [85].

Given the increased risk of VTE and potential contribution of abnormal coagulation to pulmonary fibrosis, the efficacy of warfarin treatment was evaluated in IPF patients treated with prednisolone compared to prednisolone alone in Japan and was found to reduce the risk of death at 1 year (58 % vs. 78 %) [8].

Although randomization was attempted, the study was not blinded, and there was withdrawal of a substantial number of patients from the warfarin arm as compared to controls (~25 %) secondary to intolerance of frequent lab monitoring. A follow-up, double-blind, randomized IPF-Net study involving 145 patients treated with warfarin versus placebo was stopped after interim review found an increased risk of death in those assigned to warfarin therapy (14 deaths vs. 3) [91]. The administration of anticoagulation therapy in an attempt to inhibit disease progression in IPF is not supported. Such therapy can only be recommended for patients if diagnosed with VTE.

## Cardiovascular Disease

Several population-based, cross-sectional, and case–control studies have found an increased association of cardiovascular disease with interstitial lung disease and lung fibrosis [83, 92–95]. Panos et al. first reported that cardiovascular disease and its related vascular complications accounted for nearly 27 % of deaths associated with IPF [2]. Olson et al. subsequently reported data from the National Center for Health Statistics between 1992 and 2003 indicating nearly 9.6 % of annual deaths in IPF were secondary to ischemic heart disease and congestive heart failure [96]. A study out of the United Kingdom suggested an increased risk of both cardiovascular disease and DVT in IPF patients twice that of the normal or control population [83]. Additionally, three studies of patients undergoing cardiac catheterization [92–94] prior to lung transplantation found a significantly higher incidence of coronary artery disease (defined as greater than 50 % blockage in one or more coronary vessels) in patients with IPF and lung fibrosis when compared to their non-fibrotic counterparts despite a higher prevalence of smoking history in COPD controls. Even when controlled for baseline cardiovascular risk factors, the presence of idiopathic pulmonary fibrosis appeared predictive of underlying coronary disease [94], and baseline cardiovascular risk factors did not differ between the two groups in one study [92]. Finally, Ponnuswamy et al. were unable to find an association between statin use and ILD, but noted an increased association of ILD with ischemic heart disease [95]. They did not find a difference in baseline cardiovascular risk factors between patients with lung fibrosis and control patients, contrary to the findings of others who had proposed diabetes mellitus as a risk factor for lung fibrosis [97].

Mechanisms proposed by Kizer et al. for the association of cardiovascular disease with lung fibrosis include a common injury or initiation from an unknown etiology, proclivity to develop fibrosis in patients with cardiovascular disease, or a causative relationship between fibrosis and coronary disease where fibrosis may initiate or worsen atherosclerosis [93]. It is appreciated that lung fibrosis may be an inflammatory process with systemic implications despite its relatively poor response to anti-inflammatory or immunosuppressive therapy. Similarly elevated inflammatory markers such as IL-1, IL-8, and TNF-α are found in patients with IPF and atherosclerotic heart disease, and these cytokines may promote vascular or endothelial injury [98–100]. The exact mechanism between fibrosis and athero-sclerosis is unknown, and although the incidence of cardiovascular disease appears to be increased in patients with lung fibrosis, not all patients with cardiovascular disease have fibrotic lung disease. It may be more likely that the fibrotic process promotes atherosclerosis rather than both being secondary to a common but unknown inflammatory or injurious mechanism. This is supported by the observed similarity in baseline cardiac risk factors such as hypertension or diabetes among patients with IPF and COPD, but an increased incidence of coronary artery disease (CAD) is observed in IPF patients compared to those with COPD. Death or morbid-ity from cardiovascular disease in patients with IPF may also be secondary to an increased clotting tendency or prothrombotic state that is unique to IPF, as sug-gested by a prior Japanese study [8], although anticoagulant interventions have not been helpful from a fibrosis standpoint.

No specific clinical trials or studies have evaluated the impact of increased screening or aggressive management of underlying cardiovascular disease on improving morbidity and mortality in IPF. Nonetheless, it is suggested that aware-ness of an increased incidence of mild to moderate disease may lead to more aggres-sive medical management, as masking of underlying coronary disease by respiratory symptoms from lung fibrosis may frequently occur. Nathan et al. propose the practi-cal and efficient use of coronary calcium scores in non-gated diagnostic and routine chest CT scans as a means of diagnosing and correlating ischemic heart disease in IPF patients, as there is good sensitivity and specificity as well as strong kappa agreement among study radiologists [101]. No specific recommendations currently exist for the management of ischemic heart disease in IPF, and no data exist on whether mortality can be reduced with an aggressive approach to coronary disease detection and treatment.

# Lung Cancer

Previous reports suggest an increased risk of cancer in the setting of lung fibrosis, with frequencies ranging from 4.8 [102] to 48 % [103] in IPF patients. The risk of malignancy appears increased from the general population, though recent reports are conflicting with older autopsy-based reviews [103, 104]. A US population-based study found the lowest reported incidence [102], while a recent British study found a malignancy risk in IPF increased to 1.5 times that of the general population [105] as compared to a previous study quoting seven to eight times the risk [106]. There remains conflicting data on the most commonly reported histological type, with apparent equal frequency of adenocarcinoma [103, 104] and squamous cell carci-noma [107–109], while small cell carcinoma was suggested as highly frequent in one report [110], a finding dissimilar to the general population. Reported clinical risk factors include extensive smoking history, male gender [104, 107, 111], and older age at the time of diagnosis [107, 111], though baseline risk appears increased in IPF patients compared to the general population even when smoking was accounted for [106]. In particular, gender may be a confounding variable, as IPF is more common in males, and men have a higher smoking frequency in some cohorts [107]. One report suggested acute exacerbation may occur with occult lung fibrosis secondary to UIP seen incidentally with lung resection for malignancy [112].

Radiologic features of IPF-associated lung malignancy have also been conflicting. The theoretical association of malignancy with fibrosis is supported by CT findings of increased malignancy in the peripheral lower lung zones [108, 110, 113] surrounding fibrosis and honeycombing, and can present as focal amorphous consolidation or infiltrate [108, 110]. Others report a similar distribution, but more defined nodular densities with lobulation or spiculation are present [114]. In contrast, Park et al. reported nearly half of their IPF-associated lung cancers presenting with upper lobe-predominant, non-peripheral lesions on initial CT assessment [107]. Additionally, an increased specificity of positron emission tomography (PET) use as compared to CT for detecting lymph node spread in IPF-associated malignancy has been proposed, as lymphadenopathy is a common feature in IPF [115].

The presence of concomitant IPF and lung malignancy portends a significantly worse prognosis despite surgical resection of the tumor (when such resection is appropriate). Patients with IPF may have limited lung function precluding tumor resection as seen in patients with advanced COPD. Prior studies suggest actuarial survival ranging from 52 % at 2 years [116] to 54 % at 3 years [117], and reports of 5-year survival have ranged from 0 [116] to 62 % [109, 118], with cause of death equally distributed between disease progression due to pulmonary fibrosis and recurrence of malignancy. Fujimoto et al. reported an increased recurrence of cancer in IPF patients after resection as compared to the general population [116], and serious immediate postoperative complications have been reported [109, 117, 119] including acute exacerbation [109] with substantial mortality (26–64 %) [120]. Preoperative risk factors that predict operative complications or survival are conflicting. Kushibe et al. suggested that patients with low preoperative FVC (<90 %) should be assessed carefully prior to resection [120], and Fujimoto et al. endorsed ascertaining a pathological UIP diagnosis prior to tumor resection, given the substantially increased risk of morbidity when underlying fibrosis is present [116].

The exact mechanism of fibrosis-associated lung malignancy is not well established, though proposed hypotheses suggest that a number of processes (genetic deletions or mutations, uncontrolled aberrant cell growth and dysplasia, and altered cell-to-cell communication) increase the risk of fibrosis-associated malignancy [121]. Recently, autoantibodies to p53, a tumor suppressor gene, were similarly elevated in the serum of patients with lung malignancy, IPF without malignancy, and patients with IPF-associated lung cancer, suggesting that p53 mutations accumulate in both malignant and fibrotic processes [122]. Others have proposed that carcinogens are deposited in focally fibrotic regions, though this appears discordant with recent findings of malignancy outside areas of fibrosis [123]. It is suggested, nonetheless, that smokers should be encouraged to quit. No studies have looked at screening protocols to detect earlier disease in light of the noted increased malignancy risk.

# Quality of Life, Dyspnea, and End-of-Life Care

Respiratory failure remains the primary cause of death in the majority of patients with IPF [124, 125]. As the disease is progressive and unrelenting, quality-of-life (QOL) and end-of-life issues have recently gained interest as areas of study, particularly in advanced and end-stage diseases. Palliative care is defined as a systematic approach to reducing physical pain and suffering as well as addressing spiritual and psychosocial concerns of patients and their families in the setting of non-curable life-threatening disease [126–128]. Where underlying disease management is limited but symptom burden is high, appropriateness of palliation and other aspects of improving patient quality of life are not in question.

Prior reports have suggested that significantly poor QOL is experienced by patients with IPF as their disease progresses [129–132]. Specific health-related quality-of-life (HRQOL) scores used in the past include the SF-36 (an 8-domain, 36-item questionnaire used for assessment of general health) [133]; the St. George's Respiratory Quotient (SGRQ) [132], which is a three-domain COPD-specific questionnaire; and the World Health Organization Quality-of-Life Assessment (WHOQOL-100) [129]. All tests uniformly demonstrated worse quality of life in IPF patients when compared to controls or as found in disease-specific focus groups. No test has yet been designed to assess disease-specific quality of life in IPF, although prior studies have recommended the WHOQOL-100 [134] or SGRQ [132] over others. When reviewed in summary, there appears to be a correlation between QOL scores and specific physiological indicators (including pulmonary function testing and 6-min walk distance), although they appear weaker than the most correlative subjective domain of dyspnea [135, 136]. One study found positive correlations between higher $PaO_2$ and better SF-36 scores and higher $FEV_1$ values correlated with better "social functioning" and reduced bodily pain, suggesting decreased suffering [133]. When assessing improvement in HRQOL scores with treatment, one study that sought to holistically manage symptoms via cognitive behavioral therapy found worse HRQOL scores after a 6-week intervention versus baseline, although anxiety in spouses and family members was significantly improved [137]. Studies involving medical intervention have included HRQOL testing as endpoints, although the most appropriate scoring test has not been standardized, and few studies have found significant changes in overall QOL with the exception, perhaps, of an improvement in dyspnea [138]. Only pulmonary rehabilitation as nonmedical management has found promise in improving exercise capacity and overall quality of life [139, 140].

Nearly all studies report dyspnea at diagnosis in patients with IPF and note progressive severity over time. Grading dyspnea may be done with several tests, the most common of which is the Medical Research Council (MRC) scale, a five-tier scale denoting progressively worse dyspnea based on activity tolerance [138]. When assessed, dyspnea appears to correlate well with functional decline and lower $PaO_2$ and oxygen saturations. Oxygen therapy appears to improve dyspnea with little evidence for its use in the absence of hypoxemia, though overall HRQOL appears to be worse in patients requiring oxygen, perhaps suggesting oxygen use as a surrogate for overall declining health [138]. Pulmonary rehabilitation has been studied in patients with IPF and other forms of ILD [141] with noted improvement in exercise capacity and symptoms, while others have found improvement in the 6-min walk distance and SGQR as compared to baseline over an 8–10-week treatment period [140]. A smaller study found similar improvements in subjective assessments of general health and dyspnea with a home-based regimen [142], while a recent study suggested not only measurable improvements in distance walked but subjective improvement in fatigue [139]. In all, pulmonary rehabilitation appears promising in terms of improving quality of life and ameliorating the natural deconditioning associated with dyspnea-related inactivity.

Cough is a common symptom associated with progressive IPF and can be debilitating. Ten of eleven patients in an open-label study using thalidomide reported resolution of IPF-associated cough [143]. Other studies addressing the specific management of cough include the use of corticosteroids and opioids [144, 145]. No definitive conclusions specific to IPF can be made, and general cough treatment with cough suppressants both opioid and non-opioid based may be appropriate according to symptom burden and side-effect tolerance.

Depression is common with a reported prevalence of 23.5 % [129] in one cohort and 21 % in a recent study [146] involving ILD patients. Depression has been noted to be associated with dyspnea, pain severity, lower forced vital capacity (FVC), and poor sleep quality. No specific management has been recommended, but these studies suggest baseline screening for depression and perhaps supportive therapy. An American Thoracic Society guideline suggests the use of selective serotonin uptake inhibitors or benzodiazepines in these patients [128].

End-of-life management remains challenging in patients with IPF given the variable nature of the disease course [147]. Determining when to pursue pharmacologic therapy for IPF versus general symptom control may be difficult as effective disease-specific therapies are lacking and an individual patient's course is not entirely predictable. As no specific prognostic tool is in common clinical practice, the decision to offer palliation is recommended on an individualized basis. Nonetheless, many reports suggest significant morbidity and mortality in patients with acute exacerbation or those with end-stage disease requiring intensive care unit admission with or without mechanical ventilatory support [35, 86, 148]. In such situations, outcomes remain poor both acutely and in the long term. The decision to pursue invasive ventilation may best be addressed as part of early care discussion with alignment of goals and interventions prior to acute deterioration as such invasive maneuvers are unproven in extending survival or improving end-of-life comfort.

# Summary

The clinical course of IPF is generally progressive and unrelenting, though it may be highly variable in individual patients. Recognized complications and comorbidities in patients with IPF are numerous and include acute exacerbations, PH, combined presence of pulmonary fibrosis and emphysema, GERD, VTE, cardiovascular disease, and lung cancer. The optimal management of these diagnoses and their relative impact on the outcome of patients with IPF is not entirely clear at the present time. In the absence of effective therapy for the progressive pulmonary fibrosis that characterizes IPF, the identification and treatment of these problems may reduce symptom burden and improve QOL in affected patients.

# References

1. Daniels CE, Yi ES, Ryu JH. Autopsy findings in 42 consecutive patients with idiopathic pulmonary fibrosis. Eur Respir J. 2008;32(1):170–4.
2. Panos RJ, Mortenson RL, Niccoli SA, King Jr TE. Clinical deterioration in patients with idiopathic pulmonary fibrosis: causes and assessment. Am J Med. 1990;88(4):396–404.
3. Ambrosini V, Cancellieri A, Chilosi M, Zompatori M, Trisolini R, Saragoni L, et al. Acute exacerbation of idiopathic pulmonary fibrosis: report of a series. Eur Respir J. 2003;22(5):821–6.
4. Kim DS, Park JH, Park BK, Lee JS, Nicholson AG, Colby T. Acute exacerbation of idiopathic pulmonary fibrosis: frequency and clinical features. Eur Respir J. 2006;27(1):143–50.
5. Akira M, Kozuka T, Yamamoto S, Sakatani M. Computed tomography findings in acute exacerbation of idiopathic pulmonary fibrosis. Am J Respir Crit Care Med. 2008;178(4):372–8.
6. Kondoh Y, Taniguchi H, Kawabata Y, Yokoi T, Suzuki K, Takagi K. Acute exacerbation in idiopathic pulmonary fibrosis. Analysis of clinical and pathologic findings in three cases. Chest. 1993;103(6):1808–12.
7. Collard HR, Moore BB, Flaherty KR, Brown KK, Kaner RJ, King TE, et al. Acute exacerbations of idiopathic pulmonary fibrosis. Am J Respir Crit Care Med. 2007;176(7):636–43.
8. Kubo H, Nakayama K, Yanai M, Suzuki T, Yamaya M, Watanabe M, et al. Anticoagulant therapy for idiopathic pulmonary fibrosis. Chest. 2005;128(3):1475–82.
9. Azuma A, Nukiwa T, Tsuboi E, Suga M, Abe S, Nakata K, et al. Double-blind, placebo-controlled trial of pirfenidone in patients with idiopathic pulmonary fibrosis. Am J Respir Crit Care Med. 2005;171(9):1040–7.
10. Agarwal R, Jindal SK. Acute exacerbation of idiopathic pulmonary fibrosis: a systematic review. Eur J Intern Med. 2008;19(4):227–35.
11. Noble PW, Albera C, Bradford WZ, Costabel U, Glassberg MK, Kardatzke D, et al. Pirfenidone in patients with idiopathic pulmonary fibrosis (CAPACITY): two randomised trials. Lancet. 2011;377(9779):1760–9.
12. Song JW, Hong SB, Lim CM, Koh Y, Kim DS. Acute exacerbation of idiopathic pulmonary fibrosis: incidence, risk factors and outcome. Eur Respir J. 2011;37(2):356–63.
13. Sakamoto K, Taniguchi H, Kondoh Y, Ono K, Hasegawa Y, Kitaichi M. Acute exacerbation of idiopathic pulmonary fibrosis as the initial presentation of the disease. Eur Respir Rev. 2009;18(112):129–32.
14. Parambil JG, Myers JL, Ryu JH. Histopathologic features and outcome of patients with acute exacerbation of idiopathic pulmonary fibrosis undergoing surgical lung biopsy. Chest. 2005;128(5):3310–5.
15. Silva CI, Müller NL, Fujimoto K, Kato S, Ichikado K, Taniguchi H, et al. Acute exacerbation of chronic interstitial pneumonia: high-resolution computed tomography and pathologic findings. J Thorac Imaging. 2007;22(3):221–9.
16. Park IN, Kim DS, Shim TS, Lim CM, Lee SD, Koh Y, et al. Acute exacerbation of interstitial pneumonia other than idiopathic pulmonary fibrosis. Chest. 2007;132(1):214–20.
17. Hyzy R, Huang S, Myers J, Flaherty K, Martinez F. Acute exacerbation of idiopathic pulmonary fibrosis. Chest. 2007;132(5):1652–8.

18. Collard HR, Calfee CS, Wolters PJ, Song JW, Hong SB, Brady S, et al. Plasma biomarker profiles in acute exacerbation of idiopathic pulmonary fibrosis. Am J Physiol Lung Cell Mol Physiol. 2010;299(1):L3–7.

19. Selman M, Pardo A. Role of epithelial cells in idiopathic pulmonary fibrosis: from innocent targets to serial killers. Proc Am Thorac Soc. 2006;3(4):364–72.

20. Wootton SC, Kim DS, Kondoh Y, Chen E, Lee JS, Song JW, et al. Viral infection in acute exacerbation of idiopathic pulmonary fibrosis. Am J Respir Crit Care Med. 2011;183(12):1698–702.

21. Lee JS, Song JW, Wolters PJ, Elicker BM, King TE, Kim DS, et al. Bronchoalveolar lavage pepsin in acute exacerbation of idiopathic pulmonary fibrosis. Eur Respir J. 2012;39(2):352–8.

22. Churg A, Muller NL, Silva CI, Wright JL. Acute exacerbation (acute lung injury of unknown cause) in UIP and other forms of fibrotic interstitial pneumonias. Am J Surg Pathol. 2007;31(2):277–84.

23. Suda T, Kaida Y, Nakamura Y, Enomoto N, Fujisawa T, Imokawa S, et al. Acute exacerbation of interstitial pneumonia associated with collagen vascular diseases. Respir Med. 2009;103(6):846–53.

24. Dallari R, Foglia M, Paci M, Cavazza A. Acute exacerbation of idiopathic pulmonary fibrosis. Eur Respir J. 2004;23(5):792.

25. Judge EP, Fabre A, Adamali HI, Egan JJ. Acute exacerbations and pulmonary hypertension in advanced idiopathic pulmonary fibrosis. Eur Respir J. 2012;40:93–100.

26. Kondoh Y, Taniguchi H, Kitaichi M, Yokoi T, Johkoh T, Oishi T, et al. Acute exacerbation of interstitial pneumonia following surgical lung biopsy. Respir Med. 2006;100(10): 1753–9.

27. Hoshikawa Y, Kondo T. [Perioperative lung injury: acute exacerbation of idiopathic pulmonary fibrosis and acute interstitial pneumonia after pulmonary resection]. Nihon Geka Gakkai Zasshi. 2004;105(12):757–62.

28. Enomoto T, Kawamoto M, Kunugi S, Hiramatsu K, Sakakibara K, Usuki J, et al. [Clinicopathological analysis of patients with idiopathic pulmonary fibrosis which became acutely exacerbated after video-assisted thoracoscopic surgical lung biopsy]. Nihon Kokyuki Gakkai Zasshi. 2002;40(10):806–11.

29. Hiwatari N, Shimura S, Takishima T, Shirato K. Bronchoalveolar lavage as a possible cause of acute exacerbation in idiopathic pulmonary fibrosis patients. Tohoku J Exp Med. 1994;174(4):379–86.

30. Sakamoto K, Taniguchi H, Kondoh Y, Wakai K, Kimura T, Kataoka K, et al. Acute exacerbation of IPF following diagnostic bronchoalveolar lavage procedures. Respir Med. 2012;106(3):436–42.

31. Fujimoto K, Taniguchi H, Johkoh T, Kondoh Y, Ichikado K, Sumikawa H, et al. Acute exacerbation of idiopathic pulmonary fibrosis: high-resolution CT scores predict mortality. Eur Radiol. 2012;22(1):83–92.

32. Horita N, Akahane M, Okada Y, Kobayashi Y, Arai T, Amano I, et al. Tacrolimus and steroid treatment for acute exacerbation of idiopathic pulmonary fibrosis. Intern Med. 2011;50(3):189–95.

33. Inase N, Sawada M, Ohtani Y, Miyake S, Isogai S, Sakashita H, et al. Cyclosporin A followed by the treatment of acute exacerbation of idiopathic pulmonary fibrosis with corticosteroid. Intern Med. 2003;42(7):565–70.

34. Blivet S, Philit F, Sab JM, Langevin B, Paret M, Guérin C, et al. Outcome of patients with idiopathic pulmonary fibrosis admitted to the ICU for respiratory failure. Chest. 2001;120(1):209–12.

35. Fumeaux T, Rothmeier C, Jolliet P. Outcome of mechanical ventilation for acute respiratory failure in patients with pulmonary fibrosis. Intensive Care Med. 2001;27(12):1868–74.

36. Mallick S. Outcome of patients with idiopathic pulmonary fibrosis (IPF) ventilated in intensive care unit. Respir Med. 2008;102(10):1355–9.

37. Mollica C, Paone G, Conti V, Ceccarelli D, Schmid G, Mattia P, et al. Mechanical ventilation in patients with end-stage idiopathic pulmonary fibrosis. Respiration. 2010;79(3):209–15.

38. Mejía M, Carrillo G, Rojas-Serrano J, Estrada A, Suárez T, Alonso D, et al. Idiopathic pulmonary fibrosis and emphysema: decreased survival associated with severe pulmonary arterial hypertension. Chest. 2009;136(1):10–5.
39. Cottin V, Nunes H, Brillet PY, Delaval P, Devouassoux G, Tillie-Leblond I, et al. Combined pulmonary fibrosis and emphysema: a distinct underrecognised entity. Eur Respir J. 2005;26(4):586–93.
40. Brillet PY, Cottin V, Letoumelin P, Landino F, Brauner MW, Valeyre D, et al. [Combined apical emphysema and basal fibrosis syndrome (emphysema/fibrosis syndrome): CT imaging features and pulmonary function tests]. J Radiol. 2009;90(1 Pt 1):43–51.
41. Grubstein A, Bendayan D, Schactman I, Cohen M, Shitrit D, Kramer MR. Concomitant upper-lobe bullous emphysema, lower-lobe interstitial fibrosis and pulmonary hypertension in heavy smokers: report of eight cases and review of the literature. Respir Med. 2005;99(8):948–54.
42. Cottin V, Le Pavec J, Prévot G, Mal H, Humbert M, Simonneau G, et al. Pulmonary hypertension in patients with combined pulmonary fibrosis and emphysema syndrome. Eur Respir J. 2010;35(1):105–11.
43. Cottin V, Cordier JF. The syndrome of combined pulmonary fibrosis and emphysema. Chest. 2009;136(1):1–2.
44. Yousem SA. Respiratory bronchiolitis-associated interstitial lung disease with fibrosis is a lesion distinct from fibrotic nonspecific interstitial pneumonia: a proposal. Mod Pathol. 2006;19(11):1474–9.
45. Katzenstein AL, Mukhopadhyay S, Zanardi C, Dexter E. Clinically occult interstitial fibrosis in smokers: classification and significance of a surprisingly common finding in lobectomy specimens. Hum Pathol. 2010;41(3):316–25.
46. Rogliani P, Mura M, Mattia P, Ferlosio A, Farinelli G, Mariotta S, et al. HRCT and histopathological evaluation of fibrosis and tissue destruction in IPF associated with pulmonary emphysema. Respir Med. 2008;102(12):1753–61.
47. Schmidt SL, Nambiar AM, Tayob N, Sundaram B, Han MK, Gross BH, et al. Pulmonary function measures predict mortality differently in IPF versus combined pulmonary fibrosis and emphysema. Eur Respir J. 2011;38(1):176–83.
48. Simonneau G, Robbins IM, Beghetti M, Channick RN, Delcroix M, Denton CP, et al. Updated clinical classification of pulmonary hypertension. J Am Coll Cardiol. 2009;54(1 Suppl): S43–54.
49. Lettieri CJ, Nathan SD, Barnett SD, Ahmad S, Shorr AF. Prevalence and outcomes of pulmonary arterial hypertension in advanced idiopathic pulmonary fibrosis. Chest. 2006;129(3):746–52.
50. Nadrous HF, Pellikka PA, Krowka MJ, Swanson KL, Chaowalit N, Decker PA, et al. Pulmonary hypertension in patients with idiopathic pulmonary fibrosis. Chest. 2005;128(4):2393–9.
51. Zisman DA, Karlamangla AS, Kawut SM, Shlobin OA, Saggar R, Ross DJ, et al. Validation of a method to screen for pulmonary hypertension in advanced idiopathic pulmonary fibrosis. Chest. 2008;133(3):640–5.
52. Swigris JJ, Olson AL, Shlobin OA, Ahmad S, Brown KK, Nathan SD. Heart rate recovery after six-minute walk test predicts pulmonary hypertension in patients with idiopathic pulmonary fibrosis. Respirology. 2011;16(3):439–45.
53. Zisman DA, Ross DJ, Belperio JA, Saggar R, Lynch JP, Ardehali A, et al. Prediction of pulmonary hypertension in idiopathic pulmonary fibrosis. Respir Med. 2007;101(10):2153–9.
54. Zisman DA, Karlamangla AS, Ross DJ, Keane MP, Belperio JA, Saggar R, et al. High-resolution chest CT findings do not predict the presence of pulmonary hypertension in advanced idiopathic pulmonary fibrosis. Chest. 2007;132(3):773–9.
55. Nathan SD, Shlobin OA, Ahmad S, Koch J, Barnett SD, Ad N, et al. Serial development of pulmonary hypertension in patients with idiopathic pulmonary fibrosis. Respiration. 2008;76(3):288–94.
56. Papakosta D, Pitsiou G, Daniil Z, Dimadi M, Stagaki E, Rapti A, et al. Prevalence of pulmonary hypertension in patients with idiopathic pulmonary fibrosis: correlation with physiological parameters. Lung. 2011;189(5):391–9.

57. Nathan SD, Shlobin OA, Ahmad S, Urbanek S, Barnett SD. Pulmonary hypertension and pulmonary function testing in idiopathic pulmonary fibrosis. Chest. 2007;131(3):657–63.
58. Nathan SD, Shlobin OA, Barnett SD, Saggar R, Belperio JA, Ross DJ, et al. Right ventricular systolic pressure by echocardiography as a predictor of pulmonary hypertension in idiopathic pulmonary fibrosis. Respir Med. 2008;102(9):1305–10.
59. Gagermeier J, Dauber J, Yousem S, Gibson K, Kaminski N. Abnormal vascular phenotypes in patients with idiopathic pulmonary fibrosis and secondary pulmonary hypertension. Chest. 2005;128(6 Suppl):601S.
60. Farkas L, Gauldie J, Voelkel NF, Kolb M. Pulmonary hypertension and idiopathic pulmonary fibrosis: a tale of angiogenesis, apoptosis, and growth factors. Am J Respir Cell Mol Biol. 2011;45(1):1–15.
61. Parra ER, David YR, da Costa LR, Ab'Saber A, Sousa R, Kairalla RA, et al. Heterogeneous remodeling of lung vessels in idiopathic pulmonary fibrosis. Lung. 2005;183(4): 291–300.
62. King TE, Behr J, Brown KK, du Bois RM, Lancaster L, de Andrade JA, et al. BUILD-1: a randomized placebo-controlled trial of bosentan in idiopathic pulmonary fibrosis. Am J Respir Crit Care Med. 2008;177(1):75–81.
63. King Jr TE, Brown KK, Raghu G, du Bois RM, Lynch DA, Martinez F, et al. BUILD-3: a randomized, controlled trial of bosentan in idiopathic pulmonary fibrosis. Am J Respir Crit Care Med. 2011;184(1):92–9.
64. Collard HR, Anstrom KJ, Schwarz MI, Zisman DA. Sildenafil improves walk distance in idiopathic pulmonary fibrosis. Chest. 2007;131(3):897–9.
65. Ghofrani HA, Wiedemann R, Rose F, Schermuly RT, Olschewski H, Weissmann N, et al. Sildenafil for treatment of lung fibrosis and pulmonary hypertension: a randomised controlled trial. Lancet. 2002;360(9337):895–900.
66. Olschewski H, Ghofrani HA, Walmrath D, Schermuly R, Temmesfeld-Wollbruck B, Grimminger F, et al. Inhaled prostacyclin and iloprost in severe pulmonary hypertension secondary to lung fibrosis. Am J Respir Crit Care Med. 1999;160(2):600–7.
67. Saggar R, Shapiro SS, Ross DJ, Fishbein MC, Zisman DA, Lynch JP, et al. Treprostinil to reverse pulmonary hypertension associated with idiopathic pulmonary fibrosis as a bridge to single-lung transplantation. J Heart Lung Transplant. 2009;28(9):964–7.
68. Raghu G, Yang ST, Spada C, Hayes J, Pellegrini CA. Sole treatment of acid gastroesophageal reflux in idiopathic pulmonary fibrosis: a case series. Chest. 2006;129(3):794–800.
69. Tobin RW, Pope CE, Pellegrini CA, Emond MJ, Sillery J, Raghu G. Increased prevalence of gastroesophageal reflux in patients with idiopathic pulmonary fibrosis. Am J Respir Crit Care Med. 1998;158(6):1804–8.
70. Sweet MP, Patti MG, Leard LE, Golden JA, Hays SR, Hoopes C, et al. Gastroesophageal reflux in patients with idiopathic pulmonary fibrosis referred for lung transplantation. J Thorac Cardiovasc Surg. 2007;133(4):1078–84.
71. Jamieson JR, Stein HJ, DeMeester TR, Bonavina L, Schwizer W, Hinder RA, et al. Ambulatory 24-h esophageal pH monitoring: normal values, optimal thresholds, specificity, sensitivity, and reproducibility. Am J Gastroenterol. 1992;87(9):1102–11.
72. Raghu G, Freudenberger TD, Yang S, Curtis JR, Spada C, Hayes J, et al. High prevalence of abnormal acid gastro-oesophageal reflux in idiopathic pulmonary fibrosis. Eur Respir J. 2006;27(1):136–42.
73. el-Serag HB, Sonnenberg A. Comorbid occurrence of laryngeal or pulmonary disease with esophagitis in United States military veterans. Gastroenterology. 1997;113(3):755–60.
74. Raiha I, Manner R, Hietanen E, Hartiala J, Sourander L. Radiographic pulmonary changes of gastro-oesophageal reflux disease in elderly patients. Age Ageing. 1992;21(4):250–5.
75. D'Ovidio F, Singer LG, Hadjiliadis D, Pierre A, Waddell TK, de Perrot M, et al. Prevalence of gastroesophageal reflux in end-stage lung disease candidates for lung transplant. Ann Thorac Surg. 2005;80(4):1254–60.
76. Lee JS, Ryu JH, Elicker BM, Lydell CP, Jones KD, Wolters PJ, et al. Gastroesophageal reflux therapy is associated with longer survival in patients with idiopathic pulmonary fibrosis. Am J Respir Crit Care Med. 2011;184(12):1390–4.

77. Popper H, Juettner F, Pinter J. The gastric juice aspiration syndrome (Mendelson syndrome). Aspects of pathogenesis and treatment in the pig. Virchows Arch A Pathol Anat Histopathol. 1986;409(1):105–17.
78. Raghu G. Idiopathic pulmonary fibrosis: increased survival with "gastroesophageal reflux therapy": fact or fallacy? Am J Respir Crit Care Med. 2011;184(12):1330–2.
79. Raghu G, Meyer KC. Silent gastro-oesophageal reflux and microaspiration in IPF: mounting evidence for anti-reflux therapy? Eur Respir J. 2012;39(2):242–5.
80. Linden PA, Gilbert RJ, Yeap BY, Boyle K, Deykin A, Jaklitsch MT, et al. Laparoscopic fundoplication in patients with end-stage lung disease awaiting transplantation. J Thorac Cardiovasc Surg. 2006;131(2):438–46.
81. Davis Jr RD, Lau CL, Eubanks S, Messier RH, Hadjiliadis D, Steele MP, et al. Improved lung allograft function after fundoplication in patients with gastroesophageal reflux disease undergoing lung transplantation. J Thorac Cardiovasc Surg. 2003;125(3):533–42.
82. Cantu 3rd E, Appel 3rd JZ, Hartwig MG, Woreta H, Green C, Messier R, et al. J. Maxwell Chamberlain Memorial Paper. Early fundoplication prevents chronic allograft dysfunction in patients with gastroesophageal reflux disease. Ann Thorac Surg. 2004;78(4):1142–51. discussion −51.
83. Hubbard RB, Smith C, Le Jeune I, Gribbin J, Fogarty AW. The association between idiopathic pulmonary fibrosis and vascular disease: a population-based study. Am J Respir Crit Care Med. 2008;178(12):1257–61.
84. Sode BF, Dahl M, Nielsen SF, Nordestgaard BG. Venous thromboembolism and risk of idiopathic interstitial pneumonia: a nationwide study. Am J Respir Crit Care Med. 2010;181(10):1085–92.
85. Sprunger DB, Olson AL, Huie TJ, Fernandez-Perez ER, Fischer A, Solomon JJ, et al. Pulmonary fibrosis is associated with an elevated risk of thromboembolic disease. Eur Respir J. 2012;39(1):125–32.
86. Saydain G, Islam A, Afessa B, Ryu JH, Scott JP, Peters SG. Outcome of patients with idiopathic pulmonary fibrosis admitted to the intensive care unit. Am J Respir Crit Care Med. 2002;166(6):839–42.
87. Wygrecka M, Jablonska E, Guenther A, Preissner KT, Markart P. Current view on alveolar coagulation and fibrinolysis in acute inflammatory and chronic interstitial lung diseases. Thromb Haemost. 2008;99(3):494–501.
88. Chambers RC, Leoni P, Blanc-Brude OP, Wembridge DE, Laurent GJ. Thrombin is a potent inducer of connective tissue growth factor production via proteolytic activation of protease-activated receptor-1. J Biol Chem. 2000;275(45):35584–91.
89. Rizkallah J, Man SF, Sin DD. Prevalence of pulmonary embolism in acute exacerbations of COPD: a systematic review and metaanalysis. Chest. 2009;135(3):786–93.
90. Tillie-Leblond I, Marquette CH, Perez T, Scherpereel A, Zanetti C, Tonnel AB, et al. Pulmonary embolism in patients with unexplained exacerbation of chronic obstructive pulmonary disease: prevalence and risk factors. Ann Intern Med. 2006;144(6):390–6.
91. Noth I, Anstrom KJ, Calvert SB, de Andrade J, Flaherty KR, Glazer C, et al. A placebo-controlled randomized trial of warfarin in idiopathic pulmonary fibrosis. Am J Respir Crit Care Med. 2012;186:88–95.
92. Izbicki G, Ben-Dor I, Shitrit D, Bendayan D, Aldrich TK, Kornowski R, et al. The prevalence of coronary artery disease in end-stage pulmonary disease: is pulmonary fibrosis a risk factor? Respir Med. 2009;103(9):1346–9.
93. Kizer JR, Zisman DA, Blumenthal NP, Kotloff RM, Kimmel SE, Strieter RM, et al. Association between pulmonary fibrosis and coronary artery disease. Arch Intern Med. 2004;164(5):551–6.
94. Nathan SD, Basavaraj A, Reichner C, Shlobin OA, Ahmad S, Kiernan J, et al. Prevalence and impact of coronary artery disease in idiopathic pulmonary fibrosis. Respir Med. 2010;104(7):1035–41.
95. Ponnuswamy A, Manikandan R, Sabetpour A, Keeping IM, Finnerty JP. Association between ischaemic heart disease and interstitial lung disease: a case–control study. Respir Med. 2009;103(4):503–7.

96. Olson AL, Swigris JJ, Lezotte DC, Norris JM, Wilson CG, Brown KK. Mortality from pulmonary fibrosis increased in the United States from 1992 to 2003. Am J Respir Crit Care Med. 2007;176(3):277–84.

97. Enomoto T, Usuki J, Azuma A, Nakagawa T, Kudoh S. Diabetes mellitus may increase risk for idiopathic pulmonary fibrosis. Chest. 2003;123(6):2007–11.

98. Ross R. Atherosclerosis – an inflammatory disease. N Engl J Med [Research Support, US Gov't, PHS Review]. 1999;340(2):115–26.

99. Kelly M, Kolb M, Bonniaud P, Gauldie J. Re-evaluation of fibrogenic cytokines in lung fibrosis. Curr Pharm Des [Review]. 2003;9(1):39–49.

100. Gifford AH, Matsuoka M, Ghoda LY, Homer RJ, Enelow RI. Chronic inflammation and lung fibrosis: pleotropic syndromes but limited distinct phenotypes. Mucosal Immunol. 2012;5:480–4.

101. Nathan SD, Weir N, Shlobin OA, Urban BA, Curry CA, Basavaraj A, et al. The value of computed tomography scanning for the detection of coronary artery disease in patients with idiopathic pulmonary fibrosis. Respirology. 2011;16(3):481–6.

102. Wells C, Mannino DM. Pulmonary fibrosis and lung cancer in the United States: analysis of the multiple cause of death mortality data, 1979 through 1991. South Med J. 1996;89(5):505–10.

103. Matsushita H, Tanaka S, Saiki Y, Hara M, Nakata K, Tanimura S, et al. Lung cancer associated with usual interstitial pneumonia. Pathol Int. 1995;45(12):925–32.

104. Kawai T, Yakumaru K, Suzuki M, Kageyama K. Diffuse interstitial pulmonary fibrosis and lung cancer. Acta Pathol Jpn. 1987;37(1):11–9.

105. Le Jeune I, Gribbin J, West J, Smith C, Cullinan P, Hubbard R. The incidence of cancer in patients with idiopathic pulmonary fibrosis and sarcoidosis in the UK. Respir Med. 2007;101(12):2534–40.

106. Hubbard R, Venn A, Lewis S, Britton J. Lung cancer and cryptogenic fibrosing alveolitis. A population-based cohort study. Am J Respir Crit Care Med. 2000;161(1):5–8.

107. Park J, Kim DS, Shim TS, Lim CM, Koh Y, Lee SD, et al. Lung cancer in patients with idiopathic pulmonary fibrosis. Eur Respir J. 2001;17(6):1216–9.

108. Lee HJ, Im JG, Ahn JM, Yeon KM. Lung cancer in patients with idiopathic pulmonary fibrosis: CT findings. J Comp Assist Tomogr. 1996;20(6):979–82.

109. Watanabe A, Higami T, Ohori S, Koyanagi T, Nakashima S, Mawatari T. Is lung cancer resection indicated in patients with idiopathic pulmonary fibrosis? J Thorac Cardiovasc Surg. 2008;136(5):1357–63. 63.e1-2.

110. Mizushima Y, Kobayashi M. Clinical characteristics of synchronous multiple lung cancer associated with idiopathic pulmonary fibrosis. A review of Japanese cases. Chest. 1995;108(5):1272–7.

111. Hironaka M, Fukayama M. Pulmonary fibrosis and lung carcinoma: a comparative study of metaplastic epithelia in honeycombed areas of usual interstitial pneumonia with or without lung carcinoma. Pathol Int. 1999;49(12):1060–6.

112. Goto T, Maeshima A, Akanabe K, Oyamada Y, Kato R. Acute exacerbation of idiopathic pulmonary fibrosis of microscopic usual interstitial pneumonia pattern after lung cancer surgery. Ann Thorac Cardiovasc Surg. 2011;17(6):573–6.

113. Sakai S, Ono M, Nishio T, Kawarada Y, Nagashima A, Toyoshima S. Lung cancer associated with diffuse pulmonary fibrosis: CT-pathologic correlation. J Thorac Imaging. 2003;18(2):67–71.

114. Kishi K, Homma S, Kurosaki A, Motoi N, Yoshimura K. High-resolution computed tomography findings of lung cancer associated with idiopathic pulmonary fibrosis. J Comput Assist Tomogr. 2006;30(1):95–9.

115. Jeon TY, Lee KS, Yi CA, Chung MP, Kwon OJ, Kim BT, et al. Incremental value of PET/CT over CT for mediastinal nodal staging of non-small cell lung cancer: comparison between patients with and without idiopathic pulmonary fibrosis. AJR Am J Roentgenol. 2010;195(2):370–6.

116. Fujimoto T, Okazaki T, Matsukura T, Hanawa T, Yamashita N, Nishimura K, et al. Operation for lung cancer in patients with idiopathic pulmonary fibrosis: surgical contraindication? Ann Thorac Surg. 2003;76(5):1674–8. discussion 9.

117. Kumar P, Goldstraw P, Yamada K, Nicholson AG, Wells AU, Hansell DM, et al. Pulmonary fibrosis and lung cancer: risk and benefit analysis of pulmonary resection. J Thorac Cardiovasc Surg. 2003;125(6):1321–7.
118. Saito Y, Kawai Y, Takahashi N, Ikeya T, Murai K, Kawabata Y, et al. Survival after surgery for pathologic stage IA non-small cell lung cancer associated with idiopathic pulmonary fibrosis. Ann Thorac Surg. 2011;92(5):1812–7.
119. Kawasaki H, Nagai K, Yoshida J, Nishimura M, Nishiwaki Y. Postoperative morbidity, mortality, and survival in lung cancer associated with idiopathic pulmonary fibrosis. J Surg Oncol. 2002;81(1):33–7.
120. Kushibe K, Kawaguchi T, Takahama M, Kimura M, Tojo T, Taniguchi S. Operative indications for lung cancer with idiopathic pulmonary fibrosis. Thorac Cardiovasc Surg. 2007;55(8):505–8.
121. Vancheri C, Failla M, Crimi N, Raghu G. Idiopathic pulmonary fibrosis: a disease with similarities and links to cancer biology. Eur Respir J. 2010;35(3):496–504.
122. Oshikawa K, Sugiyama Y. Serum anti-p53 autoantibodies from patients with idiopathic pulmonary fibrosis associated with lung cancer. Respir Med. 2000;94(11):1085–91.
123. Ohwada H, Hayashi Y, Seki M. An experimental study on carcinogenesis related to localized fibrosis in the lung. Gann. 1980;71(3):285–91.
124. Fernández Pérez ER, Daniels CE, Schroeder DR, St Sauver J, Hartman TE, Bartholmai BJ, et al. Incidence, prevalence, and clinical course of idiopathic pulmonary fibrosis: a population-based study. Chest. 2010;137(1):129–37.
125. Martinez FJ, Safrin S, Weycker D, Starko KM, Bradford WZ, King Jr TE, et al. The clinical course of patients with idiopathic pulmonary fibrosis. Ann Intern Med. 2005;142(12 Pt 1): 963–7.
126. Borgsteede SD, Deliens L, Francke AL, Stalman WA, Willems DL, van Eijk JT, et al. Defining the patient population: one of the problems for palliative care research. Palliat Med. 2006;20(2):63–8.
127. Billings JA. What is palliative care? J Palliat Med. 1998;1(1):73–81.
128. Lanken PN, Terry PB, Delisser HM, Fahy BF, Hansen-Flaschen J, Heffner JE, et al. An official American Thoracic Society clinical policy statement: palliative care for patients with respiratory diseases and critical illnesses. Am J Respir Crit Care Med. 2008;177(8):912–27.
129. De Vries J, Kessels BL, Drent M. Quality of life of idiopathic pulmonary fibrosis patients. Eur Respir J. 2001;17(5):954–61.
130. Tomioka H, Imanaka K, Hashimoto K, Iwasaki H. Health-related quality of life in patients with idiopathic pulmonary fibrosis – cross-sectional and longitudinal study. Intern Med. 2007;46(18):1533–42.
131. Swigris JJ, Kuschner WG, Jacobs SS, Wilson SR, Gould MK. Health-related quality of life in patients with idiopathic pulmonary fibrosis: a systematic review. Thorax. 2005;60(7):588–94.
132. Chang JA, Curtis JR, Patrick DL, Raghu G. Assessment of health-related quality of life in patients with interstitial lung disease. Chest. 1999;116(5):1175–82.
133. Jastrzebski D, Kozielski J, Banaś A, Cebula T, Gumola A, Ziora D, et al. Quality of life during one-year observation of patients with idiopathic pulmonary fibrosis awaiting lung transplantation. J Physiol Pharmacol. 2005;56 Suppl 4:99–105.
134. De Vries J, Seebregts A, Drent M. Assessing health status and quality of life in idiopathic pulmonary fibrosis: which measure should be used? Respir Med. 2000;94(3):273–8.
135. Nishiyama O, Taniguchi H, Kondoh Y, Kimura T, Ogawa T, Watanabe F, et al. Health-related quality of life in patients with idiopathic pulmonary fibrosis. What is the main contributing factor? Respir Med. 2005;99(4):408–14.
136. Swigris JJ, Gould MK, Wilson SR. Health-related quality of life among patients with idiopathic pulmonary fibrosis. Chest. 2005;127(1):284–94.
137. Lindell KO, Olshansky E, Song MK, Zullo TG, Gibson KF, Kaminski N, et al. Impact of a disease-management program on symptom burden and health-related quality of life in patients with idiopathic pulmonary fibrosis and their care partners. Heart Lung. 2010;39(4): 304–13.

138. Ryerson CJ, Donesky D, Pantilat SZ, Collard HR. Dyspnea in idiopathic pulmonary fibrosis: a systematic review. J Pain Symptom Manage. 2012;43(4):771–82.
139. Swigris JJ, Fairclough DL, Morrison M, Make B, Kozora E, Brown KK, et al. Benefits of pulmonary rehabilitation in idiopathic pulmonary fibrosis. Respir Care. 2011;56(6):783–9.
140. Nishiyama O, Kondoh Y, Kimura T, Kato K, Kataoka K, Ogawa T, et al. Effects of pulmonary rehabilitation in patients with idiopathic pulmonary fibrosis. Respirology. 2008;13(3):394–9.
141. Holland AE, Hill CJ, Conron M, Munro P, McDonald CF. Short term improvement in exercise capacity and symptoms following exercise training in interstitial lung disease. Thorax. 2008;63(6):549–54.
142. Ozalevli S, Karaali HK, Ilgin D, Ucan ES. Effect of home-based pulmonary rehabilitation in patients with idiopathic pulmonary fibrosis. Multidiscip Respir Med. 2010;5:31–7.
143. Horton MR, Danoff SK, Lechtzin N. Thalidomide inhibits the intractable cough of idiopathic pulmonary fibrosis. Thorax [Clinical Trial, Phase II Letter Research Support, Non-US Gov't]. 2008;63(8):749.
144. Hope-Gill BD, Hilldrup S, Davies C, Newton RP, Harrison NK. A study of the cough reflex in idiopathic pulmonary fibrosis. Am J Respir Crit Care Med. 2003;168(8):995–1002.
145. Allen S, Raut S, Woollard J, Vassallo M. Low dose diamorphine reduces breathlessness without causing a fall in oxygen saturation in elderly patients with end-stage idiopathic pulmonary fibrosis. Palliat Med. 2005;19(2):128–30.
146. Ryerson CJ, Berkeley J, Carrieri-Kohlman VL, Pantilat SZ, Landefeld CS, Collard HR. Depression and functional status are strongly associated with dyspnea in interstitial lung disease. Chest. 2011;139(3):609–16.
147. Ley B, Collard HR, King Jr TE. Clinical course and prediction of survival in idiopathic pulmonary fibrosis. Am J Respir Crit Care Med. 2011;183(4):431–40.
148. Stern JB, Mal H, Groussard O, Brugière O, Marceau A, Jebrak G, et al. Prognosis of patients with advanced idiopathic pulmonary fibrosis requiring mechanical ventilation for acute respiratory failure. Chest. 2001;120(1):213–9.

# Chapter 16

# The Role of Pulmonary Rehabilitation and Supplemental Oxygen Therapy in the Treatment of Patients with Idiopathic Pulmonary Fibrosis

**Anne E. Holland and Jeffrey J. Swigris**

**Abstract** Pulmonary rehabilitation and supplemental oxygen therapy are two interventions commonly employed in the treatment of patients with idiopathic pulmonary fibrosis (IPF). Results from a number of studies reveal that pulmonary rehabilitation is associated with several beneficial effects in patients with IPF, including increased exercise capacity and improved quality of life. In fact, the data appear robust enough to support participation in a pulmonary rehabilitation program as standard of care for patients with IPF. Supplemental oxygen therapy is universally prescribed for IPF patients with hypoxemia at rest, with exertion, or during sleep, but few studies have been performed to assess its effectiveness in these patients.

**Keywords** Idiopathic pulmonary fibrosis • Pulmonary rehabilitation • Exercise • Supplemental oxygen • Dyspnea • Quality of life

## Introduction

In patients with idiopathic pulmonary fibrosis (IPF), pulmonary physiological restriction and hypoxemia induce dyspnea, and it is primarily dyspnea that drives impairments in functional capacity and quality of life (QOL) [1–4]. Another bothersome yet often overlooked symptom plaguing IPF patients is fatigue or low

A.E. Holland, B.App.Sc., Ph.D.
Department of Physiotherapy, Alfred Health and La Trobe University,
Melbourne, VIC, Australia

J.J. Swigris, D.O., M.S. (✉)
Autoimmune Lung Center and Interstitial Lung Disease Program, National Jewish Health,
1400 Jackson Street, Denver, CO 80238, USA
e-mail: swigrisj@njc.org

K.C. Meyer and S.D. Nathan (eds.), *Idiopathic Pulmonary Fibrosis: A Comprehensive Clinical Guide*, Respiratory Medicine 9, DOI 10.1007/978-1-62703-682-5_16,
© Springer Science+Business Media New York 2014

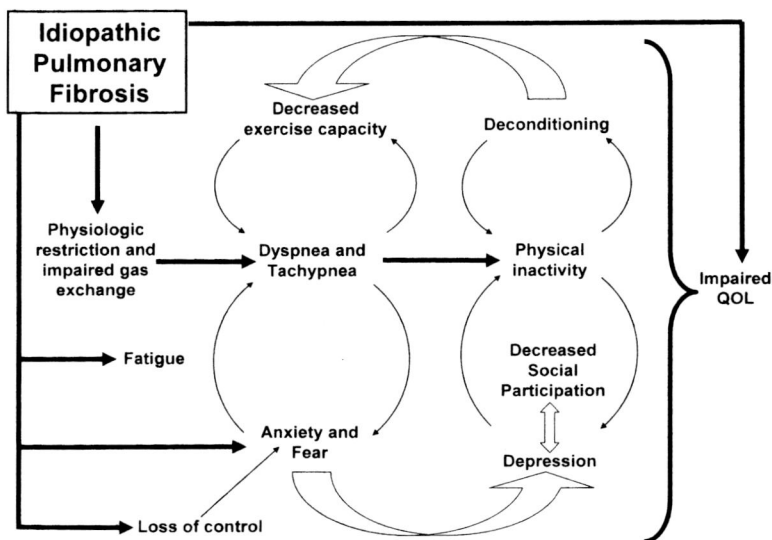

**Fig. 16.1** Conceptual framework for how IPF affects various life domains. Reprinted from Respiratory Medicine, 102/12, Jeffrey J. Swigris, Kevin K. Brown, Barry J. Make, Frederick S. Wamboldt, Pulmonary rehabilitation in idiopathic pulmonary fibrosis: a call for continued investigation, 1675–80, Copyright 2008, with permission from Elsevier

energy—or even more precisely, "exhaustion"—which may or may not be attributed entirely to episodic or continuous blood oxygen desaturation [3, 4]. Psychological distress is common, with clinically significant depression detected in 23 % of patients with IPF [5] and higher levels of anxiety than healthy controls [6]. As fibrosis advances, resting and exertional hypoxemia, dyspnea, and exhaustion worsen, patients become less and less physically active, and they are unable to perform even the most basic physical activities (e.g., dressing and bathing) without becoming severely short of breath. A number of detrimental downstream effects (Fig. 16.1) are put into motion, including aerobic and skeletal muscle deconditioning, social isolation, and impaired emotional well-being [7].

Pulmonary rehabilitation is a program that combines exercise training, disease-specific education, and psychosocial support in an attempt to reduce symptoms, optimize functional status, and increase participation in daily life activities [8]. Pulmonary rehabilitation programs were traditionally designed for people with chronic obstructive pulmonary disease (COPD) in whom completion of pulmonary rehabilitation has been observed to induce a number of beneficial effects. Respiratory rate decreases (by prolonging expiration), tidal volume and oxygen saturation increase [9], cardiac conditioning improves, lean body mass increases [10], the quadriceps become more fatigue resistant [11], and the efficiency of skeletal muscle function is enhanced at the cellular and molecular levels [8]. These effects translate to statistically significant and clinically meaningful improvements in exercise capacity, QOL, and dyspnea [8].

Because of the lack of effective drug therapy for IPF, and building on the vast data supporting the benefits of PR in COPD, there is growing enthusiasm for recommending that IPF patients participate in a pulmonary rehabilitation program. Although research into the effects of pulmonary rehabilitation on patients with IPF has only recently taken off [12–15], early results are promising.

Another nonmedicinal intervention commonly prescribed for IPF patients is supplemental oxygen. Like pulmonary rehabilitation, it seems obvious that supplemental oxygen would help IPF patients in a number of ways, including increasing physical activity and staving off pulmonary hypertension, but little research has been conducted to inform these intuitions. In this chapter, we discuss the use of pulmonary rehabilitation and supplemental oxygen therapy in patients with IPF.

## Pulmonary Rehabilitation

At the time of writing, only two randomized, controlled trials have been conducted to evaluate the effectiveness of pulmonary rehabilitation for people with IPF [14, 15]. A combined total of 62 participants with IPF and mean transfer capacity of the lung for carbon monoxide (TLCO) of 52 % predicted underwent 8–9 weeks of twice-weekly supervised exercise training consisting of aerobic and strengthening exercises. Supplemental oxygen was used, when required, to maintain peripheral oxyhemoglobin saturation above 85–90 %. Pooled data from these trials indicate that immediately after the training period there were significant improvements in 6-minute walk distance (mean improvement 27 m, 95 % confidence interval 3–50 m) [13]. There were also improvements in QOL, with a trend towards reduction in dyspnea. Effect sizes for these outcomes were moderate, with slightly larger effects for exercise tolerance and QOL compared to dyspnea (Fig. 16.2). In one trial, investigators followed participants for an additional 6 months after completion of pulmonary rehabilitation. Disappointingly, they observed that the benefits in exercise capacity, symptoms, and QOL that were evident immediately after completion of the program were not maintained [14]. As part of the trial, subjects were asked (but not required) to exercise at home, but subjects' activity levels were not systematically followed after completion of the formal pulmonary rehabilitation program.

Pulmonary rehabilitation may also positively impact other domains in people with IPF. Two non-randomized trials in people with interstitial lung disease (ILD), some of whom had IPF, suggest that 6–8 weeks of pulmonary rehabilitation may reduce depression [12, 16]. A trend towards reduced anxiety has been documented following rehabilitation in people with IPF [17]. Importantly, pulmonary rehabilitation reduces fatigue [14, 17], a very disabling symptom for many people with IPF. Recent studies suggest that people with IPF may not achieve the same degree of improvement in certain clinical outcomes from pulmonary rehabilitation that have been observed in patients with other chronic lung diseases, [18] and in IPF, the beneficial effects may not last as long. However, the magnitude of changes in exercise capacity and QOL is clinically significant (Table 16.1), especially in the context of

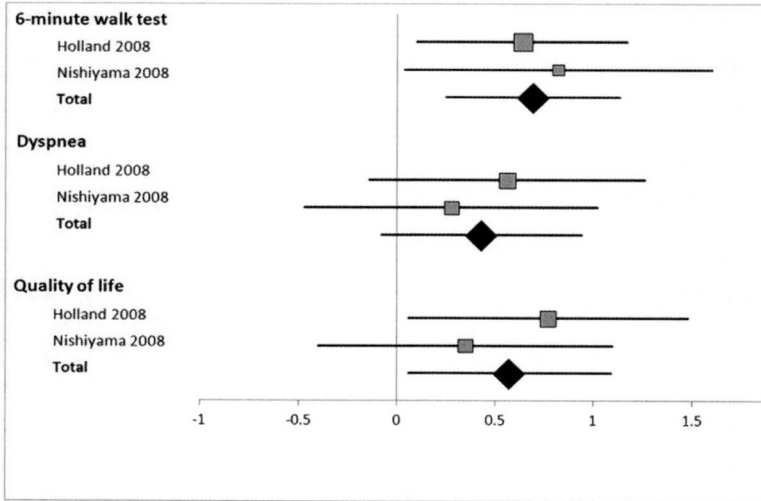

**Fig. 16.2** Effect sizes for pulmonary rehabilitation outcomes in randomized controlled trials in patients with IPF. Data are mean effect size and 95 % confidence intervals, based on Holland and Hill [13]

**Table 16.1** Significance of changes in clinical outcomes following pulmonary rehabilitation for IPF

| Outcome | Measure | Study | Design | Mean change following PR (95 % CI) | Exceeds minimal important difference |
|---|---|---|---|---|---|
| Exercise tolerance | 6-minute walk test | Holland et al. [14] | RCT | 16 m (−13 to 46 m) | No |
| | 6-minute walk test | Nishiyama et al. [15] | RCT | 46 m (6 to 80 m) | Yes |
| Quality of life | Chronic Respiratory Disease Questionnaire | Holland et al. [14] | RCT | 14.1 units (2.1–26.0 units) | Yes |
| | St George's Respiratory Questionnaire | Nishiyama et al. [15] | RCT | −6.0 units (−11.7 to −0.5 units) | Yes |
| Dyspnea | Modified Medical Research Council Scale | Holland et al. [14] | RCT | 0.7 units (0.1–1.3 units) | No |
| | Baseline Dyspnea Index | Nishiyama et al. [15] | RCT | 0.4 units (−0.6 to 1.4 units) | No |
| Fatigue | Chronic Respiratory Disease Questionnaire Fatigue Domain | Holland et al. [14] | RCT | 3.0 units (0.13 to 5.9 units) | Yes |
| | Fatigue Severity Scale | Swigris et al. [17] | OBS | −1.5 units (−2.5 to −0.5 units) | Yes |
| Anxiety | General anxiety disorder-7 | Swigris et al. [17] | OBS | −1.4 units (−3.4 to 0.6 units) | NS |

*PR* pulmonary rehabilitation, *RCT* randomized controlled trial, *OBS* observational study, *NS* not specified

a disease with few treatment options. The current multinational consensus guidelines on the management of IPF contain a weak recommendation for enrolling IPF patients in formal pulmonary rehabilitation programs [19]. This indicates that the consensus writers believe that the majority of IPF patients would want to enroll in pulmonary rehabilitation but that some patients would not. The lack of strength (i.e., weakness) of the recommendation stems from the lack of data surrounding durable, longer-term effects of pulmonary rehabilitation [19]. Because pulmonary rehabilitation is now considered by many experts to be part of standard treatment for most people with IPF, it is important that patients have access to a pulmonary rehabilitation program at a time when they are likely to benefit.

## When Should Pulmonary Rehabilitation Be Offered to People with IPF?

The natural history of IPF is variable, but the median survival from the time of diagnosis is between 3 and 5 years in the majority of studies. Most individuals experience a gradually progressive disease course; however, some remain stable for long periods, while others experience rapid clinical decline [19]. The burden of attending rehabilitation must be offset by likely benefits, especially for those individuals with severe or rapidly progressing disease.

Investigators have conducted studies in an attempt to identify the best time to refer IPF patients to a pulmonary rehabilitation program so that short- and longer-term benefits are maximized. The data are somewhat conflicting: two studies suggest that greater improvements are gained from pulmonary rehabilitation when it is offered earlier in the disease course. For example, greater 6-minute walk distances were associated with higher forced vital capacity (FVC), less severe exercise-induced peripheral oxygen desaturation, and a lesser degree of disability at baseline [20, 21]. Subjects with higher nadir peripheral oxygen saturations during a baseline 6-minute walk test were more likely to experience sustained improvements in exercise tolerance at 6 months following the program [20]. Interestingly, subjects with more dyspnea at baseline achieved greater long-term relief of dyspnea after completing pulmonary rehabilitation [20]. These studies indicate that individuals with less advanced, but highly symptomatic, disease are particularly likely to experience benefits from pulmonary rehabilitation, possibly due to a greater degree of physical deconditioning or mood disturbance—features that can be addressed successfully in a rehabilitation program. In another study, baseline dyspnea, oxygen use, FVC, and diffusing capacity of the lung for carbon dioxide were not predictors of beneficial response to pulmonary rehabilitation, but baseline 6-minute walk distance was [12]. And although nearly every subject improved their 6-minute walk distance after pulmonary rehabilitation, there was an inverse relationship between baseline 6-minute walk distance and post-pulmonary rehabilitation 6-minute walk distance [12].

In our opinion, people with IPF should be afforded the opportunity to participate in pulmonary rehabilitation programs as early as practicable in order to maximize the likelihood of achieving clinically important gains. However, we believe that even patients with more severe disease should be considered for participation and encouraged to participate in pulmonary rehabilitation. An exercise prescription that is tailored to the needs of individuals with high disability or severe exercise-induced oxygen desaturation (e.g., interval training rather than continuous training) may provide a better training stimulus and a greater chance to achieve benefits in this group. Because no data exist on which method of exercise is most beneficial in patients with IPF, this statement is purely speculative. Clearly, this is an area that is ripe for research.

## Components of Pulmonary Rehabilitation for IPF

Exercise training is a core component of pulmonary rehabilitation programs for IPF and makes an important contribution to rehabilitation outcomes [14]. Typical exercise programs for people with IPF have been conducted in the outpatient setting. Programs are from 6 to 8 weeks in duration, with 2 or 3 supervised sessions each week [14, 15, 17, 21]. Participants undertake 20–30 min of endurance exercise (treadmill or hallway walking, stationary bike, or elliptical-type trainer), with intensity and duration escalated as tolerated over the course of the program. If a patient has recently completed a maximal cardiopulmonary exercise test (CPET), then data from it can be used to set the starting point and exercise goals for the program. For example, some programs use 60 % of the maximum workload from the CPET as a starting point, with intensity increased gradually if the duration goal is met. When CPET data are not available, 60 % of the age-predicted maximum heart rate can be used instead of workload to set the starting point. Most programs also include light resistance exercises—using either weights, resistance bands, or Pilates machines—for the upper and lower limbs. Heart rate and $SpO_2$ are usually monitored during each session, and supplemental oxygen is used to maintain normoxia. Some programs also incorporate breathing training (or retraining) exercises and instruction in pacing [12, 17, 21]. Although there are no data to support the benefits of pursed-lip breathing—and it really makes no physiological sense—in IPF, our anecdotal experience is that IPF patients routinely use and rave about pursed-lip breathing. Rather than promoting lung emptying, as in COPD, in IPF, the use of PLB likely only encourages diaphragmatic breathing and a greater sense of calm and control by getting patients to focus more on controlled respiration.

Education sessions to improve disease management are commonly included in pulmonary rehabilitation programs. Because the majority of existing pulmonary rehabilitation programs were designed for and may predominantly enroll patients with COPD, their educational components may need to be modified to meet the unique requirements of people with IPF. Suggested topics include symptom management, oxygen use, prevention and treatment of IPF exacerbations, energy conservation, managing mood, medication management including side effects, preparation for lung transplantation, and advanced care planning [22]. The impact of such educational and psychosocial interventions for IPF is not clear. In one randomized, controlled trial, investigators found that six weekly sessions of a disease management intervention, focusing on symptom management and mood, had a negative impact on the physical aspects of health-related QOL, along with a trend for greater anxiety [23]. However, subjects valued the opportunity to meet others with IPF. These findings suggest that peer support may be an important component of pulmonary rehabilitation, but that educational topics should be individualized to meet patient needs.

A comprehensive patient assessment is a key element of pulmonary rehabilitation. At the commencement of the program, all participants should undertake a medical assessment and an objective measure of exercise tolerance. This should include measurement of exercise-induced oxyhemoglobin desaturation so that supplemental oxygen can be used appropriately during training. Evaluation of symptoms and health-related QOL should be undertaken using standardized measurement tools that are sensitive to change in IPF. The multidisciplinary nature of pulmonary rehabilitation provides a unique opportunity to evaluate the presence and impact of mood disorders such as anxiety, panic, and depression. These may respond to the usual components of pulmonary rehabilitation [16, 17] or may require individualized therapies. Because patients with IPF are at risk for coronary artery disease (CAD) [24], either due entirely to their age or, perhaps, because of circulating factors that promote CAD, consideration should be given to having patients undergo cardiac stress testing prior to starting pulmonary rehabilitation. All participants should be reevaluated after the pulmonary rehabilitation program to establish its effects on exercise capacity, symptoms, QOL, and mood and to plan for the ongoing care needs of the individual.

## *Special Considerations for Pulmonary Rehabilitation in IPF*

People with IPF often exhibit marked hypoxemia during exercise, which is known to limit exercise performance [25]. Pulmonary rehabilitation facilities must have the capacity to provide supplemental oxygen during all aspects of exercise training for people with IPF, including provision of high-flow oxygen if needed to prevent significant desaturation. Pulmonary hypertension is common in people with IPF [26] and may worsen during exercise. Patients with pulmonary hypertension may require modifications to the standard exercise prescription, including a reduction in intensity of endurance and resistance exercises [27]. Clinicians should be trained to detect important signs and symptoms requiring cessation of exercise, including dizziness, hypotension, pre-syncope, excessive fatigue, palpitations, tachycardia, or chest pain. Finally, it must be recognized that some people with advanced IPF will require close supervision and support during all phases of exercise in order to achieve a sufficient training stimulus while maintaining adequate oxygenation and symptom control.

## Supplemental Oxygen

Because large-scale, systematic investigations of supplemental oxygen in IPF have never been performed, the field's knowledge of this therapy is based predominantly on scientific rationale, anecdote, and inferences formulated by extrapolation of data published in the COPD literature. However, even in COPD, the data on the beneficial effects of supplemental oxygen are limited and surprisingly controversial [28]. Although there is strong, yet dated [29, 30], evidence that supplemental oxygen improves survival in COPD patients with severe hypoxemia at rest, for those patients with mild to moderate resting hypoxemia or blood oxygen desaturation only during exertion or sleep, the data are far less compelling and even contradictory [28].

Very little research has been conducted on the merits and pitfalls of supplemental oxygen in patients with IPF. In two small studies, investigators observed that supplemental oxygen improved exercise endurance and other exercise-specific outcome measures (e.g., maximal oxygen uptake) in patients with ILD, at least some of whom likely had IPF as it is currently defined [31, 32]. In a more recent study, Visca and colleagues examined the effects of supplemental oxygen on outcomes collected in relation to a timed walk test (6MWT) [33]. They found that among 52 subjects with ILD (including 34 with a fibrotic interstitial pneumonia of whom some had IPF) compared with baseline values collected while subjects breathed ambient air, the use of supplemental oxygen during the 6-minute walk test led to improvements in mean walk distance, end-test peripheral oxygen saturation ($SpO_2$), dyspnea, and $SpO_2$ recovery time.

In a few studies conducted in patients with ILD (some with IPF), investigators found that supplemental oxygen led to immediate improvements in either 6-minute walk distance or certain variables collected during a maximal cardiopulmonary exercise test [31–33]. Almost entirely unknown is how durable those benefits are and whether supplemental oxygen has any beneficial effects on patient-reported outcomes (e.g., cough, dyspnea, or QOL) or survival. Swinburn and colleagues studied 10 inpatients with ILD who were hypoxemic at rest and found that supplemental oxygen reduced dyspnea as measured by a visual analog scale. However, it is not mentioned why these patients were hospitalized or whether any of them had IPF.

Despite an absence of data to suggest that supplemental oxygen improves how patients with IPF feel, function, or survive, most clinicians caring for IPF patients believe that supplemental oxygen is warranted [34] and prescribe it when resting, during exercise, or when nocturnal peripheral oxygen saturation ($SpO_2$) falls below 89 %. This belief is likely driven by clinicians' unwillingness to leave uncorrected something ($SpO_2$) that can be remedied when so many other aspects of the disease are untreatable.

In Denver (altitude 5,280 ft above sea level), IPF patients generally require higher flows of supplemental oxygen than they do at sea level to maintain a $SpO_2$ >89 %, and it is not uncommon for IPF patients to require concentrators and delivery devices capable of delivering high oxygen flows (i.e., >6 L/min). Using these flows causes portable tanks to run out of oxygen relatively quickly and leads to significant drying of the nasal passages. Because production of copious, thick sputum is not the norm for patients with IPF, oxygen delivery via a transtracheal catheter is an attractive option for some patients, and intratracheal oxygen delivery can lower flow rates required to attain a target $SpO_2$ level. Although transtracheal catheter has been associated with a number of beneficial effects [35], there are no published studies of this mode of oxygen delivery in IPF patients specifically.

## Summary

Pulmonary rehabilitation is a promising intervention for patients with IPF that can lead to clinically important improvements in dyspnea, QOL, and mood. Current IPF treatment guidelines support the inclusion of pulmonary rehabilitation in the treatment plan of the majority of people with IPF. Although not entirely clear, there are data to suggest that patients with less severe disease but significant symptoms may achieve the greatest and most sustained benefit. Thus, individuals with IPF should be encouraged to participate in pulmonary rehabilitation as early as possible. There are a number of unanswered questions about pulmonary rehabilitation for IPF patients. For example, what is the ideal format for exercise training? What is the optimal duration for pulmonary rehabilitation programs? Although clinicians have a strong intuition that supplemental oxygen should be prescribed for IPF patients if $SpO_2$ falls below 89 % at rest, with activity, or during sleep, there are few data supporting this practice. Like pulmonary rehabilitation, there is a great deal to learn about the benefits of supplemental oxygen for patients with IPF.

## References

1. Nishiyama O, Taniguchi H, Kondoh Y, Kimura T, Ogawa T, Watanabe F, et al. Factors in maintaining long-term improvements in health-related quality of life after pulmonary rehabilitation for COPD. Qual Life Res. 2005;14:2315–21.
2. Nishiyama O, Taniguchi H, Kondoh Y, Kimura T, Kato K, Ogawa T, et al. Dyspnoea at 6-min walk test in idiopathic pulmonary fibrosis: comparison with COPD. Respir Med. 2007;101:833–8.
3. Swigris JJ, Stewart AL, Gould MK, Wilson SR. Patients' perspectives on how idiopathic pulmonary fibrosis affects the quality of their lives. Health Qual Life Outcomes. 2005;3:61.
4. Swigris JJ, Kuschner WG, Jacobs SS, Wilson SR, Gould MK. Health-related quality of life in patients with idiopathic pulmonary fibrosis: a systematic review. Thorax. 2005;60:588–94.
5. Ryerson CJ, Berkeley J, Carrieri-Kohlman VL, Pantilat SZ, Landefeld CS, Collard HR. Depression and functional status are strongly associated with dyspnea in interstitial lung disease. Chest. 2011;139:609–16.
6. Tzanakis N, Samiou M, Lambiri I, Antoniou K, Siafakas N, Bouros D. Evaluation of health-related quality-of-life and dyspnea scales in patients with idiopathic pulmonary fibrosis. Correlation with pulmonary function tests. Eur J Intern Med. 2005;16:105–12.
7. Swigris JJ, Brown KK, Make BJ, Wamboldt FS. Pulmonary rehabilitation in idiopathic pulmonary fibrosis: a call for continued investigation. Respir Med. 2008;102:1675–80.

8. Nici L, Donner C, Wouters E, Zuwallack R, Ambrosino N, Bourbeau J, et al. American Thoracic Society/European Respiratory Society statement on pulmonary rehabilitation. Am J Respir Crit Care Med. 2006;173:1390–413.

9. Bianchi R, Gigliotti F, Romagnoli I, Lanini B, Castellani C, Binazzi B, et al. Impact of a rehabilitation program on dyspnea intensity and quality in patients with chronic obstructive pulmonary disease. Respiration. 2011;81:186–95.

10. Bernard S, Whittom F, Leblanc P, Jobin J, Belleau R, Berube C, et al. Aerobic and strength training in patients with chronic obstructive pulmonary disease. Am J Respir Crit Care Med. 1999;159:896–901.

11. Mador MJ, Kufel TJ, Pineda LA, Steinwald A, Aggarwal A, Upadhyay AM, et al. Effect of pulmonary rehabilitation on quadriceps fatiguability during exercise. Am J Respir Crit Care Med. 2001;163:930–5.

12. Ferreira A, Garvey C, Connors GL, Hilling L, Rigler J, Farrell S, et al. Pulmonary rehabilitation in interstitial lung disease: benefits and predictors of response. Chest. 2009;135:442–7.

13. Holland A, Hill C. Physical training for interstitial lung disease. Cochrane Database Syst Rev. 2008;4, CD006322.

14. Holland AE, Hill CJ, Conron M, Munro P, McDonald CF. Short term improvement in exercise capacity and symptoms following exercise training in interstitial lung disease. Thorax. 2008;63:549–54.

15. Nishiyama O, Kondoh Y, Kimura T, Kato K, Kataoka K, Ogawa T, et al. Effects of pulmonary rehabilitation in patients with idiopathic pulmonary fibrosis. Respirology. 2008;13:394–9.

16. Naji NA, Connor MC, Donnelly SC, McDonnell TJ. Effectiveness of pulmonary rehabilitation in restrictive lung disease. J Cardiopulm Rehabil. 2006;26:237–43.

17. Swigris JJ, Fairclough DL, Morrison M, Make B, Kozora E, Brown KK, et al. Beneficial effects of pulmonary rehabilitation in idiopathic pulmonary fibrosis. Respir Care. 2011;56(6):783–9.

18. Lacasse Y, Goldstein R, Lasserson TJ, Martin S. Pulmonary rehabilitation for chronic obstructive pulmonary disease. Cochrane Database Syst Rev. 2006;4, CD003793.

19. Raghu G, Collard HR, Egan JJ, Martinez FJ, Behr J, Brown KK, et al. An official ats/ers/jrs/alat statement: idiopathic pulmonary fibrosis: evidence-based guidelines for diagnosis and management. Am J Respir Crit Care Med. 2011;183:788–824.

20. Holland AE, Hill CJ, Glaspole I, Goh N, McDonald CF. Predictors of benefit following pulmonary rehabilitation for interstitial lung disease. Respir Med. 2012;106:429–35.

21. Kozu R, Jenkins S, Senjyu H. Effect of disability level on response to pulmonary rehabilitation in patients with idiopathic pulmonary fibrosis. Respirology. 2011;16:1196–202.

22. Garvey C. Interstitial lung disease and pulmonary rehabilitation. J Cardiopulm Rehabil Prev. 2010;30:141–6.

23. Lindell KO, Olshansky E, Song MK, Zullo TG, Gibson KF, Kaminski N, et al. Impact of a disease-management program on symptom burden and health-related quality of life in patients with idiopathic pulmonary fibrosis and their care partners. Heart Lung. 2010;39:304–13.

24. Nathan SD, Basavaraj A, Reichner C, Shlobin OA, Ahmad S, Kiernan J, et al. Prevalence and impact of coronary artery disease in idiopathic pulmonary fibrosis. Respir Med. 2010;104:1035–41.

25. Miki K, Maekura R, Hiraga T, Okuda Y, Okamoto T, Hirotani A, et al. Impairments and prognostic factors for survival in patients with idiopathic pulmonary fibrosis. Respir Med. 2003;97:482–90.

26. Glaser S, Noga O, Koch B, Opitz CF, Schmidt B, Temmesfeld B, et al. Impact of pulmonary hypertension on gas exchange and exercise capacity in patients with pulmonary fibrosis. Respir Med. 2009;103:317–24.

27. Mereles D, Ehlken N, Kreuscher S, Ghofrani S, Hoeper MM, Halank M, et al. Exercise and respiratory training improve exercise capacity and quality of life in patients with severe chronic pulmonary hypertension. Circulation. 2006;114:1482–9.

28. Make B, Krachman S, Panos RJ, Doherty DE, Stoller JK. Oxygen therapy in advanced copd: in whom does it work? Semin Respir Crit Care Med. 2010;31:334–42.

29. Continuous or nocturnal oxygen therapy in hypoxemic chronic obstructive lung disease: a clinical trial. Nocturnal Oxygen Therapy Trial Group. Ann Intern Med. 1980;93:391–98.
30. Long term domiciliary oxygen therapy in chronic hypoxic cor pulmonale complicating chronic bronchitis and emphysema. Report of the Medical Research Council Working Party. Lancet. 1981;1:681–86.
31. Bye PT, Anderson SD, Woolcock AJ, Young IH, Alison JA. Bicycle endurance performance of patients with interstitial lung disease breathing air and oxygen. Am Rev Respir Dis. 1982;126:1005–12.
32. Harris-Eze AO, Sridhar G, Clemens RE, Gallagher CG, Marciniuk DD. Oxygen improves maximal exercise performance in interstitial lung disease. Am J Respir Crit Care Med. 1994;150:1616–22.
33. Visca D, Montgomery A, de Lauretis A, Sestini P, Soteriou H, Maher TM, Wells AU, Renzoni EA. Ambulatory oxygen in interstitial lung disease. Eur Respir J. 2011;38:987–90.
34. Nathan SD, Noble PW, Tuder RM. Idiopathic pulmonary fibrosis and pulmonary hypertension: connecting the dots. Am J Respir Crit Care Med. 2007;175:875–80.
35. Christopher KL, Schwartz MD. Transtracheal oxygen therapy. Chest. 2011;139:435–40.

# Chapter 17
# Acute Exacerbation of Idiopathic Pulmonary Fibrosis

**Joyce S. Lee and Harold R. Collard**

**Abstract** Acute exacerbation of idiopathic pulmonary fibrosis (IPF) is a clinically important complication of IPF that carries a high morbidity and mortality. In the last decade, we have learned much about this event, but there are many remaining questions: What is it? Why does it happen? How can we prevent it? How can we treat it? This chapter attempts to summarize our current understanding of the epidemiology, etiology, and management of acute exacerbation of IPF and point out areas where additional data are sorely needed.

**Keywords** Acute exacerbation • Risk factors • Pathobiology • Diagnosis • Prognosis • Management

## A Case

A 78-year-old man was referred for surgical lung biopsy in the evaluation of his interstitial lung disease (ILD). At baseline, he reported mild dyspnea on exertion and a chronic, dry cough. His past medical history was significant for hypertension and gastroesophageal reflux (GER) disease. His medications included an antihypertensive medication and a proton pump inhibitor. He was a lifelong nonsmoker and worked as a dentist. He had no family history of ILD. His physical exam was significant for dry inspiratory crackles at both bases and normal resting oxygen saturation. His pulmonary function was abnormal with a forced vital capacity of 57 %

J.S. Lee, M.D. (✉)
Department of Medicine, Interstitial Lung Disease Program, University of California,
San Francisco, 505 Parnassus Ave, Campus Box 0111, San Francisco, CA 94143, USA
e-mail: joyce.lee@ucsf.edu

H.R. Collard, M.D.
Department of Medicine, University of California, San Francisco, San Francisco, CA, USA

K.C. Meyer and S.D. Nathan (eds.), *Idiopathic Pulmonary Fibrosis: A Comprehensive Clinical Guide*, Respiratory Medicine 9, DOI 10.1007/978-1-62703-682-5_17,
© Springer Science+Business Media New York 2014

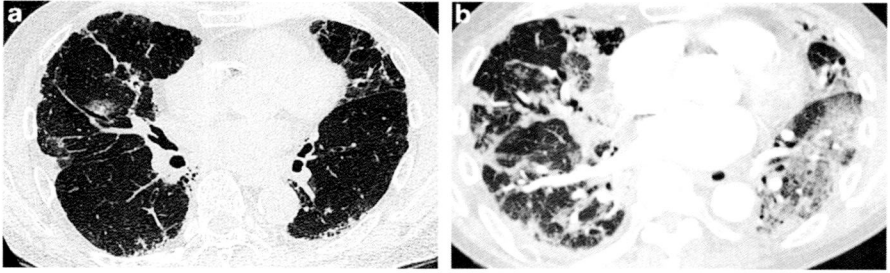

Fig. 17.1 *Bottom left* image is presurgery demonstrating peripheral reticulation and traction bronchiectasis without honeycombing. *Upper right* image is 5 days postoperatively, demonstrating diffuse ground-glass opacities, most prominent in the left lung

predicted and a diffusing capacity for carbon monoxide of 67 % predicted. His high-resolution computed tomography (HRCT) scan demonstrated peripheral, subpleural predominant reticulation and traction bronchiectasis without honeycombing.

He was referred for surgical lung biopsy and had a video-assisted thoracic surgery procedure with biopsies obtained from the right lung. His perioperative course was uncomplicated. His pathology was reviewed and was consistent with a usual interstitial pneumonia (UIP) pattern, confirming the diagnosis of IPF. His initial postoperative course was uncomplicated, but approximately 5 days postoperatively, he developed increased dyspnea and cough with occasional production of clear sputum. He had new-onset hypoxemia (88 % on room air) with diffuse crackles to auscultation that were more prominent in the left chest. A repeat HRCT demonstrated new ground-glass opacities in the left lung (Fig. 17.1). All microbiologic data were negative, and there was no evidence of cardiac dysfunction or ischemia.

This case was thought to be due to an acute exacerbation (AEx) of IPF triggered by surgical lung biopsy possibly due to single lung ventilation of the left lung. Unfortunately, the patient progressively worsened despite supportive care and subsequently died from his AEx of IPF.

## Epidemiology, Clinical Features, and Risk Factors

Our view of the natural history of IPF has changed over the last decade with the recognition that there are several distinct clinical courses that patients may follow [1]. Although most patients with IPF experience a steady decline in lung function over time, some will decline quickly, while others seem stable for many years. Increasingly, we recognize that some patients may also have a more unpredictable course [2]. These patients experience periods of relative stability followed by acute episodes of worsening in their respiratory status [3]. Episodes of acute respiratory decline in IPF can be secondary to complications such as infection, pulmonary embolism, pneumothorax, or heart failure [3, 4]. Such episodes of acute respiratory deterioration have been termed AEx of IPF when the cause for the acute worsening cannot be identified. Acute exacerbations likely comprise almost 50 % of these acute respiratory events, and the clinical characteristics and prognosis are indistinguishable from acute exacerbations of known cause. This chapter will discuss only AEx of IPF.

The phenomenon of AEx has been recognized since the late 1980s, when it was initially reported in the Japanese literature [5–8]. A survey of providers in the USA suggests that most clinicians believe AEx to be somewhat or very common [9]. The true incidence of AEx remains unknown, and the incidence may vary by country due to different genetic and environmental factors. Largely due to differences in case definition, patient population, sample size, and duration of follow-up, the range of AEx incidence in clinical studies ranges anywhere from 1 % to 24 % [3, 4]. The largest and probably most robust study of 461 patients with IPF that were followed longitudinally over 3 years found a 1- and 3-year incidence of 14.2 % and 20.7 %, respectively [4].

The clinical presentation of AEx is generally quite dramatic and characterized by acute to subacute worsening of dyspnea over days to weeks [3]. Some patients experience symptoms of worsening cough, sputum production, and fever mimicking a respiratory tract infection [10, 11]. Most reported cases of AEx have required unscheduled medical attention (emergency room or hospital care), but there may well be less severe cases that do not get noted by patients and providers and, therefore, are not documented.

The occurrence of AEx is unpredictable and can sometimes be the presenting manifestation of IPF [11–13]. A few risk factors have been identified, including lower baseline forced vital capacity (FVC) % predicted and having been a nonsmoker [4]. It seems likely that patients with more severe IPF are more likely to develop clinically significant AEx of disease, and this perception is supported by the increased incidence of AEx that was observed in the only study of advanced disease reported in the literature to date, namely, STEP-IPF [14]. Precipitating factors such as surgical lung biopsy and bronchoalveolar lavage (BAL) have also been reported [11, 15–20]. The occurrence of AEx after videoscopic-assisted surgical lung biopsy is particularly intriguing, as the exacerbation appears to be more pronounced in the lung that was ventilated (i.e., the nonsurgical side receiving single lung ventilation) [19]. However, the precise relationship between these precipitating factors and AEx remains unclear.

Acute exacerbations have also been described in non-IPF ILD, including nonspecific interstitial pneumonia (NSIP) [21], connective tissue disease-associated ILD [21–23], and hypersensitivity pneumonitis [24, 25]. Compared to IPF AEx, patients with an underlying NSIP pattern appeared to have a better prognosis following their AEx [21]. A UIP pattern may be a risk factor for AEx in the context of connective tissue disease-associated ILD and hypersensitivity pneumonitis, as the presence of a UIP pattern appeared to be a risk factor in some case series [21, 25]. Whether AEx of non-IPF forms of ILD shares a similar pathobiology as AEx of IPF is unknown.

## Etiology and Pathobiology

The etiology of AEx of IPF remains unknown. Several hypotheses have been proposed, including the following: (1) AEx of IPF represents an abrupt acceleration of the patients underlying disease; (2) AEx is a collection of occult, pathobiologically distinct conditions (e.g., infection, heart failure); or (3) AEx is a combination of both processes that can serve as an occult trigger that leads to acceleration of the underlying fibroproliferative process.

Occult aspiration of gastric contents has been suggested as a possible trigger or cause of AEx of IPF. GER is nearly universal in patients with IPF [26, 27] and is thought to be a risk factor for aspiration [28, 29]. BAL pepsin levels, a biomarker for aspiration of gastric secretions, were shown to be elevated in a subset of patients with AEx of IPF [30]. In addition, patients with asymmetric IPF on HRCT scan had a higher rate of GER and AEx compared to patients with non-asymmetric disease, suggesting a role for GER and occult aspiration in a subset of patients with IPF [31].

Infection has also been suggested as a cause of AEx of IPF. Data in support of this hypothesis include animal studies [32] as well as some human studies [33, 34]. In one case series, 75.7 % of 37 AEx cases occurred between December and May [10], lending further support to occult infection as a cause of AEx. However, in a prospective study of AEx of IPF ($n = 47$), acute viral infection, as determined by the most current genomics-based methodologies, was found in only 9 % of this cohort [35]. While some cases may well have been missed (i.e., the virus had come and gone by the time testing was obtained), these data suggest that there are many cases of AEx that are not primarily due to occult infection.

An alternative explanation is that AEx of IPF is caused by an inherent acceleration of the pathobiology of IPF [3]. There is indirect evidence for this in several studies that evaluated serum biomarkers and gene expression in AEx. Serum biomarkers of alveolar epithelial cell injury/proliferation have been shown to be increased in AEx, in a pattern that is qualitatively distinct from what is seen in acute lung injury (Table 17.1).

Gene expression studies performed in patients with AEx of IPF [37] have shown that patients have increased expression of genes encoding proteins involved in epithelial injury and proliferation including CCNA2 and alpha-defensins. Interestingly, there was no evidence from the same study for upregulation of genes commonly expressed in viral infection.

## Work-Up and Diagnostic Criteria

### Laboratory Evaluation

There are no specific laboratory tests that aid in the evaluation and diagnosis of AEx of IPF. Often, patients are found to have impaired gas exchange with a decrease in

Table 17.1  Potential biomarkers in acute exacerbation of IPF

| Biomarker | Mechanism of action | Association with AEx of IPF | References |
| --- | --- | --- | --- |
| Alpha defensin | Cationic proteins with antimicrobial activity found in neutrophils | Plasma levels higher in AEx compared to stable and seemed to correlate with disease course | [36, 37] |
| Annexin 1 | Anti-inflammatory, antiproliferative, and pro-apoptotic calcium and phospholipid-binding protein that regulates differentiation; found in alveolar type II cells and alveolar macrophages | Associated with antibody production and CD4+ T-cell response in AEx | [38] |
| Circulating fibrocytes | Circulating mesenchymal cell progenitors involved in tissue repair and fibrosis | Increased levels of circulating fibrocytes in AEx compared to stable IPF | [39] |
| High-mobility group protein B1 (HMGB1) | Nuclear nonhistone protein and involved in endogenous danger signaling and a mediator of systemic inflammation; can bind to RAGE to promote chemotaxis and production of cytokines via NF-kB activation | Serum HMGB1 levels are higher in AEx requiring mechanical ventilation compared to stable IPF; BAL HMGB1 gradually increases during AEx, which correlated with monocyte chemotactic protein-1 (MCP-1) | [40, 41] |
| IL-6 | Cytokine involved in a broad range of cellular responses including inflammation | Higher levels in AEx vs. stable | [42] |
| KL-6 | Marker of alveolar type II cell injury and/or proliferation | Plasma levels higher in AEx of IPF compared to stable; serial serum KL-6 levels increased in patients who died of their AEx | [42, 43] |
| PAI-1 | Principal inhibitor of tissue plasminogen activator and urokinase | Higher plasma levels in AEx compared to stable | [42] |
| Protein C | The activated form regulates blood clotting, inflammation, and cell death | Higher plasma % in AEx compared to stable | [42] |
| RAGE | Marker of alveolar type I cell injury and/or proliferation | No difference in plasma levels between stable and AEx of IPF | [42] |
| ST2 | Predominantly expressed in Th2 cells and induced by proinflammatory cytokines | Higher serum levels in AEx compared to stable with a sensitivity of 71 % and specificity of 92 % | [44] |
| SP-D | Marker of alveolar type II cell injury and/or proliferation | Plasma levels higher in AEx compared to stable | [42] |
| Thrombomodulin | Membrane protein expressed on the surface of endothelial cells which serves as a receptor for thrombin | Plasma levels higher in AEx compared to stable and log change in thrombomodulin was predictive of survival | [42] |
| von Willebrand factor | Marker of endothelial cell injury and is involved in hemostasis | Higher plasma % in AEx compared to stable | [42] |

AEx acute exacerbation, IPF idiopathic pulmonary fibrosis, KL-6 Krebs von den Lungen-6, PAI-1 plasminogen activator inhibitor-1, RAGE receptor for advanced glycation end products, NF-kB nuclear factor-kB, ST2, SP-D surfactant protein D

their arterial oxygen tension [10]. In patients that can tolerate bronchoscopy with lavage, an increase in BAL neutrophils has been reported [11, 45]. Nonspecific elevations in serum lactate dehydrogenase (LDH) and C-reactive protein (CRP) have also been observed [10]. Serial levels of serum KL-6 and baseline thrombomodulin may help identify patients at increased risk for death from AEx [42, 43]. Although many experimental biomarkers have been investigated, as shown in Table 17.1, none are routinely used in clinical practice.

## Radiologic Evaluation

High-resolution CT scans are often obtained during AEx of IPF. The findings include new, generally bilateral, ground-glass opacities and/or consolidation superimposed on the underlying UIP pattern [46]. The pattern of ground-glass changes during an AEx may have prognostic significance, with more diffuse abnormality correlating with worse outcomes [46].

## Histopathologic Evaluation

Surgical lung biopsy is not frequently obtained during AEx of IPF. A small case series of seven patients who had a surgical lung biopsy during their AEx demonstrated primarily diffuse alveolar damage (DAD) associated with underlying changes typical for UIP (Fig. 17.2) [47]. One case had organizing pneumonia and UIP and another case had DAD without underlying UIP. Autopsy series and other case series have demonstrated similar findings [6, 11, 45, 48–50].

## Diagnostic Criteria

Several definitions have been used over the last decade to define AEx of IPF [3, 6, 50]. In order to standardize these criteria, a consensus definition was proposed by the National Institutes of Health-funded US IPF Network (IPFNet) in 2007 (Table 17.2) [3]. Other definitions that have been described are generally similar; however, they often include a reduction in $PaO_2$ as one of their criteria as well as bilateral chest x-ray abnormalities (instead of a HRCT scan) [6, 50].

The IPFNet criteria have helped to standardize the definition of AEx of IPF, but satisfaction of all criteria is quite difficult to achieve in many clinical settings. Specifically, it is not infrequent that in patients who appear to have AEx of IPF, microbiologic data and occasionally radiologic data are not collected due to the severity of illness or because the clinician does not feel the tests will change clinical management. By maximizing specificity at the cost of sensitivity, these criteria

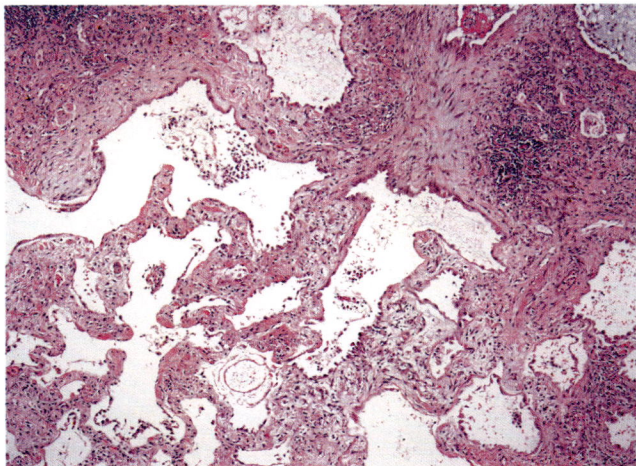

**Fig. 17.2** Section from lung explant shows subpleural fibrosis with honeycombing typical of usual interstitial pneumonia. The central lung tissue shows diffuse alveolar septal thickening by edema and type II pneumocyte hyperplasia, and airspace consolidation by edema and fibrin (H&E, ×100). Figure courtesy of Kirk Jones, MD

**Table 17.2** IPFNet consensus criteria for acute exacerbation of idiopathic pulmonary fibrosis[a]

Previous or concurrent diagnosis of idiopathic pulmonary fibrosis

Unexplained development or worsening of dyspnea within 30 days

High-resolution computed tomography with new bilateral ground-glass abnormality and/or consolidation superimposed on a background reticular or honeycomb pattern consistent with usual interstitial pneumonia

No evidence of pulmonary infection by endotracheal aspirate or bronchoalveolar lavage

Exclusion of alternative causes, including left heart failure, pulmonary embolism, and other identifiable causes of acute lung injury

[a]Patients who do not meet all five criteria should be termed "suspected acute exacerbation"

(along with the selection of only mild to moderate patients for enrollment) have likely contributed to the low prevalence of AEx observed in recent clinical trials [51–53]. The choice of definition has significant implications for outcome analyses in clinical trials and should be a focus for further discussion among clinical trialists.

## Management and Prognosis

There is no known effective treatment for preventing or improving outcomes in AEx of IPF.

## Prevention

While there are no data to support efficacy, vaccination and treatment of comorbidities like heart disease and GER seem prudent as measures that could prevent episodes of acute decline in respiratory function due to known causes such as infection, heart failure, and aspiration. Some novel therapies have suggested a reduction in AEx in clinical trials; these include warfarin [54], pirfenidone [55], and, most recently, BIBF 1120 [56]. Unfortunately, both warfarin and pirfenidone have subsequently been shown to have no impact on the rate of AEx, suggesting that the initial observations were inaccurate [51, 57].

## Medical Therapy During AEx

Although commonly prescribed for the treatment of AEx of IPF, there have been no controlled trials assessing the efficacy of high-dose corticosteroids. Recent international guidelines on IPF management suggested that the majority of IPF patients with AEx could be treated with corticosteroids [58]; however, approaches to dosing, route, and duration of therapy were not provided.

Although most clinicians would treat patients who develop an AEx of IPF with high-dose corticosteroids, the efficacy of this treatment is unclear. Perhaps we should be more critical of the use of corticosteroids to treat AEx of IPF. There are two distinct viewpoints regarding the role of corticosteroids in AEx of IPF. The first viewpoint is that AEx of IPF is histopathologically similar to acute respiratory distress syndrome (ARDS) characterized by DAD and acute lung injury [59] and should, therefore, be treated similarly to ARDS. In the ARDS literature, the mortality benefit of corticosteroids is unclear [60–65]. In one study, increased mortality was observed in ARDS patients treated with delayed corticosteroids (after 14 days) [65]. If we were to follow the ARDS paradigm, most clinicians would not use corticosteroids in the treatment of AEx of IPF. A second viewpoint for the role of corticosteroids in IPF is that some patients with AEx of IPF have organizing pneumonia on biopsy [49]. Organizing pneumonia is generally thought to be steroid responsive, and it may be that the pathobiology is different enough between ARDS and AEx of IPF to warrant continued use of corticosteroids. There remains equipoise on the efficacy of corticosteroids in AEx of IPF, and this treatment intervention should be studied more carefully [42].

The use of another immunosuppressant, cyclosporine A, to treat AEx of IPF has been reported. These studies suggest some benefit to the use of cyclosporine A plus corticosteroids [66–68]. However, conclusions that can be made from these data are limited by problems with study design and small sample size, and benefit has not yet been validated in a randomized controlled trial.

Other experimental therapies that have reported possible efficacy to treat AEx of IPF include tacrolimus [69], hemoperfusion with polymyxin B-immobilized fiber column [70–72], and sivelestat [73]. These investigations were all limited by small numbers and suboptimal study design.

## Supportive Therapy During AEx

Supportive therapy is the standard of care in AEx of IPF. Supportive care for respiratory failure almost always requires higher oxygen supplementation and consideration of additional means of ventilatory support, including mechanical ventilation (see discussion below) and noninvasive positive-pressure ventilation (NIPPV). Yokoyama et al. described the outcomes of patients with AEx of IPF treated with NIPPV to avoid intubation in acute respiratory failure [74]. In this retrospective case series of 11 patients, 6 patients failed a NIPPV trial and went subsequently succumbed to respiratory failure. The other five patients survived more than 3 months after the onset of their AEx. However, the use of ventilatory support in AEx (both mechanical ventilation and NIPPV) has never been studied in a randomized controlled trial.

## Lung Transplantation

A few select centers have experience with emergent transplantation for AEx of IPF [75–78]. These critically ill IPF patients have generally been bridged to lung transplant with extracorporeal membrane oxygenation (ECMO) and/or mechanical ventilation [76]. Outcomes of patients who have undergone emergent transplantation have been mixed [77, 78]. Emergent lung transplantation requires careful patient selection and is not done at all transplant centers.

## Prognosis

The prognosis of AEx of IPF is poor, with most case series reporting very high short-term mortality rates [11, 79–83]. This is particularly true for those patients requiring mechanical ventilation. A systematic review of mechanical ventilation in IPF and respiratory failure ($n = 135$), including AEx, reported a hospital mortality of 87 % [81]. Short-term mortality (within 3 months of hospital discharge) was 94 %. The routine use of mechanical ventilation in patients with AEx of IPF is not recommended in the international consensus guidelines because of its low likelihood of benefit and high risk of complications and further suffering [58]. Careful consideration regarding intubation and goals of care must be made, given the poor prognosis associated with this condition. Ideally, a discussion concerning end-of-life issues should be held between the patient and their provider in the outpatient setting with the inclusion of the patient's family, if applicable.

# Summary

Acute exacerbation of IPF is responsible for substantial morbidity and mortality in patients with IPF. We suggest that AEx of IPF represents an acute acceleration of the fibroproliferative process (i.e., the underlying pathobiology of IPF) that is triggered by some generally occult stress or insult to the lung (e.g., infection, aspiration, mechanical stretch from ventilation or lavage, high inspired oxygen concentration during surgery). As many patients with AEx of IPF will not meet the current consensus criteria due to missing data, it may be more useful clinically to define AEx by less stringent criteria. It seems likely that the prevention and treatment of AEx of IPF must focus on both disease-specific (e.g., anti-fibrotic therapies) and non-disease-specific (e.g., vaccination, prevention of stress) areas. The next decade will hopefully answer many of the unresolved questions concerning AEx of IPF.

# References

1. Kim DS, Collard HR, King Jr TE. Classification and natural history of the idiopathic interstitial pneumonias. Proc Am Thorac Soc. 2006;3(4):285–92.
2. Ley B, Collard HR, King Jr TE. Clinical course and prediction of survival in idiopathic pulmonary fibrosis. Am J Respir Crit Care Med. 2011;183(4):431–40.
3. Collard HR, Moore BB, Flaherty KR, Brown KK, Kaner RJ, King Jr TE, et al. Acute exacerbations of idiopathic pulmonary fibrosis. Am J Respir Crit Care Med. 2007;176(7):636–43.
4. Song JW, Hong SB, Lim CM, Koh Y, Kim DS. Acute exacerbation of idiopathic pulmonary fibrosis: incidence, risk factors and outcome. Eur Respir J. 2011;37(2):356–63.
5. Suga T, Sugiyama Y, Ohno S, Kitamura S. [Two cases of IIP which developed acute exacerbation after bronchoalveolar lavage]. Nihon Kyobu Shikkan Gakkai Zasshi. 1994;32(2):174–8.
6. Kondoh Y, Taniguchi H, Kawabata Y, Yokoi T, Suzuki K, Takagi K. Acute exacerbation in idiopathic pulmonary fibrosis. Analysis of clinical and pathologic findings in three cases. Chest. 1993;103(6):1808–12.
7. Kondo A, Saiki S. Acute exacerbation in idiopathic interstitial pneumonia (IIP). In: Harasawa M, Fukuchi Y, Morinari H, editors. Interstitial pneumonia of unknown etiology. Tokyo: University of Tokyo Press; 1989.
8. Horio H, Nomori H, Morinaga S, Fuyuno G, Kobayashi R, Iga R. [Exacerbation of idiopathic interstitial pneumonia after lobectomy for lung cancer]. Nihon Kyobu Shikkan Gakkai Zasshi. 1996;34(4):439–43.
9. Collard HR, Loyd JE, King Jr TE, Lancaster LH. Current diagnosis and management of idiopathic pulmonary fibrosis: a survey of academic physicians. Respir Med. 2007;101(9):2011–6.
10. Simon-Blancal V, Freynet O, Nunes H, Bouvry D, Naggara N, Brillet PY, et al. Acute exacerbation of idiopathic pulmonary fibrosis: outcome and prognostic factors. Respiration. 2012;83(1):28–35.
11. Kim DS, Park JH, Park BK, Lee JS, Nicholson AG, Colby T. Acute exacerbation of idiopathic pulmonary fibrosis: frequency and clinical features. Eur Respir J. 2006;27(1):143–50.
12. Sakamoto K, Taniguchi H, Kondoh Y, Ono K, Hasegawa Y, Kitaichi M. Acute exacerbation of idiopathic pulmonary fibrosis as the initial presentation of the disease. Eur Respir Rev. 2009;18(112):129–32.

13. Kondoh Y, Taniguchi H, Katsuta T, Kataoka K, Kimura T, Nishiyama O, et al. Risk factors of acute exacerbation of idiopathic pulmonary fibrosis. Sarcoidosis Vasc Diffuse Lung Dis. 2010;27(2):103–10.
14. Zisman DA, Schwarz M, Anstrom KJ, Collard HR, Flaherty KR, Hunninghake GW. A controlled trial of sildenafil in advanced idiopathic pulmonary fibrosis. N Engl J Med. 2010;363(7):620–8.
15. Zegdi R, Azorin J, Tremblay B, Destable MD, Lajos PS, Valeyre D. Videothoracoscopic lung biopsy in diffuse infiltrative lung diseases: a 5-year surgical experience. Ann Thorac Surg. 1998;66(4):1170–3.
16. Yuksel M, Ozyurtkan MO, Bostanci K, Ahiskali R, Kodalli N. Acute exacerbation of interstitial fibrosis after pulmonary resection. Ann Thorac Surg. 2006;82(1):336–8.
17. Utz JP, Ryu JH, Douglas WW, Hartman TE, Tazelaar HD, Myers JL, et al. High short-term mortality following lung biopsy for usual interstitial pneumonia. Eur Respir J. 2001;17(2):175–9.
18. Kumar P, Goldstraw P, Yamada K, Nicholson AG, Wells AU, Hansell DM, et al. Pulmonary fibrosis and lung cancer: risk and benefit analysis of pulmonary resection. J Thorac Cardiovasc Surg. 2003;125(6):1321–7.
19. Kondoh Y, Taniguchi H, Kitaichi M, Yokoi T, Johkoh T, Oishi T, et al. Acute exacerbation of interstitial pneumonia following surgical lung biopsy. Respir Med. 2006;100(10):1753–9.
20. Hiwatari N, Shimura S, Takishima T, Shirato K. Bronchoalveolar lavage as a possible cause of acute exacerbation in idiopathic pulmonary fibrosis patients. Tohoku J Exp Med. 1994;174(4):379–86.
21. Park IN, Kim DS, Shim TS, Lim CM, Lee SD, Koh Y, et al. Acute exacerbation of interstitial pneumonia other than idiopathic pulmonary fibrosis. Chest. 2007;132(1):214–20.
22. Tachikawa R, Tomii K, Ueda H, Nagata K, Nanjo S, Sakurai A, et al. Clinical features and outcome of acute exacerbation of interstitial pneumonia: collagen vascular diseases-related versus idiopathic. Respiration. 2012;83(1):20–7.
23. Suda T, Kaida Y, Nakamura Y, Enomoto N, Fujisawa T, Imokawa S, et al. Acute exacerbation of interstitial pneumonia associated with collagen vascular diseases. Respir Med. 2009;103(6):846–53.
24. Olson AL, Huie TJ, Groshong SD, Cosgrove GP, Janssen WJ, Schwarz MI, et al. Acute exacerbations of fibrotic hypersensitivity pneumonitis: a case series. Chest. 2008;134(4):844–50.
25. Miyazaki Y, Tateishi T, Akashi T, Ohtani Y, Inase N, Yoshizawa Y. Clinical predictors and histologic appearance of acute exacerbations in chronic hypersensitivity pneumonitis. Chest. 2008;134(6):1265–70.
26. Tobin RW, Pope 2nd CE, Pellegrini CA, Emond MJ, Sillery J, Raghu G. Increased prevalence of gastroesophageal reflux in patients with idiopathic pulmonary fibrosis. Am J Respir Crit Care Med. 1998;158(6):1804–8.
27. Raghu G, Freudenberger TD, Yang S, Curtis JR, Spada C, Hayes J, et al. High prevalence of abnormal acid gastro-oesophageal reflux in idiopathic pulmonary fibrosis. Eur Respir J. 2006;27(1):136–42.
28. Marik PE. Aspiration pneumonitis and aspiration pneumonia. N Engl J Med. 2001;344(9):665–71.
29. Lee JS, Collard HR, Raghu G, Sweet MP, Hays SR, Campos GM, et al. Does chronic microaspiration cause idiopathic pulmonary fibrosis? Am J Med. 2010;123(4):304–11.
30. Lee JS, Song JW, Wolters PJ, Elicker BM, King Jr TE, Kim DS, et al. Bronchoalveolar lavage pepsin in acute exacerbation of idiopathic pulmonary fibrosis. Eur Respir J. 2012;39(2):352–8.
31. Tcherakian C, Cottin V, Brillet PY, Freynet O, Naggara N, Carton Z, et al. Progression of idiopathic pulmonary fibrosis: lessons from asymmetrical disease. Thorax. 2011;66(3):226–31.
32. McMillan TR, Moore BB, Weinberg JB, Vannella KM, Fields WB, Christensen PJ, et al. Exacerbation of established pulmonary fibrosis in a murine model by gammaherpesvirus. Am J Respir Crit Care Med. 2008;177(7):771–80.
33. Tomioka H, Sakurai T, Hashimoto K, Iwasaki H. Acute exacerbation of idiopathic pulmonary fibrosis: role of Chlamydophila pneumoniae infection. Respirology. 2007;12(5):700–6.

34. Huie TJ, Olson AL, Cosgrove GP, Janssen WJ, Lara AR, Lynch DA, et al. A detailed evaluation of acute respiratory decline in patients with fibrotic lung disease: aetiology and outcomes. Respirology. 2010;15(6):909–17.
35. Wootton SC, Kim DS, Kondoh Y, Chen E, Lee JS, Song JW, et al. Viral infection in acute exacerbation of idiopathic pulmonary fibrosis. Am J Respir Crit Care Med. 2011;183(12):1698–702.
36. Mukae H, Iiboshi H, Nakazato M, Hiratsuka T, Tokojima M, Abe K, et al. Raised plasma concentrations of alpha-defensins in patients with idiopathic pulmonary fibrosis. Thorax. 2002;57(7):623–8.
37. Konishi K, Gibson KF, Lindell KO, Richards TJ, Zhang Y, Dhir R, et al. Gene expression profiles of acute exacerbations of idiopathic pulmonary fibrosis. Am J Respir Crit Care Med. 2009;180(2):167–75.
38. Kurosu K, Takiguchi Y, Okada O, Yumoto N, Sakao S, Tada Y, et al. Identification of annexin 1 as a novel autoantigen in acute exacerbation of idiopathic pulmonary fibrosis. J Immunol. 2008;181(1):756–67.
39. Moeller A, Gilpin SE, Ask K, Cox G, Cook D, Gauldie J, et al. Circulating fibrocytes are an indicator of poor prognosis in idiopathic pulmonary fibrosis. Am J Respir Crit Care Med. 2009;179(7):588–94.
40. Ebina M, Taniguchi H, Miyasho T, Yamada S, Shibata N, Ohta H, et al. Gradual increase of high mobility group protein b1 in the lungs after the onset of acute exacerbation of idiopathic pulmonary fibrosis. Pulm Med. 2011;2011:916486.
41. Abe S, Hayashi H, Seo Y, Matsuda K, Kamio K, Saito Y, et al. Reduction in serum high mobility group box-1 level by polymyxin B-immobilized fiber column in patients with idiopathic pulmonary fibrosis with acute exacerbation. Blood Purif. 2011;32(4):310–6.
42. Collard HR, Calfee CS, Wolters PJ, Song JW, Hong SB, Brady S, et al. Plasma biomarker profiles in acute exacerbation of idiopathic pulmonary fibrosis. Am J Physiol Lung Cell Mol Physiol. 2010;299(1):L3–7.
43. Yokoyama A, Kohno N, Hamada H, Sakatani M, Ueda E, Kondo K, et al. Circulating KL-6 predicts the outcome of rapidly progressive idiopathic pulmonary fibrosis. Am J Respir Crit Care Med. 1998;158(5 Pt 1):1680–4.
44. Tajima S, Oshikawa K, Tominaga S, Sugiyama Y. The increase in serum soluble ST2 protein upon acute exacerbation of idiopathic pulmonary fibrosis. Chest. 2003;124(4):1206–14.
45. Ambrosini V, Cancellieri A, Chilosi M, Zompatori M, Trisolini R, Saragoni L, et al. Acute exacerbation of idiopathic pulmonary fibrosis: report of a series. Eur Respir J. 2003;22(5):821–6.
46. Akira M, Kozuka T, Yamamoto S, Sakatani M. Computed tomography findings in acute exacerbation of idiopathic pulmonary fibrosis. Am J Respir Crit Care Med. 2008;178(4):372–8.
47. Parambil JG, Myers JL, Ryu JH. Histopathologic features and outcome of patients with acute exacerbation of idiopathic pulmonary fibrosis undergoing surgical lung biopsy. Chest. 2005;128(5):3310–5.
48. Rice AJ, Wells AU, Bouros D, du Bois RM, Hansell DM, Polychronopoulos V, et al. Terminal diffuse alveolar damage in relation to interstitial pneumonias. An autopsy study. Am J Clin Pathol. 2003;119(5):709–14.
49. Churg A, Muller NL, Silva CI, Wright JL. Acute exacerbation (acute lung injury of unknown cause) in UIP and other forms of fibrotic interstitial pneumonias. Am J Surg Pathol. 2007;31(2):277–84.
50. Akira M, Hamada H, Sakatani M, Kobayashi C, Nishioka M, Yamamoto S. CT findings during phase of accelerated deterioration in patients with idiopathic pulmonary fibrosis. AJR Am J Roentgenol. 1997;168(1):79–83.
51. Noble PW, Albera C, Bradford WZ, Costabel U, Glassberg MK, Kardatzke D, et al. Pirfenidone in patients with idiopathic pulmonary fibrosis (CAPACITY): two randomised trials. Lancet. 2011;377(9779):1760–9.
52. King Jr TE, Brown KK, Raghu G, du Bois RM, Lynch DA, Martinez F, et al. BUILD-3: a randomized, controlled trial of bosentan in idiopathic pulmonary fibrosis. Am J Respir Crit Care Med. 2011;184(1):92–9.

53. Fernandez Perez ER, Daniels CE, Schroeder DR, St Sauver J, Hartman TE, Bartholmai BJ, et al. Incidence, prevalence, and clinical course of idiopathic pulmonary fibrosis: a population-based study. Chest. 2010;137(1):129–37.
54. Kubo H, Nakayama K, Yanai M, Suzuki T, Yamaya M, Watanabe M, et al. Anticoagulant therapy for idiopathic pulmonary fibrosis. Chest. 2005;128(3):1475–82.
55. Azuma A, Nukiwa T, Tsuboi E, Suga M, Abe S, Nakata K, et al. Double-blind, placebo-controlled trial of pirfenidone in patients with idiopathic pulmonary fibrosis. Am J Respir Crit Care Med. 2005;171(9):1040–7.
56. Richeldi L, Costabel U, Selman M, Kim DS, Hansell DM, Nicholson AG, et al. Efficacy of a tyrosine kinase inhibitor in idiopathic pulmonary fibrosis. N Engl J Med. 2011;365(12):1079–87.
57. Noth I, Anstrom KJ, Calvert SB, de Andrade J, Flaherty KR, Glazer C, et al. A Placebo-controlled randomized trial of warfarin in idiopathic pulmonary fibrosis. Am J Respir Crit Care Med. 2012;186(1):89–95.
58. Raghu G, Collard HR, Egan JJ, Martinez FJ, Behr J, Brown KK, et al. An Official ATS/ERS/JRS/ALAT statement: idiopathic pulmonary fibrosis: evidence-based guidelines for diagnosis and management. Am J Respir Crit Care Med. 2011;183(6):788–824.
59. Ware LB, Matthay MA. The acute respiratory distress syndrome. N Engl J Med. 2000;342(18):1334–49.
60. Weigelt JA, Norcross JF, Borman KR, Snyder 3rd WH. Early steroid therapy for respiratory failure. Arch Surg. 1985;120(5):536–40.
61. Peter JV, John P, Graham PL, Moran JL, George IA, Bersten A. Corticosteroids in the prevention and treatment of acute respiratory distress syndrome (ARDS) in adults: meta-analysis. BMJ. 2008;336(7651):1006–9.
62. Meduri GU, Golden E, Freire AX, Taylor E, Zaman M, Carson SJ, et al. Methylprednisolone infusion in early severe ARDS: results of a randomized controlled trial. Chest. 2007;131(4):954–63.
63. Luce JM, Montgomery AB, Marks JD, Turner J, Metz CA, Murray JF. Ineffectiveness of high-dose methylprednisolone in preventing parenchymal lung injury and improving mortality in patients with septic shock. Am Rev Respir Dis. 1988;138(1):62–8.
64. Bernard GR, Luce JM, Sprung CL, Rinaldo JE, Tate RM, Sibbald WJ, et al. High-dose corticosteroids in patients with the adult respiratory distress syndrome. N Engl J Med. 1987;317(25):1565–70.
65. Steinberg KP, Hudson LD, Goodman RB, Hough CL, Lanken PN, Hyzy R, et al. Efficacy and safety of corticosteroids for persistent acute respiratory distress syndrome. N Engl J Med. 2006;354(16):1671–84.
66. Sakamoto S, Homma S, Miyamoto A, Kurosaki A, Fujii T, Yoshimura K. Cyclosporin A in the treatment of acute exacerbation of idiopathic pulmonary fibrosis. Intern Med. 2010;49(2):109–15.
67. Inase N, Sawada M, Ohtani Y, Miyake S, Isogai S, Sakashita H, et al. Cyclosporin A followed by the treatment of acute exacerbation of idiopathic pulmonary fibrosis with corticosteroid. Intern Med. 2003;42(7):565–70.
68. Homma S, Sakamoto S, Kawabata M, Kishi K, Tsuboi E, Motoi N, et al. Cyclosporin treatment in steroid-resistant and acutely exacerbated interstitial pneumonia. Intern Med. 2005;44(11):1144–50.
69. Horita N, Akahane M, Okada Y, Kobayashi Y, Arai T, Amano I, et al. Tacrolimus and steroid treatment for acute exacerbation of idiopathic pulmonary fibrosis. Intern Med. 2011;50(3):189–95.
70. Seo Y, Abe S, Kurahara M, Okada D, Saito Y, Usuki J, et al. Beneficial effect of polymyxin B-immobilized fiber column (PMX) hemoperfusion treatment on acute exacerbation of idiopathic pulmonary fibrosis. Intern Med. 2006;45(18):1033–8.
71. Miyamoto K, Tasaka S, Hasegawa N, Kamata H, Shinoda H, Kimizuka Y, et al. [Effect of direct hemoperfusion with a polymyxin B immobilized fiber column in acute exacerbation of interstitial pneumonia and serum indicators]. Nihon Kokyuki Gakkai Zasshi. 2009;47(11):978–84.

72. Enomoto N, Suda T, Uto T, Kato M, Kaida Y, Ozawa Y, et al. Possible therapeutic effect of direct haemoperfusion with a polymyxin B immobilized fibre column (PMX-DHP) on pulmonary oxygenation in acute exacerbations of interstitial pneumonia. Respirology. 2008;13(3):452–60.
73. Nakamura M, Ogura T, Miyazawa N, Tagawa A, Kozawa S, Watanuki Y, et al. [Outcome of patients with acute exacerbation of idiopathic interstitial fibrosis (IPF) treated with sivelestat and the prognostic value of serum KL-6 and surfactant protein D]. Nihon Kokyuki Gakkai Zasshi. 2007;45(6):455–9.
74. Yokoyama T, Kondoh Y, Taniguchi H, Kataoka K, Kato K, Nishiyama O, et al. Noninvasive ventilation in acute exacerbation of idiopathic pulmonary fibrosis. Intern Med. 2010;49(15): 1509–14.
75. Gottlieb J, Warnecke G, Hadem J, Dierich M, Wiesner O, Fuhner T, et al. Outcome of critically ill lung transplant candidates on invasive respiratory support. Intensive Care Med. 2012;38(6):968–75.
76. Fuehner T, Kuehn C, Hadem J, Wiesner O, Gottlieb J, Tudorache I, et al. Extracorporeal membrane oxygenation in awake patients as bridge to lung transplantation. Am J Respir Crit Care Med. 2012;185(7):763–8.
77. Boussaud V, Mal H, Trinquart L, Thabut G, Danner-Boucher I, Dromer C, et al. One-year experience with high-emergency lung transplantation in france. Transplantation. 2012;93(10): 1058–63.
78. Bermudez CA, Rocha RV, Zaldonis D, Bhama JK, Crespo MM, Shigemura N, et al. Extracorporeal membrane oxygenation as a bridge to lung transplant: midterm outcomes. Ann Thorac Surg. 2011;92(4):1226–31. discussion 31-2.
79. Saydain G, Islam A, Afessa B, Ryu JH, Scott JP, Peters SG. Outcome of patients with idiopathic pulmonary fibrosis admitted to the intensive care unit. Am J Respir Crit Care Med. 2002;166(6):839–42.
80. Mollica C, Paone G, Conti V, Ceccarelli D, Schmid G, Mattia P, et al. Mechanical ventilation in patients with end-stage idiopathic pulmonary fibrosis. Respiration. 2010;79(3):209–15.
81. Mallick S. Outcome of patients with idiopathic pulmonary fibrosis (IPF) ventilated in intensive care unit. Respir Med. 2008;102(10):1355–9.
82. Blivet S, Philit F, Sab JM, Langevin B, Paret M, Guerin C, et al. Outcome of patients with idiopathic pulmonary fibrosis admitted to the ICU for respiratory failure. Chest. 2001;120(1):209–12.
83. Stern JB, Mal H, Groussard O, Brugiere O, Marceau A, Jebrak G, et al. Prognosis of patients with advanced idiopathic pulmonary fibrosis requiring mechanical ventilation for acute respiratory failure. Chest. 2001;120(1):213–9.

# Chapter 18
# Lung Transplantation for Idiopathic Pulmonary Fibrosis

**Daniela J. Lamas and David J. Lederer**

**Abstract** Despite advances in the development of novel pharmaceutical agents to treat idiopathic pulmonary fibrosis (IPF), there are no medical therapies known to resolve fibrosis or improve lung function in IPF. Therefore, lung transplantation remains the only life-saving therapy available to treat patients with IPF. However, a shortage of suitable donor organs limits the number of affected individuals who can undergo this procedure, and this shortage highlights the need to allocate donor lungs to those who are in the greatest need of a life-saving therapy yet ensure that those who undergo transplantation will have a reasonable expectation of long-term survival.

Publications based on SRTR/OPTN 2010 Annual Report data [3] should include the following statement: The data and analyses reported in the 2010 Annual Data Report of the Organ Procurement and Transplantation Network and the US Scientific Registry of Transplant Recipients have been supplied by the Minneapolis Medical Research Foundation and UNOS under contract with HHS/HRSA. The authors of the Annual Data Report alone are responsible for reporting and interpreting these data; the viewed expressed in the Annual Data Report are those of the authors of the Report and not necessarily those of the US Government.

The use of the term idiopathic pulmonary fibrosis (IPF) in transplant registries has historically referred to a variety of forms of interstitial lung disease rather than IPF alone. In this chapter, usage of the term IPF may occasionally include interstitial lung diseases other than IPF.

D.J. Lamas, M.D.
Pulmonary and Critical Care Medicine, Harvard University, Massachusetts General Hospital, Boston, MA, USA

D.J. Lederer, M.D., M.S. (✉)
Lung Transplantation Program, Columbia University Medical Center, New York, NY, USA

Interstitial Lung Disease Program, Columbia University Medical Center, New York, NY, USA

Division of Pulmonary, Allergy, and Critical Care Medicine, Columbia University Medical Center, New York, NY, USA
e-mail: dl427@columbia.edu

K.C. Meyer and S.D. Nathan (eds.), *Idiopathic Pulmonary Fibrosis: A Comprehensive Clinical Guide*, Respiratory Medicine 9, DOI 10.1007/978-1-62703-682-5_18,
© Springer Science+Business Media New York 2014

Still, outcomes remain relatively poor for many patients after lung transplantation, although a sizable minority of patients can enjoy long-term survival after lung transplantation.

**Keywords** Lung transplantation • Idiopathic pulmonary fibrosis • Lung allocation score • Transplant candidate selection • Deceased donor organ allocation

# Background

Lung transplantation is a surgical procedure during which one or both diseased lungs are replaced by organs from a deceased organ donor (or, less commonly, by lobes from living donors) (Table 18.1). Although survival time after lung transplantation is typically limited, transplantation can confer substantial benefits, including prolongation of life, to selected candidates with advanced lung diseases such as idiopathic pulmonary fibrosis (IPF) [1]. Between 1988 and 2011, there were 23,652 lung transplant procedures performed in the USA, of which 5,565 (24 %) were performed for IPF [2]. In recent years, the proportion of lung transplant procedures performed for IPF in the USA has increased, and in 2007, IPF surpassed chronic obstructive pulmonary disease as the leading indication for lung transplantation in the USA (Fig. 18.1) [3]. In 2011, 36 % of US lung transplant procedures were performed for IPF [2]. In this chapter, we will review the role of lung transplantation for patients with IPF, including candidate selection criteria, the evaluation process, organ allocation in the USA, and outcomes and complications of transplantation.

**Table 18.1** Types of lung transplant procedures

| Procedure | Description | Number performed in the USA in 2010[a] |
|---|---|---|
| Single lung transplantation | Replacement of a single lung with a deceased donor lung | 539 |
| Bilateral sequential lung transplantation | Replacement of both lungs with deceased donor lungs with two main stem bronchial anastomoses | 1,212 |
| En bloc bilateral lung transplantation | Replacement of both lungs with deceased donor lungs with a single tracheal anastomosis | 19 |
| Heart-lung transplantation | Replacement of both lungs and the heart with deceased donor lungs and heart | 41 |
| Living-donor lung transplantation | Replacement of both lungs with lobes from two living donors | 0 |

[a]*Source*: OPTN data as of May 4, 2012

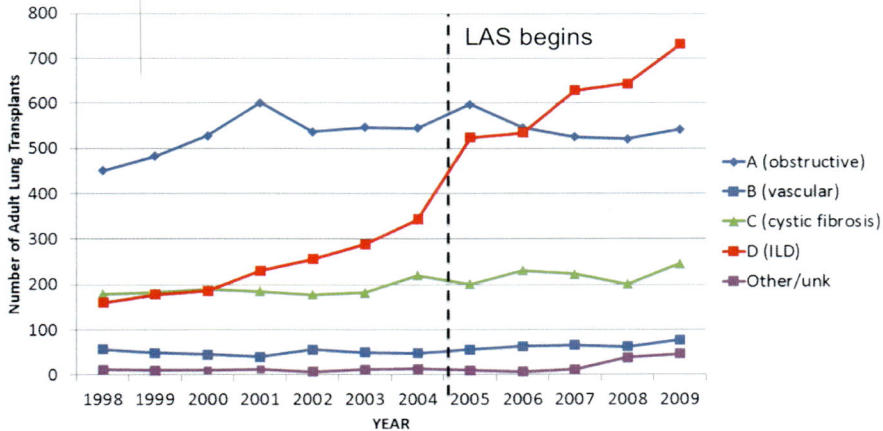

**Fig. 18.1** Number of patients undergoing lung transplantation in the USA stratified by LAS diagnostic group, 1998–2009. *Group A*, obstructive lung disease. *Group B*, pulmonary vascular disease. *Group C*, cystic fibrosis. *Group D*, restrictive lung disease including IPF. Adapted from data provided in Organ Procurement and Transplantation Network (OPTN) and Scientific Registry of Transplant Recipients (SRTR). OPTN/SRTR 2010 Annual Data Report. Rockville, MD: Department of Health and Human Services, Health Resources and Services Administration, Healthcare Systems Bureau, Division of Transplantation; 2011. Available at http://srtr.transplant. hrsa.gov/annual_reports/2010/chapter_index.htm. Accessed 31 May 2012

# Timing of Referral of IPF Patients for Lung Transplant Evaluation

IPF has been estimated to affect as many as 89,000 Americans [4]. Yet, in 2011 only 666 adults underwent lung transplantation for IPF in the USA [2]. While some patients with IPF do not meet criteria for lung transplantation or may be too well for the procedure, the surprisingly small number of patients with IPF undergoing transplantation annually largely reflects the scarcity of suitable lungs from deceased organ donors. While there were in excess of 12,000 deceased donor kidney transplants performed in the USA in 2011, only 3,160 lungs from deceased organ donors were used for transplantation. This discrepancy is largely due to unsuitable pulmonary conditions at the time of death in the majority of donors, such as pneumonia, ARDS, and pulmonary contusion [2].

In the face of this organ shortage, lung transplant providers must not only balance the risks and benefits of lung transplantation for individual patients but must also attempt to allocate deceased donor organs in a fashion that maximizes the overall public good achieved through transplantation (a utilitarian approach to the principle of distributive justice) [5]. Therefore, patients who stand to benefit from transplantation, but who are also at exceedingly high risk of early death after transplantation, should not undergo lung transplantation in geographic regions where a donor shortage exists. Stated simply, a patient must be "sick enough" to warrant transplantation, but also "well enough" to tolerate the procedure and potentially enjoy many years of additional life after transplantation.

For these reasons, the selection of appropriate candidates for lung transplantation is challenging. In 2006, the International Society for Heart and Lung Transplantation (ISHLT) published guidelines to aid in the selection of candidates for lung transplantation [6]. In general, these guidelines recommend that patients be referred for transplant evaluation when it is estimated that a patient has only a 50 % chance of surviving the next 2–3 years or has New York Heart Association class III or IV symptoms [6]. Given the poor prognosis of patients with IPF, the guidelines specifically recommend that patients with IPF be referred for lung transplantation upon identification of "histologic or radiographic evidence of UIP irrespective of vital capacity" [6]. In a joint statement, the American Thoracic Society, the European Respiratory Society, the Japanese Respiratory Society, and the Latin American Thoracic Association have recommended that IPF patients undergo transplant evaluation "at the first sign of objective deterioration," but details or specific criteria for "deterioration" were not provided in this guideline document [7].

While these recommendations have strong face validity, current evidence suggests that many patients are not referred for subspecialty or transplant care early in the course of their disease. Two prior studies have shown that the median delay between symptom onset and accessing subspecialty pulmonary care (by an ILD expert or transplant pulmonologist) is 2 years [8, 9] and that longer delays are associated with a higher risk of death independent of lung function and age [9].

While some clinicians have used failure of a trial of corticosteroids as an indication for transplant referral (as prior guidelines have suggested [10]), one arm of a recent clinical trial of immunosuppressive therapy for IPF was halted early when an interim efficacy analysis indicated that increased mortality, hospitalizations, and adverse events were observed among study participants allocated to a combination of prednisone, azathioprine, and $n$-acetylcysteine [11]. In the absence of the availability of an effective medical therapy for IPF, a trial of medical therapy should not delay referral of patients with IPF for transplant evaluation.

One recent study demonstrated that a higher titrated oxygen requirement (TOR) was associated with greater mortality in IPF, independent of forced vital capacity and 6-minute walk test results, with higher TOR values having greater specificity to predict the risk of death [12]. It may be reasonable to include TOR in clinical decision making, but there are insufficient data to support TOR as a sole criterion to delay referral for transplantation.

Early referral for lung transplant evaluation allows sufficient time for a thorough evaluation of the medical, surgical, and psychosocial candidacy of the patient, permits longitudinal evaluation of progression by the transplant team, ensures adequate transplant-specific education, and avoids high-risk emergent transplantation of patients with severe hypoxemic respiratory failure. It is our recommendation that patients with IPF be referred for lung transplantation as soon as the diagnosis is made. In cases in which delayed referral is favored by providers, it is our opinion that referral should occur no later than upon determination that supplemental oxygen is required during ambulation and/or exercise.

## Contraindications to Lung Transplantation

ISHLT-recommended contraindications to lung transplantation are listed in Table 18.2 [6]. There is general agreement that malignancy, severe chronic comorbid illness, psychosocial barriers, and the other absolute contraindications in Table 18.2 should prohibit lung transplantation for most candidates. On the other hand, the barrier that each of the relative contraindications listed in Table 18.2 poses to transplantation will vary according to candidate- and center-specific characteristics. These relative contraindications are largely factors reflecting body composition and surgical suitability that increase the risk of complications after lung transplantation.

Older age is associated with shorter survival time after lung transplantation [13]. The median survival time for adults over age 65 is only 3.5 years compared to 6.7 years for those age 35–49 (Fig. 18.2) [14]. Despite this increased risk, the proportion of lung transplants performed for older individuals has increased over time: in 2011, 26 % of all lung transplant procedures in the USA were performed for adults 65 years of age and older [2]. The ISHLT guidelines state that age alone should not be used as the sole criterion to deny lung transplantation, but instead should be considered as one of the many factors when determining suitability for transplantation.

Obesity, defined as a body mass index (BMI) >30 kg/m², is an independent risk factor for increased early mortality and primary graft dysfunction after lung

**Table 18.2** Contraindications to lung transplantation

Absolute contraindications
- Malignancy in the last 2 years, with the exception of cutaneous squamous and basal cell tumors. In general, a 5-year disease-free interval is prudent
- Untreatable advanced dysfunction of another major organ system (e.g., heart, liver, or kidney)
- Non-curable chronic extrapulmonary infection including chronic active viral hepatitis B, hepatitis C, and human immunodeficiency virus
- Significant chest wall or spinal deformity
- Documented nonadherence or inability to follow through with medical therapy or office follow-up, or both
- Untreatable psychiatric or psychological condition associated with the inability to cooperate or comply with medical therapy
- Absence of a consistent or reliable social support system
- Substance addiction (e.g., alcohol, tobacco, or narcotics) that is either active or within the last 6 months

Relative contraindications
- Age older than 65 years
- Critical or unstable clinical condition (e.g., shock, mechanical ventilation, or extracorporeal membrane oxygenation)
- Severely limited functional status with poor rehabilitation potential
- Colonization with highly resistant or highly virulent bacteria, fungi, or mycobacteria
- Obesity defined as a body mass index (BMI) exceeding 30 kg/m²
- Severe or symptomatic osteoporosis
- Mechanical ventilation
- Suboptimal treatment of other medical conditions that have not resulted in end-stage organ damage, such as diabetes mellitus, systemic hypertension, peptic ulcer disease, or gastroesophageal reflux

Table created with data from [6]

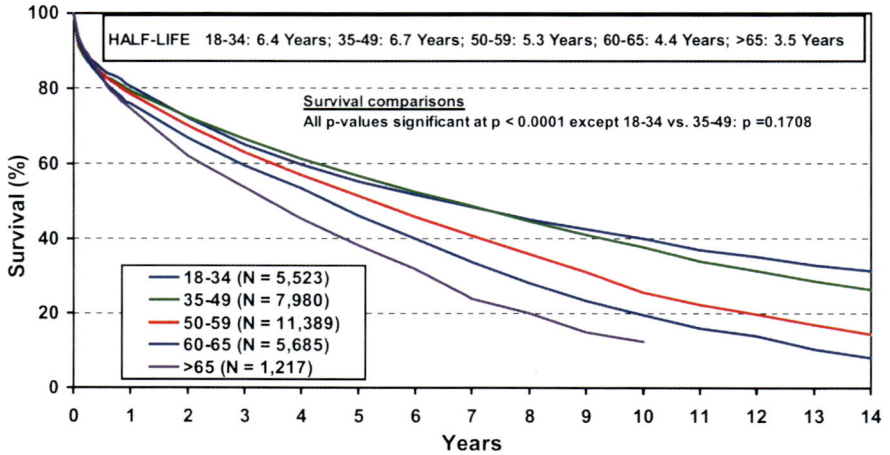

**Fig. 18.2** Unadjusted survival of adult lung transplant recipients in the ISHLT registry stratified by age group, 1990–June 2009. The median survival time for lung transplant recipients over the age of 65 years is 3.5 years compared to a median survival time of 6.7 years for lung transplant recipients age 35–49. Reprinted from The Journal of Heart and Lung Transplantation, 30/10, Christie JD, Edwards LB, Kucheryavaya AY, Benden C, Dobbels F, Kirk R, et al., The Registry of the International Society for Heart and Lung Transplantation: Twenty-eighth Adult Lung and Heart-Lung Transplant Report—2011, 1104–1122, 2011, with permission from Elsevier

transplantation in IPF [15, 16]. The mechanisms underlying these findings are not yet clear, but may involve secretion of pro-inflammatory mediators from macrophages in adipose tissue [17]. The magnitude of harm from obesity in IPF may be substantial, with an estimated twofold increased risk of primary graft dysfunction and a 30 % increased risk of death, and it appears that obesity might account for as many as 20 % of all deaths in the first year after transplantation for IPF [15, 16]. Based on these risks, mild elevations in BMI should not prohibit lung transplantation in all candidates, but instead the risks associated with obesity should be balanced with other risk factors and the potential benefit of transplantation for each individual candidate. In some cases, it may be reasonable to withhold lung transplantation from obese candidates (particularly with severe forms of obesity) until weight loss has been achieved. Healthcare providers should provide counseling, and, when indicated, interventions in order to achieve a healthy weight for all patients with IPF should be recommended, regardless of disease severity. For a discussion of the impact of age and obesity in lung transplantation, we refer the reader to a recent review on this topic [18].

## Candidate Evaluation and Timing of Listing for Lung Transplantation

Once referred for lung transplant evaluation, patients with IPF should undergo a thorough evaluation to determine if they are suitable candidates for lung transplantation based on the selection criteria described above and in Table 18.2. There are

**Table 18.3** Suggested evaluation of lung transplant candidates

Radiologic and functional studies
- Chest radiograph and high-resolution chest computed tomography scan
- Quantitative ventilation/perfusion lung scan
- Complete pulmonary function tests with arterial blood gas
- Cardiopulmonary exercise testing (if deemed necessary)
- 6-minute walk test
- Echocardiogram and electrocardiogram
- Right heart catheterization
- Left heart catheterization with coronary angiography in patients above age 45 or with risk factors for CAD
- Bone densitometry
- Barium esophagram

Laboratory evaluation
- Complete blood count, electrolytes, BUN/creatinine, liver function studies, fasting lipid profile, quantitative immunoglobulin levels, viral serologies (HIV, HBsAg, HBsAb, HBcAb, HCV, HSV, CMV, EBV, VZV), toxoplasma antibody, aspergillus antibodies, blood type and screen, urinalysis, MDRD calculation of creatinine clearance, prostate-specific antigen (males over the age of 40), panel reactive antibody testing, and identification of specific anti-HLA antibodies
- PPD testing

Consultations
- Psychosocial evaluation is completed by a transplant social worker and, if deemed necessary, supplemented by psychiatric evaluation
- Rehabilitation medicine
- Nutritionist, if deemed necessary on the initial nutritional screening
- Dental evaluation
- Ophthalmologic evaluation

Age- and gender-appropriate cancer screening

few published descriptions of the required elements of the evaluation of a lung transplant candidate, making the evaluation largely center specific. Candidate evaluation typically begins with a review of medical records to determine if any absolute contraindications exist. If none are identified, the candidate meets with a transplant pulmonologist, thoracic surgeon, and/or a transplant coordinator during which an extensive history and physical examination is performed, and the patient and his or her family are educated about the evaluation process, the transplant procedure, postoperative expectations, complications, post-transplant lifestyle changes, and survival statistics. In addition, this opportunity is taken to individualize the discussion of risks and benefits of transplantation and to discuss the patient's specific barriers to transplantation (such as obesity, underweight, poor functional status, and comorbidities), and recommendations to improve candidacy are made.

Following the initial consultation, patients typically undergo an extensive evaluation to determine their suitability for lung transplantation (Table 18.3). Once the evaluation has been completed, the patient's case is discussed at a multidisciplinary team selection meeting. If deemed a suitable candidate for transplantation, the patient is placed on the active waiting list for transplantation. Commonly, patients will not be deemed candidates until they complete miss components of the evaluation, achieve strict health-related goals (such as weight loss and participation in pulmonary

| **Table 18.4** ISHLT recommendations for the timing of listing for lung transplantation in IPF | Diffusing capacity of carbon monoxide of less than 39 % predicted |
| --- | --- |
| | A 10 % or greater decrement in forced vital capacity during 6 months of follow-up |
| | A decrease in pulse oximetry below 88 % during 6-minute walk testing |
| | Honeycombing on HRCT (fibrosis score of > 2) |
| | Table created with data from [6] |

rehabilitation), or until additional follow-up shows signs of disease progression. The timing of listing for lung transplantation is based largely on the estimated risk of respiratory failure and death for patients with IPF. Table 18.4 shows known predictors of an increased risk of death in IPF that are recommended by the ISHLT as thresholds for listing patients with IPF for lung transplantation [6]. In addition to these criteria, patients with IPF who have an interval increase in oxygen requirements or develop pulmonary hypertension should also be considered for active listing for lung transplantation. Additional factors that might favor earlier listing for lung transplantation (depending on local donor availability) include pre-sensitization to human leukocyte antigens, need for bilateral transplantation, and short stature.

## Deceased Donor Lung Allocation in the USA

Prior to 2005, allocation of deceased donor lungs in the USA was based on waiting time, with the highest priority given to those with the longest waiting time. Aside from a 90-day credit for patients with IPF, disease severity was not a factor in determining waiting list priority. In 1999, the US Department of Health and Human Services issued the "Final Rule," which requires that deceased organ allocation systems de-emphasize waiting time and instead allocate organs based on "objective and measureable medical criteria… ordered from most to least medically urgent…" [19]. In response, UNOS/OPTN and the SRTR developed the Lung Allocation Score (LAS) system, which was put into place on May 4, 2005 [20]. The LAS system prioritizes waiting list candidates based on two criteria: medical urgency (the predicted risk of dying within 1 year) and estimated transplant benefit (the number of additional days of life expected from lung transplantation during the next year). Transplant benefit is calculated as the difference between expected survival time after lung transplantation and expected waiting list survival time (medical urgency). Medical urgency and expected survival after lung transplantation are estimated from multivariable regression models that contain the predictors given in Table 18.5. The LAS, which varies from 0 to 100, is then derived from output of these models. Those with the greater medical urgency and expected transplant benefit receive higher LAS scores. After accounting for other criteria (geographic proximity to the donor, pediatric age, and blood type), deceased donor lungs are offered first to those with higher LAS scores. The LAS has been updated since its inception to include

**Table 18.5**   Variables included in the LAS calculation

| Category | Waiting list urgency | Post-transplant survival |
|---|---|---|
| Disease severity | Forced vital capacity | Forced vital capacity |
| | Mechanical ventilation | Mechanical ventilation |
| | Diagnosis | Diagnosis |
| | Oxygen requirement | Pulmonary capillary wedge pressure |
| | Pulmonary artery pressure | |
| | Partial pressure of carbon dioxide in arterial blood | |
| Physiologic reserve | Age | Age |
| | Functional status | Functional status |
| | Diabetes mellitus | Serum creatinine |
| | Body mass index | |
| | 6-minute walk distance | |

the addition of the partial pressure of carbon dioxide in arterial blood, and the addition of serum bilirubin is planned (to aid the estimation of medical urgency for those with right heart failure due to pulmonary arterial hypertension). In addition, extensive modifications to the LAS calculation are currently undergoing public comment and will likely be instituted in the near future.

The LAS system has had a number of notable consequences overall and for patients with IPF in particular. First, the transplantation rate for actively listed patients has increased dramatically with the greatest increase observed among those with IPF (Fig. 18.3), leading to IPF becoming the leading indication for lung transplantation in the USA (see Fig. 18.1) [3]. Second, waiting list mortality rates, which were decreasing prior to institution of the LAS system, have begun to increase, particularly for patients with IPF (Fig. 18.4) [3]. Whether this increase in waiting list mortality is due to removal of healthier patients from the waiting list, due to listing of more severely affected patients, and/or an inadequate number of donors remains to be determined. Third, as discussed above, older patients are now being considered more commonly for transplantation, opening up this treatment modality to a wider pool of patients with IPF.

While the LAS score appears to have increased the availability of transplantation for patients with IPF, concern remains that the scoring system—by preferentially emphasizing pre-transplant urgency—may be prioritizing those at highest risk for poor post-transplant outcomes. Indeed, one study suggested there might be higher rates of primary graft dysfunction and longer intensive care unit stays under the LAS system [21]. Two studies have also suggested that higher LAS scores are associated with higher mortality rates after lung transplantation [22, 23]. These studies raise questions about the utility of a system that grants organs to the sickest patients, increasing the likelihood of performing "futile" transplantation (i.e., transplantation of a donor organ without a consequent prolongation of life). Development of innovative methods to predict perioperative and post-transplant risk is under way and may ultimately lead to improved allocation methods and may aid in optimizing the timing of lung transplantation.

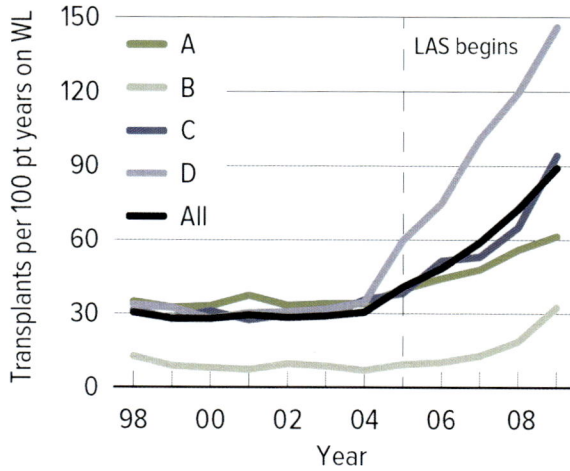

**Fig. 18.3** Rate of lung transplantation for waiting list candidates in the USA stratified by LAS diagnostic group, 1998–2009. *Group A*, obstructive lung disease. *Group B*, pulmonary vascular disease. *Group C*, cystic fibrosis. *Group D*, restrictive lung disease including IPF. Adapted from Organ Procurement and Transplantation Network (OPTN) and Scientific Registry of Transplant Recipients (SRTR). OPTN/SRTR 2010 Annual Data Report. Rockville, MD: Department of Health and Human Services, Health Resources and Services Administration, Healthcare Systems Bureau, Division of Transplantation; 2011. Available at http://srtr.transplant.hrsa.gov/annual_reports/2010/chapter_index.htm. Accessed 31 May 2012

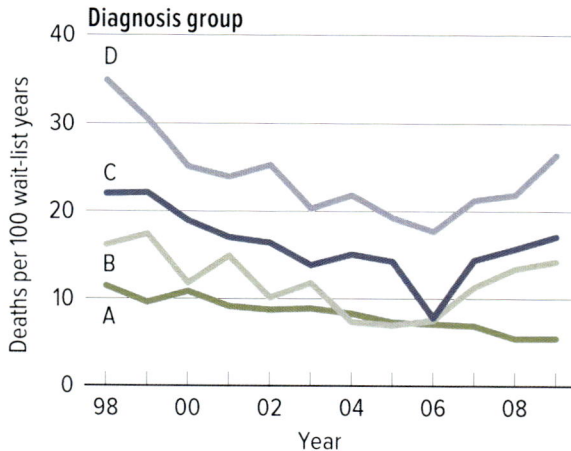

**Fig. 18.4** Mortality rate of adults on the lung transplant waiting list, by LAS diagnosis group, 1998–2009. *Group A*, obstructive lung disease. *Group B*, pulmonary vascular disease. *Group C*, cystic fibrosis. *Group D*, restrictive lung disease including IPF. Adapted from Organ Procurement and Transplantation Network (OPTN) and Scientific Registry of Transplant Recipients (SRTR). OPTN/SRTR 2010 Annual Data Report. Rockville, MD: Department of Health and Human Services, Health Resources and Services Administration, Healthcare Systems Bureau, Division of Transplantation; 2011. Available at http://srtr.transplant.hrsa.gov/annual_reports/2010/chapter_index.htm. Accessed 31 May 2012

## Types of Transplant Procedures

While five different lung transplant procedures have been developed (see Table 18.1), the vast majority of lung transplant procedures performed in the modern era are either bilateral sequential lung transplantation or single lung transplantation. In general, bilateral lung transplantation is indicated for patients with septic lung disease (such as bronchiectasis) and is preferred in patients with moderate-to-severe pulmonary hypertension. In IPF, many patients are candidates for either a bilateral or single lung transplant procedure, and there are advantages to each procedure: bilateral transplantation confers greater improvement in lung mechanics and avoids native lung complications (such as malignancy), while single lung transplantation is a simpler, shorter operation with a shorter waiting time that leaves the recipient with native lung function that may aid gas exchange during allograft complications, such as primary graft dysfunction [24].

The first isolated lung transplant procedures were single lung transplant procedures for IPF and other interstitial lung diseases [25, 26]. Over time, bilateral lung transplantation has become the preferred procedure for IPF in the USA (Fig. 18.5) [27], yet controversy remains regarding whether one procedure confers a survival benefit over the other. The earliest report comparing single to bilateral lung transplantation came from Washington University and found that among 45 patients with IPF who underwent lung transplantation between 1988 and 1998, single lung transplantation was associated with longer survival time than bilateral lung transplantation [28]. An analysis of OPTN data comprising 821 patients with IPF who underwent lung transplantation between 1994 and 2000 also found that single lung transplantation was associated with improved survival compared to double lung transplantation only among patients younger than 50 (which may reflect a population enriched for ILDs other than IPF) [29]. In contrast, a report from Cleveland of

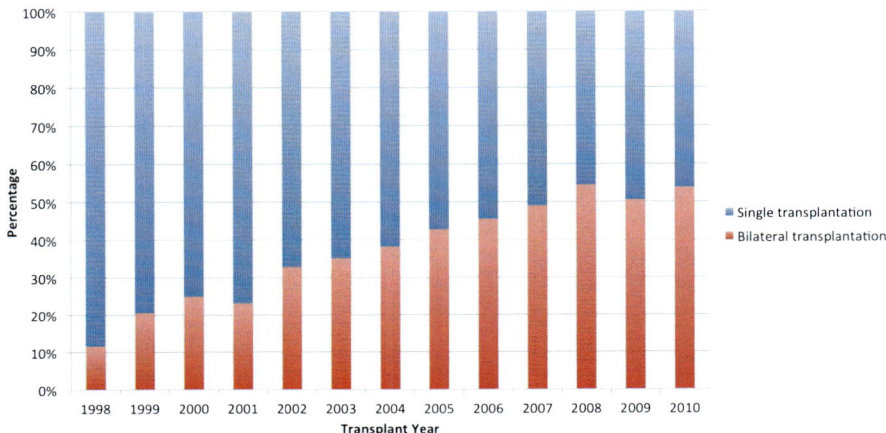

**Fig. 18.5** Distribution of single and bilateral lung transplantation for IPF in the USA, 1998–2010. Data from the Organ Procurement and Transplantation Network

82 patients with IPF transplanted between 1990 and 2005 suggested that bilateral lung transplantation was associated with improved survival compared to single lung transplantation [30]. ISHLT registry data suggest that patients who have undergone single or bilateral lung transplantation for IPF have fared similarly over the first 2 years after lung transplantation, but that single lung transplant recipients have had higher risks of death after that time period [14].

Observational studies of treatments are typically confounded by the indication for the treatment itself [31], making interpretation of these studies problematic. One group attempted to overcome this issue by performing an observational comparative effective study of single versus bilateral lung transplantation for IPF using OPTN data [27]. In propensity-matched analyses, single and bilateral lung transplant recipients with IPF fared equally well, suggesting that earlier studies did not adequately take confounding factors (such as disease severity) into account. The authors did note a small increase in early mortality among bilateral recipients (perhaps related to surgical factors) and a small increase in late mortality (perhaps related to malignancy) among single recipients.

In clinical practice, the decision to offer single or bilateral lung transplantation to patients with IPF is often informed by the presence of pulmonary hypertension and the candidate's perceived surgical suitability for one procedure or the other. For candidates thought to be eligible for either procedure, single lung transplantation should be preferred, since the other lung could be used to transplant a second candidate, and available data suggest that overall outcomes are similar between procedures. Indeed, patients with IPF listed for single lung transplantation have higher transplantation rates and lower waiting list mortality rates than those listed for bilateral lung transplantation [32].

## Outcomes and Complications of Lung Transplantation

Overall survival after lung transplantation has improved over time, with the median survival time improving from 4.7 years in the 1988 to 1994 ISHLT cohort to 5.9 years in the 2000–2009 ISHLT cohort [14]. For patients with IPF, the historical median survival time is 4.5 years (see Fig. 18.2), and unfortunately patients with IPF have the lowest 5- and 10-year survival rates compared to patients with other diagnoses [14]. Risk factors for 1-year mortality after lung transplantation for patients with IPF include older age, mechanical ventilation or hospitalization at the time of listing, prior pregnancy, elevated bilirubin, and elevated creatinine [14]. Despite these risks, observational studies suggest that, on average, lung transplantation prolongs life for patients with IPF [1, 33].

Most lung transplant recipients have improved functional status, with over 80 % of surviving lung transplant recipients having no activity limitation at 1, 3, or 5 years after transplantation, and approximately 50 % of 5-year survivors work full or part time (or are retired) [14], suggesting a significant personal benefit of lung transplantation to many recipients.

**Table 18.6** Bronchiolitis obliterans syndrome (BOS) staging

| BOS stage | FEV$_1$ criterion | FEF25-75 criterion |
|---|---|---|
| BOS 0 | 90 % or more of baseline | >75 % of baseline |
| BOS 0-p | 81–90 % of baseline | ≤75 % of baseline |
| BOS 1 | 66–80 % of baseline | Any |
| BOS 2 | 51–65 % of baseline | Any |
| BOS 3 | ≤50 % of baseline | Any |

Adapted from The Journal of Heart and Lung Transplantation, 21/3, Estenne M, Maurer JR, Boehler A, Egan JJ, Frost A, Hertz M, et al., Bronchiolitis obliterans syndrome 2001: an update of the diagnostic criteria, 297–310, 2002, with permission from Elsevier

Despite these benefits, lung transplantation carries significant risk. During the first post-transplant year, approximately 30 % of lung transplant recipients experience an episode of acute rejection and 60 % are re-hospitalized, most commonly for infection or rejection [14]. Metabolic and cardiovascular complications are also common, with 54 % developing systemic hypertension, 24 % developing chronic kidney disease, 29 % developing hyperlipidemia, and 30 % developing diabetes within 1 year of lung transplantation [14]. The leading causes of death in the first year after transplantation are graft failure and non-CMV infection [14].

The most feared complication of lung transplantation is bronchiolitis obliterans syndrome (BOS), a disorder recognized clinically as an irreversible reduction in FEV$_1$ below the post-transplant baseline (Table 18.6) that occurs in approximately 50 % of lung transplant recipients by 5 years and 75 % by 10 years [14, 34]. BOS is often due to obliterative bronchiolitis and manifests as airflow obstruction, but alternative causes have been described [35] and a restrictive allograft syndrome without airflow obstruction is increasingly recognized [36]. BOS is likely a final common pathway of multiple causes of airway injury, including alloimmune-mediated inflammation, infection, and gastroesophageal reflux [37], suggesting a variety of methods to potentially prevent BOS. Nevertheless, once BOS is present, there are (by definition) no known methods to improve lung function. BOS is often progressive and is the leading cause of death after the first year of transplantation [14].

# Summary

Lung transplantation is an effective therapy for highly selected patients with advanced IPF. Early referral to a lung transplant program should be considered for all patients with IPF. Because selection criteria continue to evolve, referring clinicians should consider referral of patients who may not have been candidates in past years, such as adults over the age of 70 and those with acute illness.

# References

1. Hosenpud JD, Bennett LE, Keck BM, Edwards EB, Novick RJ. Effect of diagnosis on survival benefit of lung transplantation for end-stage lung disease. Lancet. 1998;351(9095):24–7.
2. Organ Procurement and Transplantation Network data as of May 4, 2012. http://optn.transplant. hrsa.gov/data/
3. Organ Procurement and Transplantation Network (OPTN) and Scientific Registry of Transplant Recipients (SRTR). OPTN/SRTR 2010 Annual Data Report. Rockville, MD: Department of Health and Human Services, Health Resources and Services Administration, Healthcare Systems Bureau, Division of Transplantation; 2011. http://srtr.transplant.hrsa.gov/annual_ reports/2010/chapter_index.htm. Accessed 31 May 2012.
4. Raghu G, Weycker D, Edelsberg J, Bradford WZ, Oster G. Incidence and prevalence of idiopathic pulmonary fibrosis. Am J Respir Crit Care Med. 2006;174(7):810–6.
5. Persad G, Wertheimer A, Emanuel EJ. Principles for allocation of scarce medical interventions. Lancet. 2009;373(9661):423–31.
6. Orens JB, Estenne M, Arcasoy S, Conte JV, Corris P, Egan JJ, et al. International guidelines for the selection of lung transplant candidates: 2006 update–a consensus report from the Pulmonary Scientific Council of the International Society for Heart and Lung Transplantation. J Heart Lung Transplant. 2006;25(7):745–55.
7. Raghu G, Collard HR, Egan JJ, Martinez FJ, Behr J, Brown KK, et al. An official ATS/ERS/ JRS/ALAT statement: idiopathic pulmonary fibrosis: evidence-based guidelines for diagnosis and management. Am J Respir Crit Care Med. 2011;183(6):788–824.
8. King Jr TE, Tooze JA, Schwarz MI, Brown KR, Cherniack RM. Predicting survival in idiopathic pulmonary fibrosis: scoring system and survival model. Am J Respir Crit Care Med. 2001;164(7):1171–81.
9. Lamas DJ, Kawut SM, Bagiella E, Philip N, Arcasoy SM, Lederer DJ. Delayed access and survival in idiopathic pulmonary fibrosis: a cohort study. Am J Respir Crit Care Med. 2011;184(7):842–7.
10. Maurer JR, Frost AE, Estenne M, Higenbottam T, Glanville AR. International guidelines for the selection of lung transplant candidates. The International Society for Heart and Lung Transplantation, the American Thoracic Society, the American Society of Transplant Physicians, the European Respiratory Society. J Heart Lung Transplant. 1998;17(7):703–9.
11. Raghu G, Anstrom KJ, King Jr TE, Lasky JA, Martinez FJ. Prednisone, azathioprine, and N-acetylcysteine for pulmonary fibrosis. N Engl J Med. 2012;366(21):1968–77.
12. Hook JL, Arcasoy SM, Zemmel D, Bartels MN, Kawut SM, Lederer DJ. Titrated oxygen requirement and prognostication in idiopathic pulmonary fibrosis. Eur Respir J. 2012;39(2): 359–65.
13. Gutierrez C, Al-Faifi S, Chaparro C, Waddell T, Hadjiliadis D, Singer L, et al. The effect of recipient's age on lung transplant outcome. Am J Transplant. 2007;7(5):1271–7.
14. Christie JD, Edwards LB, Kucheryavaya AY, Benden C, Dobbels F, Kirk R, et al. The registry of the international society for heart and lung transplantation: twenty-eighth adult lung and heart-lung transplant report–2011. J Heart Lung Transplant. 2011;30(10):1104–22.
15. Lederer DJ, Wilt JS, D'Ovidio F, Bacchetta MD, Shah L, Ravichandran S, et al. Obesity and underweight are associated with an increased risk of death after lung transplantation. Am J Respir Crit Care Med. 2009;180(9):887–95.
16. Lederer DJ, Kawut SM, Wickersham N, Winterbottom C, Bhorade S, Palmer SM, et al. Obesity and primary graft dysfunction after lung transplantation: the Lung Transplant Outcomes Group Obesity Study. Am J Respir Crit Care Med. 2011;184(9):1055–61.
17. Weisberg SP, McCann D, Desai M, Rosenbaum M, Leibel RL, Ferrante Jr AW. Obesity is associated with macrophage accumulation in adipose tissue. J Clin Invest. 2003;112(12): 1796–808.
18. Hook JL, Lederer DJ. Selecting lung transplant candidates: where do current guidelines fall short? Expert Rev Respir Med. 2012;6(1):51–61.

19. "Allocation of Organs" Code of Federal Regulations Title 42, Pt. 121.8, 1999 ed.
20. Egan TM, Murray S, Bustami RT, Shearon TH, McCullough KP, Edwards LB, et al. Development of the new lung allocation system in the United States. Am J Transplant. 2006;6(5 Pt 2):1212–27.
21. Kozower BD, Meyers BF, Smith MA, De Oliveira NC, Cassivi SD, Guthrie TJ, et al. The impact of the lung allocation score on short-term transplantation outcomes: a multicenter study. J Thorac Cardiovasc Surg. 2008;135(1):166–71.
22. Russo MJ, Iribarne A, Hong KN, Davies RR, Xydas S, Takayama H, et al. High lung allocation score is associated with increased morbidity and mortality following transplantation. Chest. 2010;137(3):651–7.
23. Liu V, Zamora MR, Dhillon GS, Weill D. Increasing lung allocation scores predict worsened survival among lung transplant recipients. Am J Transplant. 2010;10(4):915–20.
24. Hadjiliadis D, Angel LF. Controversies in lung transplantation: are two lungs better than one? Semin Respir Crit Care Med. 2006;27(5):561–6.
25. Unilateral lung transplantation for pulmonary fibrosis. Toronto Lung Transplant Group. N Engl J Med. 1986;314(18):1140–5.
26. Grossman RF, Frost A, Zamel N, Patterson GA, Cooper JD, Myron PR, et al. Results of single-lung transplantation for bilateral pulmonary fibrosis. The Toronto Lung Transplant Group. N Engl J Med. 1990;322(11):727–33.
27. Thabut G, Christie JD, Ravaud P, Castier Y, Dauriat G, Jebrak G, et al. Survival after bilateral versus single-lung transplantation for idiopathic pulmonary fibrosis. Ann Intern Med. 2009;151(11):767–74.
28. Meyers BF, Lynch JP, Trulock EP, Guthrie T, Cooper JD, Patterson GA. Single versus bilateral lung transplantation for idiopathic pulmonary fibrosis: a ten-year institutional experience. J Thorac Cardiovasc Surg. 2000;120(1):99–107.
29. Meyer DM, Edwards LB, Torres F, Jessen ME, Novick RJ. Impact of recipient age and procedure type on survival after lung transplantation for pulmonary fibrosis. Ann Thorac Surg. 2005;79(3):950–7.
30. Mason DP, Brizzio ME, Alster JM, McNeill AM, Murthy SC, Budev MM, et al. Lung transplantation for idiopathic pulmonary fibrosis. Ann Thorac Surg. 2007;84(4):1121–8.
31. Mauri L. Why we still need randomized trials to compare effectiveness. N Engl J Med. 2012;366(16):1538–40.
32. Nathan SD, Shlobin OA, Ahmad S, Burton NA, Barnett SD, Edwards E. Comparison of wait times and mortality for idiopathic pulmonary fibrosis patients listed for single or bilateral lung transplantation. J Heart Lung Transplant. 2010;29(10):1165–71.
33. Titman A, Rogers CA, Bonser RS, Banner NR, Sharples LD. Disease-specific survival benefit of lung transplantation in adults: a national cohort study. Am J Transplant. 2009;9(7): 1640–9.
34. Estenne M, Maurer JR, Boehler A, Egan JJ, Frost A, Hertz M, et al. Bronchiolitis obliterans syndrome 2001: an update of the diagnostic criteria. J Heart Lung Transplant. 2002;21(3): 297–310.
35. Martinu T, Howell DN, Davis RD, Steele MP, Palmer SM. Pathologic correlates of bronchiolitis obliterans syndrome in pulmonary retransplant recipients. Chest. 2006;129(4):1016–23.
36. Sato M, Waddell TK, Wagnetz U, Roberts HC, Hwang DM, Haroon A, et al. Restrictive allograft syndrome (RAS): a novel form of chronic lung allograft dysfunction. J Heart Lung Transplant. 2011;30(7):735–42.
37. Bowdish ME, Arcasoy SM, Wilt JS, Conte JV, Davis RD, Garrity ER, et al. Surrogate markers and risk factors for chronic lung allograft dysfunction. Am J Transplant. 2004;4(7):1171–8.

# Chapter 19
# Evolving Genomics of Pulmonary Fibrosis

**Jose D. Herazo-Maya and Naftali Kaminski**

**Abstract** Genomic-scale transcript profiling approaches provide an unbiased view of the transcriptome of organs, tissues, and cells. Such technologies have been applied to the study of lungs and cells of patients with fibrotic lung disease and animal models of lung disease with the goal of detecting key molecules that play a significant role in pathogenesis, identifying potential drug targets, and developing biomarkers of disease presence, progression, and outcome. Genomic profiling studies have also been used to classify and distinguish different interstitial lung diseases such as IPF, nonspecific interstitial pneumonia (NSIP), lung fibrosis associated with scleroderma, and hypersensitivity pneumonitis (HP). In this chapter, we describe the progress and insights derived from applying genomic-scale transcript profiling approaches to fibrotic lung diseases as well as the potential impact of new technologies and NIH-funded projects on the field of genomics.

**Keywords** Interstitial lung diseases (ILD) • Idiopathic pulmonary fibrosis (IPF) • Genome-scale transcript profiling

## Introduction

The central dogma of gene expression in eukaryote cells assumes that a process is initiated by a signal that triggers the transcription of a DNA sequence into messenger RNA (mRNA), which is then translated to create a protein. Recent analyses suggest that this initial dogma may have been oversimplified. Many other factors

J.D. Herazo-Maya, M.D. • N. Kaminski, M.D. (✉)
Pulmonary, Critical Care and Sleep Medicine, Yale School of Medicine,
New Haven, CT, USA

K.C. Meyer and S.D. Nathan (eds.), *Idiopathic Pulmonary Fibrosis: A Comprehensive Clinical Guide*, Respiratory Medicine 9, DOI 10.1007/978-1-62703-682-5_19,
© Springer Science+Business Media New York 2014

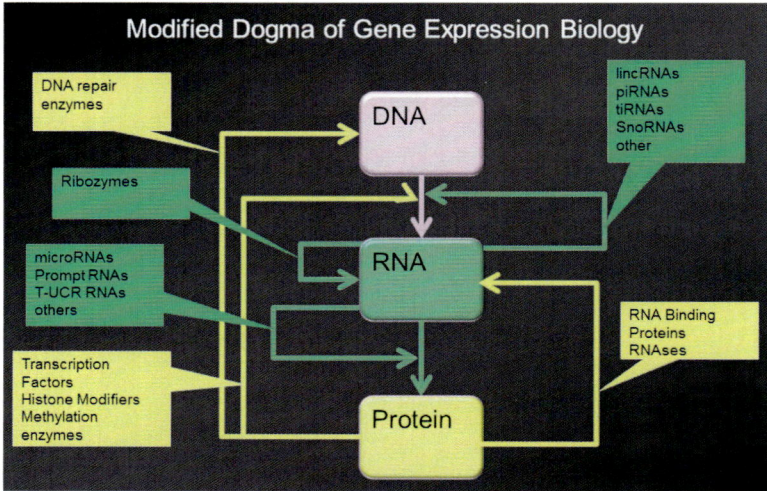

**Fig. 19.1** The new dogma of gene expression regulation has shifted from a linear view of DNA leading to RNA leading to protein synthesis to a complex model in which proteins and nonprotein coding RNAs act as regulators of genome expression potential on multiple levels

may be involved that have a significant role for epigenetic modification of DNA by large and small noncoding RNA molecules and posttranslational mechanisms (Fig. 19.1). This new and complex image of gene expression is a direct result of genomics, a discipline that emerged out of the Human Genome Project [1], and the rapid spread of technologies that allowed for genome-scale transcript profiling and variant calling, as well as the advanced computational and analytical methods that are required for this approach. This discipline, which is dedicated to the study of the sequence, expression, and function of multiple genes in parallel with the goal of understanding their biological function and interactions in health and disease, is rapidly becoming a key component of twenty-first-century medical research and represents an important component of efforts to redesign the practice of medicine such that a more precise and personalized approach can be offered to patients. While genomics includes both genome-scale studies of genetic code (DNA) and transcripts (RNA), because the DNA variant profiling approaches fit more readily into a discussion of the genetic sources of disease, we will mainly focus on advances in applying genome-scale transcript profiling approaches in this chapter.

## Genome-Scale Transcript Profiling

The concept of genome-scale transcript profiling was initially developed as a slide hybridization-based gene expression detection technology. Gene expression microarrays were originally developed by Fodor and colleagues [2] and based on the principle of light-directed, in situ oligonucleotide synthesis with the later development of cDNA and oligonucleotide arrays [3, 4]. More recently, novel methods that utilize high-throughput sequencing technologies have been applied to genome-scale transcript profiling. Such technologies, which will soon render gene arrays obsolete, provide transcript-level information that can be combined with gene structure information such as alternative splicing, information about noncoding RNAs, and posttranscriptional modifications, as well as genomic variants at the base-level resolution [5].

Regardless of the technology, experiments are performed with RNA extracted from the tissue or cell of interest and depend on the purity and integrity of the RNA. Genome-scale transcript profiling experiments measure the expression of a large number of transcripts (typically around 40,000–50,000), which generates a large amount of information that has to be preprocessed, analyzed, and validated before the results can be used. Obtaining the right information out of these large datasets represents the major challenge when analyzing such large genomic datasets. Before describing the most significant results obtained from genomic studies in lung fibrosis, it is critical to understand the steps required after the completion of microarray experiments. These steps can be summarized as comprising three broad categories: quality assessment, normalization, and statistical analysis. Because quality assessment and normalization approaches vary greatly with technology, they will not be discussed here.

Once the genomic dataset is (1) assessed for quality and normalized and (2) outliers and batch effects (if present) are handled satisfactorily, investigators can then proceed to perform statistical analyses. Different algorithms for statistical analyses can be used for genome-scale transcriptome data, and their use depends on the objectives of the study. Typically, the statistical algorithms used for gene expression profiling in human disease can be grouped into four major study objectives as defined by Simon and colleagues [6]: class comparison, class prediction, class discovery, and pathway analysis. Two additional study objectives may also be considered for inclusion in this group: outcome analysis and meta-analysis. Table 19.1 provides a description of the types of transcriptome study objectives and lists some of the available algorithms that can be applied to each type of objective. Some of these algorithms can be used independently, be part of a computational software program (such as GeneSpring GX, Bioconductor [43], and BRB array tools [44]), or be used in a statistical environment, the most widely used being the R statistical environment [45]. However, regardless of the tools, attention to testing multiple hypotheses and using effective visualization are critically important.

After the statistical analysis is completed, the number of differentially expressed transcripts may still be too large to validate and study in depth. Traditionally, two different approaches have been used to deal with this issue. One can use the reductionist or "cherry picking" approach versus the global or

**Table 19.1** Summary of the type of transcript profiling experimental objectives and relevant algorithms for statistical analysis

| Study objectives | Description | Statistical algorithms for each category |
|---|---|---|
| Class comparison | Class comparison analyses focus on the identification of differentially expressed genes among predefined classes of samples | $t$-test<br>• Analysis of variance (ANOVA) [7]<br>• Significance analysis of microarrays (SAM) [8, 9]<br>• Random variance model (RVM) [10]<br>• Lassoed principal component (LPC) [11] |
| Class prediction | Class prediction studies are also based on predefined classes of samples, although its goal is to develop a statistical prediction model based on the expression of a group of genes to allow the prediction of the class in each sample | • Threshold number of misclassifications (TNoM) [12, 13]<br>• Compound covariate predictor [14, 15]<br>• Partial least square [16]<br>• k-Nearest neighbor (KNN) [17, 18]<br>• Support vector machine (SVM) [19]<br>• Nearest shrunken centroid (PAM) [20]<br>• Top scoring pairs [21] |
| Class discovery | Class discovery emphasizes on the detection of an unidentified class based on the co-expression of genes. Typically these studies are performed to characterize an unknown clinical disease subphenotype based on the expression of clusters of genes | • K-Means clustering [22]<br>• Hierarchical clustering [23]<br>• Biclustering [24]<br>• Self-organizing maps (SOM) [25]<br>• Model-based clustering [26]<br>• Gene expression dynamic inspector (GEDI) [27] |
| Pathway analysis | Pathway analysis studies focuses on the identification of differentially expressed genes that occur in the same molecular pathway in predefined classes of samples | • Global test for groups of genes [28]<br>• Gene set enrichment analysis (GSEA) [29]<br>• SAM-GS [30]<br>• Gene set analysis (GSA) [31]<br>• Integrative microarray analysis of pathways (IMAP) [31]<br>• Gene set expression comparison [32] |
| Outcome analysis | Outcome analysis studies explore the association of gene expressions with a predefined outcome (i.e., survival, transplant-free survival, disease progression) | • Cox model [33]<br>• Partial least squares proportional hazard regression [34]<br>• Multiple random validation [35]<br>• Prediction by supervised principal component (SuperPC) [36] |
| Meta-analysis | Gene expression meta-analysis studies combine multiple and similar gene expression datasets to increase the statistical power and accuracy of the results | • Truncated product method for combining $P$-values [37]<br>• $t$-based modeling [38]<br>• RankProd [39]<br>• Meta-analysis based on control of false discovery rate [40]<br>• Predictor-based approach [41]<br>• MetaOmics [42] |

"systems" approach [46]. In the "cherry picking" approach, researchers select differentially expressed transcripts for which there is prior biological knowledge. Such transcripts are validated at the RNA and protein level if a given transcript is a coding RNA. Following this validation, in-depth in vitro and in vivo studies are required to determine its relevance to the disease. The findings are then translated back to humans to confirm an association with the disease of interest, and the transcripts' potential use as a biomarker or as a therapeutic target is assessed. When using the global or "systems" approach, researchers try to study gene expression profiles as a unit by using the concept that differentially expressed genes belong to a common pathway that is relevant to disease or that a number of genes can interact with each other depending on their pattern of expression. The global approach has been made possible with the use of gene ontology annotations, previously published knowledge of gene interactions, and pathway analysis with a focus on the identification of differentially expressed genes occurring in the same molecular pathway.

Finally, the selection of relevant genes for validation can be facilitated with the integration of patient clinical information with the analysis of gene expression data, which can facilitate the identification of profiles that characterize a clinical variable of interest. This is typically used to study gene profiles associated with response to drug therapy, disease severity and progression, and subsequent outcomes.

In summary, the analysis of genome-scale transcript profiling experiments requires dedicated quality control, data normalization, and statistical analysis that are based on the objectives of the study. The selection of gene(s) for validation and potential translation to patient care can be facilitated using a reductionist approach, a global approach, or both. In addition, depending on the ultimate goal of the study, clinical variables could be introduced to the analysis of gene expression to ensure an easier translation to clinical practice.

# The Contribution of Genomics to Our Mechanistic Understanding of Lung Fibrosis

In contrast to hypothesis-driven experimental approaches that are based on what is known, the results of genome-scale transcript profiling experiments often contain results that were unforeseen or even contrary to currently accepted paradigms. When one considers that many breakthroughs in modern medicine were the result of serendipity [47, 48], one could consider large-scale genomic profiling experiments as a means that can introduce serendipity into pulmonary research and thereby identify new hypotheses and provide new insights.

## *The Lung Phenotype in IPF Is Not a Result of Passive Accumulation of Extracellular Matrix*

A passive accumulation of extracellular matrix was the dominant paradigm that was perceived to explain pulmonary fibrosis in the last decade of the twentieth century, and this explanation assumed that fibrosis and accumulation of extracellular matrix were the result of a protease–antiprotease imbalance. This concept was accompanied by an apparent increase in the activity of naturally occurring inhibitors of metalloproteases accompanied by an associated reduction in the activity of matrix metalloproteases that was thought to lead to the accumulation of extracellular matrix [49]. This paradigm was supported by observations from a limited set of hypothesis based, albeit carefully designed experiments, but it was never tested in a global non-biased analysis of the lung environment in IPF.

When Zuo et al. [50] analyzed lung tissue of patients with IPF and compared them with healthy controls, they immediately noticed that multiple members of the matrix metalloproteinase (MMP) family (including MMP 1, 7, and 9) were upregulated at the mRNA and protein level in IPF lungs. Among the overexpressed genes in IPF, MMP-7 was the most informative and was localized to the alveolar epithelium, a finding that suggested an active role of the alveolar epithelium in the lung remodeling that characterizes IPF. Interestingly, MMP-7 knockout mice were relatively protected from bleomycin-induced fibrosis, suggesting the potential role of this protease as a regulator of fibrosis. Indeed, it is impressive that despite the fact that these original observations were obtained on a very small number of tissues, they have been repeatedly verified [51–53].

The proteolytic effects of MMP-7 can mediate the cleavage of molecules such as collagen type IV, aggrecan, laminin, fibronectin, gelatin, entactin, decorin, tenascin, vitronectin, osteonectin, elastin, and SPP1 (among others) [54]. MMP-7 is also an example of a metalloprotease that may have regulatory effects that can be inferred by looking at its bioactive substrates that potentially include fibrosis-relevant proteins such as FAS ligand, $\beta$4 integrin, E-cadherin, pro-HB-epidermal growth factor, plasminogen, pro-TNF-$\alpha$, pro-$\alpha$-defensin, endostatin, syndecan, and insulin growth factor-binding protein-3 (IGFBP-3) [55]. While the local effects of MMP-7 overexpression in the alveolar epithelium in humans are not clear, evidence from mice concerning its regulation of neutrophil egress, regulation of dendritic cells, and activation of defensins [56–58] suggests that it may have a significant role in regulating the local inflammatory milieu. Its effect on SPP1 provides additional support in this regard [59].

Other MMPs, including MMP 1, 2, 3, 9, 10, and 19 [49, 60–62], have been consistently found to be increased in IPF lungs, and some of these proteins have been shown to be relevant to the pathogenesis of pulmonary fibrosis. As an example, Yamashita et al. demonstrated that rats transfected with an adeno-MMP-3 vector developed transient pulmonary fibrosis, and in vitro treatment of lung epithelial cells with MMP-3 resulted in activation of the $\beta$-catenin signaling pathway followed by subsequent induction of epithelial-mesenchymal transition (EMT), which is one of the proposed mechanisms for the development of lung fibrosis [61]. More recently, after performing microarray expression studies of the lung microenvironment obtained by laser capture microdissected lung tissue from IPF patients, our group identified MMP-19 overexpression in hyperplastic epithelial cells from patients with IPF when compared with normal appearing epithelial cells. The presence of MMP-19 was confirmed by immunohistochemistry in hyperplastic epithelial cells that were overlying fibrotic areas, but in contrast to what was observed with MMP-7, MMP-19 knockout mice developed worse fibrosis when exposed to bleomycin, suggesting that MMP19 overexpression failed to provide protection. Thus, genome-scale transcript profiling studies have led to a paradigm shift in the perception of the role of proteases in lung fibrosis, and instead of the simplistic protease–antiprotease imbalance paradigm, we now have a more complex understanding that suggests that proteases have multiple and sometimes opposing roles in lung fibrosis. The roles of these MMPs depend on their temporal expression, the MMP-producing cell type and spatial distribution, and the availability of substrates [63].

Genome-scale transcript profiling studies have not only generated relevant information regarding the presence and potential role of some of the MMP family members in IPF but also opened a new biomarker field for their use in IPF diagnosis, disease monitoring, and mortality prediction. Based on our previous findings [50], our group applied a targeted proteomic approach and identified a protein signature that includes MMP-1, MMP-7, MMP-8, IGFBP-1, and TNFRSA1F [53], and this signature was able to distinguish IPF from healthy controls with a sensitivity of 98.6 % and specificity of 98.1 %. Two members of this signature, MMP-1 and MMP-7, differentiated IPF patients from those with subacute/chronic hypersensitivity pneumonitis (HP) with a sensitivity of 96.3 % and specificity of 87.2 %. Increased concentrations of MMPs, including MMP-7, have also been shown in the bronchoalveolar lavage (BAL) of IPF patients [53, 64], confirming that these molecules not only participate in disease pathogenesis but can also be used as makers of disease presence. More recently, we also demonstrated that increased plasma concentrations of MMP-7 at the initial clinical presentation were predictive of subsequent increased mortality in IPF [65], especially when MMP-7 was used along with clinical variables. These findings have potential implications for risk stratification, patient counseling, and prioritization for lung transplantation in the future.

Thus, the emergence of MMPs as mechanistically important in determining the lung phenotype in IPF and other interstitial lung diseases (as well as their role as new peripheral blood biomarker candidates) can be fully attributed to unbiased genome-scale transcript profiling.

## The Wnt Pathway in IPF

As previously discussed, one of the advantages of the "systems" approach over the "cherry picking" approach for genome-scale transcript profiling is that by grouping differentially expressed genes in gene sets based on their attributes, researchers are allowed to identify pathways (and genes within the pathways) that characterize the differences between the analyzed groups. This procedure enables the generation of new hypotheses regarding disease pathogenesis by focusing on pathways that were not considered relevant to the disease. This also helps researchers to focus on differentially expressed genes within a pathway that might otherwise have been missed.

Following a "systems" approach, we reanalyzed the microarray datasets generated by our group using more powerful pathway analysis tools and, surprisingly, identified a large number of developmental pathway genes [66]. Some of the development-related genes that were found overexpressed in IPF included members of transcription factor families (such as the Sry-related high-mobility group box and forkhead box) and genes related to the Wnt/β-catenin pathway [67]. In our analysis, the Wnt pathway was one of the most significantly overexpressed pathways in IPF, and, interestingly, this was not the case in HP.

The Wnt pathway consists of a network of glycoproteins that are involved in embryogenesis and development, and this pathway was especially characterized after the identification that a mutation in one of its genes, "Wingless," was associated with the development of wingless *Drosophila melanogaster* flies (fruit fly) [68]. The key player of the canonical Wnt signaling is β-catenin, which, after it accumulates in the cytoplasm, eventually translocates into the nucleus and interacts with transcription factors of the LEF/TCF family, which affects gene transcription [69]. Most Wnt proteins bind to the frizzled family of receptors and LRP5/6 co-receptors, and these, in turn, inhibit the phosphorylation and degradation of β-catenin, which allows its translocation into the nucleus [70]. Without Wnt signaling, β-catenin is degraded by its destruction complex.

Experiments in mice have demonstrated that β-catenin is required for the normal differentiation of the bronchiolar and alveolar epithelium [71]. Wnt7b-deficient mice exhibit impaired alveolar type I cell differentiation, have hypoplastic lungs, and die at birth of respiratory failure [72]. Similarly, Wnt5a-deficient mice exhibit increased proliferation of lung epithelial and mesenchymal compartments and die shortly after birth due to respiratory failure [73, 74]. In humans, mutations and genetic variations in genes of the Wnt pathway have been associated with conditions such as cancer, neuropsychiatric disorders, cardiac diseases, and bone disorders [75]. Several reports that appeared following publication of our microarray findings validated the increase of functional Wnt in IPF. Chilosi et al. demonstrated β-catenin accumulation in fibroblastic foci of IPF lungs and its expression co-localized with two Wnt downstream target genes (cyclin-D1 and MMP-7) in proliferative bronchiolar lesions [76]. This report was followed by the findings of Königshoff et al. who demonstrated the overexpression of Wnt1, 7b and 10b, Fzd2 and 3, beta-catenin, and Lef1 expression in IPF lungs by qRT-PCR and localized Wnt1, Wnt3a, β-catenin, and Gsk-3β expression to alveolar and bronchial epithelium by immunohistochemistry [77]. Along with the discovery of increased functional Wnt in IPF, there is evidence of reversal of pulmonary fibrosis after the inhibition of Wnt/β-catenin [78]. Interestingly, MMP7, which was recently mentioned as both a mechanistically relevant molecule and a peripheral blood biomarker, is a repeatedly validated Wnt pathway target gene [79].

In summary, the observation of overexpression of Wnt signaling in IPF suggests an aberrant activation of developmental pathways that are not usually involved in normal lung health. A better understanding of these mechanisms could lead to potentially effective therapeutic strategies for this devastating lung disease.

## *Apoptosis in Lung Fibrosis from a Genomic Perspective*

Two studies using genomics-based approaches (and published only a month apart) confirmed the role of apoptosis in IPF pathogenesis. Bridges et al. [80] performed microarray gene expression experiments with cells obtained from normal lung samples and compared them with cells from IPF lungs (including samples obtained from microdissected fibroblastic foci). They used class discovery (unsupervised clustering) and class comparison (t-test) analyses and identified Twist 1 as one of the most consistently up-regulated transcription factors in the IPF lung. In this study, researchers determined that overexpression of Twist1 led to increased viability of rat lung fibroblasts exposed to pro-apoptotic molecules (lipid 4-HNE and thapsigargin). However, lower concentrations of these proapoptotic stimuli resulted in a reduction of Twist1, which in turn resulted in increased activity of caspase-3, which is a marker of apoptosis.. They also demonstrated that profibrotic growth factors such as platelet derived growth factor (PDGF) induced Twist1 expression in rat lung fibroblasts, which was necessary to protect these cells from apoptosis, particularly in the continued presence of these growth factors. In summary, the results demonstrated an anti-apoptotic role of Twist1 by promoting fibroblast viability when these cells where exposed to growth factors.

Our group corroborated the findings confirming the role of apoptosis in the pathogenesis of acute exacerbations of IPF [81]. We performed microarray experiments and compared lung tissue of IPF patients with acute exacerbation of IPF, lung tissue from IPF subjects with stable disease, and non-IPF lungs with normal histology using a class comparison approach (significance analysis of microarrays). A total of 579 genes were found to be differentially expressed between the lungs of patients with acute exacerbations of IPF versus patients with stable IPF; specifically, cyclin A2 (CCNA2), a cell cycle regulatory gene, was one of the top overexpressed genes in this signature and was localized to alveolar epithelial cells in subjects with acute exacerbations of IPF. Increased CCNA2 protein expression was localized to proliferating epithelial cells, and this finding suggests the presence of accelerated epithelial cell proliferation, which could potentially reflect a compensatory response to injured epithelium. The finding that lungs of IPF patients showed widespread apoptosis by in situ TUNEL assay was of even greater interest. Taken together, these observations suggest an aberrant proliferative response of the alveolar epithelium in reaction to apoptosis during acute exacerbations of IPF.

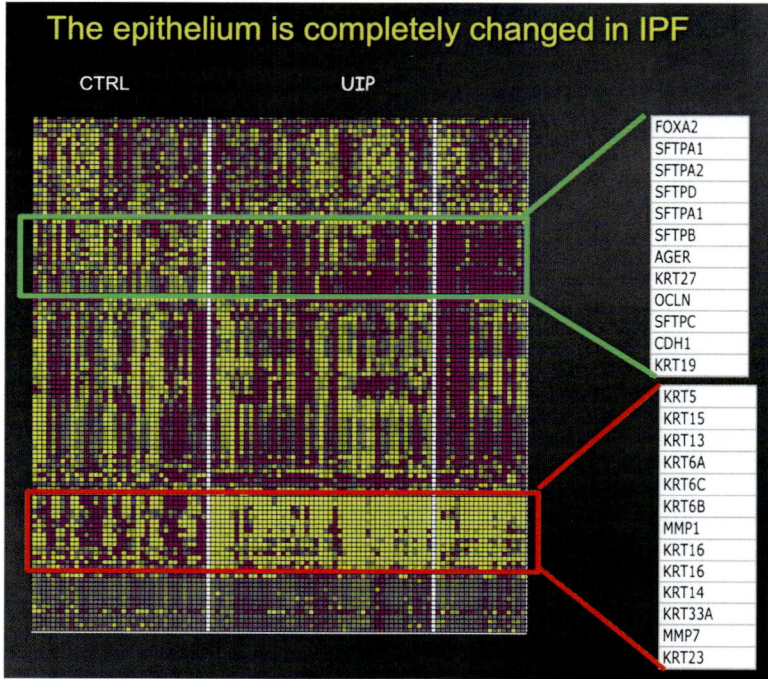

**Fig. 19.2** Illustrative figure of changes in epithelial gene expression in IPF lungs. Genes known to be expressed in the epithelium were extracted from a larger microarray dataset. Increased shades of *yellow* mean increased gene expression, *gray* means unchanged, and increased shades of *purple* decreased. Note the reduction in genes known to be expressed in type II cells and the change in the cytokeratin profile of IPF lungs

## Global Analysis of IPF Lungs Reveals Dramatic Changes in Epithelial Cell Phenotype

While the histopathologic hallmark of IPF is the presence of fibroblastic foci, there is growing evidence of the role of the alveolar epithelium in the pathogenesis of IPF [82, 83], and the observation that a large number of differentially expressed genes in IPF are localized to the alveolar epithelium supports this concept. We have demonstrated that MMP-1, MMP-7, and MMP-19 localize to the alveolar epithelium as do SPP1, N-cadherin, IGFBP-4, and CCNA2. Similarly, the Wnt pathway genes Wnt1, Wnt3a, β-catenin, and Gsk-3β have also been localized to the alveolar and bronchial epithelium as well as HIF1A and VEGF [50, 59, 76, 77, 84–86]. Impressively, a global view of known epithelial cells in IPF (Fig. 19.2) demonstrates a shift in epithelial cell markers with a decline in traditional epithelial markers and an increase in markers that are not normally expressed. Many other genes that may be associated with preservation of a normal epithelial cell phenotype are differentially expressed in IPF, suggesting that key transcriptional events in IPF occur in an injured alveolar epithelium, which, in turn, responds with the expression of profibrotic markers.

## Gene Expression Profiling and the Classification of Interstitial Lung Diseases

The diagnosis of interstitial lung diseases in clinical practice can be challenging at times given the fact that some of the patients can present with radiological patterns that are inconclusive [87–89]. Further, in some cases, lung histology may show discordant patterns such as a usual interstitial pneumonia (UIP) pattern in one lobe and a nonspecific interstitial pneumonia (NSIP) pattern in a different lobe from the same patient [90, 91].

The diagnostic dilemma usually is more common when comparing cases of chronic HP, NSIP, and ILD associated with collagen vascular disease from those with IPF. One of the goals of genomic studies in ILD has been to find transcript profiles that could differentiate these entities in order to develop more accurate diagnostic strategies. We will discuss the gene expression studies addressing these issues in the following section.

## Differences in Gene Expression Between IPF and HP

To study gene expression differences in lung tissue from patients with IPF versus patients with HP, our group performed gene expression microarrays and compared transcript levels using a class comparison (*t*-test) and class prediction (threshold number of misclassifications—TNoM) approach and identified 407 genes that accurately distinguished IPF from HP [84]. The pathway analysis of this signature confirmed the prior knowledge regarding the pathogenesis of these two entities. While the HP signature is characterized by enrichment of pathways associated with cytokine and T-cell activation, inflammation, and humoral immune responses, the IPF signature is characterized by cell adhesion, extracellular matrix, and smooth muscle differentiation as well as genes associated with lung development, heparin binding, enzyme inhibitor activity, and insulin growth factor binding [46]. It is clear after looking at the gene pathway differences between these two conditions that gene expression associated with inflammation is more pronounced in HP, while increased expression of genes involved in matrix turnover and developmental pathways is more characteristic of IPF. These findings are consistent with the knowledge that evidence of inflammation in IPF is not as prominent as initially thought [92].

## IPF and Familial Pulmonary Fibrosis (FPF) Are Unexpectedly Different While IPF and NSIP Are Unexpectedly Similar

Yang et al. [93] performed gene expression microarrays of lung tissue from patients with sporadic IPF, FPF, NSIP, and normal controls. However, because these investigators were unable to identify statistically significant differences between IPF and NSIP, the results were considered somewhat disappointing but were in agreement with our prior observations [84]. An interesting finding was the identification of differentially expressed genes between sporadic IPF and FPF, diseases that have considerably more similarities than differences. While the genes distinguishing familial cases from the sporadic ones were part of the same functional pathways as genes distinguishing IPF from normal samples, they seemed to exhibit larger changes. One conclusion was that familial pulmonary fibrosis may represent a more extreme molecular phenotype of the same disease process as sporadic IPF. However, while this is certainly possible, we suggest that the stage in the natural history of the disease when tissue sampling was performed may have played a role in these differences [94], because 50 % of the familial samples were obtained from open lung biopsies, whereas 90 % of sporadic cases were collected from explant or autopsy, suggesting that the differences may be due to differences in disease stage.

## Different Forms of UIP Share Very Similar Gene Expression Patterns

The UIP pattern in lung biopsies of patients with systemic sclerosis (SSc) can be indistinguishable from the UIP pattern of IPF patients [95], a finding that contrasts with the major clinical differences between these two entities. In an attempt to better elucidate the molecular mechanisms behind the differences in SSc and IPF, Hsu and colleagues [96] performed gene expression profiling in patients with SSc and classified patients as having a predominance of pulmonary fibrosis (with a UIP pattern) or as a pulmonary arterial hypertension (PAH) phenotype and compared them with lung tissue from IPF and idiopathic pulmonary arterial hypertension (IPAH) patients. Using a class comparison approach (efficiency analysis and significance analysis of microarrays), they identified 242 differentially expressed genes between the studied subclasses of SSc patients. Focusing on the comparison that is relevant to our discussion and similar to what was observed between IPF and NSIP, the gene expression profile of the UIP lung of IPF patients was very similar to the UIP lung of systemic SSc patients, with only 25 genes being uniquely expressed in IPF lung tissue and 20 genes uniquely expressed in the UIP lung tissue of SSc patients.

The authors of this study acknowledge that one of their limitations was the use of explanted lung tissue of patients undergoing lung transplant, which could represent end-stage disease, suggesting that comparisons in gene expression between SSc and IPF at earlier stages could potentially provide a better molecular characterization of these two entities.

## Identification of Gene Expression Profiles Associated with Disease Severity in the IPF Lung and Peripheral Blood

It has been shown that IPF patients have different patterns of disease progression. Although some patients can be stable for long period of time, others can quickly deteriorate or have an acute exacerbation and die as a consequence of an accelerated disease course [97]. The recognition of this erratic clinical behavior of some IPF patients prompted Selman et al. [85] to study gene expression profiles of IPF patients with evidence of rapid progression (defined as symptoms starting 6 months prior to initial presentation) and compare them with IPF patients with slow progression (defined as symptoms present for more than 24 months) using a class comparison and class prediction approach. The investigators identified a group of 437 differentially expressed genes between these two patient groups. When a pathway analysis was performed, patients with evidence of rapid progression had overexpression of genes involved in morphogenesis, cancer, oxidative stress, cell proliferation, apoptosis, and genes from fibroblast/smooth muscle cells. The discovery of overexpression of genes associated with cell proliferation and apoptosis preceded the findings by Konishi et al. [81] who demonstrated evidence of overexpression of cyclins (cell cycle regulators) along with overwhelming apoptosis in the lung of patients with an acute exacerbation. This observation again suggested the potential presence of aberrant proliferative responses in response to apoptosis in patients with rapid progression of their IPF.

Konishi et al. [81] discovered another interesting finding in the lung tissue of IPF patients with acute exacerbations; alpha-defensins, particularly defensin alpha 3 (DEFA3) and 4 (DEFA4), were overexpressed, and these authors also demonstrated increased levels in the serum of these natural antimicrobial peptides, which are a component of innate immunity and participate in host defense [98]. Interestingly, defensins released in response to microbial invasion can activate an adaptive immune response [99], a mechanism that has been described in IPF [100], by attracting antigen-presenting dendritic cells to the site of invasion. Defensins are mostly expressed by neutrophils, epithelial cells, and paneth cells, and, interestingly, they are activated via proteolytic cleavage by MMP-7 [58]. In summary, these findings support the notion that defensins are not only surrogates of disease activity and severity, but they may also be closely associated with IPF pathogenesis.

The overexpression of defensins has been validated in the peripheral blood transcriptome of IPF patients with evidence of advanced disease by Yang et al. [101]. These investigators performed gene expression profiling of patients with IPF who were stratified according to disease severity. They defined severe disease as DLCO ≤35 % or FVC ≤50 % and compared them with IPF patients with mild disease that was defined as DLCO ≥65 % or FVC ≥75 %. They also compared these two subclasses of IPF patients with age and gender-matched healthy controls using a class comparison approach (significance analysis of microarrays). When comparing patients categorized by percent-predicted DLCO ≥65 % with patients with DLCO ≤35 %, the authors identified 13 differentially expressed transcripts including DEFA3 and DEFA4. DEFA3 also differentiated mild and severe IPF cases from healthy controls, confirming the relevance of defensins in IPF progression.

The functional analysis performed in the study by Yang et al. [101] using the 13 differentially expressed transcripts differentiating mild and severe cases of IPF revealed a finding that is contradictory to our prior observations in lung tissue of IPF individuals. Specifically, they reported overexpression of genes associated with inflammatory responses and immune trafficking in the severe IPF group. While this could represent evidence that inflammatory responses are indeed potentially relevant in IPF, it can also indicate that a more inflammatory phenotype is present in patients with more rapid disease progression.

Boon and colleagues [102] also studied and compared gene expression profiles from lung tissue of IPF patients with evidence of disease progression or relatively stable disease, defined respectively as FVC% and DLCO% decline $\geq$10 % and $\geq$15 % versus decline of <10 % and <15 % over a 12-month period. For this study, the investigators used serial analysis of gene expression (SAGE), a technique that has the same goal of microarrays with the difference that SAGE sampling is based on sequencing of short tags of mRNA, while microarrays are based on hybridization of mRNAs to probes. Using a class comparison (*t*-test) and class discovery (hierarchical clustering) approach, 134 differentially expressed transcripts distinguished the two cohorts. While this study is also limited by the small number of samples (six in each group), it certainly provided interesting findings, because some of the overexpressed genes in the group of patients with evidence of IPF progression included surfactant protein A1 (SFTPA1), SPP1, and heat shock 70 KDa protein 1A (HSPA1A) among others. These findings correlated with previously noted associations of surfactant protein A levels in serum and autoantibodies against heat shock protein 70 (HSP70) with worse survival in IPF [103, 104]. We have previously reported consistent overexpression of SPP1 when analyzing gene expression profiles of IPF lung tissue compared to normal controls [59] and have also demonstrated increased SPP1 levels in BAL of IPF patients. We also found evidence suggesting that SPP1 activates MMP-7 and co-localizes with this molecule in alveolar epithelial cells of IPF patients, resulting in a profibrotic effect on lung fibroblasts and epithelial cells. Others have demonstrated the relative protection to bleomycininduced fibrosis in SPP1 knockout mice and increased SPP1 levels in serum of patients with interstitial lung disease. In summation, this body of evidence suggests that SPP1 is not only relevant to the pathogenesis of IPF but could also be a potential biomarker for disease progression. Table 19.2 includes a summary of some of the most relevant molecules identified in IPF (based on gene expression studies).

## Noncoding RNAs in IPF

One of the direct results of the Human Genome Project and the large next-generation sequencing studies that followed, including ENCODE [108], was the recognition that noncoding RNAs are critically important in determining cell and organ phenotype through their effects on gene and protein expression (see Fig. 19.1). While the data are only now emerging, it is already obvious that at least one family of noncoding RNAs, that of microRNAs, is critically important in IPF. MicroRNAs are small, noncoding RNAs (21–25 nucleotides) that bind via base pairing to the 3′ untranslated region of their target mRNAs. In most cases they repress gene expression by increasing mRNA degradation or by disrupting translation initiation [109]. In two recent studies that utilized different generations of

**Table 19.2** Summary of relevant genes in IPF identified by transcript profiling

| Gene/pathway | Gene name | Direction of expression | Compartment identified | Relevant pathway | References |
|---|---|---|---|---|---|
| MMP-7 | Matrix metallopeptidase 7 | Overexpressed | Lung, peripheral blood, and BAL | Extracellular matrix degradation | [50, 51, 53, 65, 84] |
| MMP-3 | Matrix metallopeptidase 3 | Overexpressed | Lung | Extracellular matrix degradation | [61] |
| MMP-19 | Matrix metallopeptidase 19 | Overexpressed | Lung—hyperplastic epithelial cells | Extracellular matrix degradation | [62] |
| SERPINF1 (PEDF) | Pigment epithelium-derived factor | Overexpressed | Lung | Angiogenesis | [105] |
| SPP1 | Osteopontin | Overexpressed | Lung | Extracellular matrix degradation | [59, 102] |
| HIF1A | Hypoxia-inducible factor-1alpha | Overexpressed | Lung | Hypoxia | [86] |
| Wnt | Wingless and others | Overexpressed | Lung | WNT signaling | [66, 77] |
| CXCL12 | Chemokine ligand 12 | Overexpressed | Lung | Inflammation | [93] |
| TWIST1 | Twist basic helix-loop-helix transcription factor 1 | Overexpressed | Lung—fibroblastic foci | Apoptosis | [80] |
| CCNA2 | Cyclin A2 | Overexpressed | Lung | Cell cycle regulation | [81] |
| DEFA3–4 | Defensin alpha 3 and 4 | Overexpressed | Lung and peripheral blood | Host defense | [81, 101] |
| CAV1 | Caveolin 1 | Underexpressed | Lung | Cell cycle regulation | [106] |
| AGER (RAGE) | Advanced glycosylation end product-specific receptor | Underexpressed | Lung and peripheral blood | Inflammation | [53, 107] |

microRNA profiling technologies, we determined that approximately 10 % of the microRNAs measured were differentially expressed in IPF [110, 111]. Our first report focused on let-7d microRNA [110], an epithelial microRNA that is down-regulated in IPF lungs, and found evidence that let7d is a modulator of transforming growth factor-β signaling and a sustainer of epithelial cell phenotype. Thus, when we inhibited let-7 microRNAs in vitro and in vivo, we found a change in epithelial cell phenotype with increased expression of mesenchymal markers and a phenotype consistent with EMT. We then focused on microRNAs increased in IPF lungs and identified 43 significantly upregulated microRNAs [111]. Over half of them were localized to chromosome 14q32. Among the increased microRNAs, mir-154, which was increased in IPF fibroblasts, emerged as a regulator of fibroblast proliferation and migration through its permissive effect on WNT pathway activation in lung fibroblasts. This provides further supportive, evidence of aberrant WNT pathway activation in IPF. Several other studies suggested roles for mir-21 [112], mir-200 [113], mir-31 [114], and the mir-17-92 cluster [115] and even suggested a defect in microRNA processing in IPF [116]. Taken together, these studies indicate a profound dysregulation of microRNAs in IPF that may have significant mechanistic roles and potentially therapeutic implications in IPF [117]. The recent recognition of the expression of microRNAs in the peripheral blood in other disease entities [118, 119] in addition to their potential role in the pathogenesis of lung fibrosis should encourage investigators to extend their studies to the blood. Finally, considering that microRNAs are only one family of microRNAs, it is highly likely that other noncoding RNAs, such as large intergenic, noncoding RNAs (lincRNAs), are also probably aberrantly expressed and functionally relevant [120, 121].

## Epigenomic Changes in IPF Lungs

Epigenetic mechanisms, such as DNA methylation and histone modifications, are key adaptive mechanisms by which lasting changes in cell or organism phenotypes are induced in response to environmental or other stresses without changes in DNA content [122]. In addition to several reports of changes in the promoter methylation state in specific genes in IPF [123–125], two recent reports have suggested that global methylation changes occur in IPF lungs [126, 127].

Rabinovich et al. [127] employed Agilent human CpG Islands Microarrays and methylated DNA immunoprecipitation (MEDIP) to characterize both IPF and control lungs (this method applies antibodies to methylated cytosine to identify differential methylation). They identified 625 differentially methylated CpG islands, some of which they then validated. Interestingly, they compared IPF methylation patterns to lung cancer or control samples and discovered that IPF lungs displayed an intermediate methylation profile between lung cancer and controls with 402 differentially methylated CpG islands overlapping between IPF and cancer. Sanders et al. [128] utilized the bisulfite conversion assay that converts unmethylated cytosine into uracil and determined that 870 genes were differentially methylated. These authors identified 16 genes with inversely related significant changes in gene methylation and expression, 8 of which were previously shown to be associated with fibrosis. While at this stage it is impossible to draw any final conclusions from the small number of samples [129], both studies suggest that the changes in methylation, which represents one aspect of epigenetics, are indeed relatively significant and justify additional forays into genome-scale profiling of epigenetic changes in IPF.

## Summary and Future Direction

In this chapter, we discussed the discipline of genomics and its impact on our understanding of fibrotic lung diseases with a focus on IPF, the most common and lethal idiopathic interstitial lung disease. Of genomic technologies, the technique that has had the greatest impact to date is genome-scale transcript profiling using microarrays. Indeed, most of the significant findings (including the role of matrix metalloproteases, the role of developmental pathways such as the Wnt pathway and apoptosis, and the role of the alveolar epithelium) that have emerged from microarray experiments have fostered a paradigm shift in our understanding of the pathogenesis of IPF.

The contribution of genomic studies in fibrotic lung disease is not limited to pathogenesis. The transcript profiling findings also led to the identification of MMP-7, one of the emerging peripheral blood biomarkers for IPF diagnosis and outcome prediction, as well as many other markers. Similarly, we reviewed the differences and similarities in gene expression profiling between IPF and other forms of ILD as well as the identification of gene expression profiles associated with disease severity in lung tissue and the peripheral blood of IPF patients. Although these results are less developed, they still highlight the depth of information that is relevant to this disease and can be gleaned from genome-scale transcript profiles, and these exciting findings should serve to encourage larger and more detailed studies.

While the field of genomics is continuously evolving and new discoveries in ILD are constantly appearing, extensively analysis and review of the available data, and at least from a "systems" perspective, has greatly advanced our knowledge of what characterizes abnormalities in the IPF lung. It is clear that new studies are required to provide an in-depth look into other less common forms of ILD and to explore the differences between the two physiologic extremes of pulmonary ailments, namely, the obstructive versus the restrictive lung diseases. Future study designs that may potentially impact the care of patients should include the use of large transcriptomic analyses of peripheral blood on a serial basis, because this could lead to the development of biomarkers that provide a closer representation of disease activity and progression at the molecular level [130]. Additionally, it is also important to develop studies that integrate clinical data as well as other regulatory portions of the genome such as microRNAs and long intergenic noncoding RNAs. This integration has already started with the financial support of the National Institute of Health (NIH) through their funding of the Lung Tissue Research Consortium (http://www. ltrcpublic.com/) and the Lung Genomics Research Consortium (http://www. lung-genomics.org/), which have generated genetic and genomic information of more than 700 lung tissues that are available to the public for data analysis.

Finally, it is critical for investigators and clinicians to push the integration of the genetic and genomic information into patient care. In addition to the findings described within this chapter, several recent studies have applied genome-wide association studies to identify novel variants associated with IPF [131, 132]. So that the progress achieved in the discipline of genomics can materialize into meaningful change in how we manage ILD patients, it is essential that a concerted effort is undertaken, including "buy-in" and collaboration among clinicians, the scientific community, industry, and regulatory agencies. This chapter presents strong evidence of the importance of the genomic field to the study of lung fibrosis, its potential for translation into patient care, and the potential for ongoing development and discovery. However, all these efforts will be for naught if they are not focused on a specific cause and goal, which remains the optimal evaluation and treatment of patients with fibrotic lung diseases.

# References

1. Yang IV, Schwartz DA. The next generation of complex lung genetic studies. Am J Respir Crit Care Med. 2012;186(11):1087–94.
2. Fodor SP, Read JL, Pirrung MC, Stryer L, Lu AT, Solas D. Light-directed, spatially addressable parallel chemical synthesis. Science. 1991;251(4995):767–73.
3. Lipshutz RJ, Morris D, Chee M, Hubbell E, Kozal MJ, Shah N, et al. Using oligonucleotide probe arrays to access genetic diversity. Biotechniques. 1995;19(3):442–7.
4. Schena M, Heller RA, Theriault TP, Konrad K, Lachenmeier E, Davis RW. Microarrays: biotechnology's discovery platform for functional genomics. Trends Biotechnol. 1998;16(7):301–6.
5. Cloonan N, Grimmond SM. Transcriptome content and dynamics at single-nucleotide resolution. Genome Biol. 2008;9(9):234.
6. Simon R, Korn E, McShane L, Radmacher M, Wright G, Zhao Y. Design and analysis of DNA microarray investigations. New York, NY: Springer; 2003.
7. Churchill GA. Using ANOVA to analyze microarray data. Biotechniques. 2004;37(2):173–5. 177.
8. Consortium M, Shi L, Reid LH, Jones WD, Shippy R, Warrington JA, et al. The MicroArray Quality Control (MAQC) project shows inter- and intraplatform reproducibility of gene expression measurements. Nat Biotechnol. 2006;24(9):1151–61.
9. Tusher VG, Tibshirani R, Chu G. Significance analysis of microarrays applied to the ionizing radiation response. Proc Natl Acad Sci USA. 2001;98(9):5116–21.
10. Wright GW, Simon RM. A random variance model for detection of differential gene expression in small microarray experiments. Bioinformatics. 2003;19(18):2448–55.
11. Witten DM, Tibshirani R. Testing significance of features by lassoed principal components. Ann Appl Stat. 2008;2(3):986–1012.
12. Bittner M, Meltzer P, Chen Y, Jiang Y, Seftor E, Hendrix M, et al. Molecular classification of cutaneous malignant melanoma by gene expression profiling. Nature. 2000;406(6795): 536–40.

13. Ben-Dor A, Bruhn L, Friedman N, Nachman I, Schummer M, Yakhini Z. Tissue classification with gene expression profiles. J Comput Biol. 2000;7(3–4):559–83.
14. Tukey JW. Tightening the clinical trial. Control Clin Trials. 1993;14(4):266–85.
15. Hedenfalk I, Duggan D, Chen Y, Radmacher M, Bittner M, Simon R, et al. Gene-expression profiles in hereditary breast cancer. N Engl J Med. 2001;344(8):539–48.
16. Nguyen DV, Rocke DM. Tumor classification by partial least squares using microarray gene expression data. Bioinformatics. 2002;18(1):39–50.
17. Cover TM, Hart PE. Nearest neighbor pattern classification. IEEE Trans Inf Theory. 1967;13:21–7.
18. Parry RM, Jones W, Stokes TH, Phan JH, Moffitt RA, Fang H, et al. k-Nearest neighbor models for microarray gene expression analysis and clinical outcome prediction. Pharmacogenomics J. 2010;10(4):292–309.
19. Brown MP, Grundy WN, Lin D, Cristianini N, Sugnet CW, Furey TS, et al. Knowledge-based analysis of microarray gene expression data by using support vector machines. Proc Natl Acad Sci USA. 2000;97(1):262–7.
20. Tibshirani R, Hastie T, Narasimhan B, Chu G. Diagnosis of multiple cancer types by shrunken centroids of gene expression. Proc Natl Acad Sci USA. 2002;99(10):6567–72.
21. Geman D, d'Avignon C, Naiman DQ, Winslow RL. Classifying gene expression profiles from pairwise mRNA comparisons. Stat Appl Genet Mol Biol. 2004;3:19.
22. Hartigan JA, Wong MA. Algorithm AS 136: a K-means clustering algorithm. J R Stat Soc Ser C Appl Stat. 1979;28(1):100–8.
23. Eisen MB, Spellman PT, Brown PO, Botstein D. Cluster analysis and display of genome-wide expression patterns. Proc Natl Acad Sci USA. 1998 Dec 8;95(25):14863–8.
24. Cheng Y, Church GM. Biclustering of expression data. Proc Int Conf Intell Syst Mol Biol. 2000;8:93–103.
25. Tamayo P, Slonim D, Mesirov J, Zhu Q, Kitareewan S, Dmitrovsky E, et al. Interpreting patterns of gene expression with self-organizing maps: methods and application to hematopoietic differentiation. Proc Natl Acad Sci USA. 1999;96(6):2907–12.
26. Yeung KY, Fraley C, Murua A, Raftery AE, Ruzzo WL. Model-based clustering and data transformations for gene expression data. Bioinformatics. 2001;17(10):977–87.
27. Eichler GS, Huang S, Ingber DE. Gene Expression Dynamics Inspector (GEDI): for integrative analysis of expression profiles. Bioinformatics. 2003;19(17):2321–2.
28. Goeman JJ, van de Geer SA, de Kort F, van Houwelingen HC. A global test for groups of genes: testing association with a clinical outcome. Bioinformatics. 2004;20(1):93–9.
29. Subramanian A, Tamayo P, Mootha VK, Mukherjee S, Ebert BL, Gillette MA, et al. Gene set enrichment analysis: a knowledge-based approach for interpreting genome-wide expression profiles. Proc Natl Acad Sci USA. 2005;102(43):15545–50.
30. Dinu I, Potter JD, Mueller T, Liu Q, Adewale AJ, Jhangri GS, et al. Improving gene set analysis of microarray data by SAM-GS. BMC Bioinformatics. 2007;8:242.
31. Setlur SR, Royce TE, Sboner A, Mosquera JM, Demichelis F, Hofer MD, et al. Integrative microarray analysis of pathways dysregulated in metastatic prostate cancer. Cancer Res. 2007;67(21):10296–303.
32. Xu X, Zhao Y, Simon R. Gene set expression comparison kit for BRB-ArrayTools. Bioinformatics. 2008;24(1):137–9.
33. Cox DR. Regression models and life-tables. J R Stat Soc Series B. 1972;34(2):187–220.
34. Nguyen DV, Rocke DM. Partial least squares proportional hazard regression for application to DNA microarray survival data. Bioinformatics. 2002;18(12):1625–32.
35. Michiels S, Koscielny S, Hill C. Prediction of cancer outcome with microarrays: a multiple random validation strategy. Lancet. 2005;365(9458):488–92.
36. Bair E, Hastie T, Paul D, Tibshirani R. Prediction by supervised principal components. J Am Stat Assoc. 2006;101(473):119–37.
37. Zaykin DV, Zhivotovsky LA, Westfall PH, Weir BS. Truncated product method for combining P-values. Genet Epidemiol. 2002;22(2):170–85.

38. Choi JK, Yu U, Kim S, Yoo OJ. Combining multiple microarray studies and modeling interstudy variation. Bioinformatics. 2003;19 Suppl 1:i84–90.
39. Hong F, Breitling R, McEntee CW, Wittner BS, Nemhauser JL, Chory J. RankProd: a bioconductor package for detecting differentially expressed genes in meta-analysis. Bioinformatics. 2006;22(22):2825–7.
40. Pyne S, Futcher B, Skiena S. Meta-analysis based on control of false discovery rate: combining yeast ChIP-chip datasets. Bioinformatics. 2006;22(20):2516–22.
41. Fishel I, Kaufman A, Ruppin E. Meta-analysis of gene expression data: a predictor-based approach. Bioinformatics. 2007;23(13):1599–606.
42. Wang X, Kang DD, Shen K, Song C, Lu S, Chang LC, et al. An R package suite for microarray meta-analysis in quality control, differentially expressed gene analysis and pathway enrichment detection. Bioinformatics. 2012;28(19):2534–6.
43. Reimers M, Carey VJ. Bioconductor: an open source framework for bioinformatics and computational biology. Methods Enzymol. 2006;411:119–34.
44. Simon R, Lam A, Li MC, Ngan M, Menenzes S, Zhao Y. Analysis of gene expression data using BRB-ArrayTools. Cancer Inform. 2007;3:11–7.
45. Raponi M, Zhang Y, Yu J, Chen G, Lee G, Taylor JM, et al. Gene expression signatures for predicting prognosis of squamous cell and adenocarcinomas of the lung. Cancer Res. 2006;66(15):7466–72.
46. Kaminski N, Rosas IO. Gene expression profiling as a window into idiopathic pulmonary fibrosis pathogenesis: can we identify the right target genes? Proc Am Thorac Soc. 2006;3(4):339–44.
47. Ban TA. The role of serendipity in drug discovery. Dialogues Clin Neurosci. 2006;8(3):335–44.
48. Steinberg D. Chance and serendipity in science: two examples from my own career. J Biol Chem. 2011;286(44):37895–904.
49. Selman M, Ruiz V, Cabrera S, Segura L, Ramirez R, Barrios R, et al. TIMP-1, -2, -3, and -4 in idiopathic pulmonary fibrosis. A prevailing nondegradative lung microenvironment? Am J Physiol Lung Cell Mol Physiol. 2000;279(3):L562–74.
50. Zuo F, Kaminski N, Eugui E, Allard J, Yakhini Z, Ben-Dor A, et al. Gene expression analysis reveals matrilysin as a key regulator of pulmonary fibrosis in mice and humans. Proc Natl Acad Sci USA. 2002;99(9):6292–7.
51. Cosgrove GP, Schwarz MI, Geraci MW, Brown KK, Worthen GS. Overexpression of matrix metalloproteinase-7 in pulmonary fibrosis. Chest. 2002;121(3 Suppl):25S–6.
52. Fujishima S, Shiomi T, Yamashita S, Yogo Y, Nakano Y, Inoue T, et al. Production and activation of matrix metalloproteinase 7 (matrilysin 1) in the lungs of patients with idiopathic pulmonary fibrosis. Arch Pathol Lab Med. 2010;134(8):1136–42.
53. Rosas IO, Richards TJ, Konishi K, Zhang Y, Gibson K, Lokshin AE, et al. MMP1 and MMP7 as potential peripheral blood biomarkers in idiopathic pulmonary fibrosis. PLoS Med. 2008;5(4):e93.
54. Pardo A, Selman M. Matrix metalloproteases in aberrant fibrotic tissue remodeling. Proc Am Thorac Soc. 2006;3(4):383–8.
55. Pardo A, Selman M. Role of matrix metaloproteases in idiopathic pulmonary fibrosis. Fibrogenesis Tissue Repair. 2012;5 Suppl 1:S9.
56. Manicone AM, Huizar I, McGuire JK. Matrilysin (Matrix Metalloproteinase-7) regulates anti-inflammatory and antifibrotic pulmonary dendritic cells that express CD103 (alpha(E) beta(7)-integrin). Am J Pathol. 2009;175(6):2319–31.
57. Swee M, Wilson CL, Wang Y, McGuire JK, Parks WC. Matrix metalloproteinase-7 (matrilysin) controls neutrophil egress by generating chemokine gradients. J Leukoc Biol. 2008;83(6):1404–12.
58. Wilson CL, Schmidt AP, Pirila E, Valore EV, Ferri N, Sorsa T, et al. Differential processing of {alpha}- and {beta}-defensin precursors by matrix metalloproteinase-7 (MMP-7). J Biol Chem. 2009;284(13):8301–11.
59. Pardo A, Gibson K, Cisneros J, Richards TJ, Yang Y, Becerril C, et al. Up-regulation and profibrotic role of osteopontin in human idiopathic pulmonary fibrosis. PLoS Med. 2005;2(9):e251.

60. Checa M, Ruiz V, Montano M, Velazquez-Cruz R, Selman M, Pardo A. MMP-1 polymorphisms and the risk of idiopathic pulmonary fibrosis. Hum Genet. 2008;124(5):465–72.
61. Yamashita CM, Dolgonos L, Zemans RL, Young SK, Robertson J, Briones N, et al. Matrix metalloproteinase 3 is a mediator of pulmonary fibrosis. Am J Pathol. 2011;179(4): 1733–45.
62. Yu G, Kovkarova-Naumovski E, Jara P, Parwani A, Kass D, Ruiz V, et al. Matrix metalloproteinase-19 is a key regulator of lung fibrosis in mice and humans. Am J Respir Crit Care Med. 2012;186(8):752–62.
63. Pardo A, Selman M, Kaminski N. Approaching the degradome in idiopathic pulmonary fibrosis. Int J Biochem Cell Biol. 2008;40(6–7):1141–55.
64. McKeown S, Richter AG, O'Kane C, McAuley DF, Thickett DR. Matrix metalloproteinase expression and abnormal lung permeability are important determinants of outcome in IPF. Eur Respir J. 2009;33(1):77–84.
65. Richards TJ, Kaminski N, Baribaud F, Flavin S, Brodmerkel C, Horowitz D, et al. Peripheral blood proteins predict mortality in idiopathic pulmonary fibrosis. Am J Respir Crit Care Med. 2012;185(1):67–76.
66. Studer SM, Kaminski N. Towards systems biology of human pulmonary fibrosis. Proc Am Thorac Soc. 2007;4(1):85–91.
67. Selman M, Pardo A, Kaminski N. Idiopathic pulmonary fibrosis: aberrant recapitulation of developmental programs? PLoS Med. 2008;5(3):e62.
68. Sharma RP, Chopra VL. Effect of the Wingless (wg1) mutation on wing and haltere development in Drosophila melanogaster. Dev Biol. 1976;48(2):461–5.
69. Rao TP, Kuhl M. An updated overview on Wnt signaling pathways: a prelude for more. Circ Res. 2010;106(12):1798–806.
70. Blankesteijn WM, van de Schans VA, ter Horst P, Smits JF. The Wnt/frizzled/GSK-3 beta pathway: a novel therapeutic target for cardiac hypertrophy. Trends Pharmacol Sci. 2008;29(4):175–80.
71. Stripp BR, Reynolds SD. Maintenance and repair of the bronchiolar epithelium. Proc Am Thorac Soc. 2008;5(3):328–33.
72. Rajagopal J, Carroll TJ, Guseh JS, Bores SA, Blank LJ, Anderson WJ, et al. Wnt7b stimulates embryonic lung growth by coordinately increasing the replication of epithelium and mesenchyme. Development. 2008;135(9):1625–34.
73. Behrens J. The role of the Wnt signalling pathway in colorectal tumorigenesis. Biochem Soc Trans. 2005;33(Pt 4):672–5.
74. Vuga LJ, Ben-Yehudah A, Kovkarova-Naumovski E, Oriss T, Gibson KF, Feghali-Bostwick C, et al. WNT5A is a regulator of fibroblast proliferation and resistance to apoptosis. Am J Respir Cell Mol Biol. 2009;41(5):583–9.
75. Luo J, Chen J, Deng ZL, Luo X, Song WX, Sharff KA, et al. Wnt signaling and human diseases: what are the therapeutic implications? Lab Invest. 2007;87(2):97–103.
76. Chilosi M, Poletti V, Zamo A, Lestani M, Montagna L, Piccoli P, et al. Aberrant Wnt/beta-catenin pathway activation in idiopathic pulmonary fibrosis. Am J Pathol. 2003;162(5): 1495–502.
77. Konigshoff M, Balsara N, Pfaff EM, Kramer M, Chrobak I, Seeger W, et al. Functional Wnt signaling is increased in idiopathic pulmonary fibrosis. PLoS One. 2008;3(5):e2142.
78. Henderson Jr WR, Chi EY, Ye X, Nguyen C, Tien YT, Zhou B, et al. Inhibition of Wnt/beta-catenin/CREB binding protein (CBP) signaling reverses pulmonary fibrosis. Proc Natl Acad Sci USA. 2010;107(32):14309–14.
79. Schmalhofer O, Spaderna S, Brabletz T. Native promoter reporters validate transcriptional targets. Methods Mol Biol. 2008;468:111–28.
80. Bridges RS, Kass D, Loh K, Glackin C, Borczuk AC, Greenberg S. Gene expression profiling of pulmonary fibrosis identifies Twist1 as an antiapoptotic molecular "rectifier" of growth factor signaling. Am J Pathol. 2009;175(6):2351–61.
81. Konishi K, Gibson KF, Lindell KO, Richards TJ, Zhang Y, Dhir R, et al. Gene expression profiles of acute exacerbations of idiopathic pulmonary fibrosis. Am J Respir Crit Care Med. 2009;180(2):167–75.

82. Selman M, Pardo A. Role of epithelial cells in idiopathic pulmonary fibrosis: from innocent targets to serial killers. Proc Am Thorac Soc. 2006;3(4):364–72.

83. Selman M, Pardo A. Idiopathic pulmonary fibrosis: an epithelial/fibroblastic cross-talk disorder. Respir Res. 2002;3:3.

84. Selman M, Pardo A, Barrera L, Estrada A, Watson SR, Wilson K, et al. Gene expression profiles distinguish idiopathic pulmonary fibrosis from hypersensitivity pneumonitis. Am J Respir Crit Care Med. 2006;173(2):188–98.

85. Selman M, Carrillo G, Estrada A, Mejia M, Becerril C, Cisneros J, et al. Accelerated variant of idiopathic pulmonary fibrosis: clinical behavior and gene expression pattern. PLoS One. 2007;2(5):e482.

86. Tzouvelekis A, Harokopos V, Paparountas T, Oikonomou N, Chatziioannou A, Vilaras G, et al. Comparative expression profiling in pulmonary fibrosis suggests a role of hypoxia-inducible factor-1alpha in disease pathogenesis. Am J Respir Crit Care Med. 2007;176(11):1108–19.

87. MacDonald SL, Rubens MB, Hansell DM, Copley SJ, Desai SR, du Bois RM, et al. Nonspecific interstitial pneumonia and usual interstitial pneumonia: comparative appearances at and diagnostic accuracy of thin-section CT. Radiology. 2001;221(3):600–5.

88. Sverzellati N, Wells AU, Tomassetti S, Desai SR, Copley SJ, Aziz ZA, et al. Biopsy-proved idiopathic pulmonary fibrosis: spectrum of nondiagnostic thin-section CT diagnoses. Radiology. 2010;254(3):957–64.

89. Silva CI, Muller NL, Lynch DA, Curran-Everett D, Brown KK, Lee KS, et al. Chronic hypersensitivity pneumonitis: differentiation from idiopathic pulmonary fibrosis and nonspecific interstitial pneumonia by using thin-section CT. Radiology. 2008;246(1):288–97.

90. Flaherty KR, Travis WD, Colby TV, Toews GB, Kazerooni EA, Gross BH, et al. Histopathologic variability in usual and nonspecific interstitial pneumonias. Am J Respir Crit Care Med. 2001;164(9):1722–7.

91. Monaghan H, Wells AU, Colby TV, du Bois RM, Hansell DM, Nicholson AG. Prognostic implications of histologic patterns in multiple surgical lung biopsies from patients with idiopathic interstitial pneumonias. Chest. 2004;125(2):522–6.

92. Selman M, King TE, Pardo A, American Thoracic Society, European Respiratory Society, American College of Chest Physicians. Idiopathic pulmonary fibrosis: prevailing and evolving hypotheses about its pathogenesis and implications for therapy. Ann Intern Med. 2001;134(2):136–51.

93. Yang IV, Burch LH, Steele MP, Savov JD, Hollingsworth JW, McElvania-Tekippe E, et al. Gene expression profiling of familial and sporadic interstitial pneumonia. Am J Respir Crit Care Med. 2007;175(1):45–54.

94. Rosas IO, Kaminski N. When it comes to genes–IPF or NSIP, familial or sporadic–they're all the same. Am J Respir Crit Care Med. 2007;175(1):5–6.

95. Lamblin C, Bergoin C, Saelens T, Wallaert B. Interstitial lung diseases in collagen vascular diseases. Eur Respir J Suppl. 2001;32:69s–80.

96. Hsu E, Shi H, Jordan RM, Lyons-Weiler J, Pilewski JM, Feghali-Bostwick CA. Lung tissues in patients with systemic sclerosis have gene expression patterns unique to pulmonary fibrosis and pulmonary hypertension. Arthritis Rheum. 2011;63(3):783–94.

97. Martinez FJ, Safrin S, Weycker D, Starko KM, Bradford WZ, King Jr TE, et al. The clinical course of patients with idiopathic pulmonary fibrosis. Ann Intern Med. 2005;142(12 Pt 1):963–7.

98. Oppenheim JJ, Biragyn A, Kwak LW, Yang D. Roles of antimicrobial peptides such as defensins in innate and adaptive immunity. Ann Rheum Dis. 2003;62 Suppl 2:ii17–21.

99. Lillard Jr JW, Boyaka PN, Chertov O, Oppenheim JJ, McGhee JR. Mechanisms for induction of acquired host immunity by neutrophil peptide defensins. Proc Natl Acad Sci USA. 1999 Jan 19;96(2):651–6.

100. Feghali-Bostwick CA, Tsai CG, Valentine VG, Kantrow S, Stoner MW, Pilewski JM, et al. Cellular and humoral autoreactivity in idiopathic pulmonary fibrosis. J Immunol. 2007;179(4):2592–9.

101. Yang IV, Luna LG, Cotter J, Talbert J, Leach SM, Kidd R, et al. The peripheral blood transcriptome identifies the presence and extent of disease in idiopathic pulmonary fibrosis. PLoS One. 2012;7(6):e37708.

102. Boon K, Bailey NW, Yang J, Steel MP, Groshong S, Kervitsky D, et al. Molecular phenotypes distinguish patients with relatively stable from progressive idiopathic pulmonary fibrosis (IPF). PLoS One. 2009;4(4):e5134.

103. Greene KE, King Jr TE, Kuroki Y, Bucher-Bartelson B, Hunninghake GW, Newman LS, et al. Serum surfactant proteins-A and -D as biomarkers in idiopathic pulmonary fibrosis. Eur Respir J. 2002;19(3):439–46.

104. Kahloon RA, Xue J, Bhargava A, Csizmadia E, Otterbein L, Kass DJ, et al. Idiopathic pulmonary fibrosis patients with antibodies to heat shock protein 70 have poor prognoses. Am J Respir Crit Care Med. 2013;187(7):768–75.

105. Cosgrove GP, Brown KK, Schiemann WP, Serls AE, Parr JE, Geraci MW, et al. Pigment epithelium-derived factor in idiopathic pulmonary fibrosis: a role in aberrant angiogenesis. Am J Respir Crit Care Med. 2004;170(3):242–51.

106. Wang XM, Zhang Y, Kim HP, Zhou Z, Feghali-Bostwick CA, Liu F, et al. Caveolin-1: a critical regulator of lung fibrosis in idiopathic pulmonary fibrosis. J Exp Med. 2006;203(13):2895–906.

107. Englert JM, Hanford LE, Kaminski N, Tobolewski JM, Tan RJ, Fattman CL, et al. A role for the receptor for advanced glycation end products in idiopathic pulmonary fibrosis. Am J Pathol. 2008;172(3):583–91.

108. Consortium EP, Dunham I, Kundaje A, Aldred SF, Collins PJ, Davis CA, et al. An integrated encyclopedia of DNA elements in the human genome. Nature. 2012;489(7414):57–74.

109. Bazzini AA, Lee MT, Giraldez AJ. Ribosome profiling shows that miR-430 reduces translation before causing mRNA decay in zebrafish. Science. 2012;336(6078):233–7.

110. Pandit KV, Corcoran D, Yousef H, Yarlagadda M, Tzouvelekis A, Gibson KF, et al. Inhibition and role of let-7d in idiopathic pulmonary fibrosis. Am J Respir Crit Care Med. 2010;182(2):220–9.

111. Milosevic J, Pandit K, Magister M, Rabinovich E, Ellwanger DC, Yu G, et al. Profibrotic role of miR-154 in pulmonary fibrosis. Am J Respir Cell Mol Biol. 2012;47(6):879–87.

112. Liu G, Friggeri A, Yang Y, Milosevic J, Ding Q, Thannickal VJ, et al. miR-21 mediates fibrogenic activation of pulmonary fibroblasts and lung fibrosis. J Exp Med. 2010;207(8):1589–97.

113. Yang S, Banerjee S, de Freitas A, Sanders YY, Ding Q, Matalon S, et al. Participation of miR-200 in pulmonary fibrosis. Am J Pathol. 2012;180(2):484–93.

114. Yang S, Xie N, Cui H, Banerjee S, Abraham E, Thannickal VJ, et al. miR-31 is a negative regulator of fibrogenesis and pulmonary fibrosis. FASEB J. 2012;26(9):3790–9.

115. Dakhlallah D, Batte K, Wang Y, Cantemir-Stone CZ, Yan P, Nuovo G, et al. Epigenetic regulation of miR-17 92 contributes to the pathogenesis of pulmonary fibrosis. Am J Respir Crit Care Med. 2013;187(4):397–405.

116. Oak SR, Murray L, Herath A, Sleeman M, Anderson I, Joshi AD, et al. A micro RNA processing defect in rapidly progressing idiopathic pulmonary fibrosis. PLoS One. 2011;6(6):e21253.

117. Pandit KV, Milosevic J, Kaminski N. MicroRNAs in idiopathic pulmonary fibrosis. Translational Res. 2011;157(4):191–9.

118. Dai Y, Huang YS, Tang M, Lv TY, Hu CX, Tan YH, et al. Microarray analysis of microRNA expression in peripheral blood cells of systemic lupus erythematosus patients. Lupus. 2007;16(12):939–46.

119. Hausler SF, Keller A, Chandran PA, Ziegler K, Zipp K, Heuer S, et al. Whole blood-derived miRNA profiles as potential new tools for ovarian cancer screening. Br J Cancer. 2010;103(5):693–700.

120. Cabili MN, Trapnell C, Goff L, Koziol M, Tazon-Vega B, Regev A, et al. Integrative annotation of human large intergenic noncoding RNAs reveals global properties and specific subclasses. Genes Dev. 2011;25(18):1915–27.

121. Rinn JL, Chang HY. Genome regulation by long noncoding RNAs. Annu Rev Biochem. 2012;81:145–66.
122. Yang IV. Epigenomics of idiopathic pulmonary fibrosis. Epigenomics. 2012;4(2):195–203.
123. Sanders YY, Pardo A, Selman M, Nuovo GJ, Tollefsbol TO, Siegal GP, et al. Thy-1 promoter hypermethylation: a novel epigenetic pathogenic mechanism in pulmonary fibrosis. Am J Respir Cell Mol Biol. 2008;39(5):610–8.
124. Coward WR, Watts K, Feghali-Bostwick CA, Jenkins G, Pang L. Repression of IP-10 by interactions between histone deacetylation and hypermethylation in idiopathic pulmonary fibrosis. Mol Cell Biol. 2010;30(12):2874–86.
125. Cisneros J, Hagood J, Checa M, Ortiz-Quintero B, Negreros M, Herrera I, et al. Hypermethylation-mediated silencing of p14ARF in fibroblasts from idiopathic pulmonary fibrosis. Am J Physiol Lung Cell Mol Physiol. 2012;303(4):L295–303.
126. Sanders YY, Tollefsbol TO, Varisco BM, Hagood JS. Epigenetic regulation of thy-1 by histone deacetylase inhibitor in rat lung fibroblasts. Am J Respir Cell Mol Biol. 2011;45(1):16–23.
127. Rabinovich EI, Kapetanaki MG, Steinfeld I, Gibson KF, Pandit KV, Yu G, et al. Global methylation patterns in idiopathic pulmonary fibrosis. PLoS One. 2012;7(4):e33770.
128. Sanders YY, Ambalavanan N, Halloran B, Zhang X, Liu H, Crossman DK, et al. Altered DNA methylation profile in idiopathic pulmonary fibrosis. Am J Respir Crit Care Med. 2012;186(6):525–35.
129. Rabinovich EI, Selman M, Kaminski N. Epigenomics of idiopathic pulmonary fibrosis: evaluating the first steps. Am J Respir Crit Care Med. 2012;186(6):473–5.
130. Herazo-Maya JD, Kaminski N. Personalized medicine: applying 'omics' to lung fibrosis. Biomark Med. 2012;6(4):529–40.
131. Fingerlin TE, Murphy E, Zhang W, Peljto AL, Brown KK, Steele MP, et al. Genome-wide association study identifies multiple susceptibility loci for pulmonary fibrosis. Nat Genet. 2013;45(6):613–20.
132. Noth I, Zhang Y, Ma S-F, Flores C, Barber M, Huang Y, et al. Genetic variants associated with idiopathic pulmonary fibrosis susceptibility and mortality: a genome-wide association study. Lancet. 2013;1(4):309–17.

# Chapter 20
# Idiopathic Pulmonary Fibrosis Clinical Trials: Evolving Concepts

Fernando J. Martinez

**Abstract** Idiopathic pulmonary fibrosis (IPF) is a progressive disorder with variable rates of disease progression (Raghu et al., Am J Respir Crit Care Med 183:788–824, 2011). Development of therapeutic interventions has proven quite challenging, which, in part, reflects the complex underlying biology, the difficult nature of identifying the optimal endpoints for pivotal studies, and the varying rate of disease progression (Raghu et al., Am J Respir Crit Care Med 185:1044–8, 2012). Over the past 10 years, significant advances have occurred in the conduct of clinical trials in IPF (Luppi et al., Curr Opin Pulm Med 18:428–32, 2012). Table 20.1 enumerates published trials over this time period with characteristics of the individual studies. The advances included in these trials include the adoption of guideline-based diagnostic criteria, standard approaches to initial evaluation and characterization of study subjects, and a robust methodology to study conduct. Numerous challenges remain, however, including identifying the optimal primary endpoint(s) for late-stage development, the role of biomarkers or intermediate markers in clinical trials, defining disease progression in individual study subjects to allow study enrichment, and targeting novel pathways in future clinical trials. This chapter will describe the approach to diagnosis and characterization of study subjects, the approach to physiological assessment, and the modalities that are needed to design and conduct proof of concept (POC), early-phase, and late-phase therapeutic trials.

**Keywords** Biomarkers • Clinical practice guideline • Clinical trial • Endpoint determination • Idiopathic pulmonary fibrosis • Therapeutics

Idiopathic pulmonary fibrosis (IPF) is a progressive disorder with variable rates of disease progression [1]. Development of therapeutic interventions has proven quite

F.J. Martinez, M.D., M.S. (✉)
Division of Pulmonary and Critical Care Medicine, Department
of Internal Medicine, University of Michigan Health System, 1500 E Medical
Center Drive, Room 3916 TC, Ann Arbor, MI 48109-5360, USA
e-mail: fmartine@umich.edu

K.C. Meyer and S.D. Nathan (eds.), *Idiopathic Pulmonary Fibrosis: A Comprehensive Clinical Guide*, Respiratory Medicine 9, DOI 10.1007/978-1-62703-682-5_20,
© Springer Science+Business Media New York 2014

challenging, which, in part, reflects the complex underlying biology, the difficult nature of identifying the optimal endpoints for pivotal studies, and the varying rate of disease progression [2]. Over the past 10 years significant advances have occurred in the conduct of clinical trials in IPF [3]. Table 20.1 enumerates published trials over this time period with characteristics of the individual studies. The advances included in these trials include the adoption of guideline-based diagnostic criteria, standard approaches to initial evaluation and characterization of study subjects, and a robust methodology to study conduct. Numerous challenges remain, however, including identifying the optimal primary endpoint(s) for late-stage development, the role of biomarkers or intermediate markers in clinical trials, defining disease progression in individual study subjects to allow study enrichment, and targeting novel pathways in future clinical trials. This chapter will describe the approach to diagnosis and characterization of study subjects, the approach to physiological assessment, and the modalities that are needed to design and conduct proof of concept (POC), early-phase, and late-phase therapeutic trials.

## Diagnostic Approach to IPF in Therapeutic Studies

The diagnostic approach to the idiopathic interstitial pneumonias and IPF in particular has been standardized by international respiratory societies over the past decade [1, 4]. These groups generally recommend the definition of the usual interstitial pneumonia (UIP) pattern with either imaging (high-resolution computed tomography, HRCT) or surgical biopsy (Table 20.2). In principle, these approaches have been incorporated in therapeutic trials conducted over the past 10 years (see Table 20.1). The earlier methodological approaches (see Table 20.1) included combinations of HRCT and SLB findings that were made operational in numerous therapeutic trials (see Table 20.1). The more recent revisions have combined HRCT and SLB findings, creating categories of definite, probable, or possible IPF. This latter approach has recently been incorporated into a series of therapeutic trials (see Table 20.1). Some therapeutic trials required minor HRCT abnormalities and surgical biopsy confirmation of a definite UIP pattern [5, 6].

The overall approach to IPF diagnosis has proven challenging, with only modest interobserver agreements between expert clinicians, radiologists, and pathologists [7, 8]. The level of interobserver agreement is even lower when comparing academic experts with community-based clinicians, radiologists, and pathologists [9], and the interpretation of HRCT can be particularly challenging in the setting of concomitant emphysema and lead to a decrease in interobserver agreement [10]. International consensus statements support the use of an iterative, interactive approach that includes all of these specialties [1]. One early study demonstrated reasonable concordance between study-site and core radiologists [11]. A separate multicenter group included central review of HRCT by a panel of three expert radiologists and lung biopsy by three expert pathologists [8], and a prospective study has confirmed that such an approach improves diagnostic agreement among participating physicians [7]. The therapeutic trials listed in Table 20.1 have taken varying approaches to the implementation of guideline criteria for IPF diagnosis.

**Table 20.1** Randomized, controlled trials in IPF published since 2004

| Citation | Comparators | N | Trial duration | Selected inclusion criteria; *diagnostic assurance* | Primary endpoint | Age (year) | FVC (% pred) | DLCO (% pred) | Primary result |
|---|---|---|---|---|---|---|---|---|---|
| Raghu et al. [66] | Interferon gamma-1b<br>Placebo | 162<br>168 | 383 days<br>374 days | HRCT definite or probable UIP<br>SLB with UIP or nondiagnostic TBBx<br>Disease progression<br>Prednisone allowed<br>*Local diagnosis* | PFS [FVC, P(A-a) O₂, death] | 63.6<br>63.4 | 63.9<br>64.1 | 37.2<br>36.8 | Negative |
| Strieter et al. [67] | Interferon gamma-1b<br>Placebo | 17<br>15 | 26 weeks | HRCT and tissue diagnosis<br>FVC 50–90<br>Disease progression<br>*Local diagnosis* | Lung molecular markers | 64.1<br>63.0 | 67.0<br>67.6 | 43.8<br>40.1 | Positive for some markers |
| Azuma et al. [68] | Pirfenidone<br>Placebo | 72<br>35 | 6 months | HRCT definite or probable UIP<br>Adequate exertional PaO₂<br>*Central radiology review* | 6MWT trough SpO₂ | 64.0<br>64.3 | 81.6<br>78.4 | 57.6<br>57.7 | Negative; stopped by DSMB due to AE IPF imbalance favoring pirfenidone |
| Kubo et al. [69] | Prednisolone + Warfarin<br>Prednisolone alone[a] | 33<br>23 | NA | HRCT and/or tissue diagnosis<br>Admitted to hospital<br>Prednisolone allowed<br>*Local pathology; independent radiology review* | Survival and hospitalization-free period | 68.1<br>71.3 | 71<br>69 | 63<br>59 | Improved survival but post-randomization/ pre-therapy imbalance |

(continued)

**Table 20.1** (continued)

| Citation | N | Trial duration | Selected inclusion criteria; *diagnostic assurance* | Primary endpoint | Age (year) | FVC (% pred) | DLCO (% pred) | Primary result |
|---|---|---|---|---|---|---|---|---|
| Demedts et al. [70] Prednisone/azathioprine/ NAC<br>Prednisone/azathioprine/ placebo | 80<br>75 | 12 months | HRCT and SLB (particularly if age <50)<br>Dyspnea, VC<80 % or TLC<90 %, and DLCO<80 %<br>*Central review of HRCT and SLB* | Absolute change in FVC and DLCO | 62<br>64 | 80<br>75 | 79<br>74 | Positive for lesser deterioration in FVC and DLCO with added NAC |
| Antoniou et al. [71] Interferon gamma-1γ<br>Colchicine[a] | 32<br>18 | 2 years | HRCT or tissue diagnosis<br>FVC 55 %–90 %, DLCO ≥35 %, PAO$_2$ >7.3 kPa<br>*Local diagnosis* | Molecular markers | 66<br>69 | 71.8<br>70.7 | 54.5<br>51.1 | Positive for FVC and symptoms |
| King et al. [5] Bosentan<br>Placebo | 74<br>84 | 12 months | HRCT or tissue diagnosis<br>6MWD 150–499 m<br>*Local diagnosis* | 6MWD | 65.3<br>65.1 | 65.9<br>69.5 | 42.3<br>41.4 | Negative |
| Raghu et al. [72] Etanercept<br>Placebo | 46<br>41 | 48 weeks | HRCT or tissue diagnosis<br>Disease progression<br>FVC ≥45 %, DLCO ≥25 %, PaO$_2$ ≥55 mmHg<br>*Local diagnosis* | Δ FVC, DLCO, and p(A-a)O$_2$ | 65.2<br>65.1 | 64.7<br>63.0 | 36.3<br>36.9 | Negative |
| Daniels et al. [73] Imatinib<br>Placebo | 59<br>60 | 96 weeks | HRCT or tissue diagnosis<br>Disease progression<br>FVC ≥55 %, DLCO ≥35 %, PaO$_2$ ≥60 mmHg<br>*Local diagnosis* | PFS[b] [FVC, death] | 66<br>67.8 | 64.4<br>65.6 | 39.8<br>39.3 | Negative |

| Study | Treatment | N | Duration | Inclusion criteria | Primary endpoint | | | | Result |
|---|---|---|---|---|---|---|---|---|---|
| King et al. [47] | Interferon gamma-1γ<br>Placebo | 551<br>275 | 64 weeks | HRCT definite/probable UIP<br>SLB with UIP or nondiagnostic TBBx<br>Disease progression<br>*Central review of HRCT and SLB* | Survival | 66.0<br>65.9 | 72.2<br>73.1 | 47.4<br>47.3 | Negative (DSMB stopped due to futility) |
| IPFnet [20] | Sildenafil<br>Placebo | 89<br>91 | 12 weeks blinded; 12 weeks open label | HRCT definite UIP with SLB definite/probable UIP or HRCT consistent with UIP and SLB definite/probable UIP<br>DLCO<35 %<br>6MWD>50 m and <15 % variability<br>*Local diagnosis/random sample HRCT and SLB review* | 6MWD | 69.8<br>68.2 | 54.9<br>58.7 | 25.8<br>26.7 | Negative |
| Jackson et al. [74] | Sildenafil<br>Placebo | 14<br>15 | 6 months | HRCT definite/probable UIP and SLB definite/probable UIP<br>FVC 40–90 %, DLCO 30–90 %, 6MWD 150–500 m<br>RVSP or $PA_{sys}$ 25–50 mmHg<br>*Local diagnosis* | 6MWD | 70<br>71 | 62.2<br>62.7 | 40.4<br>43.5 | Negative |

(continued)

**Table 20.1** (continued)

| Citation | Comparators | N | Trial duration | Selected inclusion criteria; diagnostic assurance | Primary endpoint | Age (year) | FVC (% pred) | DLCO (% pred) | Primary result |
|---|---|---|---|---|---|---|---|---|---|
| Taniguchi et al. [75] | Pirfenidone 1,800 mg/day | 108 | 52 weeks | HRCT definite UIP or HRCT probable UIP and SLB definite UIP 6MWT SpO$_2$ desaturation ≥5% trough SpO$_2$ ≥85% | Initially 6MWT trough SpO$_2$; changed to VC pre-unblinding | 65.4 | 77.3 | 52.1 | Positive for revised primary endpoint |
|  | Pirfenidone 1,200 mg/day | 55 |  |  |  | 63.9 | 76.2 | 53.6 |  |
|  | Placebo | 104 |  |  |  | 64.7 | 79.1 | 55.2 |  |
|  | *Central HRCT review* |  |  |  |  |  |  |  |  |
| King et al. [6] | Bosentan | 407 | 52 weeks | SLB definite UIP <5% HRCT honeycomb change | PFS [FVC, DLCO, AEIPF, death] | 63.8 | 74.9 | 47.7 | Negative |
|  | Placebo | 209 |  |  |  | 63.2 | 73.1 | 47.9 |  |
| Noble et al. [63] | Pirfenidone 2,403 mg/day | 174 | 72 weeks | HRCT definite UIP or if <50 year age/probable UIP required SLB UIP FVC 50–90%, DLCO 35–90%, 6MWD>150 m | ΔFVC | 66.8 | 74.9 | 47.8 | Study 004—positive Study 006—negative |
|  | Pirfenidone 1,197 mg/day | 87 |  |  |  | 68.0 | 76.4 | 46.4 |  |
|  | Placebo[b] | 174 |  |  |  | 66.3–67[b] | 73.1–76.2[b] | 46.1–47.4[b] |  |
| Richeldi et al. [76] | BIBF 1120 50 mg qd | 86 | 52 weeks | FVC≥50%, DLCO 30–79% PaO2≥50/55 mmHg | ΔFVC | 65.3 | 79.8 | 3.5[c] | Negative (p=0.06) |
|  | BIBF 1120 50 mg bd | 86 |  |  |  | 64.9 | 80.4 | 3.6[c] |  |
|  | BIBF 1120 100 mg bd | 86 |  |  |  | 65.1 | 83.0 | 3.7[c] |  |
|  | BIBF 1120 150 mg bd | 85 |  |  |  | 65.4 | 78.1 | 3.5[c] |  |
|  | Placebo | 85 |  |  |  | 64.8 | 77.6 | 3.7[c] |  |
| Malouf et al. [77] | Everolimus | 44 | 3 years | SLB confirmed | Time to ΔFVC/TLC≥10% or DLCO≥15% or ≥4% SaO$_2$ | 59 | 65 | 39 | Negative |
|  | Placebo | 45 |  |  |  | 60 | 69 | 42 |  |

| Study | Intervention | n | Duration | Inclusion criteria | Primary endpoint | Age | FVC | DLCO | Result |
|---|---|---|---|---|---|---|---|---|---|
| Noth et al. [49] | Warfarin<br>Placebo | 72<br>73 | 28 weeks | HRCT definite UIP with SLB definite/probable UIP or HRCT consistent with UIP and SLB definite/probable UIP<br>Disease progression<br>Standard concomitant therapy allowed | Time to all-cause mortality, nonelective, nonbleeding hospitalization, Δ FVC ≥ 10 % | 67.3<br>66.7 | 58.9<br>58.7 | 33.8<br>34.6 | Negative (DSMB stopped due to harm) |
| IPFnet [32] | Prednisone/azathioprine/<br>NAC<br>Placebo | 77<br>78 | 32 weeks | HRCT definite UIP with SLB definite/probable UIP or HRCT consistent with UIP and SLB definite/probable UIP<br>FVC ≥ 50 %, DLCO ≥ 30 % | Δ FVC | 68.8<br>67.9 | 69.3<br>72.1 | 42.1<br>45.3 | Negative (DSMB stopped due to harm) |
| Horton et al. [78] | Thalidomide[d] | 23 | 12 weeks | HRCT or SLB consistent with UIP<br>FVC 40–90 %, DLCO 30–90 %, chronic cough | Cough-specific quality of life | 67.6 | 70.4 | 57.4 | Positive |

*HRCT* high-resolution computed tomography of chest, *SLB* surgical lung biopsy, *UIP* usual interstitial pneumonia, *TBBx* transbronchial biopsy, *PFS* progression-free survival, *6MWT* 6-minute walk test, *DSMB* data safety monitoring board, *NA* not available, *6MWD* 6-minute walk distance, *NAC* N-acetyl cysteine

[a] Open-label
[b] Two separate studies
[c] mmol(min kPa)
[d] Double-blind, crossover

**Table 20.2** ATS/ERS criteria for IPF diagnosis evolution over time

| Version ATS/ERS international multidisciplinary consensus classification of the idiopathic interstitial pneumonias [4] | ATS/ERS/JRS/ALAT statement on idiopathic pulmonary fibrosis [1] |
|---|---|
| *In absence of surgical biopsy* | *Criteria for diagnosis of IPF* |
| Major criteria: | Exclusion of other known causes of interstitial lung disease |
| Exclusion of other known cause of interstitial lung disease | Presence of UIP pattern on HRCT if not subjected to SLB |
| Abnormal pulmonary function | Combination of HRCT and SLB in those subjected to SLB: |
| Bibasilar reticular abnormalities with minimal ground glass on HRCT | HRCT UIP pattern with SLB UIP, probable UIP, possible |
| Transbronchial biopsy or BAL documenting no alternate diagnosis | UIP, nonclassifiable—definite IPF |
| Minor criteria: | HRCT possible UIP with SLB UIP, probable UIP—definite |
| Age >50 year | IPF |
| Insidious onset of dyspnea on exertion | HRCT possible UIP with SLB possible UIP, nonclassifiable— |
| Duration of illness >3 months | probable IPF |
| Bibasilar, inspiratory crackles | HRCT inconsistent with SLB UIP—possible IPF |
| *HRCT findings* | *HRCT findings* |
| Basal-predominant reticular abnormality with volume loss | UIP pattern (all four features): |
| Peripheral, subpleural, basal | Subpleural, basal predominance |
| Reticular, honeycombing, traction bronchiectasis/bronchiolectasis, architectural distortion, | Reticular abnormality |
| focal ground glass | Honeycombing with/without traction bronchiectasis |
|  | Absence of inconsistent features (see below) |
|  | Possible UIP pattern (all three features): |
|  | Subpleural, basal predominance |
|  | Reticular abnormality |
|  | Absence of inconsistent features (see below) |
|  | Inconsistent with UIP pattern (any of these): |
|  | Upper or mid-lung predominance |
|  | Peribronchovascular predominance |
|  | Extensive ground-glass abnormality |
|  | Profuse micronodules |
|  | Discrete cysts |
|  | Diffuse mosaic attenuation/air-trapping |
|  | Consolidation in bronchopulmonary segments/lobes |

*Surgical histological findings*

Key findings:

Dense fibrosis causing remodeling of lung architecture with frequent "honeycomb" fibrosis

Fibroblastic foci typically scattered at edges of dense scars

Patchy lung involvement

Frequent subpleural and paraseptal distribution

Pertinent negative findings:

Lack of active lesions of other interstitial diseases

Lack of marked interstitial chronic inflammation

Granulomas are inconspicuous or absent

Lack of substantial inorganic dust deposits

Lack of marked eosinophilia

*Surgical histological findings*

UIP pattern (all four criteria):

Marked distortion fibrosis/architectural distortion, ± honeycombing in a predominantly subpleural/paraseptal distribution

Patchy involvement of lung parenchyma by fibrosis

Presence of fibroblastic foci

Absence of features suggesting alternate diagnosis (see below)

Probable UIP pattern:

Marked fibrosis/architectural distortion, ± honeycombing

Absence of either patchy involvement or fibroblastic foci, but not both

Absence of features suggesting alternate diagnosis

Honeycomb changes only

Possible UIP pattern (all three criteria):

Patchy or diffuse involvement of parenchyma, with or without interstitial inflammation

Absence of UIP criteria (see above)

Absence of alternate diagnosis

Not UIP pattern (any of the criteria):

Hyaline membranes

Organizing pneumonia

Granulomas

Marked interstitial inflammatory cell infiltrate away from honeycombing

Predominant airway centered changes

Features of alternate diagnosis

**Table 20.3** Combining HRCT and pathology interpretation to determine if IPF is present in the IPFnet[a]

| HRCT diagnosis | Pathology diagnosis | Diagnosis of IPF |
|---|---|---|
| Definite UIP | Definite UIP | Yes |
| Definite UIP | Probable UIP | Yes |
| Definite UIP | Possible UIP | Yes |
| Definite UIP | Not UIP | No |
| Definite UIP | Unavailable | Yes |
| Consistent with UIP | Definite UIP | Yes |
| Consistent with UIP | Probable UIP | Yes |
| Consistent with UIP | Possible UIP | No |
| Consistent with UIP | Not UIP | No |
| Consistent with UIP | Unavailable | No |
| Suggests alternative diagnosis | Any | No |

[a]Adapted from [32]

Future studies should ensure that a systematic approach to diagnostic criteria is adopted for inclusion of patients in clinical trials. A central approach that utilizes review of imaging and histopathological data enhances the likelihood that subjects will have a diagnosis that follows international guidelines, but this creates the issues of operational challenges and lesser generalizability. An approach that allows local interpretation and assessment of diagnostic criteria is easier to implement, but it will likely suffer from an increased rate of enrolling patients with inconsistent diagnoses. A hybrid model (as used by the IPFnet) is likely the best approach and utilizes intense training and retraining of local investigators (including radiologists and pathologists), central reading of primary data from the initially enrolled subjects at each site, and subsequent central reading of diagnostic tests from a random number of enrolled subjects. This approach to diagnosis in multicenter trials has proven straightforward and adaptable (Table 20.3).

## Characterization of Disease Severity in Clinical Trials

The approach to characterizing disease severity has varied in accordance with the intended target(s) of the therapeutic trial. In general, physiological severity classification includes spirometric measurement (principally FVC; forced vital capacity) and assessment of gas exchange [12]. The former has been traditionally utilized as a measure of abnormal lung compliance and may be reflective of the extent of fibroproliferation and matrix deposition [13]. A lower baseline FVC has been associated with impaired mortality in cohort studies [12] and in several clinical trials [14]. Ley and colleagues, in a three-center study, identified a decreased FVC as independently predictive of survival with thresholds of 50–75 % predicted and <50 % predicted, suggesting increasing risk of death [15]. Du Bois and colleagues examined results from two large IPF clinical trials and defined a risk prediction model for mortality at 1 year [14]. Baseline FVC was predictive in multivariate modeling (thresholds of <50, 51–65, and 66–79 % associated with progressively impaired survival). Numerous clinical trials have included FVC to confirm "milder" disease. Future clinical trials should include this measurement to provide a simple measure of physiological severity and to allow comparison to other clinical trials.

Gas exchange is most frequently assessed by recording the diffusing capacity for carbon monoxide (DLCO). This parameter tracks with the extent of parenchymal abnormality [13] as well as pulmonary vasculopathy [16]. Numerous cohort studies [12] and analyses from clinical trials [14] have suggested that lower baseline DLCO is associated with worse mortality. The work of Ley and Collard suggests that a DLCO <36–65 % predicted and ≤35 % are associated with increasing mortality [17]. Similar (but less predictive) results have been reported in the post hoc analyses of two large IPF therapeutic trials [14]. Difficulty in the interpretation of this physiological parameter is seen in the setting of IPF when coexistent emphysema is present; the DLCO is disproportionately decreased in this setting [18]. Several clinical trials have utilized DLCO thresholds to define "milder" disease (see Table 20.1), and some investigators have suggested that the composite physiological index (CPI), which includes FVC, DLCO, the $FEV_1$ and the extent of HRCT abnormality, allows a composite approach to address physiological severity in IPF patients with concomitant emphysema [19]. One recent IPF clinical trial that tested the role of sildenafil in IPF used the DLCO as a key inclusion criterion (DLCO <35 % predicted) to enrich the population for subjects who were likely to have pulmonary vasculopathy [20]. Interestingly, an independent analysis of echocardiography in this study suggested that pulmonary hypertension, as defined by increased right ventricular systolic pressure or abnormal right ventricular structure or function, was only present in a minority of study participants [21]. Despite these limitations DLCO should routinely be measured at baseline to provide additional physiological assessment.

An additional physiological measure that serves as a measure of disease severity is assessment of exercise capacity. Early studies confirmed that complex cardiopulmonary exercise testing could be used to define subjects with interstitial pneumonias at risk of poor outcome [13, 22]. A more recent cohort study using the latest diagnostic criteria for IPF confirmed that a maximal $VO_2$ less than 8.3 ml/(kg min) was independently associated with worse prognosis [23]. In an effort to utilize a simpler and more widely available measure, the 6-minute walk test has been used by numerous groups to assess disease severity. Several groups have suggested that this test is reproducible over a 1-week interval in fibrotic interstitial pneumonias [24] and that the distance walked can predict survival [25, 26]. Some groups have extended this to demonstrate that exertional desaturation portends a particularly poor prognosis [27, 28]. Although there appears to be a trough and ceiling to 6-minute walk distance [29], this parameter has generally been utilized in IPF clinical trials when the walk distance has been used as a key outcome (see Table 20.1).

As noted earlier the HRCT has been shown to be instrumental for the diagnosis of IPF, but its role for defining disease severity has proven controversial. One group has suggested that the typical HRCT features of UIP are associated with an impaired prognosis (median survival 2.08 years) compared to IPF patients with a nondiagnostic HRCT whose diagnosis was confirmed by histopathological assessment of surgical lung biopsies (median survival 5.81 years) [30]. In contrast, two other groups have not confirmed that typical HRCT features are associated with impaired survival in a clinical trial [11] or in multicenter cohorts [31]. In clinical trials that have been reported to date, HRCT is generally utilized for its diagnostic value (see Table 20.1) and not usually as a measure of disease severity. A post hoc analysis in one therapeutic trial suggested that very mild HRCT disease (<5 % honeycomb change) was associated with a beneficial response to bosentan [5]. A subsequent trial using this HRCT criterion did not confirm this beneficial effect [6]. In other therapeutic trials, HRCT has been utilized to exclude significant concomitant emphysema because of its potential confounding effect given the inclusion of an antioxidant agent in the active drug combination [32].

## Molecular Markers in Clinical Trials

Biomarkers are "characteristics that are objectively measured and evaluated as indicators of normal biological processes, pathogenic processes, or pharmacological responses to an intervention" [33]. Biomarkers may (1) define populations that respond to therapeutic interventions, (2) improve drug development, (3) predict disease progression and clinical outcomes, (4) document therapeutic effects, and (5) identify new biological pathways [34]. With regard to drug development, the Food and Drug Administration (FDA) will accept qualification of a biomarker for several specific contexts of use, including (1) to stratify patient populations, (2) for dose ranging, and (3) as a measure of disease outcome. The availability of molecular biomarkers that enhance diagnostic criteria, define individuals at risk of disease progression, and serve to define therapeutic response or disease activity could revolutionize the management of IPF patients and alter the design and conduct of clinical trials [35, 36]. The development process for these molecular biomarkers has been facilitated by regulatory actions. The FDA and the Institute of Medicine provided a clear guideline for the identification and development of relevant biomarkers. The evaluation framework includes (1) analytical validation, (2) qualification, and (3) utilization [33]. The qualification process has been facilitated by a clear guidance for industry by global regulatory authorities [37] (http://www.ema.europa.eu/ema/index.jsp?curl=pages/regulation/document_listing/document_listing_000319.jsp&murl=menus/regulations/regulations.jsp&MCID=WC0b01ac058 0022bb0#). Qualification means that regulatory bodies will accept results of clinical trial that use the biomarker within the context approved.

The development of biological markers in IPF has been the subject of much investigation, particularly circulating molecular biomarkers [35, 36]. However, diagnostic molecular biomarkers have been less robust, particularly when used to separate IPF from other diffuse parenchymal lung disorders [35]. Table 20.4 enumerates selected cohort studies that have studied a variety of circulating molecular

**Table 20.4** Selected studies of circulating molecular markers in IPF[a]

| Circulating marker | Diagnostic | Disease severity | Disease progression | Mortality | References |
|---|---|---|---|---|---|
| IL-8 | Y | FVC, TLC, DLCO, $PaO_2$ | Disease progression | – | [79] |
|  | Y | FEV1, FVC | – | – | [80] |
| KL-6 | N | – | – | Y | [81] |
|  | N | – | – | – | [82] |
|  | Y | – | – | – | [83] |
|  | Y | – | – | – | [84] |
| SP-A | N | – | – | – | [82] |
|  | Y | – | – | – | [83] |
|  | – | N | – | Y | [85] |
|  | – | N | N | Y | [86] |
|  | – | N | N | Y | [87] |
|  | Y | – | – | – | [84] |
| SP-D | Y | – | – | – | [82] |
|  | Y | – | – | – | [83] |
|  | – | – | – | – | [85] |
|  | – | N | N | Y | [86] |
|  | – | N | Δ FVC/TLC | Y | [87] |
|  | Y | – | – | – | [84] |
| MMP-1 | Y | N | – | – | [38] |
| MMP-7 | Y | FVC/DLCO | – | – | [38] |
|  | – | – | – | Y | [88] |
| CCL 18 | – | TLC, DLCO | Δ TLC | – | [89] |
|  | – | – | Δ FVC/TLC | Y | [89] |
| VEGF | – | N | Δ VC | – | [90] |
| YKL-40 | – | N | – | Y | [91] |
|  | – | DLCO, $AaDO_2$, $PaO_2$ | – | – | [92] |
| Osteopontin | N | $PaO_2$ | – | – | [93] |
| Periostin | Y | NA | Δ FVC/TLC | – | [94] |
|  | – | – | Disease progression | – | [95] |
| Napsin A | Y | FVC | – | – | [84] |
| cCK-18 | Y | – | – | – | [96] |
| CEA | – | FVC/DLCO | – | – | [97] |
| CCN2 (CTGF) | Y | – | Δ FVC | – | [98] |
| Fibrocytes | – | N | – | Y | [99] |
| CD4:CD28+ T cells | – | FVC | Δ FVC/TLC | Y | [100] |
| Regulatory T cells | Y | FVC, DLCO | Δ FVC/TLC | – | [101] |
| Semaphorin 7a+regulatory T cells | – | – | Disease progression | – | [102] |
| Red cell width | – | $FEV_1$, DLCO | – | Y | [103] |
| Blood transcriptome | Y | DLCO | – | – | [104] |

NA, not available

[a]Adapted from [36]

biomarkers in IPF. Those markers that aid in the diagnostic approach to IPF are the most limited, as the majority of series compare diseased subjects with normal controls. Rosas and colleagues applied a targeted proteomic approach and identified MMP-1 and MMP-7 among a series of circulating proteins that segregated IPF from controls and hypersensitivity pneumonitis; MMP-7 was also increased in subclinical ILD as well as patients with clinically evident IPF [38]. Further work is required to determine if such a biomarker-driven approach improves diagnostic ability in future IPF clinical trials.

The ability to define disease course in individual IPF patients would significantly enhance clinical care and improve our ability to define subjects in clinical trials who are most likely to experience disease progression. Such subjects would represent those who are most likely to benefit from therapeutic interventions, and focusing on this patient subset would improve the efficiency of clinical trials, particularly earlier phase studies. As such, there has been intensive investigation that seeks to identify molecular biomarkers in the peripheral circulation that prove to be predictive of disease course. Table 20.3 enumerates the extensive work reported in the field. It is evident that a series of circulating molecular biomarkers have been associated with varying physiological measures of disease severity, varying definitions of disease progression, and mortality. KL-6, SP-A, and SP-D have been studied for the longest time, but their acceptance has been limited by relatively small study cohorts and lack of robust replication [35]. Circulating CCL 18, YKL 40, and periostin have been related to disease progression, including mortality. Various circulating cells (including T cells, fibrocytes, and monocytes) have been associated with disease progression and/or mortality. Unfortunately, the lack of extensive validation in multiple cohorts has limited the broad acceptance of these markers in the clinical setting or in therapeutic trials, and none of these measures have been utilized as stratification or enrichment modalities in clinical trials. It is clear that a concerted approach that includes investigators, trial sponsors, and regulatory authorities is vitally important to extend these concepts and biomarker use into future clinical trials.

## Endpoints in Clinical Trials

Table 20.1 supports the increasing interest among federal and industry sponsors in supporting clinical trials of novel therapeutic approaches in IPF. Also notable is the range in endpoints utilized by the various investigative groups and the predominantly negative results of the published trials. The reasons for the negative results have been discussed by others [3, 39], but these may reflect ineffective therapies, the heterogeneity of the IPF population, or problems with the endpoints used to define treatment response. The latter has led to an ongoing debate in the published literature [2, 39–42].

There has been extensive guidance in the literature regarding the approach to defining the nature of endpoints in clinical trials. The ideal endpoint should be reliable, responsive to change in disease status, clinically meaningful, predictive of clinical outcome, and responsive to an intervention [40]. The most important characteristic of an endpoint has been suggested to be that effects on the endpoint provide "reliable evidence about whether the intervention provides clinically meaningful benefit" [43]. To extend this concept, the primary outcome measure in a definitive trial should be "a clinical event relevant to the patient" [44] or one that "measures directly how a patient feels, functions, or survives" [45]. Within this construct endpoints can be considered as primary, clinically meaningful endpoints, or surrogate endpoints [43]. The latter have been defined as outcomes that are "used as a substitute for a clinically meaningful endpoint" [45]. An abbreviated list of outcome measures characterized as a four-point hierarchy in cardiovascular, infectious disease, or pulmonary disorders is enumerated in Table 20.5.

**Table 20.5** Categorization of outcome measures, according to the level of evidence regarding efficacy in selected cardiovascular, infectious disease, and pulmonary disorders[a]

| |
| --- |
| Level 1. A true clinical efficacy measure |
| Death |
| {Death or hospitalization}, in heart failure |
| (Death, lung transplantation, or hospitalization for pulmonary arterial hypertension) in PAH |
| (Cardiovascular death, stroke, or symptomatic myocardial infarction) in acute coronary syndrome |
| (Stroke or systemic embolic event) in atrial fibrillation |
| (Cough, dyspnea, chest pain, or fever [if defined as symptomatic warmth and chills]) in community-acquired pneumonia |
| Pain at the area of skin lesions in acute bacterial skin and skin structure infections |
| Level 2. A validated surrogate (for a specific disease setting and class of interventions) (when interventions are safe, with strong evidence that risks from off-target effects are acceptable) |
| Systolic and diastolic blood pressure, in multiple classes of antihypertensives |
| >40-m improvements in 6-minute walk distance, in pulmonary arterial hypertension |
| Human immunodeficiency virus (HIV) infection, if the mechanism of the HIV prevention intervention only reduces susceptibility rather than impacting disease progression or infectiousness should infection occur |
| Level 3. A non-validated surrogate, yet one established to be "reasonably likely to predict clinical benefit" (for a specific disease setting and class of interventions when interventions are safe, with evidence that risks from off-target effects are acceptable) |
| Large and durable effects on viral load, in some treatment of HIV infection settings |
| Level 4. A correlate that is a measure of biological activity, but not established to be at a higher level |
| CD-4 in HIV-infected patients |
| Fever (if defined as elevated body temperature) in community-acquired bacterial pneumonia |
| Decolonization of vancomycin-resistant enterococcus (VRE) in the gastrointestinal tract to prevent VRE bacteremia |
| Decolonization of *Staphylococcus aureus* in preventing wound or bloodstream infections |
| Antibody levels and cell mediated immune responses in vaccines for prevention of HIV |
| $FEV_1$ and FVC, in pulmonary diseases |
| Silent myocardial infarction in cardiovascular diseases |
| Negative cultures and polymerase chain reaction tests in treating various infectious diseases |

Composite endpoints are denoted by {*brackets*}
[a]Adapted from [43]

The approach to the definition and validation of surrogate endpoints has been described by various investigators [43–45]. A guiding principle in these discussions includes the concept that "a correlate does not a surrogate make" [43]. Challenges in applying this principle include an understanding that biomarkers that are strongly correlated with clinical efficacy but are not in the causal pathway of disease processes may provide misleading information. Similarly, the multidimensionality of causal mechanisms in disease may prove challenging to the interpretation and application of surrogate endpoints. The lack of knowledge about the magnitude and duration of effect on a disease pathway required to achieve a particular effect size also limits the ability to interpret and decreases reliability of trials designed with surrogate endpoints [43]. Ideally, one would have confidence in the validity of a specific surrogate if there is a comprehensive understanding of (1) the principal pathways through which the disease process affects how a patient feels, functions, or survives; (2) the extent to which the biomarker captures "on target" effects of an intervention; and (3) the nature of "off-target" effects not captured by the biomarker [43, 46]. The application of these concepts to definition and validation of surrogate measures in IPF has proven particularly challenging. This, in part, reflects a difference of opinion as to the meaning of the term "clinically meaningful" for IPF surrogate endpoints and the level of validation required [2, 42].

It is generally accepted that improving mortality with a therapeutic intervention would be seen as a robust clinical effect [2]. In fact, one therapeutic trial has been conducted with all-cause mortality as the primary endpoint [47]. The results of this groundbreaking study definitively answered ongoing controversy at the time concerning the clinical effect and role of interferon gamma-$\gamma$ as a novel therapeutic agent for IPF. In addition, the recent IPFnet STEP study failed to meet its primary endpoint, but it approached significance on improving mortality, a predefined secondary endpoint [20]. The main difficulty in requiring mortality as the primary endpoint in future therapeutic trials in IPF reflects concerns raised by some investigators regarding the practicality of conducting such trials, particularly in patients with earlier-stage disease and lower rates of mortality events [41, 42].

Hospitalization is considered an alternate, "clinically meaningful," endpoint in IPF clinical trials [2]. The negative implications of these events are easy to interpret for patients and their caregivers. Furthermore, respiratory hospitalizations have been frequently reported in IPF patients participating in a clinical trial [48], and these events have been demonstrated to be predictive of 1-year mortality in the pooled data from two large clinical trials [14]. Critics have highlighted the limited data regarding the response to therapy of this clinical event in clinical trials and the variability in hospitalization use across a range of healthcare systems [42]. Importantly, hospitalizations have already been incorporated as primary endpoints in several clinical trials (see Table 20.1), and this endpoint has demonstrated negative treatment effects with active therapy in IPF in two recent clinical trials [32, 49].

Patient-reported outcomes (PROs) are "any report of the status of a patient's health condition that comes directly from the patient, without interpretation of the patient's response by a clinician or anyone else" [50]. As such, these parameters would be relevant to defining how a patient "feels" and would be considered clinically meaningful. Unfortunately, there are no validated PROs for use in IPF clinical trials. Two IPF-specific PROs have been developed (ATAQ-IPF and the SGRQi) but have not yet been validated for use in clinical trials [39]. Interestingly, instruments developed for use in the COPD patient population have demonstrated treatment responsiveness in an IPF therapeutic trial of sildenafil [20].

The major controversy revolves around the role of physiological tests as measures of treatment responsiveness. Some have considered these to be "clinically meaningful," [41, 42] while others have considered these to be correlates of disease severity but not validated surrogate endpoints [2]. The FVC has been the most widely used physiological measure in clinical trials (see Table 20.1). The FVC has proven to be reliable with acceptable variation over time during short-term testing in the same IPF subjects [51, 52]. Several groups have demonstrated that serial changes in FVC are predictive of mortality in the clinical setting [29, 53–55], and a 10 % decrement in this variable has proven particularly predictive. A recent analysis of data from two clinical trials supports these concepts [14, 52], and an additional analysis suggests that a relative change $\geq 10$ % was more predictive of 2-year transplant-free survival than an absolute change in FVC [56]. In addition, several groups have suggested that changes in FVC as little as 5 % are predictive of survival in IPF patients [14, 52, 57]. FVC has proven responsive in some, but not all, recent therapeutic trials (see Table 20.1), including one with a threshold of 5 % [58]. The totality of these data has compelled some to consider FVC as a "clinically meaningful" measure and an appropriate primary endpoint [41, 42].

Unfortunately, there are limitations to the use of FVC in clinical trials, which has tempered the views of other investigators [2]. The robustness of the FVC as a measure of progressive disease is highly dependent on the presence of concomitant emphysema. Several groups have demonstrated that the combination of emphysema and IPF attenuates the change in FVC over time [59] and impairs the ability of longitudinal change in FVC to predict survival [60]. The lack of consistent therapeutic responsiveness of FVC to therapy has been highlighted by the markedly different responses noted in the two CAPACITY trials comparing pirfenidone to placebo. In two recent IPFnet studies, there was a marked imbalance in mortality between active treatment and matched placebo groups with no difference in FVC change between the study groups [32, 49]. Similarly, sildenafil therapy resulted in little change in FVC in the IPFnet STEP trial, while sildenafil improved health status and symptoms, and treatment with sildenafil also showed a trend towards improved mortality [20]. These data argue against the FVC as a robust measure of therapeutic effect in the IPF patient. Although overinterpretation of the data as indicating an inability to detect a negative impact of therapy has been cautioned [41], it is notable that the deaths in the IPFnet studies were predominantly respiratory in nature, and this makes one unsure of the ability of the FVC to identify "off-target" effects of therapy in IPF patients.

The 6-minute walk distance has been advocated as a measure of functional capacity in the IPF patient [61]. As noted above, baseline distance and the presence of desaturation are predictive of mortality in clinical IPF cohorts. Longitudinal change in 6-minute walk distance and desaturation during testing has been shown to be predictive of outcomes in the clinical setting [29]. Using data from clinical trials, the minimum important difference in distance walked has been suggested to range from 28 [62] to 45 m [61]. Unfortunately, responsiveness in IPF therapeutic trials has ranged from negative [5, 20] to, at best, inconsistent benefit [63]. As noted earlier, the IPFnet sildenafil study demonstrated improvement in health status and symptoms despite showing little change in 6-minute walk distance [20].

Composite endpoints have increasingly been touted as having the potential to serve as robust alternate measures of treatment efficacy in clinical trials [40, 64]. Although this is an attractive approach, it must be noted that composites are limited by the components that comprise the endpoint. These components should be clinically meaningful as individual endpoints and have similar clinical relevance. A robust literature has developed that highlights the limitation of composites in study design, conduct, and interpretation in a variety of settings [65]. Composites have been incorporated as primary endpoints in several IPF therapeutic trials (see Table 20.1) with inconclusive results.

## Summary

Tremendous advances have occurred in understanding IPF biology and in developing promising therapeutic targets. Clinical trial design has advanced accompanied by a keen understanding of the diagnostic process among a range of clinical sites. Similarly, the approach to baseline characterization has been standardized among numerous trials. Major questions remain regarding the optimal endpoints in future clinical trials. It is likely that FVC serves as a reasonable endpoint for smaller phase II studies, particularly if biomarker strategies allow enrichment for subjects who are likely to experience disease progression over short-time frames. The optimal endpoint for pivotal, advanced-phase studies remains highly controversial with clinically meaningful endpoints favored.

## References

1. Raghu G, Collard HR, Egan JJ, Martinez FJ, Behr J, Brown KK, et al. An official ATS/ERS/JRS/ALAT statement: idiopathic pulmonary fibrosis: evidence-based guidelines for diagnosis and management. Am J Respir Crit Care Med. 2011;183(6):788–824.
2. Raghu G, Collard HR, Anstrom KJ, Flaherty KR, Fleming TR, King Jr TE, et al. Idiopathic pulmonary fibrosis: clinically meaningful primary endpoints in phase 3 clinical trials. Am J Respir Crit Care Med. 2012;185(10):1044–8.
3. Luppi F, Spagnolo P, Cerri S, Richeldi L. The big clinical trials in idiopathic pulmonary fibrosis. Curr Opin Pulm Med. 2012;18(5):428–32.
4. Travis WD, Hunninghake G, King Jr TE, Lynch DA, Colby TV, Galvin JR, et al. Idiopathic nonspecific interstitial pneumonia: report of an American Thoracic Society project. Am J Respir Crit Care Med. 2008;177(12):1338–47.

5. King Jr TE, Behr J, Brown KK, du Bois RM, Lancaster L, de Andrade JA, et al. BUILD-1: A randomized placebo-controlled trial of bosentan in idiopathic pulmonary fibrosis. Am J Respir Crit Care Med. 2008;177:75–81.

6. King Jr TE, Brown KK, Raghu G, du Bois RM, Lynch DA, Martinez F, et al. BUILD-3: A randomized, controlled trial of bosentan in idiopathic pulmonary fibrosis. Am J Respir Crit Care Med. 2011;184:92–9.

7. Flaherty KR, King Jr TE, Raghu G, Lynch 3rd JP, Colby TV, Travis WD, et al. Idiopathic interstitial pneumonia: what is the effect of a multidisciplinary approach to diagnosis? Am J Respir Crit Care Med. 2004;170(8):904–10.

8. Thomeer M, Demedts M, Behr J, Buhl R, Costabel U, Flower CD, et al. Multidisciplinary interobserver agreement in the diagnosis of idiopathic pulmonary fibrosis. Eur Respir J. 2008;31(3):585–91.

9. Flaherty KR, Andrei AC, King Jr TE, Raghu G, Colby TV, Wells A, et al. Idiopathic interstitial pneumonia: do community and academic physicians agree on diagnosis? Am J Respir Crit Care Med. 2007;175(10):1054–60.

10. Mueller-Mang C, Grosse C, Schmid K, Stiebellehner L, Bankier AA. What every radiologist should know about idiopathic interstitial pneumonias. Radiographics. 2007;27(3):595–615.

11. Lynch DA, Godwin JD, Safrin S, Starko KM, Hormel P, Brown KK, et al. High-resolution computed tomography in idiopathic pulmonary fibrosis. Diagnosis and Prognosis. Am J Respir Crit Care Med. 2005;172:488–93.

12. Ley B, Collard HR, King Jr TE. Clinical course and prediction of survival in idiopathic pulmonary fibrosis. Am J Respir Crit Care Med. 2011;183(4):431–40.

13. Fulmer J, Roberts WC, von Gal ER, Crystal RG. Morphologic-physiologic correlates of the severity of fibrosis and degree of cellularity in idiopathic pulmonary fibrosis. J Clin Invest. 1979;63:665–76.

14. Du Bois RM, Weycker D, Albera C, Bradford WZ, Costabel U, Kartashov A, et al. Ascertainment of individual risk of mortality for patients with idiopathic pulmonary fibrosis. Am J Respir Crit Care Med. 2011;184(4):459–66.

15. Ley B, Ryerson CJ, Vittinghoff E, Ryu JH, Tomassetti S, Lee JS, et al. A multidimensional index and staging system for idiopathic pulmonary fibrosis. Ann Intern Med. 2012;156(10):684–91.

16. Lama V, Martinez F. Resting and exercise physiology in interstitial lung diseases. Clin Chest Med. 2004;25:435–53.

17. Ley B, Collard HR. Risk prediction in idiopathic pulmonary fibrosis. Am J Respir Crit Care Med. 2012;185(1):6–7.

18. Fell CD. Idiopathic pulmonary fibrosis: phenotypes and comorbidities. Clin Chest Med. 2012;33(1):51–7.

19. Wells AU, Desai SR, Rubens MB, Goh NS, Cramer D, Nicholson AG, et al. Idiopathic pulmonary fibrosis: a composite physiologic index derived from disease extent observed by computed tomography. Am J Respir Crit Care Med. 2003;167(7):962–9.

20. Idiopathic Pulmonary Fibrosis Clinical Research Network, Zisman DA, Schwarz M, Anstrom KJ, Collard HR, Flaherty KR, et al. A controlled trial of sildenafil in advanced idiopathic pulmonary fibrosis. N Engl J Med. 2010;363(7):620–8.

21. Han MK, Bach DS, Hagan P, Yow E, Flaherty K, Toews GB, et al. Sildenafil preserves exercise capacity in IPF patients with right ventricular dysfunction. Chest. 2013;143(6):1699–708.

22. King Jr TE, Tooze JA, Schwarz MI, Brown KR, Cherniack RM. Predicting survival in idiopathic pulmonary fibrosis. Scoring system and survival model. Am J Respir Crit Care Med. 2001;164:1171–81.

23. Fell CD, Liu LX, Motika C, Kazerooni EA, Gross BH, Travis WD, et al. The prognostic value of cardiopulmonary exercise testing in idiopathic pulmonary fibrosis. Am J Respir Crit Care Med. 2009;179(5):402–7.

24. Eaton T, Young P, Milne D, Wells AU. Six-minute walk, maximal exercise tests: reproducibility in fibrotic interstitial pneumonia. Am J Respir Crit Care Med. 2005;171(10):1150–7.
25. Lederer DJ, Arcasoy SM, Wilt JS, D'Ovidio F, Sonett JR, Kawut SM. Six-minute-walk distance predicts waiting list survival in idiopathic pulmonary fibrosis. Am J Respir Crit Care Med. 2006;174(6):659–64.
26. Caminati A, Bianchi A, Cassandro R, Mirenda MR, Harari S. Walking distance on 6-MWT is a prognostic factor in idiopathic pulmonary fibrosis. Respir Med. 2009;103(1):117–23.
27. Lama VN, Flaherty KR, Toews GB, Colby TV, Travis WD, Long Q, et al. Prognostic value of desaturation during a 6-minute walk test in idiopathic interstitial pneumonia. Am J Respir Crit Care Med. 2003;168(9):1084–90.
28. Hallstrand TS, Boitano LJ, Johnson WC, Spada CA, Hayes JG, Raghu G. The timed walk test as a measure of severity and survival in idiopathic pulmonary fibrosis. Eur Respir J. 2005;25(1):96–103.
29. Flaherty KR, Andrei AC, Murray S, Fraley C, Colby TV, Travis WD, et al. Idiopathic pulmonary fibrosis: prognostic value of changes in physiology and six-minute-walk test. Am J Respir Crit Care Med. 2006;174(7):803–9.
30. Flaherty KR, Thwaite EL, Kazerooni EA, Gross BH, Toews GB, Colby TV, et al. Radiological versus histological diagnosis in UIP and NSIP: survival implications. Thorax. 2003;58(2):143–8.
31. Sumikawa H, Johkoh T, Colby TV, Ichikado K, Suga M, Taniguchi H, et al. Computed tomography findings in pathological usual interstitial pneumonia: relationship to survival. Am J Respir Crit Care Med. 2008;177(4):433–9.
32. The Idiopathic Pulmonary Fibrosis Clinical Research Network, Raghu G, Anstrom KJ, King Jr TE, Lasky JA, Martinez FJ. Prednisone, azathioprine, and N-acetylcysteine for pulmonary fibrosis. N Engl J Med. 2012;366:1968–77.
33. Micheel C, Ball J, editors. Evaluation of biomarkers and surrogate endpoints in chronic disease. Washington, DC: The National Academic Press; 2010.
34. Cazzola M, Novelli G. Biomarkers in COPD. Pulm Pharmacol Ther. 2010;23:493–500.
35. Zhang Y, Kaminski N. Biomarkers in idiopathic pulmonary fibrosis. Curr Opin Pulm Med. 2012;18(5):441–6.
36. Vij R, Noth I. Peripheral blood biomarkers in idiopathic pulmonary fibrosis. Transl Res. 2012;159(4):218–27.
37. Center for Drug Evaluation and Research (CDER). Qualification process for drug development tools. U.S.D.o.H.a.H. Services, editor. Rockville, MD: Food and Drug Administration; 2010.
38. Rosas IO, Richards TJ, Konishi K, Zhang Y, Gibson K, Lokshin AE, et al. MMP1 and MMP7 as potential peripheral blood biomarkers in idiopathic pulmonary fibrosis. PLoS Med. 2008;5(4):e93.
39. Olson AL, Swigris JJ, Brown KK. Clinical trials and tribulations–lessons from pulmonary fibrosis. QJM. 2012;105(11):1043–7.
40. Albera C. Challenges in idiopathic pulmonary fibrosis trials: the point on end-points. Eur Respir Rev. 2011;20(121):195–200.
41. Wells AU, Behr J, Costabel U, Cottin V, Poletti V, Richeldi L, European IPF Consensus Group. Hot of the breath: mortality as a primary end-point in IPF treatment trials: the best is the enemy of the good. Thorax. 2012;67(11):938–40.
42. du Bois RM, Nathan SD, Richeldi L, Schwarz MI, Noble PW. Idiopathic pulmonary fibrosis: lung function is a clinically meaningful endpoint for phase III trials. Am J Respir Crit Care Med. 2012;186(8):712–5.
43. Fleming TR, Powers JH. Biomarkers and surrogate endpoints in clinical trials. Stat Med. 2012;31:2973–84.
44. Fleming TR, DeMets DL. Surrogate end points in clinical trials: are we being misled? Ann Intern Med. 1996;125(7):605–13.

45. Temple R. A regulatory authority's opinion about surrogate endpoints. In: Nimmo W, Tucker G, editors. Clinical Measurement in Drug Evaluation. New York: John Wiley and Sons; 1995. p. 790.
46. Prentice RL. Surrogate endpoints in clinical trials: definition and operational criteria. Stat Med. 1989;8(4):431–40.
47. King Jr TE, Albera C, Bradford WZ, Costabel U, Hormel P, Lancaster L, et al. Effect of interferon gamma-1b on survival in patients with idiopathic pulmonary fibrosis (INSPIRE): a multicentre, randomised, placebo-controlled trial. Lancet. 2009;374:222–8.
48. Martinez FJ, Safrin S, Weycker D, Starko KM, Bradford WZ, King Jr TE, et al. The clinical course of patients with idiopathic pulmonary fibrosis. Ann Intern Med. 2005;142(12 Pt 1):963–7.
49. Noth I, Anstrom KJ, Calvert SB, de Andrade J, Flaherty KR, Glazer C, et al. A placebo-controlled randomized trial of warfarin in idiopathic pulmonary fibrosis. Am J Respir Crit Care Med. 2012;186(1):88–95.
50. Center for Drug Evaluation and Research (CDER), Center for Biologics Evaluation and Research (CBER), Center for Devices and Radiological Health (CDRH). Patient-reported outcome measures: Use in medical product development to support labeling claims. U.S.D.o.H.a.H. Services, editor. Rockville, MD: Food and Drug Administration; 2009.
51. King Jr TE, Safrin S, Starko KM, Brown KK, Noble PW, Raghu G, et al. Analyses of efficacy end points in a controlled trial of interferon-gamma1b for idiopathic pulmonary fibrosis. Chest. 2005;127(1):171–7.
52. Du Bois RM, Weycker D, Albera C, Bradford WZ, Costabel U, Kartashov A, et al. Forced vital capacity in patients with idiopathic pulmonary fibrosis: test properties and minimal clinically important difference. Am J Respir Crit Care Med. 2011;184(12):1382–9.
53. Collard HR, King Jr TE, Bartelson BB, Vourlekis JS, Schwarz MI, Brown KK. Changes in clinical and physiologic variables predict survival in idiopathic pulmonary fibrosis. Am J Respir Crit Care Med. 2003;168(5):538–42.
54. Latsi PI, du Bois RM, Nicholson AG, Colby TV, Bisirtzoglou D, Nikolakopoulou A, et al. Fibrotic idiopathic interstitial pneumonia: the prognostic value of longitudinal functional trends. Am J Respir Crit Care Med. 2003;168(5):531–7.
55. Hanson D, Winterbauer RH, Kirtland SH, Wu R. Changes in pulmonary function test results after 1 year of therapy as predictors of survival in patients with idiopathic pulmonary fibrosis. Chest. 1995;108(2):305–10.
56. Richeldi L, Ryerson CJ, Lee JS, Wolters PJ, Koth LL, Ley B, et al. Relative versus absolute change in forced vital capacity in idiopathic pulmonary fibrosis. Thorax. 2012;67(5):407–11.
57. Zappala CJ, Latsi PI, Nicholson AG, Colby TV, Cramer D, Renzoni EA, et al. Marginal decline in forced vital capacity is associated with a poor outcome in idiopathic pulmonary fibrosis. Eur Respir J. 2010;35(4):830–6.
58. Taniguchi H, Kondoh Y, Ebina M, Azuma A, Ogura T, Taguchi Y, et al. The clinical significance of 5% change in vital capacity in patients with idiopathic pulmonary fibrosis: extended analysis of the pirfenidone trial. Respir Res. 2011;12:93.
59. Akagi T, Matsumoto T, Harada T, Tanaka M, Kuraki T, Fujita M, et al. Coexistent emphysema delays the decrease of vital capacity in idiopathic pulmonary fibrosis. Respir Med. 2009;103(8):1209–15.
60. Schmidt SL, Nambiar AM, Tayob N, Sundaram B, Han MK, Gross BH, et al. Pulmonary function measures predict mortality differently in IPF versus combined pulmonary fibrosis and emphysema. Eur Respir J. 2011;38(1):176–83.
61. Du Bois RM, Weycker D, Albera C, Bradford WZ, Costabel U, Kartashov A, et al. Six-minute-walk test in idiopathic pulmonary fibrosis: test validation and minimal clinically important difference. Am J Respir Crit Care Med. 2011;183(9):1231–7.
62. Swigris JJ, Wamboldt FS, Behr J, du Bois RM, King TE, Raghu G, et al. The 6 minute walk in idiopathic pulmonary fibrosis: longitudinal changes and minimum important difference. Thorax. 2010;65(2):173–7.

63. Noble PW, Albera C, Bradford WZ, Costabel U, Glassberg MK, Kardatzke D, et al. Pirfenidone in patients with idiopathic pulmonary fibrosis (CAPACITY): two randomised trials. Lancet. 2011;377:1760–9.
64. Vancheri C, Du Bois RM. A progression-free end point for idiopathic pulmonary fibrosis trials: lessons from cancer. Eur Respir J. 2013;41(2):262–9.
65. Ferreira-Gonzalez I, Busse JW, Heels-Ansdell D, Montori VM, Akl EA, Bryant DM, et al. Problems with use of composite end points in cardiovascular trials: systematic review of randomised controlled trials. BMJ. 2007;334(7597):786.
66. Raghu G, Brown KK, Bradford WZ, Starko K, Noble PW, Schwartz DA, et al. A placebo-controlled trial of interferon gamma-1b in patients with idiopathic pulmonary fibrosis. N Engl J Med. 2004;350:125–33.
67. Strieter R, Starko KM, Enelow RI, Noth I, Valentine VG, Idiopathic Pulmonary Fibrosis Biomarkers Study Group. Effects of Interferon-γ 1b on biomarker expression in patients with idiopathic pulmonary fibrosis. Am J Respir Crit Care Med. 2004;170:133–40.
68. Azuma A, Nukiwa T, Tsuboi E, Suga M, Abe S, Nakata K, et al. Double-blind, placebo-controlled trial of pirfenidone in patients with idiopathic pulmonary fibrosis. Am J Respir Crit Care Med. 2005;171:1040–7.
69. Kubo H, Nakayama K, Yanai M, Suzuki T, Yamaya M, Watanabe M, et al. Anticoagulant therapy for idiopathic pulmonary fibrosis. Chest. 2005;128:1475–82.
70. Demedts M, Behr J, Buhl R, Costabel U, Dekhuijzen R, Jansen HM, et al. High-dose acetylcysteine in idiopathic pulmonary fibrosis. N Engl J Med. 2005;353(21):2229–42.
71. Antoniou KM, Nicholson AG, Dimadi M, Malagari K, Latsi P, Rapti A, et al. Long-term clinical effects of interferon gamma-1b and colchicine in idiopathic pulmonary fibrosis. Eur Respir J. 2006;28(3):496–504.
72. Raghu G, Brown KK, Costabel U, Cottin V, du Bois RM, Lasky JA, et al. Treatment of idiopathic pulmonary fibrosis with etanercept. An exploratory, placebo-controlled trial. Am J Respir Crit Care Med. 2008;178:948–55.
73. Daniels C, Lasky JA, Limper AH, Mieras K, Gabor E, Schroeder DR, et al. Imatinib treatment for idiopathic pulmonary fibrosis. Randomized placebo-controlled trial results. Am J Respir Crit Care Med. 2009;181:604–10.
74. Jackson R, Glassberg MK, Ramos CF, Bejarano PA, Butrous G, Gómez-Marín O. Sildenafil therapy and exercise tolerance in idiopathic pulmonary fibrosis. Lung. 2010;188:115–23.
75. Taniguchi H, Ebina M, Kondoh Y, Ogura T, Azuma A, Suga M, et al. Pirfenidone in idiopathic pulmonary fibrosis. Eur Respir J. 2010;35:821–9.
76. Richeldi L, Costabel U, Selman M, Kim DS, Hansell DM, Nicholson AG, et al. Efficacy of a tyrosine kinase inhibitor in idiopathic pulmonary fibrosis. N Engl J Med. 2011;365(12):1079–87.
77. Malouf M, Hopkins P, Snell G, Glanville AR, Everolimus in IPF Study Investigators. An investigator-driven study of everolimus in surgical lung biopsy confirmed idiopathic pulmonary fibrosis. Respirology. 2011;16(5):776–83.
78. Horton M, Santopietro V, Mathew L, Horton KM, Polito AJ, Liu MC, et al. Thalidomide for the treatment of cough in idiopathic pulmonary fibrosis. A randomized trial. Ann Intern Med. 2012;157:398–406.
79. Ziegenhagen MW, Zabel P, Zissel G, Schlaak M, Müller-Quernheim J. Serum level of interleukin 8 is elevated in idiopathic pulmonary fibrosis and indicates disease activity. Am J Respir Crit Care Med. 1998;157(3 Pt 1):762–8.
80. Tsoutsou PG, Gourgoulianis KI, Petinaki E, Germenis A, Tsoutsou AG, Mpaka M, et al. Cytokine levels in the sera of patients with idiopathic pulmonary fibrosis. Respir Med. 2006;100(5):938–45.
81. Satoh H, Kurishima K, Ishikawa H, Ohtsuka M. Increased levels of KL-6 and subsequent mortality in patients with interstitial lung diseases. J Intern Med. 2006;260(5):429–34.
82. Ohnishi H, Yokoyama A, Kondo K, Hamada H, Abe M, Nishimura K, et al. Comparative study of KL-6, surfactant protein-A, surfactant protein-D, and monocyte chemoattractant protein-1 as serum markers for interstitial lung diseases. Am J Respir Crit Care Med. 2002;165(3):378–81.

83. Ishii H, Mukae H, Kadota J, Kaida H, Nagata T, Abe K, et al. High serum concentrations of surfactant protein A in usual interstitial pneumonia compared with non-specific interstitial pneumonia. Thorax. 2003;58(1):52–7.
84. Samukawa T, Hamada T, Uto H, Yanagi M, Tsukuya G, Nosaki T, et al. The elevation of serum napsin A in idiopathic pulmonary fibrosis, compared with KL-6, surfactant protein-A and surfactant protein-D. BMC Pulm Med. 2012;12:55.
85. Kinder BW, Brown KK, McCormack FX, Ix JH, Kervitsky A, Schwarz MI, et al. Serum surfactant protein-A is a strong predictor of early mortality in idiopathic pulmonary fibrosis. Chest. 2009;135(6):1557–63.
86. Greene KE, King Jr TE, Kuroki Y, Bucher-Bartelson B, Hunninghake GW, Newman LS, et al. Serum surfactant proteins-A and -D as biomarkers in idiopathic pulmonary fibrosis. Eur Respir J. 2002;19(3):439–46.
87. Takahashi H, Fujishima T, Koba H, Murakami S, Kurokawa K, Shibuya Y, et al. Serum surfactant proteins A and D as prognostic factors in idiopathic pulmonary fibrosis and their relationship to disease extent. Am J Respir Crit Care Med. 2000;162(3 Pt 1):1109–14.
88. Richards TJ, Kaminski N, Baribaud F, Flavin S, Brodmerkel C, Horowitz D, et al. Peripheral blood proteins predict mortality in idiopathic pulmonary fibrosis. Am J Respir Crit Care Med. 2012;185(1):67–76.
89. Prasse A, Probst C, Bargagli E, Zissel G, Toews GB, Flaherty KR, et al. Serum CC-chemokine ligand 18 concentration predicts outcome in idiopathic pulmonary fibrosis. Am J Respir Crit Care Med. 2009;179(8):717–23.
90. Ando M, Miyazaki E, Ito T, Hiroshige S, Nureki SI, Ueno T, et al. Significance of serum vascular endothelial growth factor level in patients with idiopathic pulmonary fibrosis. Lung. 2010;188(3):247–52.
91. Korthagen NM, van Moorsel CH, Barlo NP, Ruven HJ, Kruit A, Heron M, et al. Serum and BALF YKL-40 levels are predictors of survival in idiopathic pulmonary fibrosis. Respir Med. 2011;105(1):106–13.
92. Furuhashi K, Suda T, Nakamura Y, Inui N, Hashimoto D, Miwa S, et al. Increased expression of YKL-40, a chitinase-like protein, in serum and lung of patients with idiopathic pulmonary fibrosis. Respir Med. 2010;104(8):1204–10.
93. Kadota J, Mizunoe S, Mito K, Mukae H, Yoshioka S, Kawakami K, et al. High plasma concentrations of osteopontin in patients with interstitial pneumonia. Respir Med. 2005;99(1):111–7.
94. Okamoto M, Hoshino T, Kitasato Y, Sakazaki Y, Kawayama T, Fujimoto K, et al. Periostin, a matrix protein, is a novel biomarker for idiopathic interstitial pneumonias. Eur Respir J. 2011;37(5):1119–27.
95. Naik PK, Bozyk PD, Bentley JK, Popova AP, Birch CM, Wilke CA, et al. Periostin promotes fibrosis and predicts progression in patients with idiopathic pulmonary fibrosis. Am J Physiol Lung Cell Mol Physiol. 2012;303(12):L1046–56.
96. Cha SI, Ryerson CJ, Lee JS, Kukreja J, Barry SS, Jones KD, et al. Cleaved cytokeratin-18 is a mechanistically informative biomarker in idiopathic pulmonary fibrosis. Respir Res. 2012;13:105.
97. Fahim A, Crooks MG, Wilmot R, Campbell AP, Morice AH, Hart SP. Serum carcinoembryonic antigen correlates with severity of idiopathic pulmonary fibrosis. Respirology. 2012;17(8):1247–52.
98. Kono M, Nakamura Y, Suda T, Kato M, Kaida Y, Hashimoto D, et al. Plasma CCN2 (connective tissue growth factor; CTGF) is a potential biomarker in idiopathic pulmonary fibrosis (IPF). Clin Chim Acta. 2011;412(23–24):2211–5.
99. Moeller A, Gilpin SE, Ask K, Cox G, Cook D, Gauldie J, et al. Circulating fibrocytes are an indicator of poor prognosis in idiopathic pulmonary fibrosis. Am J Respir Crit Care Med. 2009;179(7):588–94.
100. Gilani SR, Vuga LJ, Lindell KO, Gibson KF, Xue J, Kaminski N, et al. CD28 down-regulation on circulating CD4 T-cells is associated with poor prognoses of patients with idiopathic pulmonary fibrosis. PLoS One. 2010;5(1):e8959.

101. Kotsianidis I, Nakou E, Bouchliou I, Tzouvelekis A, Spanoudakis E, Steiropoulos P, et al. Global impairment of CD4+CD25+FOXP3+ regulatory T cells in idiopathic pulmonary fibrosis. Am J Respir Crit Care Med. 2009;179(12):1121–30.
102. Reilkoff RA, Peng H, Murray LA, Peng X, Russell T, Montgomery R, et al. Semaphorin 7a+regulatory T cells are associated with progressive idiopathic pulmonary fibrosis and are implicated in transforming growth factor-beta1-induced pulmonary fibrosis. Am J Respir Crit Care Med. 2013;187(2):180–8.
103. Nathan SD, Reffett T, Brown AW, Fischer CP, Shlobin OA, Ahmad S, et al. The red cell distribution width as a prognostic indicator in IPF. Chest. 2013;143:1692–8.
104. Yang IV, Luna LG, Cotter J, Talbert J, Leach SM, Kidd R, et al. The peripheral blood transcriptome identifies the presence and extent of disease in idiopathic pulmonary fibrosis. PLoS One. 2012;7(6):e37708.

# Chapter 21
# Future Directions in Basic and Clinical Science

**Carmen Mikacenic and Ganesh Raghu**

**Abstract** Idiopathic pulmonary fibrosis (IPF) is a fibrotic interstitial pneumonia of unclear etiology, and there is wide variability in clinical phenotype and rate of disease progression among patients who meet criteria for this diagnosis. In this chapter, we highlight the remaining challenges posed to basic and clinical researchers and discuss how these challenges might be best addressed in order to ultimately direct future care that leads to improved patient outcomes. We begin by describing avenues of future research in terms of biologic pathogenesis and genetics. From the clinical standpoint, we emphasize pathways that may lead to better classification of distinct clinical phenotypes, studies that will define more accurate clinical endpoints for clinical research, and interventions (including potentially preventive measures) that may decrease the tempo of disease progression. Lastly, novel therapies, including monoclonal antibodies in early clinical trials and regenerative strategies, are discussed. In this way, we encompass what is on the horizon for IPF research and treatment.

**Keywords** Idiopathic pulmonary fibrosis • Pathogenesis • Genetics • Biomarkers • Monoclonal antibodies • Clinical endpoint • Mesenchymal stem cells • Gastroesophageal reflux

C. Mikacenic, M.D.
Division of Pulmonary and Critical Care Medicine, University of Washington Medical Center, 1959, NE Pacific Ave, Seattle, WA 98195, USA

G. Raghu, M.D. (✉)
Division of Pulmonary and Critical Care Medicine, University of Washington Medical Center, 1959, NE Pacific Ave, Seattle, WA 98195, USA

The Center for Interstitial Lung Diseases, University of Washington Medical Center, 1959, NE Pacific Ave, Seattle, WA 98195, USA

Scleroderma Clinic, University of Washington Medical Center, 1959, NE Pacific Ave, Seattle, WA 98195, USA
e-mail: graghu@uw.edu; graghu@u.washington.edu

K.C. Meyer and S.D. Nathan (eds.), *Idiopathic Pulmonary Fibrosis: A Comprehensive Clinical Guide*, Respiratory Medicine 9, DOI 10.1007/978-1-62703-682-5_21,
© Springer Science+Business Media New York 2014

## Introduction

Idiopathic pulmonary fibrosis (IPF) is currently defined as a chronic and progressive fibrotic interstitial pneumonia of unclear etiology. In the appropriate clinical setting, a precise pattern of "definite" usual interstitial pneumonia (UIP) is a required feature in high-resolution computed tomography (HRCT) images of the lung and/or in surgical lung biopsy for an accurate diagnosis of IPF [1]. A multidisciplinary discussion among experts in interstitial lung disease (pulmonologists-radiologists-pathologists) can arrive at an accurate diagnosis using clinical and radiographic data with various combinations of defined patterns of UIP on HRCT and pathology [1].

While the recent evidence-based guidelines have provided criteria to arrive at an accurate diagnosis of IPF, the heterogeneity of the patient population that includes sporadic and familial IPF and diversity in the rate of disease progression is evident. Currently, there are no predictable biomarkers that can be reliably used in clinical practice to identify the subpopulations of patients with IPF. Efforts to further subclassify patients with distinct phenotypes and to enhance diagnostic specificity are warranted. This will be largely dependent on further understanding of the pathogenesis of the disease, how environmental and genetic factors confer risk to disease development, and how these variables affect prognosis. On the basis of this knowledge, new treatment strategies may be developed for a disease in which the median survival is only 2–3 years from the time of diagnosis with the limited current management options [2]. In this chapter, we discuss prospects to pursue future avenues for both basic science and clinical science research with the hopes of enhancing clinical management and improving outcomes for patients with IPF.

## New Directions in Basic Science: Disease Pathogenesis and Genetics

The pathologic hallmark of IPF, usual interstitial pneumonia (UIP), is characterized by temporal heterogeneity of histologic abnormalities with the abrupt transition of fibrosis, sub-epithelial fibrotic foci, and microscopic honeycombing to adjacent areas of normal pulmonary parenchyma. This occurs mainly in the sub-pleural areas, especially in the lower lobes. Often the fibrotic foci are made up of activated myofibroblasts and are located adjacent to areas of apparent epithelial damage. This has led to the hypothesis that recurrent micro-injuries to the epithelial barrier of the alveolar wall trigger aberrant mesenchymal changes leading to fibrosis and loss of gas exchange units. Restoration of the structural integrity and functional status of the alveolar wall requires epithelial cell regeneration, remodeling of the basement membrane of the alveolar wall in the damaged lung, switching the proliferating mesenchymal cells to quiescent stages of the cell cycle, decreasing synthesis of extracellular matrix, and degrading the excessive extracellular matrix deposited in the pulmonary parenchyma. From our perspective, we believe that considering

IPF as a neo-proliferative disorder of the lung will provide a platform for fruitful scientific research that will lead to the development of novel anti-fibrotic agents for patients with this devastating disease. Indeed, IPF and cancer both share fundamental pathogenic hallmarks including genetic alterations, response to growth and inhibitory signals, resistance to apoptosis, myofibroblast origin and behavior, altered cellular communications, and intracellular signaling pathways [3].

## Genetics

Recent genetic approaches have been focused on large-scale unbiased association studies to identify genes that may affect risk and epigenetic changes that may represent lasting genetic modifications of environmental exposure. The future lies in validation of these genetic markers, understanding the mechanisms behind their associations, and further development of epigenetics as a method that leads to a better understanding of the interaction between genes and the environment.

Genetic associations with the development of sporadic IPF thus far are few and include *TERT* mutations and *MUC5B* [4, 5]. Genome-wide association studies to identify genes important to the development of IPF have thus far been underpowered and the mechanisms of the associations only putative. Future studies should include genome-wide association studies with larger sample sizes to facilitate and enhance the detection of significant gene aberrations. Additionally, exome sequencing could be employed, since this technology sequences only the coding regions of the genome and enhances the ability to capture lower frequency variants that may have larger effects.

In addition to more detailed genetic studies, the future of understanding gene-environment interactions may rely on epigenetics. Epigenetic regulation takes place with changes in DNA methylation, histone modification, or microRNA (miRNA) expression that can lead to heritable changes without causing changes in DNA content. However, environmental factors can also result in epigenetic changes that are long lasting and may lead to changes in gene expression. To date, two large epigenetic studies in an IPF population have found several genes with differential methylation [6, 7]. However, there was no significant overlap in gene methylation patterns between the two studies. Future research must focus on whether there are notable changes in corresponding gene expression and how this mechanistically relates to the pathogenesis of IPF.

## Myofibroblast Origin and Behavior

The activated myofibroblast drives extracellular matrix deposition and remodeling, which is key to the pathogenesis and pathobiology of IPF. Understanding which cells transition to this damaging phenotype is important to our understanding of the basic biology of IPF. Importantly, preventing or reversing this transition could provide a therapeutic strategy for IPF patients. There is evidence that a diversity of cell types may contribute to the activated myofibroblasts in these fibroblastic foci, including alveolar epithelial cells, mesenchymal cells, mesothelial cells, and circulating stem cells [8].

Alveolar epithelial cells may be a source of activated myofibroblasts through a process called epithelial-mesenchymal transition (EMT). While in vitro data are strong, studies in vivo have yet to show that alveolar epithelial cells can acquire a full mesenchymal phenotype. Further research will need to delineate whether type I or type II alveolar epithelial cells have differing transitional potential, which may depend, at least in part, on variable mesenchymal gene expression amongst the alveolar epithelial cells. Additional studies will also need to address whether these cell types occur in vivo in IPF patients.

Mesenchymal cells themselves may take on a more aggressive phenotype. Patients with IPF have been found to have an invasive fibroblast present that was dependent on the hyaluronan-producing enzyme, hyaluronan synthase 2 (HAS2) [9]. While this is one potential mechanism, other means by which mesenchymal cells may be activated or induced into a more proliferative and invasive phenotype are not known. Another type of mesenchymal cell, the pericyte, may play a role in IPF. Pericytes have been more extensively studied in kidney fibrosis, where they are felt to be a major source of collagen production. Future research is needed to better characterize this cell type and explore its role in IPF.

Given the sub-pleural location of fibrosis in UIP, the ability of mesothelial cells to contribute to the activated myofibroblast population is currently under investigation. These pleural-derived cells are able to migrate into lung parenchyma, and sections of lung from IPF patients show mesothelial cells in fibrotic areas [10]. Future research will need to validate and further delineate to what extent this cell type plays a mechanistic role in the development of pulmonary fibrosis.

Much of our understanding described above has been derived from studies using bleomycin-induced lung injury models in mice or rats. While it is well recognized that bleomycin-induced "pulmonary fibrosis" is by no means a model for IPF, one of the essential future avenues of research will be to establish an improved model that demonstrates histological features of UIP. This should incorporate new knowledge of genetic susceptibility and include the use of aging mice or, potentially, aged relaxin-deficient mice, which acquire a phenotype that is similar to IPF [11]. In this way, future research efforts can be focused on a model of pathogenesis that more closely mimics human disease, thereby enhancing its relevance.

## Altered Signaling Pathways and Gene Expression

One of the interesting recent discoveries in IPF pathogenesis has been the recognition of reactivation of developmental signaling pathways—again mimicking cancer biology. These pathways include Sonic hedgehog (SHH) [12], Notch [13, 14], and

Wingless protein (Wnt) [15], which are all variably involved in lung development. Activation of these pathways has been suggested to contribute to the pathologic processes of fibroblast activation and EMT. Although these signaling pathways are complex, further delineation of which facets of these pathways lead to accumulating fibrosis will be important and may lead to additional therapeutic targets.

Additionally, soluble mediators of fibrosis have been discovered and have led to the development of new therapeutic targets. Lysophosphatidic acid (LPA) is one of these soluble mediators that inhibits apoptosis in fibroblasts and mediates fibroblast recruitment [16, 17]. Another soluble mediator, lysyl oxidase-like 2 (LOXL2), is an amine oxidase that participates in cross-linking of the extracellular matrix components, collagen, and elastin. A monoclonal antibody to LOXL2 has been shown to inhibit lung fibrosis in mice [18]. Connective tissue growth factor (CTGF) is a peptide mitogen that promotes the production and deposition of collagen and fibronectin. Bronchoalveolar lavage cells from patients with idiopathic pulmonary fibrosis showed higher expression of CTGF as compared to controls, while CTGF has also been shown to accumulate in murine bleomycin models [19, 20]. Lastly, serotonin induces fibroblast proliferation via its receptors specific to the lung [21]. Dissecting the roles of these mediators is key to future research, as they make excellent potential therapeutic targets that might modify the activation and recruitment of fibroblasts and extracellular matrix deposition. Humanized monoclonal antibodies to LPA, LOXL2, and CTGF are in clinical development and are discussed further in the treatment section below.

Altered intracellular signaling may also be affected by miRNAs. These are very small, noncoding RNAs that regulate the translation of messenger RNAs (mRNAs) by translational suppression or transcript degradation. In IPF, several miRNAs have been associated with the modulation of fibrosis by either enhancing [22, 23] or suppressing the fibrotic process [24, 25]. Whole lung tissue RNA samples comparing 10 IPF patients and control subjects on a miRNA microarray showed that 18 miRNAs were significantly decreased in IPF [22]. These authors showed that one of these miRNAs, let-7D, was downregulated by TGF-β(beta). Additionally, inhibition of let-7D led to increases in multiple mesenchymal markers, and in vivo inhibition of let-7D caused alveolar septal thickening and increases in collagen, ACTA2, and S100A4 expression in an alveolar epithelial cell line. Other miRNAs have been shown to be decreased in IPF fibroblasts and to negatively regulate fibrosis, including miR-200 and miR-31 [24, 25]. These studies suggest that miRNAs may be important regulators of many of the pathways known to be involved in IPF, and further insight into their effects may also lead to novel therapeutic possibilities.

## Altered Cellular Communication

Integrins are transmembrane glycoprotein receptors that mediate adhesion to a variety of extracellular matrix proteins. One of these integrins is α(alpha)Vβ6, which is expressed by lung epithelial cells and induces TGF-β in cultured lung epithelial cells [26]. A monoclonal antibody against αVβ6 has been shown to prevent radiation-induced pulmonary fibrosis [27] and to reduce bleomycin-induced collagen deposition [28]. Interestingly, knockout mice for the β(beta)6 subunit have enhanced pulmonary inflammation in response to bleomycin [26]. Targeting αVβ6 as a therapeutic strategy is currently under investigation in IPF clinical trials.

One of the yet unstudied pathways in IPF pathogenesis is the ability of ongoing cellular damage to seemingly evade the adaptive immune response, which is similar to a neoplastic state. T regulatory cells, a lymphocyte key to immune homeostasis, have been shown to be impaired in limiting inflammation when obtained from BAL fluid from patients with IPF [29], and there is also evidence that extracellular matrix components can modulate T regulatory cell responses [30, 31]. Additionally, circulating CD4[+] T cells with downregulated CD28 [32] have been associated with a poor prognosis in IPF. Potentially harnessing the immune response to detect aberrant matrix production could lead to future therapeutic strategies, but research in this area has yet to be pursued.

# New Directions in Clinical Science of IPF: Clinical Management

## Diagnosis and Identification of Phenotypes

There are relatively new data suggesting that serum proteins and peripheral blood cell populations may be able to detect disease risk, onset, and progression, although these have not yet been validated in clinical populations. Not only would the identification of accurate biomarkers be an advance for patient care, it would offer the possibility for monitoring disease progression or potentially provide a surrogate endpoint in research studies. The biomarkers established thus far as candidates can be separated into those that identify disease susceptibility, facilitate diagnosis, or provide a prognosis. Ideally, useful and validated biomarkers could be used in the future to more accurately predict slow progressors versus rapid decliners as well as to identify those at high risk to have an acute exacerbation of IPF.

## Biomarkers: Personalized Molecular Approaches with Signature Signals

Biomarkers that provide signatures for the presence of IPF have been found when these patients are compared to healthy control subjects. However, many of these proteins are also increased in smokers and other forms of ILD, which limits their utility. To truly identify a signature for IPF or subcategorize patients with IPF, it may be necessary to combine serum markers with genetic or expression profiles.

One example of this next-generation approach using proteomics found a protein signature to distinguished IPF from other lung diseases, including COPD, sarcoidosis, and hypersensitivity pneumonitis [33]. The proteins MMP-8, IGFBP-1 and TNFRSA1F, MMP-1, and MMP-7 were identified as part of this protein signature [33]. Using combinations of these biomarkers and clinical factors may help with prognostication for individual patients. For example, one study combined MMP-7 levels with gender, % predicted FVC, and % predicted diffusion capacity for carbon monoxide (DLCO) to create a personal clinical and molecular mortality prediction index that had a C-index for early mortality of 84 [34]. It will be essential to study these biomarkers longitudinally in patients over time, as these proteins may or may not be related to the pathology of IPF and may not fluctuate appropriately with disease activity.

In an attempt to find biomarkers that can differentiate individuals with stable disease versus progressive disease, gene expression profiles using both transcriptome and targeted approaches have been used. The first transcriptome was developed by comparing lung biopsies at the time of IPF diagnosis between those with stable disease versus progressive disease [35]. This study was able to develop a molecular signature, but given the small sample size of original subjects used to develop the signature and the small number of subjects in an independent cohort used to test the signature, the utility remains unknown. Another transcriptome was developed using gene expression profiles from peripheral blood RNA collected from IPF patients with mild or severe disease and healthy controls [36]. When severity of disease was classified as % predicted DLCO, 13 differentially expressed gene transcripts were found. Again, utility of this signature requires future validation in larger cohorts. Using a more targeted approach, Toll-like receptor 9 (TLR9) expression was studied on the basis of its ability to promote myofibroblast differentiation in lung fibroblasts cultured from biopsies of patients with IPF [37]. TLR9 expression distinguished between rapidly versus slowly progressive forms of IPF. These studies suggest that differential expression of genes in IPF patients may predict disease progression. However, for clinical utility, larger cohorts will need to be studied in a longitudinal manner with validation in independent patient populations.

## Monitoring and Assessment of Treatment Response by Clinically Meaningful Endpoints for Phase III Clinical Trials

Ideally, a clinically meaningful endpoint should directly measure how a patient feels, functions, or survives [38]. For IPF, measures of patient-related outcomes, such as quality of life or how the patient perceives and reports his or her own symptoms (e.g., dyspnea/cough), are not frequently incorporated into clinical studies. Much of this may be because tools to measure these outcomes that are specific for IPF patients have not been validated. Because this is fundamental to our ability to improve the quality of a patient's life, these tools should be developed and validated in the near future.

In terms of functional assessment of IPF patients, the 6-minute walk distance (6MWD) has been used in some clinical trials. However, the variability in conducting this test amongst various treatment centers is a problem and limits its practical use as a meaningful endpoint. An absolute need to develop surrogate endpoints for a clinically meaningful endpoint such as survival continues to persist for this patient population. However, simple correlation of a surrogate endpoint with a clinical endpoint is not adequate. Validation requires evidence that an intervention on the clinically meaningful endpoint is reliably predicted by the effect of the intervention on the surrogate endpoint. For example, it is unknown if improvement in FVC, a frequently used endpoint, reliably predicts decreased hospitalization, and this is a topic that is highly debated [39, 40]. For this reason, validation of novel surrogates that accurately predict meaningful clinical effects are necessary for the future of clinical trials and IPF research in general.

In essence, combinations of biomarkers, clinical measures, and patient-reported outcomes will be the key to the future for patients and clinical researchers to best assess meaningful predictors of prognosis. Development of accurate quality of life and other patient-reported measures and validation of surrogate endpoints are key to the future of clinical IPF research.

# Novel Treatment Strategies

Idiopathic pulmonary fibrosis is characterized by distortion of the pulmonary architecture and lung destruction. Treatment strategies, therefore, typically aim to arrest disease progression rather than to restore the lung to its normal architecture and function (Fig. 21.1). In the future, we should focus on taking a more personalized treatment approach that is based upon an improved understanding of genetics, the identification of truly useful biomarkers, and devising regenerative strategies.

## *Novel Monoclonal Antibodies*

Monoclonal antibodies may provide a patient-specific approach and are therefore an exciting future therapeutic direction. There are currently several monoclonal antibodies that are being studied in patients with IPF including anti-IL13, anti-CCL2, and anti-TGF-beta. Other novel targets for monoclonal antibodies in IPF have been found and are under investigation (including antibodies against LOXL2, CTGF, and αVβ6).

A monoclonal antibody against the LOXL2 is in early stages of entry into the pharmacologic pipeline. This enzyme cross-links collagen and has been shown to be upregulated in IPF [18] as well as in fibrotic liver diseases [41]. In a murine model, a monoclonal antibody against LOXL2 can attenuate fibrosis due to bleomycin injury [18]. A phase I trial in IPF is currently underway with this monoclonal

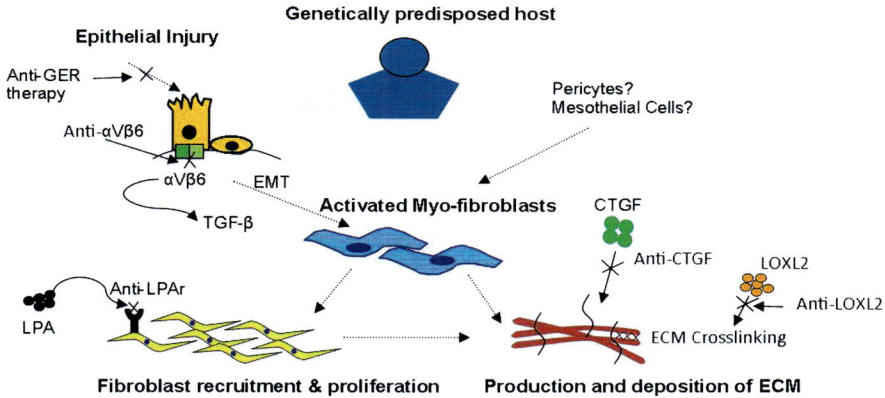

**Fig. 21.1** Future directions in IPF therapy: concepts in modulating some pathways in the pathogenesis and therapeutic strategies. In a genetically predisposed host, recurrent epithelial and basement membrane injury activates cells to produce proinflammatory and pro-fibrogenic molecules (TGF-β). Via epithelial–mesenchymal (EMT) transition or from other cell sources, activated myofibroblasts form aggregates of fibrotic foci with fibroblast recruitment, proliferation, and deposition of extracellular matrix (ECM). Anti-gastroesophageal reflux (GER) therapy or monoclonal antibodies to the integrin αVβ6, lysophosphatidic acid receptor (LIPAr), lysl oxidase-like-2 (LOXL2), and connective tissue growth factor (CTGF) may interrupt these pathogenic processes

antibody (GS-6624), to determine safety and pharmacologic properties in adult subjects (NCT01362231).

Connective tissue growth factor (CTGF), a peptide that promotes the production and deposition of collagen and fibronectin, is a relatively new target for therapy. A monoclonal antibody to CTGF has been studied in other fibrotic diseases and is now under study in IPF for safety, pharmacokinetics, and biologic activity (NCT00074698).

The integrin, αVβ6, which is highly expressed by lung epithelial cells in a state of inflammation and known to promote fibrosis, provides another novel therapeutic target [26, 27]. It is hoped that the recently initiated and ongoing phase II clinical trial using humanized monoclonal antibody against αVβ6, STX-100, will yield useful biomarkers and clinical signals that lead to phase III clinical trials. Ideally, targeting this pathway will modulate the pathobiology of IPF and improve outcomes that are clinically meaningful for patients with the disease (NCT01371305).

## Regenerative Strategies

In the fibrotic lung, the use of stem cell populations to regenerate normal, functional lung tissue is a desirable future treatment option. One of the most studied cell populations is mesenchymal stem cells (MSCs) originating from multiple tissues including bone marrow, adipose tissue, and cord blood. These cells are pleiotropic and also bear immunomodulatory properties. The ability of MSCs to fully differentiate into alveolar epithelial cells remains a subject of debate [42]. In murine studies, the ability of bone marrow-derived MSCs and cord blood MSCs to attenuate experimentally induced lung injury has been shown on multiple occasions [43–45]. However, it is unknown whether it is the immunomodulatory effects of the MSCs or the MSCs ability to differentiate that explains this attenuation.

Importantly, the safe delivery of MSCs to patients with idiopathic pulmonary fibrosis has not been demonstrated. Trials in patients with graft-versus host disease, multiple sclerosis, and Crohn's disease have suggested both safety and efficacy [46–48]. Clearly, the ability to repair and restore normal lung epithelium would be ideal, and this possibility will continue to drive future research.

## *Preventive Measures: Gastroesophageal Reflux*

Abnormal gastroesophageal reflux (GER) is highly prevalent in patients with idiopathic pulmonary fibrosis, and notably the majority of these patients have asymptomatic GER [49, 50]. Mechanistically, abnormal GER via chronic tracheobronchial aspiration is thought to induce the pathologic changes common in IPF. Animal models of gastric aspiration support this hypothesis. Furthermore, a retrospective cohort study of IPF patients suggests that the use of anti-reflux medications or fundoplication not only is associated with prolonged stabilization and lower radiologic fibrosis scores but also independently predicts survival time in patients with IPF [50, 51].

Further understanding of the pathologic mechanisms of GER is important, as this may help direct future treatment strategies. It is not known whether GER contributes to the profibrotic phenotype of alveolar epithelial and mesenchymal cells and/or contributes to epithelial-mesenchymal transition in IPF. Additionally, GER includes acidic and alkaline components as well as pepsin, *Helicobacter pylori*, and bile salts. How these various components might modify the development of fibrosis is unknown. Recent studies have demonstrated the presence of pepsin in bronchoalveolar lavage fluid obtained from patients manifesting acute exacerbations of IPF [52]. Therefore, microaspiration has been implicated in the pathogenesis of IPF as well as acute exacerbation of the disease [53].

Future clinical studies should be directed at the correlation of molecular markers of GER, including pepsin, *Helicobacter pylori*, and bile salts with differential gene expression in airway epithelial cells from patients with IPF. This might enable the identification of a molecular signature reflecting airway epithelial cell dysfunction. Importantly, human studies will need to address whether GER and the treatment of GER modulates established molecular biomarkers of IPF disease activity.

Antiacid treatment in patients with IPF epitomizes a well-known aphorism in medicine: "prevention is better than the cure." Most drugs being tested in IPF aim to slow disease progression by targeting fibroproliferation, synthesis, and deposition of extracellular matrix in the lung. In addition, most clinical trials in IPF have not demonstrated any beneficial effect on clinically meaningful outcomes such as acute exacerbations. Treatment with antiacid therapy, if effective, would be unique in that its presumed mechanism of action would be through the prevention of further insults to the IPF lung, which may be due to the attenuation of an important stimulus that can promote a fibroproliferative response. Future prospective clinical trials of anti-reflux therapies, both medical and surgical by Nissen fundoplication, should directly address whether treatment will improve survival in IPF.

## Summary

In summary, the future of IPF should be focused on better delineation of subcategories of patients so that we can best address how to improve both the quality and duration of life. In the not so distant future, our goal should be to direct the care of our patients with an integrated approach using information regarding their genetic predisposition, comorbid conditions including GER, and serum biomarker levels. We should aim to prevent manifestations of IPF in genetically susceptible individuals with measures such as avoiding exposures to known extrinsic environmental factors and/or intrinsic environmental factors such as silent GER and microaspiration. Ideally, by using novel information from genetics and biomarkers, we will be able to subcategorize IPF patients who may respond to specific targeted therapies with monoclonal antibodies. There is reason to be optimistic that significant progress will soon be made at both the bench and the bedside and that effective treatments will be discovered and made available to improve outcomes for patients with this devastating disease.

## References

1. Raghu G, Collard HR, Egan JJ, Martinez FJ, Behr J, Brown KK, et al. An official ATS/ERS/ JRS/ALAT statement: idiopathic pulmonary fibrosis: evidence-based guidelines for diagnosis and management. Am J Respir Crit Care Med. 2011;183:788–824.
2. Bjoraker JA, Ryu JH, Edwin MK, Myers JL, Tazelaar HD, Schroeder DR, et al. Prognostic significance of histopathologic subsets in idiopathic pulmonary fibrosis. Am J Respir Crit Care Med. 1998;157:199–203.
3. Vancheri C, Failla M, Crimi N, Raghu G. Idiopathic pulmonary fibrosis: a disease with similarities and links to cancer biology. Eur Respir J. 2010;35:496–504.
4. Mushiroda T, Wattanapokayakit S, Takahashi A, Nukiwa T, Kudoh S, Ogura T, et al. A genome-wide association study identifies an association of a common variant in TERT with susceptibility to idiopathic pulmonary fibrosis. J Med Genet. 2008;45:654–6.
5. Seibold MA, Wise AL, Speer MC, Steele MP, Brown KK, Loyd JE, et al. A common MUC5B promoter polymorphism and pulmonary fibrosis. N Engl J Med. 2011;364:1503–12.
6. Rabinovich EI, Kapetanaki MG, Steinfeld I, Gibson KF, Pandit KV, Yu G, et al. Global methylation patterns in idiopathic pulmonary fibrosis. PLoS One. 2012;7:e33770.
7. Sanders YY, Ambalavanan N, Halloran B, Zhang X, Liu H, Crossman DK, et al. Altered DNA methylation profile in idiopathic pulmonary fibrosis. Am J Respir Crit Care Med. 2012;186: 525–35.

8. Fernandez IE, Eickelberg O. New cellular and molecular mechanisms of lung injury and fibrosis in idiopathic pulmonary fibrosis. Lancet. 2012;380:680–8.

9. Li Y, Jiang D, Liang J, Meltzer EB, Gray A, Miura R, et al. Severe lung fibrosis requires an invasive fibroblast phenotype regulated by hyaluronan and CD44. J Exp Med. 2011;208:1459–71.

10. Mubarak KK, Montes-Worboys A, Regev D, Nasreen N, Mohammed KA, Faruqi I, et al. Parenchymal trafficking of pleural mesothelial cells in idiopathic pulmonary fibrosis. Eur Respir J. 2012;39:133–40.

11. Samuel CS, Zhao C, Bathgate RA, Bond CP, Burton MD, Parry LJ, et al. Relaxin deficiency in mice is associated with an age-related progression of pulmonary fibrosis. FASEB J. 2003;17:121–3.

12. Fitch PM, Howie SEM, Wallace WAH. Oxidative damage and TGF-β differentially induce lung epithelial cell sonic hedgehog and tenascin-C expression: implications for the regulation of lung remodelling in idiopathic interstitial lung disease. Int J Exp Pathol. 2011;92:8–17.

13. Aoyagi-Ikeda K, Maeno T, Matsui H, Ueno M, Hara K, Aoki Y, et al. Notch induces myofibroblast differentiation of alveolar epithelial cells via transforming growth factor-{beta}-Smad3 pathway. Am J Respir Cell Mol Biol. 2011;45:136–44.

14. Liu T, Hu B, Choi YY, Chung M, Ullenbruch M, Yu H, et al. Notch1 signaling in FIZZ1 induction of myofibroblast differentiation. Am J Pathol. 2009;174:1745–55.

15. Van der Velden JL, Guala AS, Leggett SE, Sluimer J, Badura EC, Janssen-Heininger YM, et al. Induction of a mesenchymal expression program in lung epithelial cells by wingless protein (Wnt)/β-catenin requires the presence of c-Jun N-terminal kinase-1 (JNK1). Am J Respir Cell Mol Biol. 2012;47:306–14.

16. Fang X, Yu S, LaPushin R, Lu Y, Furui T, Penn LZ, et al. Lysophosphatidic acid prevents apoptosis in fibroblasts via G(i)-protein-mediated activation of mitogen-activated protein kinase. Biochem J. 2000;352(Pt 1):135–43.

17. Tager AM, LaCamera P, Shea BS, Campanella GS, Selman M, Zhao Z, et al. The lysophosphatidic acid receptor LPA1 links pulmonary fibrosis to lung injury by mediating fibroblast recruitment and vascular leak. Nat Med. 2008;14:45–54.

18. Barry-Hamilton V, Spangler R, Marshall D, McCauley S, Rodriguez HM, Oyasu M, et al. Allosteric inhibition of lysyl oxidase-like-2 impedes the development of a pathologic microenvironment. Nat Med. 2010;16:1009–17.

19. Allen JT, Knight RA, Bloor CA, Spiteri MA. Enhanced insulin-like growth factor binding protein-related protein 2 (Connective tissue growth factor) expression in patients with idiopathic pulmonary fibrosis and pulmonary sarcoidosis. Am J Respir Cell Mol Biol. 1999;21:693–700.

20. Lasky JA, Ortiz LA, Tonthat B, Hoyle GW, Corti M, Athas G, et al. Connective tissue growth factor mRNA expression is upregulated in bleomycin-induced lung fibrosis. Am J Physiol. 1998;275:L365–71.

21. Königshoff M, Dumitrascu R, Udalov S, Amarie OV, Reiter R, Grimminger F, et al. Increased expression of 5-hydroxytryptamine2A/B receptors in idiopathic pulmonary fibrosis: a rationale for therapeutic intervention. Thorax. 2010;65:949–55.

22. Pandit KV, Corcoran D, Yousef H, Yarlagadda M, Tzouvelekis A, Gibson KF, et al. Inhibition and role of let-7d in idiopathic pulmonary fibrosis. Am J Respir Crit Care Med. 2010;182:220–9.

23. Milosevic J, Pandit K, Magister M, Rabinovich E, Ellwanger DC, Yu G, et al. Profibrotic role of miR-154 in pulmonary fibrosis. Am J Respir Cell Mol Biol. 2012;47(6):879–87. doi:10.1165/rcmb.2011-0377OC.

24. Yang S, Banerjee S, de Freitas A, Sanders YY, Ding Q, Matalon S, et al. Participation of miR-200 in pulmonary fibrosis. Am J Pathol. 2012;180:484–93.

25. Yang S, Xie N, Cui H, Banerjee S, Abraham E, Thannickal VJ, et al. miR-31 is a negative regulator of fibrogenesis and pulmonary fibrosis. FASEB J. 2012;26:3790–9.

26. Munger JS, Huang X, Kawakatsu H, Griffiths MJ, Dalton SL, Wu J, et al. The integrin alpha v beta 6 binds and activates latent TGF beta 1: a mechanism for regulating pulmonary inflammation and fibrosis. Cell. 1999;96:319–28.

27. Puthawala K, Hadjiangelis N, Jacoby SC, Bayongan E, Zhao Z, Yang Z, et al. Inhibition of integrin alpha(v)beta6, an activator of latent transforming growth factor-beta, prevents radiation-induced lung fibrosis. Am J Respir Crit Care Med. 2008;177:82–90.
28. Horan GS, Wood S, Ona V, Li DJ, Lukashev ME, Weinreb PH, et al. Partial inhibition of integrin alpha(v)beta6 prevents pulmonary fibrosis without exacerbating inflammation. Am J Respir Crit Care Med. 2008;177:56–65.
29. Kotsianidis I, Nakou E, Bouchliou I, Tzouvelekis A, Spanoudakis E, Steiropoulos P, et al. Global impairment of CD4+CD25+FOXP3+ regulatory T cells in idiopathic pulmonary fibrosis. Am J Respir Crit Care Med. 2009;179:1121–30.
30. Bollyky PL, Falk BA, Wu RP, Buckner JH, Wight TN, Nepom GT. Intact extracellular matrix and the maintenance of immune tolerance: high molecular weight hyaluronan promotes persistence of induced CD4+CD25+ regulatory T cells. J Leukoc Biol. 2009;86:567–72.
31. Bollyky PL, Lord JD, Masewicz SA, Evanko SP, Buckner JH, Wight TN, et al. Cutting edge: high molecular weight hyaluronan promotes the suppressive effects of CD4+CD25+ regulatory T cells. J Immunol. 2007;179:744–7.
32. Gilani SR, Vuga LJ, Lindell KO, Gibson KF, Xue J, Kaminski N, et al. CD28 down-regulation on circulating CD4 T-cells is associated with poor prognoses of patients with idiopathic pulmonary fibrosis. PLoS One. 2010;5:e8959.
33. Rosas IO, Richards TJ, Konishi K, Zhang Y, Gibson K, Lokshin AE, et al. MMP1 and MMP7 as potential peripheral blood biomarkers in idiopathic pulmonary fibrosis. PLoS Med. 2008;5:e93.
34. Richards TJ, Kaminski N, Baribaud F, Flavin S, Brodmerkel C, Horowitz D, et al. Peripheral blood proteins predict mortality in idiopathic pulmonary fibrosis. Am J Respir Crit Care Med. 2012;185:67–76.
35. Boon K, Bailey NW, Yang J, Steel MP, Groshong S, Kervitsky D, et al. Molecular phenotypes distinguish patients with relatively stable from progressive idiopathic pulmonary fibrosis (IPF). PLoS One. 2009;4:e5134.
36. Yang IV, Luna LG, Cotter J, Talbert J, Leach SM, Kidd R, et al. The peripheral blood transcriptome identifies the presence and extent of disease in idiopathic pulmonary fibrosis. PLoS One. 2012;7:e37708.
37. Trujillo G, Meneghin A, Flaherty KR, Sholl LM, Myers JL, Kazerooni EA, et al. TLR9 differentiates rapidly from slowly progressing forms of idiopathic pulmonary fibrosis. Sci Transl Med. 2010;2:57ra82.
38. Raghu G, Collard HR, Anstrom KJ, Flaherty KR, Fleming TR, King Jr TE, et al. Idiopathic pulmonary fibrosis: clinically meaningful primary endpoints in phase 3 clinical trials. Am J Respir Crit Care Med. 2012;185:1044–8.
39. Du Bois RM, Nathan SD, Richeldi L, Schwarz MI, Noble PW. Idiopathic pulmonary fibrosis: lung function is a clinically meaningful endpoint for phase III trials. Am J Respir Crit Care Med. 2012;186:712–5.
40. Wells AU, Behr J, Costabel U, Cottin V, Poletti V, Richeldi L, European IPF Consensus Group. Hot of the breath: mortality as a primary end-point in IPF treatment trials: the best is the enemy of the good. Thorax. 2012;67:938–40.
41. Vadasz Z, Kessler O, Akiri G, Gengrinovitch S, Kagan HM, Baruch Y, et al. Abnormal deposition of collagen around hepatocytes in Wilson's disease is associated with hepatocyte specific expression of lysyl oxidase and lysyl oxidase like protein-2. J Hepatol. 2005;43:499–507.
42. Tzouvelekis A, Antoniadis A, Bouros D. Stem cell therapy in pulmonary fibrosis. Curr Opin Pulm Med. 2011;17:368–73.
43. Moodley Y, Atienza D, Manuelpillai U, Samuel CS, Tchongue J, Ilancheran S, et al. Human umbilical cord mesenchymal stem cells reduce fibrosis of bleomycin-induced lung injury. Am J Pathol. 2009;175:303–13.
44. Gupta N, Su X, Popov B, Lee JW, Serikov V, Matthay MA. Intrapulmonary delivery of bone marrow-derived mesenchymal stem cells improves survival and attenuates endotoxin-induced acute lung injury in mice. J Immunol. 2007;179:1855–63.

45. Ortiz LA, Gambelli F, McBride C, Gaupp D, Baddoo M, Kaminski N, et al. Mesenchymal stem cell engraftment in lung is enhanced in response to bleomycin exposure and ameliorates its fibrotic effects. Proc Natl Acad Sci USA. 2003;100:8407–11.
46. García-Olmo D, García-Arranz M, García LG, Cuellar ES, Blanco IF, Prianes LA, et al. Autologous stem cell transplantation for treatment of rectovaginal fistula in perianal Crohn's disease: a new cell-based therapy. Int J Colorectal Dis. 2003;18:451–4.
47. Fang B, Song Y, Liao L, Zhang Y, Zhao RC. Favorable response to human adipose tissue-derived mesenchymal stem cells in steroid-refractory acute graft-versus-host disease. Transplant Proc. 2007;39:3358–62.
48. Riordan NH, Ichim TE, Min WP, Wang H, Solano F, Lara F, et al. Non-expanded adipose stromal vascular fraction cell therapy for multiple sclerosis. J Transl Med. 2009;7:29.
49. Tobin RW, Pope 2nd CE, Pellegrini CA, Emond MJ, Sillery J, Raghu G. Increased prevalence of gastroesophageal reflux in patients with idiopathic pulmonary fibrosis. Am J Respir Crit Care Med. 1998;158:1804–8.
50. Raghu G, Freudenberger TD, Yang S, Curtis JR, Spada C, Hayes J, Sillery JK, et al. High prevalence of abnormal acid gastro-oesophageal reflux in idiopathic pulmonary fibrosis. Eur Respir J. 2006;27:136–42.
51. Lee JS, Ryu JH, Elicker BM, Lydell CP, Jones KD, Wolters PJ, et al. Gastroesophageal reflux therapy is associated with longer survival in patients with idiopathic pulmonary fibrosis. Am J Respir Crit Care Med. 2011;184:1390–4.
52. Lee JS, Song JW, Wolters PJ, Elicker BM, King Jr TE, Kim DS, et al. Bronchoalveolar lavage pepsin in acute exacerbation of idiopathic pulmonary fibrosis. Eur Respir J. 2012;39:352–8.
53. Raghu G, Meyer KC. Silent gastro-oesophageal reflux and microaspiration in IPF: mounting evidence for anti-reflux therapy? Eur Respir J. 2012;39:242–5.

# Index

K.C. Meyer and S.D. Nathan (eds.), *Idiopathic Pulmonary Fibrosis: A Comprehensive*     441
*Clinical Guide*, Respiratory Medicine 9, DOI 10.1007/978-1-62703-682-5,
© Springer Science+Business Media New York 2014

Printed by Publishers' Graphics LLC
JCIMO131030.15.18.7